Methods in Molecular Medicine

Edited by Yusuf Tutar

Published in London, United Kingdom

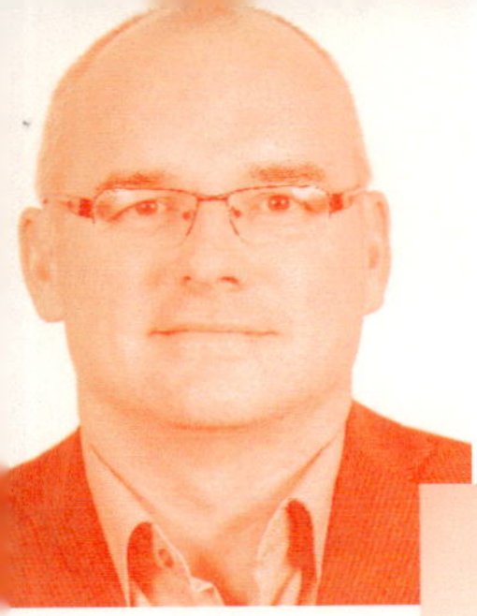
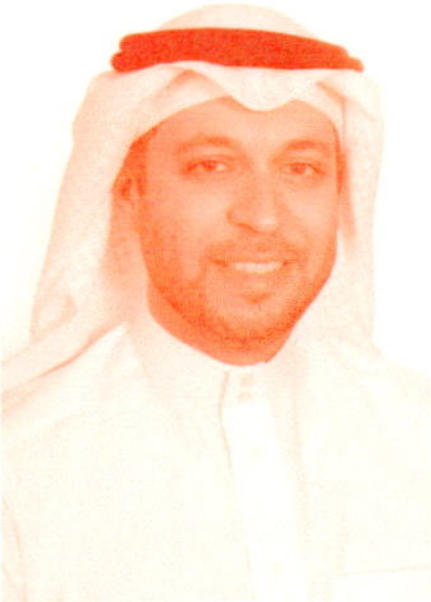
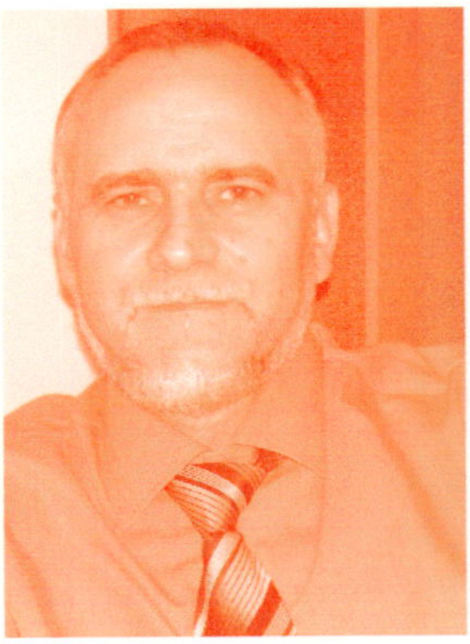
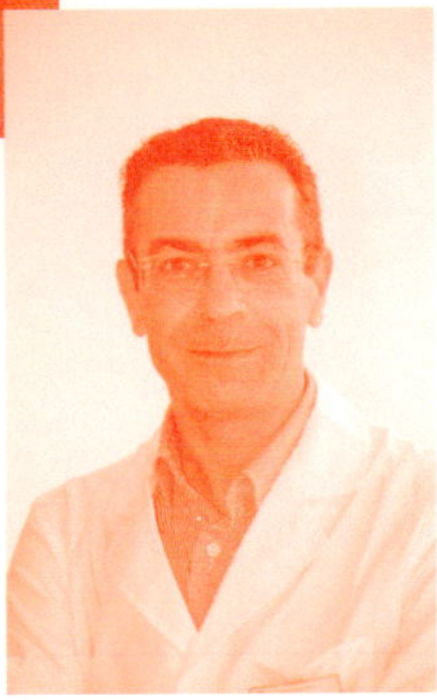
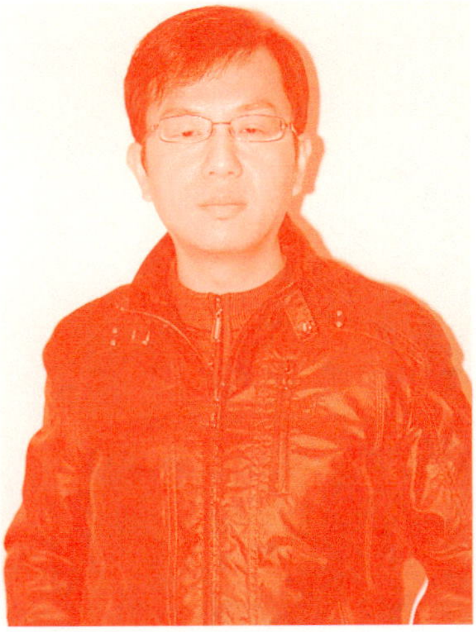
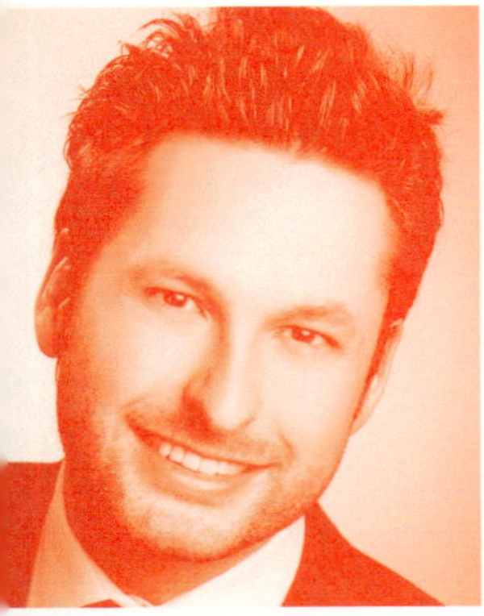
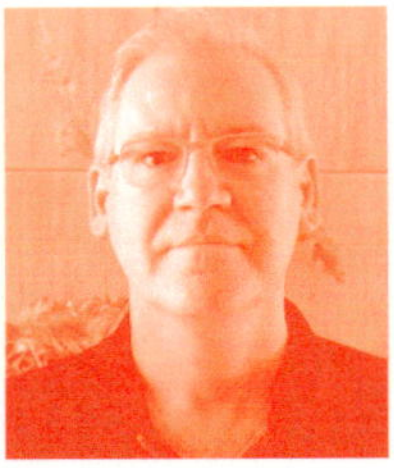

IntechOpen

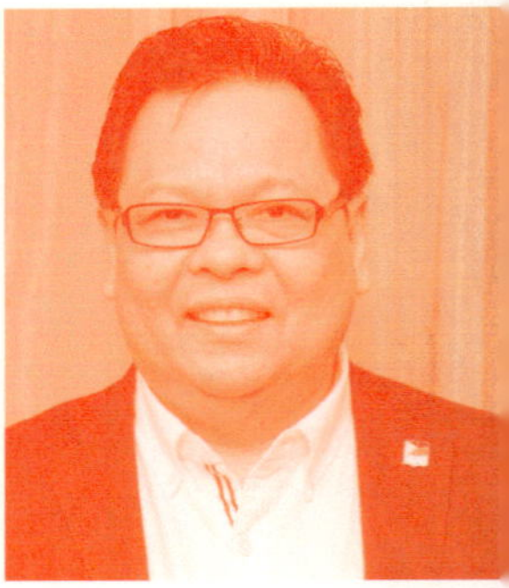
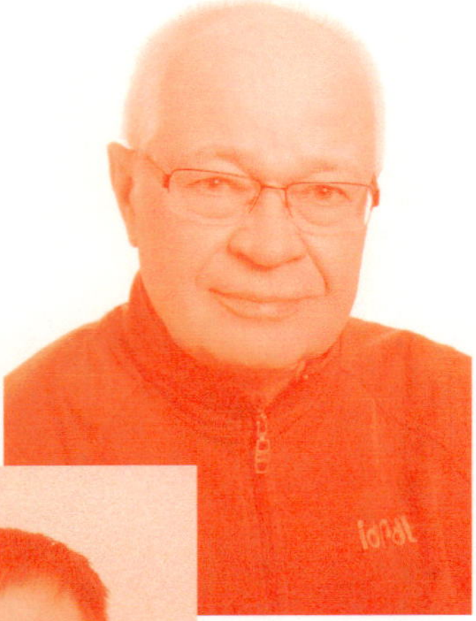
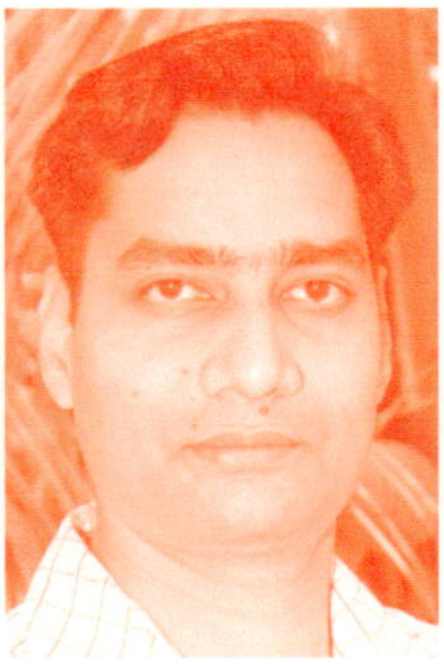
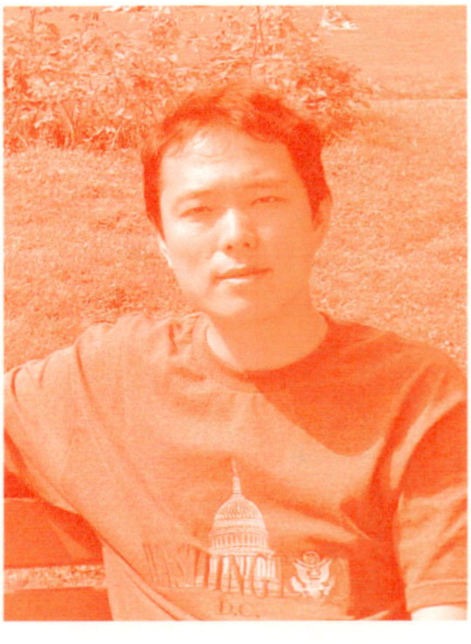
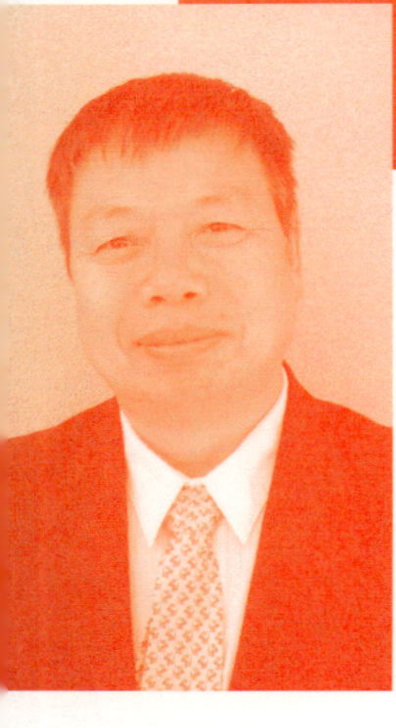
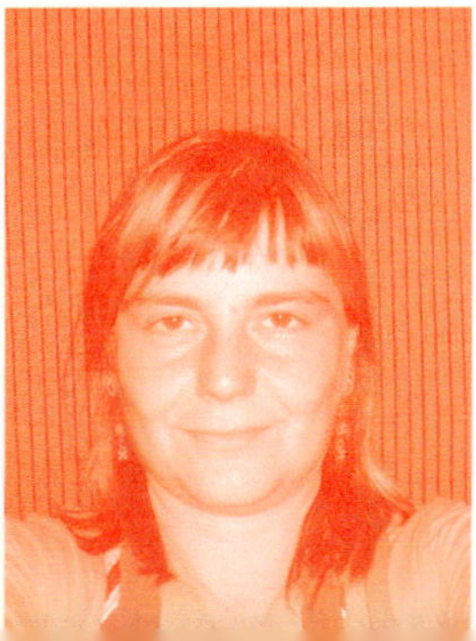

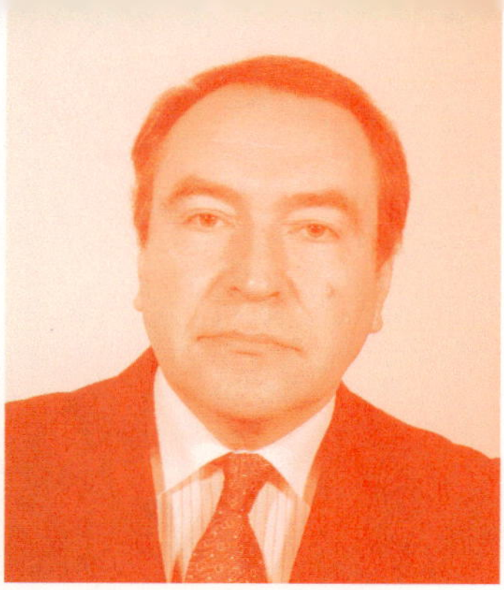
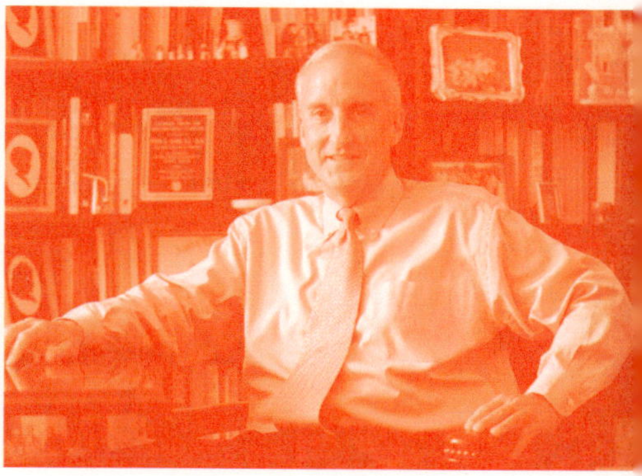
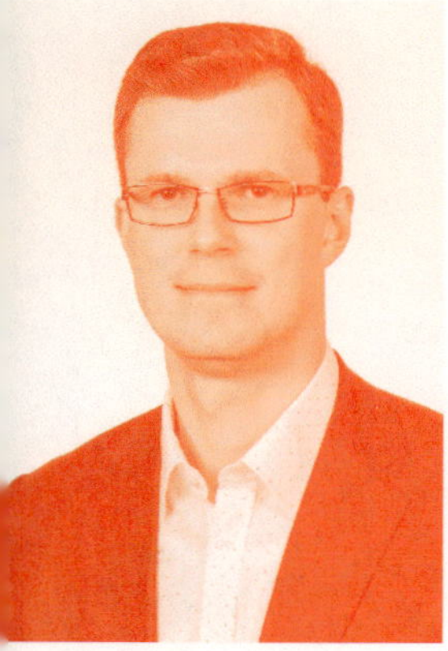
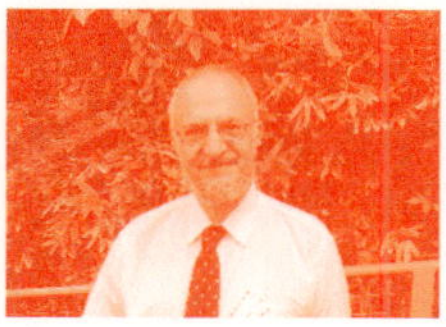
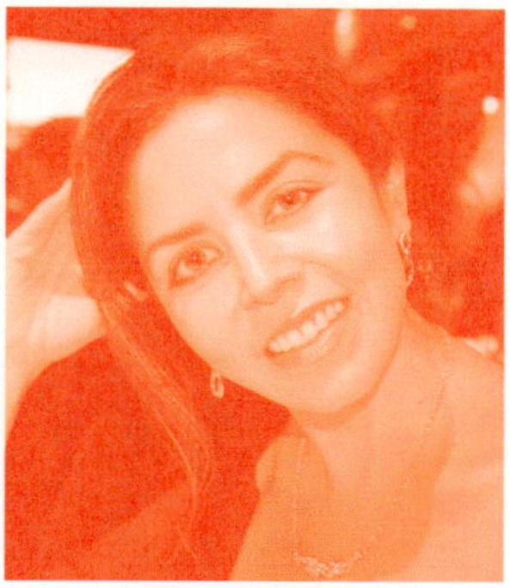

Supporting open minds since 2005

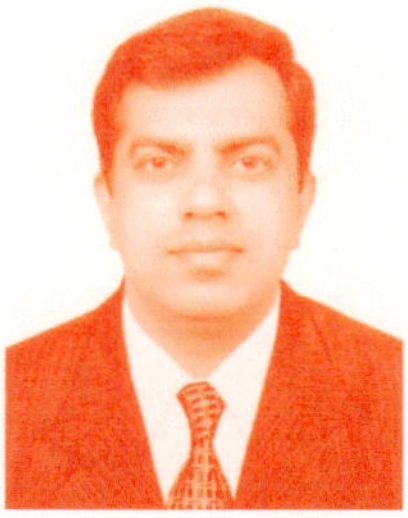
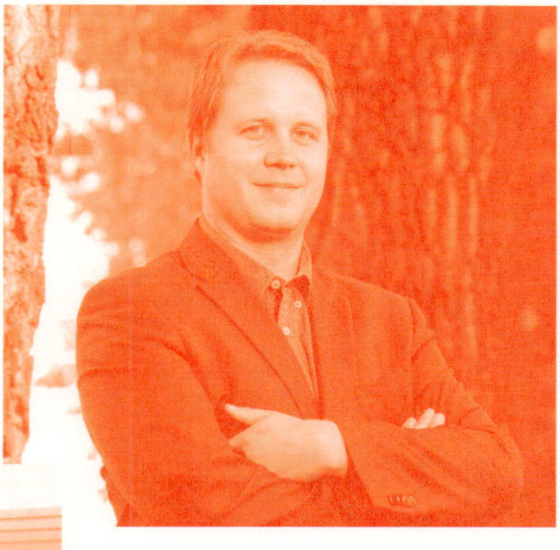
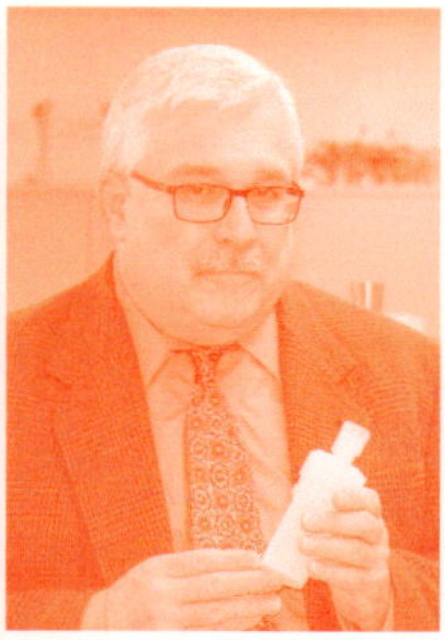
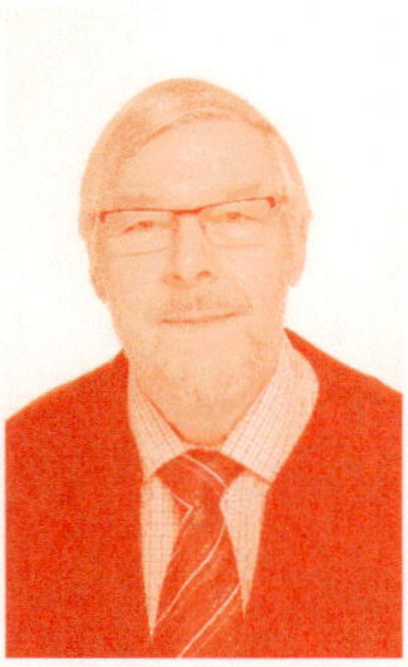
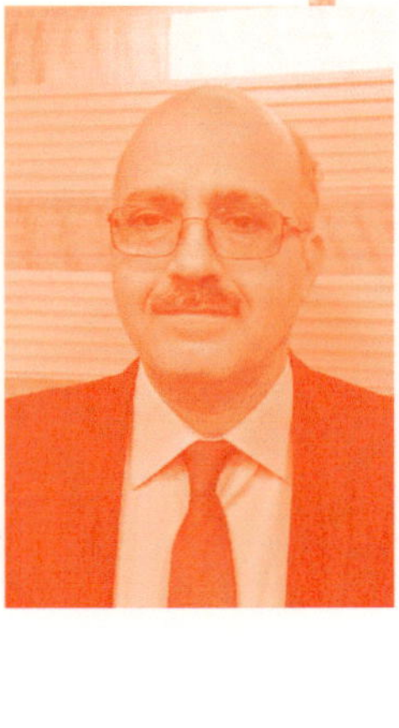
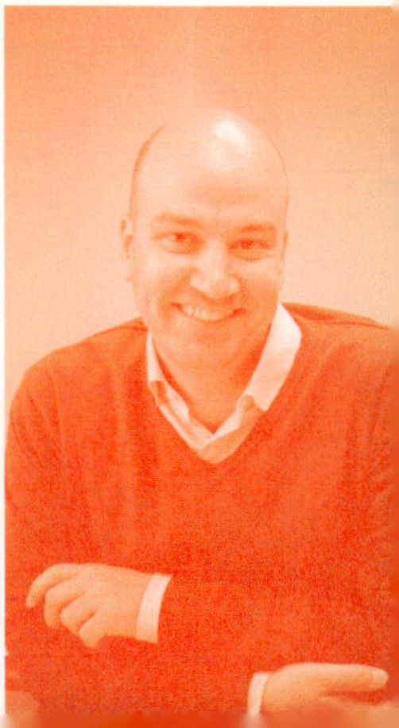
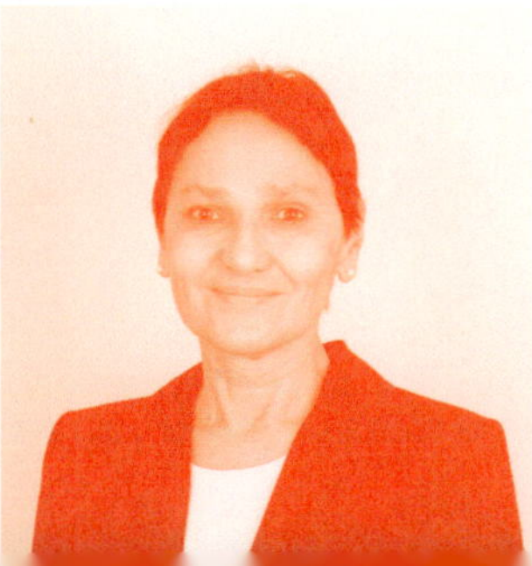

Methods in Molecular Medicine
http://dx.doi.org/10.5772/intechopen.87364
Edited by Yusuf Tutar

Contributors
Enéas Ricardo Konzen, Maria Imaculada Zucchi, Luiz Santana Da Silva, Marcella Montenegro, Carlos Amaral, Malgorzata Rogalinska, Bhawana Singh, Donald Roy Love, Debra O. Prosser, Osman Ugur Sezerman, Tugce Bozkurt, Fatma Sadife Isleyen, Je-Yoel Cho, Kang-Hoon Lee, Yusuf Tutar, Berçem Yeman Kıyak, Adnan Batman, İrem Yalım Camcı, Elif Kadıoglu, Kezban Uçar Çiftçi, Servet Tunoglu, Ezgi Nurdan Yenilmez Tunoglu, Indu Raja, Kelly Kolkiewicz, Antonio Milano

First published in London, United Kingdom, 2021 by IntechOpen
IntechOpen is the global imprint of INTECHOPEN LIMITED, registered in England and Wales, registration number: 11086078, 5 Princes Gate Court, London, SW7 2QJ, United Kingdom
Printed in Croatia

British Library Cataloguing-in-Publication Data
A catalogue record for this book is available from the British Library

Additional hard and PDF copies can be obtained from orders@intechopen.com

Methods in Molecular Medicine
Edited by Yusuf Tutar
p. cm.
Print ISBN 978-1-83962-726-2
Online ISBN 978-1-83962-727-9
eBook (PDF) ISBN 978-1-83962-728-6

For EU product safety concerns:
IN TECH d.o.o., Prolaz Marije Krucifikse Kozulić 3, 51000 Rijeka, Croatia, info@intechopen.com or visit our website at intechopen.com.

Meet the editor

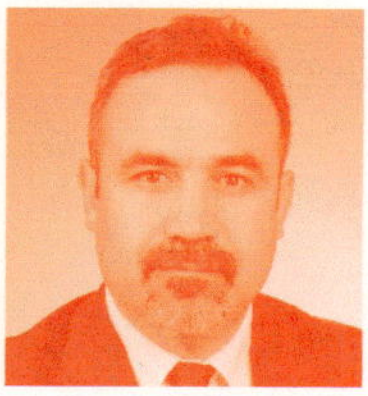

Prof. Dr. Yusuf Tutar is the Head of the Biochemistry Division in the Faculty of Pharmacy, University of Health Sciences, Turkey and he is also adjunct faculty at the Molecular Oncology Division of Health Sciences Institutes. He obtained his MSc and Ph.D. degrees at Oregon State University and Texas Tech University, respectively. He pursued his postdoctoral studies at Rutgers University Medical School and National Institutes of Health (NIH/NIDDK), USA. Dr. Tutar's research is mainly focused on biochemistry, biophysics, genetics, and molecular biology with a specialization in the fields of prion, drug design, cancer, protein structure-function, protein folding, microRNA, pseudogenes, molecular cancer, proteomics, genomics, and protein expression and characterization by spectroscopic and calorimetric methods.

Contents

Preface

Understanding disease pathology and physiological pathways depends on research that examines how certain genes become abnormal. Disease processes with personal patterns can be elucidated through molecular medicine. The crux of the cure lies in precise detection and predisposition of the disease. Revealing molecular mechanisms helps create an effective personalized treatment and minimize side effects. Treatment risk and response to therapy prediction can be forecasted through early diagnosis, which improves prognosis reliability, and the effectiveness of therapies. Using this concept, monitoring health is a way to both make predictions and devise prevention. This book covers contemporary advances in molecular markers, disease-causing variants, retroelements, and the basis of distinct diseases.

Dr. Yusuf TUTAR
Professor,
University of Health Sciences,
Turkey

Section 1

Diseases

Chapter 1

Molecular Mechanisms of Distinct Diseases

Adnan Batman, İrem Yalım Camci, Elif Kadioglu, Kezban Uçar Çifçi, Berçem Yeman Kıyak, Servet Tunoglu, Ezgi Nurdan Yenilmez Tunoglu and Yusuf Tutar

Abstract

Molecular medicine describes molecular structures and mechanisms and this chapter focuses on molecular and genetics errors of diseases. Diseases can be classified into deficiency diseases, hereditary diseases, infectious diseases and physiological diseases and to get a glimpse of the mechanisms the chapter covers the most common disease of each class.

Keywords: chromosomal diseases, cancer, neurodegenerative diseases, pulmonary diseases, obesity-induced insulin resistance, lymphoblastic leukemia, viral immunology and infectious diseases

1. Introduction

Distinct diseases have different etiology pattern and this chapter covers the chromosomal diseases, cancer, neurodegenerative diseases, pulmonary diseases, obesity-induced insulin resistance, lymphoblastic leukemia, viral immunology and infectious diseases. These communicable and non-communicable diseases negatively affect structure-function of the organism and specific symptoms are associated with these conditions. Pathogens or internal dysfunctions may lead these diseases. The chapter provides pathology of selected diseases from each class along with the molecular mechanisms.

1.1 Chromosomal diseases

1.1.1 Down syndrome

Down syndrome (DS) is the most common chromosomal genetic disorder. The disease is caused by the trisomy of human chromosome 21 (HSA21) and is also the most genetic mental disability [1]. The HSA21 mosaic can also lead to DS. Maternity age is an important aspect in the formation of an individual with DS [2]. The main cause of this disease is the absence of normal chromosome separation during meiosis and the production of gametes with two copies of chromosome copies instead of a single copy. As a result, DS individuals have trisomy 21 in some body cells, and a normal number of chromosomes in others. This is called mosaicism and is seen in approximately 4% of DS individuals. The term mosaicism was first reported in 1961

[3] and can occur in two ways: either a normal zygote is exposed to an early mitotic error following fertilization, which results in trisomy 21 in some cells, or an early mitotic error in some cells allows it to return to normal karyotype [4].

HSA21 is the most studied human chromosome, and since the long arm of chromosome 21 has been fully sequenced, a significant progress has been made in understanding its functional genomic units. HSA21 is the smallest chromosome and the overall gene density per megabase is about 15 genes per Mb (for the human genome) [5]. HSA21 is also very rich in long encoding RNA (lncRNA) genes, and, one of the poorest for genes encoding microRNA (miRNA). Also, the gene density is average for pseudogenes encoding the protein per Mb [6]. HSA21 is a weak chromosome in non-encoding RNAs (ncRNAs) and long nuclear elements (LINE). Interestingly, HSA21 shows significant enrichment for proteins found in cytoskeleton structures. These cytoskeletal proteins are known to play a role in neurological disorders, especially Alzheimer's neuropathology [7].

Individuals with DS occasionally develop the myeloproliferative disorder (TMD), a disease that is mostly unique to DS. Almost all TMD cases were found to contain somatic mutations on the X chromosome, in the GATA1 transcription factor [8]. Certain features of DS contain genes on other chromosomes causing gene and trisomy mutations and working together to reveal the disorder in HSA21. Studies have shown that the formation of Trisomy 21 precedes the formation of GATA1 mutations [1]. This may indicate that Trisomy 21 either increases genomic discrepancy leading to GATA1 mutations, or it supplies a selected medium for hematopoietic cells containing GATA1 mutations.

1.1.2 Molecular mechanism

Many hypotheses have been proposed to explain the genotype–phenotype relationship in DS. One of these is the 'gene dosage effect' hypothesis putting forward that the phenotypes arise directly from the dosage imbalance of the genes. Overlapping this hypothesis, the 'DS Critical Region' (DSCR) was announced in the 1990s. [9, 10]. Many of the DS features can be called into a subset of the critical genes in the DSCR region, suggesting that DS phenotypes are mainly caused by the dosage imbalance of only a few genes on HSA21. Genomic regions affecting the presence of certain DS phenotypes have been identified and high-resolution genetic maps of DS features have been created [11]. Olson et al. studied the DSCR regions in mice to test its hypothesis. They concluded that dosage imbalance of some individual genes on HSA21 directly affects certain phenotypes, but they stated that more studies are needed [12].

The "amplified developmental instability" hypothesis suggests that dosage imbalance of the HSA21 gene leads to a non-specific impairment of cellular homeostasis [10]. Extra chromosome materials may also contribute to phenotypes by disrupting chromosomal regions. Some data on monozygotic twins for TS21 suggest that differential expression between normal and trisomic twins can be regulated across chromosome domains. This study shows that some DS phenotypes can be enlightened by the modification of the chromatin structure in the nucleus [13]. Monozygotic twins affected by DS but showing incompatible phenotypes have been reported in some cases, suggesting the role of epigenetics in the phenotypic variability of DS. For example, DNA methylation (controlling gen expression) has been shown to change in Trizomy of chromosome 21 (TS21) samples [14].

1.1.3 Turner syndrome

Turner syndrome (TS) is a disorder in mosaic karyotypes associated with complete or partial loss of the X chromosome. Seen especially in women, TS is associated with short stature, delayed puberty, ovarian dysgenesis, infertility, congenital malformations of the heart, type 1 and type 2 diabetes mellitus, osteoporosis, and autoimmune disorders. It occurs in almost every 2500 live female births. Fetuses affected by TS are 99% estimated to result in fetal death. Approximately half have monosomy X (45, X) and 10% have a repeat (isochromosome) of the long arm of the X chromosome. Most of the rest has a mosaic in more cell lines for 45X. TS, which is associated with a missing X chromosome, was first identified about 100 years ago [15].

Related genes: Shox gene (short length homeobox protein-coding) located on X and Y chromosomes, it is a gene responsible for TS phenotype. This gene does not undergo X inactivation, and a decrease in the expression of SHOX explains some of the TS-related growth deficits. The gene product controls the expression of natriuretic peptide B (NPBB) and FGFR3 (fibroblast growth factor receptor 3) and regulates the proliferation and of chondrocytes, and also cooperates with SOX5, SOX6 and SOX9 and some other genes [16].

The TS genome is hypo-methylated with less hypermethylation sites and there are RNA expression changes that affect the X chromosome genes and autosomal genes compared to women who are 46 XX. Known escape genes are expressed differently in individuals with TS and other X chromosome genes such as RPS4X and JPX (CD40LG and KDM5C) in particularly, KDM5C (encoding lysine-specific demethylase 5C) can participate in the transcriptional profile of neuronal genes and play role in different neurocognitive profiles [17]. 40S ribosomal protein S_4 (RPS_4X) also plays an important role in TS, bringing together multiple protein complexes. In addition, the Y paralog of RPS4X (RPS4Y) may also have a role since it is normally expressed as duplicates [18].

Many different studies show that women with TS have increased mortality compared to the pool of a wide variety of related diseases [19]. The most obvious increase in morbidity is caused by autoimmunities like diabetes mellitus or thyroiditis, osteoporosis, cardiovascular diseases, hypertension, congenital malformations, especially endocrine diseases including heart diseases, digestive system and anemia [20].

1.1.4 Genotype-phenotype

It is still unclear which chromosomal regions or genes make up the phenotypical properties of TS. The physical symptoms of TS were thought to be due to the absence of normal sex chromosomes before inactivation of the X chromosome, or the haplo-insensitivity of the genes in the pseudo-autosomal regions of the aneuploidy [21]. It is thought that a complete phenotype results in the loss of short arm (Xp) in the X chromosome. Aneuploidy itself can cause growth failure. Loss of a region in Xp22.3 was found to be related to neurocognitive problems in TS [22]. Loss of the SRY gene locus in the short arm of the Y chromosome leads to the phenotype of TS, even if it does not cause a population of 45 X cells. It has also been suggested that an area in Xp11.4 is important for the development of lymphedema [23].

1.2 Cellular proliferation: cancer

Cancer can be defined as the uncontrolled cell growth with the most basic explanation. Cell stacks that grow uncontrollably are called tumors. Benign tumors grow much slower and usually do not metastasize, while malignant tumors can spread to other organs through metastasis, and lead to multiple organ damage and eventually death. Tumor cells acquire characteristic features such as sustaining growth signals in the process of cancer, avoiding growth suppressors, resisting cell death, ensuring replicative immortality, initiating angiogenesis, and activating invasion and metastasis [24].

Cancer cells acquire these abilities in the process due to genetic instability and inflammation caused by environmental and hereditary effects. Many studies show that viruses, in addition to many environmental factors such as radiation and chemicals, induce cancer. Chronic inflammation has been shown to trigger oncogenic mutations, genetic instability, tumor growth, and angiogenesis through angiogenesis and cause local immunosuppression [25].

Two types of gene groups involved in cancer are oncogenes, which trigger cellular growth and uncontrolled proliferation, causing increased genetic instability with increased expression and tumor suppressor genes that cause cancer as a result of decreased control of their expression, cell division, and growth. Proto-oncogenes include RAS, WNT, MYC, ERK, and TRK genes. A mutation that may occur on a proto-oncogene or a regulatory region of the gene (e.g., promoter region) can cause an increase in the amount of protein with the change in protein structure [26]. Expressions of oncogenes can also be regulated with miRNAs [27]. Mutations occurring in these regulatory miRNAs can cause activation of oncogenes [28]. Cancer cells increase cell growth-division by activation of oncogenes, as well as suppress preventive control mechanisms of tumor suppressor genes that control this process.

Mutations in tumor suppressor genes cause loss of function. Therefore, they occur in both alleles. To inactivate the gene and its protein, wide-ranging effects, such as deletions, frame-shift mutations, insertions, should be seen rather than point mutations [29]. Tumor suppressor genes include retinoblastoma (RB) [30], TP53, BRCA1, BRCA2, APC, and PTEN. Many side factors such as transcription complexes, changes in cellular metabolism, microenvironment can guide the course of cancer [31].

The development of cancer is a multi-stage process consisting of initiation, promotion, and progression. Cancer-inducing events are usually caused by genetic mutations. Mutant cell proliferates rapidly in the promotion stage and acquires features that allow malignant behavior in the progression stage. Production of telomerase and expression of p53 are examples of malignant behavior [32]. Then, the process proceeds in the form of dysplasia formation, where new blood vessels are formed (angiogenesis) with cellular transformation. Angiogenesis facilitates the intravasation of cancer cells after undergoing an epithelial-mesenchymal transition (EMT) [33]. EMT gives an invasive phenotype to cancer cells and is managed by various transcription factors (such as SNAI, SLUG, ZEB2, ETS1, TWIST) [34]. These transcription factors also regulate each other for the protection of EMT [35].

1.2.1 Cancer cell metabolism

Normal cells only use anaerobic glycolysis when oxygen is absent or limited, while cancer cells can convert glucose to lactate in the presence of oxygen. Otto Warburg discovered that cancer cells exhibit a differentiated metabolism ability [36]. Warburg effect is biochemical properties that help identify cancer cells. On the other side, cancer cells are generally highly glucose-dependent. Glucose intake of cells is enabled by overexpression of different isoforms of membrane glucose transporters in cancer cells [37]. It has been shown that the benefit of the Warburg effect for cancer cells is not just the formation of glycolytic ATP, but also the production of many glycolytic intermediates before anabolic processes such as NADPH and amino acids [38]. Cancer cells are also able to metabolize glutamine to synthesize some amino acids they need, use it as a nitrogen source and for fatty acid synthesis in hypoxic conditions [39]. Therefore, blood glutamine levels increase in some cancer cases [40]. Lactic acid is used to produce citric acid and maintain cancer progression in neighboring cancer cells. This is called the "Reverse Warburg effect" [41].

Tumor micro-environment, consisting of fibroblasts, adipocytes, endothelial cells, and macrophages, is a good source for tumor growth. Tumors "steal" energy-rich metabolites from their micro-environment [42]. Monocarboxylate carriers (MCTs) are used for L-lactate transfer between cancer cells and their microenvironment [43]. Tumors have heterogeneous structures with hypoxic and aerobic regions. A "metabolic symbiosis" behavior has recently been found between the two regions [44]. Lactate is produced by glycolysis in hypoxic tumor cells. This product is obtained by aerobic cancer cells by MCT1. Aerobic cells convert lactate to pyruvate with lactate dehydrogenase isoform B (LDH-B) enzyme.

When glucose consumption is not enough to meet the energy need of cancer cells, they begin the fatty acid oxidation (FAO) [45]. For example, prostate cancer, leukemia, and large B-cell lymphoma, increasing palmitate and FAO uptake in cells are among the most commonly used bioenergetic pathways [46–48]. Normal cells usually receive fatty acids by diet, while tumors show an increase in de novo fatty acid synthesis [45].

Pyruvate plays a pivotal role in the regulation of metabolic reprogramming, especially in tumors [49]. Pyruvate dehydrogenase (PDH) converts cytosolic pyruvate into mitochondrial acetyl-CoA, which is the first substrate of the Krebs cycle. Pyruvate dehydrogenase kinase (PDK) negatively regulates PDH. This reaction slides glucose from oxidative to glycolytic metabolism [50]. Lactate dehydrogenase (LDH) is the primary metabolic enzyme converting pyruvate into lactate. LDH plays an important role in arranging food interchange between stroma and tumor. Studies have shown that inhibition of LDH is important for treating advanced carcinomas [51]. Mitochondrial hyperpolarization is a mutual property of several tumor cells [52]. Tumor cells, which have more negative mitochondrial structures, are more selective targets in drug therapies [53].

1.2.2 Brain cancer

Brain tumors are cancer tissues that grow abnormally and prevent the brain or central spinal system from performing its normal functions. Primary brain tumors originating from brain tissue can usually spread only to other parts of the brain, and occasionally to other organs. Tumors that form in another tissue in the body migrate to the brain are called metastatic or secondary brain tumors. These types of tumors occur more frequently than primary brain tumors. They are termed after their tissue of origin [54].

The most prevalent primary tumor types in adults are glioma, astrocytomas, oligodendroglioma, meningioma, schwannoma, pituitary tumors, and central nervous system (CNS) lymphoma.

1.2.3 Genetic background of brain cancer

Retinoblastoma mutations are found in almost 75% of brain tumors and are mostly associated with glioblastoma, and Tp53 mutations are found in more than 80% of advanced gliomas [55]. Primary glioblastomas have EGFR tyrosine kinase mutations, tumor suppressor PTEN gene mutations, DNA repair protein O6-methylguanine-DNA methyltransferase (MGMT) protein abnormalities [56, 57]. While IDH1 mutations in the control mechanism of the citric acid cycle are seen in advanced glioblastomas, IDH2 mutations are usually shown in oligodendroglioma [58]. Mutations in the BRAF oncogene are common in pilocytic astrocytomas, pleomorphic xanthoastrocytomas, and gangliogliomas [55]. In some glioblastoma tumors, telomere length is maintained by mutations in the TERT promoter and ATRX gene [59].

WHO groups glioma patients based on the presence of two genetic changes; first, mutations [60] in the family of genes encoding isocitrate dehydrogenase (IDH), and second, loss of two specific parts of the genome (1p and 19q co-deletion) [61]. The presence or absence of these changes gives a clue about the patient's prognosis and appropriateness of various kinds of treatments.

Approximately 40% of people with astrocytoma, oligodendroglioma, or IDH mutation bear a hereditary variation. This variation is a single nucleotide polymorphism (SNP) in the 8q24 region of the genome [62]. There is another SNP in the 11q23 region, which enhances the risk of IDH-mutant brain cancer. Approximately 5–8% of gliomas are familial, POT1 gene mutations have been found in 6 of 300 families with glioma [63].

Non-coding RNAs (ncRNAs) play important roles in regulating tumor malignancy in glioma [64–66]. According to healthy brain tissue, mir-21 expression increases in glioma and mir-21 acts as an oncogene [67, 68]. It has been reported that mir-124 and mir-137 act as tumor suppressors in glioblastoma multiform cells [69]. Hotair, SOX2ot, CRNDE, Malat1, H19, GAS are lncRNAs that have been recently shown to regulate glioma [70, 71]. Glioma cells also express the circRNAs, for example, circBRAF, bircFBXW7, circSMARCA5. These regulate proliferation, migration, and invasion of glioma cells [72–74]. The exosomal ncRNAs, mir-21, mir-148a, lncRNA PU03F3, lncRNACCAT2 can be used as circulating biomarkers of glioma patients [75–78]. circRNAs and the exosomal ncRNAs were also reported as potential biomarkers for the diagnosis and prognosis of glioma patients.

1.3 Molecular pathology of neurodegenerative diseases with Alzheimer's disease in focus

As a characteristic of almost all neurodegenerative diseases, abnormal protein assembly gathers these diseases under the prion concept [79]. Prion protein, known as PrP, was introduced to define protein pathogens and distinguish them from viruses and was identified as a proteinaceous infectious particle known to resist inactivation. Even back at that time, its importance was foreseen in terms of shedding light on the etiologies of chronic degenerative diseases [80]. Self-propagation is an important characteristic of prions that is also observed in abnormal protein assembly in Alzheimer's Disease (AD) [81, 82]. Aggregation of proteins in neurodegenerative diseases was believed to occur spontaneously in autonomous cells, however, it was later understood that this aggregation begins in a particular region and propagates across other regions developing the disease further. Transmission of these prion proteins across neuronal cells takes place trans-synaptically [82].

As described more than a 100 years ago, abnormal protein assembly forms the basis of neurodegeneration with AD being one of the most common neurodegenerative diseases. The pathology of abnormal protein assembly starts with misfolding of native proteins that gather to form seeds which eventually lead to aggregation and development of protein fibrils. The pathophysiology of AD involves amyloid plaque inclusions of β-amyloid (Aβ) peptides and neurofibrillary lesions of tau protein. Tau inclusions may also be characteristics of other neurodegenerative diseases, which do not necessarily show the same implications. Altering the native forms of this protein may contribute to its pathology and cause damage to its host cell.

Most cases of this disease are sporadic, while dominantly inherited mutations are also seen to a lesser extent. Back in the 1990s, missense mutations of APP, encoding amyloid precursor, were shown to cause AD [83–87]. Mutations in this gene also increase the aggregation tendency of encoded proteins. Many studies have demonstrated phenotypes associated with neurodegeneration when this protein is overexpressed.

There are six isoforms of microtubule-associated protein tau ranging from 352 to 441 amino acids, encoded by the MAPT gene as a result of alternative mRNA splicing. One half has three repeats and the other has four repeats, altogether establishing the microtubule-binding domain and also the core of tau filaments in case of pathology [88]. All isoforms have been observed in the brains of AD patients. Diseases that have isoforms with only three or four repeats, but not both, lack the Aβ peptides seen in AD and therefore do not carry the symptoms specific to the disease [70]. Tau inclusions may be of a variety of conformations, which can also be caused by different mutations on the MAPT gene, explaining the existence of numerous tauopathies [89–93].

Aβ peptides are encoded by the amyloid precursor protein gene, APP, and are widely expressed as type 1 transmembrane glycoproteins. As a result of alternative mRNA splicing, there are three major transcripts named APP695, APP751, and APP770 [94, 95]. β- and γ-secretase enzymes take part in the production of Aβ peptides in sequential endoproteolytic cleavage. β-secretase is responsible for cleaving the N-terminus of the peptide thus removing the portion that remains on the extracellular side. This cleaved peptide is endocytosed and intracellular aggregation builds up which is later released into the extracellular space [79]. γ-Secretase is a membrane-embedded enzyme that is able to cleave many transmembrane proteins including C-terminus of the Aβ peptide. It a complex enzyme of four proteins; presenilin (PS) forming the catalytic core, presenilin enhancer-2 (Pen-2) enabling maturation of PS, anterior pharynx-defective (Aph-1) stabilizing the complex, and nicastrin possibly being the receptor for the enzyme's substrate [96, 97]. PS and Aph-1 each have two variants resulting in at least four different enzyme complexes, which give rise to various cleaved Aβ peptides. Additionally, γ-secretases cleave the peptide in three different sites. Different protein variants and cleavage sites produce Aβ peptides of different profiles, some of which may be more susceptible to aggregation [98].

Overall, it is important to target the pathways leading to abnormal protein assembly and only then treatments may be proposed based on these mechanisms. Once the first protein inclusion is formed, it is essential to keep an eye on the time frame until the disease symptoms come forth. When techniques sensitive enough to catch the first protein inclusion are developed, then tracking its transformation into filaments can be helpful in designing novel preventive approaches. Understanding this cascade will also contribute to planning more efficient therapeutic methods.

1.4 Cellular and molecular mechanisms of asthma and COPD

Asthma and chronic obstructive pulmonary disease (COPD) are common disorders characterized by progressive chronic inflammation in the lungs. They have unique characteristics with dissimilarly involved cells, mediators, and inflammation. They also have distinct responses to corticosteroid treatment. Roughly 15% of COPD patients have characteristics of asthma [99]. Also, a comparable ratio of asthma patients has traits of COPD that is currently the fifth leading cause of death worldwide [100]. Many risk factors are linked to COPD including smoking tobacco, air pollution, indoor cooking while tobacco smoking (including passive smoking) making up around 80% of the cases [101]. There are many types of cells and mediators that have a significant effect during the pathogenesis of asthma and COPD.

Macrophages have a crucial role in coordinating the inflammatory response activated by cigarette smoke extract in COPD cases [102]. They discharge inflammatory mediators including tumor necrosis factor (TNF)-α, IL-8, other CXC chemokines, monocyte chemotactic peptide (MCP)-1, LTB4 and reactive oxygen species (ROS) [103]. However, the role of macrophages in asthma is not certain. Allergens via low-affinity IgE receptors may activate macrophages causing an inflammatory response through the discharge of a definite arrangement of cytokines. On the other hand, macrophages also excrete anti-inflammatory mediators, such as IL-10 that is thought to decrease in subjects with intense asthma [104].

Activated neutrophils were shown to be enhanced in some subjects with severe asthma and COPD in their sputum and airways [105]. Among the serine proteases secreted by neutrophils are neutrophil elastase (NE), cathepsin G, proteinase-3, matrix metalloproteinase (MMP)-8 and MMP-9, leading to alveolar destruction [103]. The mechanisms of neutrophilic inflammation in asthma and COPD are not clear. Demonstration of priming in COPD occurs at neutrophils in the peripheral circulation. Many chemotactic signals exhibit the capacity for neutrophil recruitment in COPD. These include LTB4, IL-8 and related CXC chemokines, comprising GRO-α (growth-related oncoprotein) and ENA-78 (epithelial neutrophil activating protein of 78 kDa) which are enhanced in COPD airways [106]. Although the mentioned mediators might be sourced from alveolar macrophages and epithelial cells, neutrophils have the capacity of being a vital source of IL-8 [107].

Airway and alveolar epithelial cells in COPD can be a vital point of source of inflammatory mediators and proteases 5. Cigarette smoke activates epithelial cells which produce inflammatory mediators, including TNF-α, IL-1β, GM-CSF and IL-8 [108]. Epithelial cells play an important role in airways defense and tissue repair processes. Goblet cells, a type of epithelial cell, in mucus catch bacteria and inhaled particulates [109]. Epithelial cells release antioxidants and antiproteases. Immunoglobulin A is carried by epithelial cells, hence involved in adaptive immunity [110]. On a side note, native and adaptive immune reactions of the airway epithelium are triggered by cigarette smoke and damage by other harmful agents, increasing sensitivity to infection.

The main role of dendritic cells is to introduce innate and adaptive immune reaction by activating macrophages, neutrophils, T and B lymphocytes among others [103].

Lymphocytes are directly involved in the pathogenesis of both asthma and COPD. Both airway and parenchymal inflammation exist in asthma and COPD patients [111]. Most lung lymphocytes are T cells which are in the respiratory tract of ordinary humans. Activated T lymphocytes are characteristic in both asthma and COPD, but CD4+ type-2 T lymphocytes are the major player in asthma whereas CD8+ type-1 lymphocytes are specific to COPD [111]. CD4+ T lymphocytes can generate many cytokines involved in mediating cell functions and cell–cell communications. This is done through impressing physiologic cell properties such as proliferation, differentiation and activation of other immunocompetent cells, chemotaxis, and connective tissue metabolism [112]. On the other hand, CD8+ T lymphocytes exist in the respiratory mucosa and are activated in response to foreign antigens [111]. Specifically, the cells in the respiratory mucosa have an important role in anti-viral immunity. Another lymphocyte type is B cells which are the minority (<5%) lymphocytes. The main function of B cells located in the lungs is the production of immunoglobulins for local defense mechanisms [113].

Apart from these mentioned cells, there are crucial molecular mediators in the pathogenesis of asthma and COPD. The first family of mediators is transforming growth factor (TGF) family. The TGF-β subfamily is composed of five parts that exhibits plenty of effects pertaining to asthma and COPD. A recent study shows that overexpression of TGF-β1 in mice causes Smad3-dependent pulmonary expression of procollagen, antiproteases and fibrosis [114]. TGF-β exhibits chemotactic signatures for monocytes, macrophages and mast cells. Research shows an abnormal pulmonary expression of TGF-β1 in subjects suffering from COPD. Protein and mRNA expression of TGF- β1 are abundant in the lung tissue, including airway epithelial cells, of mild to moderate COPD patients. TGF-β1 has the role in pathogenesis of COPD because of its increased expression in parallel to the number of macrophages [115].

Another mediator family is the fibroblast growth factor (FGF) family with 23 members in humans. Their functional receptors are named from FGFR1 to FGFR5 [116]. FGFs have many functions such as development, tissue homeostasis, and repair. In addition to further growth factors, FGF-1, FGF-2, and FGF-7 and their receptors FGFR1 and FGFR2, are located abundantly in the lungs [101]. Research shows that increased expression degrees of FGF-1, FGF-2, and FGFR1 were detected in vascular and epithelial areas in the lungs of COPD patients. FGF-1 causes higher collagenase expression and lower collagen I expression in lung fibroblasts which prompt tissue remodeling.

Another family of mediators is the vascular endothelial growth factor (VEGF) family. There are seven units in this family capable of attaching to related cellular receptors. VEGFs have many functions including paracrine acting, angiogenic factors, prompting mitogenesis, emigration, and permeabilization of the vascular endothelium [101]. VEGF and its receptors assist in tissue remodeling as well as disease intensity in incessant lung diseases such as asthma [117]. COPD patients have increased pulmonary VEGF expression in bronchial and alveolar epithelial located around the vascular smooth muscle and alveolar macrophages. Additionally, unlike healthy subjects, COPD patients exhibit elevated levels of VEGFR-1 and VEGFR-2 expression inside the endothelium [118]. Furthermore, VEGFR-2 and VEGF expressions are decreased in COPD patients. Compared to VEGFR-2, VEGFR-1 has a higher affinity for VEGF which leads to VEGFR-1 scavenging VEGF from VEGFR-2. This phenomenon culminates VEGFR-1 activation and in the case of endothelial apoptosis, increased MMP activity as well as vascular and alveolar decimation [101]. This suggests the importance of harmony among VEGF, VEGFR-1, and VEGFR-2 during the pathogenesis of COPD subordinary types.

Finally, cytokines and chemokines are mediators supplying a chemotactic gradient which has the potential to activate macrophages, CD8+ T cells and neutrophils for COPD patients. It is known that inflammatory cells of both native and gained immune systems are significant in the COPD pathophysiology. This is where cytokines and chemokines are the key drivers [103, 119]. Different types of cytokines arrange chronic inflammation in asthma and COPD. T2 cytokines which are IL-4, IL-5, IL-9 and IL-13 interfere with allergic inflammation. Other types of cytokines including TNF-α and IL-1β accelerate the inflammatory response [120]. In asthma and COPD patients, chemokines are instrumental in drawing inflammatory cells from the circulation into the lungs [121].

1.5 The endocrine system

1.5.1 Molecular mechanism of obesity and obesity-induced insulin resistance

Obesity is a serious health problem that has become epidemic all over the world, especially in developed countries. It is characterized by hypertrophied adipocytes that secrete various adipokines and hormones, chronic inflammation in all tissues, and systemic insulin resistance resulting in type 2 diabetes, hypertension, and hyperlipidemia. In addition to these metabolic diseases, it can cause diseases such as cancer, atherosclerosis, obstructive sleep apnea syndrome, steatohepatitis, and musculoskeletal problems [122]. The obesity rate is 20% in women and 18% in men in developed countries [123]. It affects complex metabolic pathways in all tissues as a result of chronic and progressive inflammation, leads to insulin resistance, endothelial dysfunction and lipotoxicity.

The pathophysiology of obesity includes complex interactions of numerous adipokines, hormones and pro-inflammatory cytokines with the central nervous system and metabolic organs (such as liver, pancreas, and muscle) as a result of genetic-environmental interactions.

Genetic etiology: Obesity is generally present in a polygenic etiology. Many studies have investigated the genetic background of body mass index (BMI) and waist/hip ratio (WHR), which are the best measurements of obesity. The results of these studies have been presented collectively in genome-wide association studies (GWAS) [124]. Although, single gene defects (monogenic) are rare in obesity, including especially melanocortin-4 receptor, leptin and leptin receptor genes [125].

Dysregulation in hypothalamic control: The center of food intake and energy regulation in the central nervous system is the arcuate nucleus (ARC) in the hypothalamus besides the autonomic nervous system and brain stem. The balance between the opposing effects of orexigenic and anorexigenic neurons is important. Agouti-related protein (AgRP) and neuropeptide Y (NPY) (AgRP/NPY) neurons are orexigenic that promotes appetite and eating. Pro-opiomelanocortin–producing (POMC) peptide and cocaine-and-amphetamine–regulated transcript (CART), collectively known as POMC/CART neurons are anorexigenic that suppress appetite and eating. Oxygenic pathways that increase energy balance become more effective in obesity [126].

Adipose tissue dysfunction and systemic inflammation; The most important pathophysiological mechanisms of obesity and obesity-related insulin resistance are adipocyte dysfunction (visceral adipose tissue; VAT) and low-grade chronic systemic inflammation. In particular, white adipocyte tissue in obese subjects contributes to the regulation of food intake, energy metabolism and other functions by secreting adipokines from adipose tissue, which provide the necessary signals to the central nervous system, hypothalamus, liver, pancreas, muscle tissue, and other systems to regulate appetite, food intake, and energy balance [125]. Leptin is the most important adipokine that stimulates anorexigenic POMC/CART neurons and induces production of pro-inflammatory cytokines (TNF-alpha and IL-6) by macrophages and monocytes. In the case of hyperleptinemia, leptin resistance develops by the inhibition of the JAK2/STAT3 signaling pathway, which later increases oxidative stress and inflammation, causing insulin resistance, hyperlipidemia and hypertension [127]. Resistin is a pro-inflammatory adipokine produced by the resistin gene (RETN), which activates SOCS3, causing the insulin signaling pathway to be inhibited and consequently induces insulin resistance [128]. Other adipokines like Retinol binding protein 4 (RBP4), Angiopoietin-like protein 2 (ANGPTL2), Visfantin, Adiponectin, Lipocalin 2, Serum Amyloid A, Angiotensinogen, Renin, Angiotensin-Converting Enzyme, Acylation-Stimulating Protein, and Vaspin, are increased, and adiponectin, and Apelin are decreased in obesity, altogether stimulating inflammation, lipolysis, releasing free fatty acid (FFA) and causing insulin resistance as a result [129].

Gastrointestinal hormones and microbiota: Gastrointestinal hormones and gut microbiota play a significant role in the complex pathophysiology of obesity. Ghrelin produced in the stomach induces starvation and food intake by stimulating orexigenic AgPR/NPY neurons in the hypothalamus. Although the effect of ghrelin cannot be fully explained, it is thought to increase in obesity, stimulate growth hormone release (GH), increase gastrointestinal motility and insulin secretion [130]. Decreased GLP-1, Peptide YY, pancreatic polypeptide, and increased amylin and cholecystokinin cause appetite inhibition and gastric emptying delay, resulting in excess energy [129]. Besides hormones in the gastrointestinal tract, changes in microbiota-gut-brain axis and their effects on metabolic organs are also important. Occurring as a result of nutrition and gene–environment interactions; chronic systemic inflammation resulting from intestinal microbiota dysbiosis (increase in Firmicutes-Bacteroides ratio), microbial fermentation products, increase in short-chain fatty acid formation and intestinal permeability, decrease in butyrate-producing bacteria rate, leads to an increase in proinflammatory response in metabolic organs, impaired fat metabolism and glucose metabolism [131, 132].

İmpaired insulin sensitivity and oxidative stress; The beginning of insulin resistance is the first step in the pathophysiology of T2D. Anabolic effects such as glycogen and protein synthesis, glucose transport, adipogenesis are formed by phosphatidylinositol-3-kinase (PI3K)/Akt pathway activation as a result of insulin binding to its receptor (INSR) synthesized in the pancreas [133]. On the other hand, insulin shows mitogenic effects with mitogen-activated protein kinases/Ras pathway (MAPK/Ras).

Adipokines, FFA's, pro-inflammatory cytokines (TNF-a, IL-18, IL-1β, IL-6), synthesized as a result of inflammation in adipose tissue in obesity, also cause systemic inflammation in metabolic tissues such as liver and muscle. As a result, decreased GLUT-4 expression, activation of Ser/Thr kinases with insulin receptor substrate (IRS) phosphorylation, production of ceramides and proinflammatory cytokines, suppressing of cytokine signaling-3 (SOCS-3) expression, insulin pathways and effects. On the other hand, increased production of reactive oxygen radicals and production of toxic doses NO with inducible nitric oxide synthase (iNOS) activation, affect mitochondrial and endoplasmic reticulum functions. Activation of pro-inflammatory pathways increased oxidative stress, mitochondrial dysfunction, ER stress affects lipid metabolism, insulin mechanisms of action and other metabolic pathways, causing insulin resistance, Type 2 diabetes, hypertension, and hyperlipidemia [134].

Beta-cell dysfunction: In addition to peripheral insulin resistance in obesity, serious reductions in beta cell function are also observed. An increase in fat accumulation in islet cells due to chronic lipotoxicity disrupts the function of beta cells by blocking calcium channels. Chronic hyperglycemia due to disruption in glucose metabolism and systemic inflammation due to an increase in oxidative damage and lipotoxicity, disrupt insulin secretion pathways and cause changes in apoptosis gene expression. Hyperinsulinemia in obesity, impaired insulin signaling pathway, oxidative stress, lipotoxicity in islet cells, loss of beta-cell function and apoptosis may lead to the formation of type 2 diabetes [122, 135].

Obesity has become a pandemic all over the world as a result of rapidly changing lifestyles and genetic heritage in the last century. Despite the findings in recent studies on the development and complications of obesity, it is difficult to say that the subject of etiology and pathophysiology is still not fully understood. Especially omics technologies, big data on environmental gene interactions, neuroendocrinology, and neuropsychological studies will reveal findings that open up different horizons. However, due to its complications from deadly metabolic diseases to cancer, rapid preventive measures should be taken, and effective treatment models should be developed.

1.6 Alterations of blood cells: lymphoblastic leukemia

Acute lymphoblastic leukemia (ALL) is a heterogeneous malignancy emerging from lymphoid precursors. It is characterized by the proliferation of immature lymphoid cells with somatic mutations including chromosomal rearrangements, and aneuploidy [136]. ALL has two peak points; first point occurs at ~5 years of age (80%), and the second point occurs at the age of ~50 (20%) [137]. The basic mechanism underlying the development of ALL is similar in children and adults, while they have the frequency of different genetic subtypes. Molecular analysis of genetic changes in leukemia disease provides a great advantage in order to understand prognosis and pathogenesis of ALL [138].

The diagnosis of ALL depends on the presence of at least 20% lymphoblast in bone marrow. Immunophenotyping by flow cytometry (FCM) identifies the subtype of ALL that may be B-cell precursor (BCP), mature B-cell types, or T-cell ALL. Chromosomal abnormalities are a characteristic of lymphoblastic leukemia, which are found in B or T cell lineage. The most common abnormality found in adult B precursor ALL is the t(9;22) BCR-ABL translocation, while the t(12;21)(p13;q22) TEL-AML1 translocation is most commonly found in childhood B precursor ALL [139]. On the other hand, the discovery of mutations in the receptor tyrosine kinase FLT3 contributes to the understanding of leukemogenesis mechanism in hyperdiploid ALL (20% of cases). Based on this finding, targeting specific tyrosine kinase inhibition may be useful in the management of leukemia [140].

1.6.1 Treatment in patients with lymphoblastic leukemia

Small-molecule kinase inhibitors have a clear benefit in the treatment of many cancer types including leukemia. Imatinib mesylate, a small-molecule inhibitor of BCR-ABL kinase, is highly effective in the treatment of chronic myelogenous leukemia (CML) [141]. Although the single kinase inhibitor is a remarkable treatment option in a different type of leukemia, it will need to be combined with either other targeted therapy or chemotherapy because of the resistance to small-molecule inhibitor [142]. Unlike ALL, Chronic Lymphocytic Leukemia (CLL) is defined the accumulation of monoclonal B cell with a special immunophenotype in the bone marrow, blood, and other lymphoid organs where B lymphocytes express CD19, CD23, CD5, low-level CD20 and surface immunoglobulins [143]. The standard treatment procedure of ALL and CLL includes consolidation therapy following chemotherapy in pediatric patients. For adult patients, unlike pediatric patients, the allogeneic hematopoietic stem cell transplantation is frequently preferred as consolidation therapy [144]. Because the patients resistant to chemotherapy are not respond to treatment well enough, novel therapy approaches such as Chimeric antigen receptor-modified T cell (CAR-T) therapy have developed in order to overcome chemotherapy resistance and improving the outcome of patients [145]. CAR-T cells, as immunotherapeutic tools, are genetically engineered to express a chimeric antigen receptor recognizing an antigen that is located in the special cells such as a tumor [146]. CD19 antigen on B lymphocytes was considered the initial target for CAR-T cell therapy. However, specific antigen loss might cause the failure of CAR-T cell therapy in CLL. CD19–20 co-targeting CAR-T cells were designed to kill both CD19-positive and CD19-negative CLL and it was shown that these cells were very effective in killing CLL cells. In one of the first reported in pediatric ALL the clinical trials, CAR-T cells targeted the CD19 antigen of B cells are designed with CD3ζ and CD28 costimulatory domain [147].

1.7 Viral immunology and infectious diseases

1.7.1 The differences between HIV-1 and SARS-CoV-2 genome

The origin of a pathogen has a crucial role in developing vaccines and blocking transmission. This may last many years due to its elusiveness as seen in HIV-1, SARS, and MERS [148–150]. According to a recent report, it was emphasized that

SARS-CoV-2 is able to infect T cells, which are targeted by HIV [151]. Another report alleged that the motif insertions of spike glycoprotein, similar to HIV-1, may help increase the range of host cells of SARS-CoV-2. HIV-1 envelope glycoprotein contains mutable insertions and deletions not necessary for biological function. Only 1 and 2 insertions are matched in only a few HIV-1 strains and this reveals that four insertions are scarce. Thus, HIV-1 cannot be assumed as the source for those insertion sequences in the SARS-CoV-2 genome due to their inefficient identities and scarceness in the HIV-1 sequences [152].

1.7.2 The origin of SARS-CoV2

The reported cases showed that there have been 3,162,284 COVID-19 cases in at least 212 countries and approximately 7.1% of which was resulted in death as of April 30, 2020 [153]. It is known that SARS-CoV, MERS-CoV, and SARS-CoV-2 are the members of coronoviridae family of the Nidovirales order, which comprises a relatively positive-sense, single-stranded RNA genome of around 26–32 kb [154]. 5o-methylguanosine cap at the beginning, a 3o-poly-A tail at the end, and a total of 6–10 genes in between exist in their genome [155, 156].

This family has extremely expressive instability and recombination rate, which is similar to RNA viruses, so it is practically unfeasible to prevent their distribution among humans and animals worldwide; nevertheless, the fact that the virus is exceedingly pathogenic to humans is closely related to random genetic recombination in the host. Although there is a strict genetical relation between SARS-CoV-2 and SARS-CoV, it is explicit that SARS-CoV-2 has a unique feature providing rapidly spread worldwide [157].

SARS-CoV-2 genome sequence is much more resembles a SARS-like bat rather than SARS-CoV [158, 159]. Two open reading frames translating the replication- and transcription-related gene into two large non-structural polyproteins [156]. Ribosomal frameshifting contributes to translate two different but overlapping open reading frames. Besides these nonstructural proteins, the subgenomic RNA also encodes the viral genome packaging protein N (nucleocapsid), and the viral coating proteins M (membrane), E (envelope), and S (spike) as the structural proteins. Viral coating proteins, which interact with host surface receptors, is generally preferred as the therapeutic target blocking protein–protein interaction [160, 161]. TMPRSS2, the human serine protease, enables S Protein of both SARS-CoV and SARS-CoV-2 to prime, and these two viruses use the angiotensin-converting enzyme 2 (ACE2) receptor in order to bind the host cell as the first step of the viral entry mechanism. Unlike SARS-CoV and SARS-CoV-2, the cell entry of MERS-CoV depends on the binding of its own spike protein to DPP4 (dipeptidyl peptidase 4). The RT-PCR analysis of the throat swabs is essential to the diagnosis of COVID19 pneumonia, and it takes 3.5 h to provide the results [162].

1.7.3 Current treatment approaches

Clinical management puts emphasis on the importance of supportive care and prevention of complications due to a lack of specific treatment for COVID-19 pneumonia. On the other hand, potential antiviral therapies for the purpose of rapidly dealing with this pandemic are taking place on several clinical trials. These trials focused on three main targets that include enhancing the host immune system, blocking the virus spike protein-host cell surface receptor interaction, and vaccine development [163].

1.7.4 Human Papillomavirus genome and treatment

HPV genome, which is a double-stranded circular DNA, has the early (E) genes that are responsible for replication and transcription, and the late (L) genes that are responsible for viral capsid proteins. In the early stage of HPV infection, the highly expressed E1 and E2 proteins provide the maintaining of viral replication and transcription within the cervical cell [164].

HPVs, unlike SARS coronaviruses, are non-enveloped viruses and don't have a specific host cell receptor that initiates the viral infection. Additionally, HPVs have many different genotypes such as HPV type 16 and type 18 which are known as the reason for cervical cancer. HPV infection may cause low-grade cytological changes on Papanicolaou smears, or low-grade squamous intraepithelial lesions [165]. When malignant conversion considered, viral oncoproteins E6 and E7 attach, respectively, tumor suppressor protein p53 and Rb have a crucial role [166]. Until today, many vaccine developments studies have been carried out to protect HPV malignant type 16 and 18. For example, the clinical vaccine Gardasil 9 provides effective protection against vaginal, cervical, and vulvar diseases caused by HPV type 16,18 and also its 5 other different types [167].

2. Conclusion

The chapter outlined the unique mechanism of each disease. Depending of the origin of the disease; deficiency, hereditary, infectious and physiological diseases may be treated diversely but the perturbation effect can only be eliminated with proper intervention. Current amelioration may be improved by biochemical methods only if the molecular mechanism is clearly understood. Therefore, molecular medicine provides unique solutions to diagnose and treat disease by elucidating macromolecular interaction and abnormalities in cells and tissues. The chapter summarizes current findings and methods to alleviate and cure the diseases.

Acknowledgements

BYK, EK, KUC and ENYT acknowledge YOK100/2000 bursary and thanks to Turkish Council of Higher Education (YOK).

Conflict of interest

None.

Notes/thanks/other declarations

Thanks to Assistant Prof. Dr. Lütfi Tutar for carefully reading the manuscript.

Author details

Adnan Batman[1], İrem Yalim Camci[2], Elif Kadioglu[1], Kezban Uçar Çifçi[1], Berçem Yeman Kıyak[1], Servet Tunoglu[3], Ezgi Nurdan Yenilmez Tunoglu[1] and Yusuf Tutar[1,4*]

1 Division of Molecular Medicine, University of Health Sciences, Hamidiye Health Sciences Institute, 34668, Istanbul, Turkey

2 Department of Molecular Biology and Genetics, Gebze Technical University, Kocaeli, 41400, Turkey

3 Department of Molecular Medicine, Institute of Health Sciences, Istanbul University, 34093, Istanbul, Turkey

4 Department of Basic Pharmaceutical Sciences, Division of Biochemistry, University of Health Sciences, Hamidiye Faculty of Pharmacy, 34668, Istanbul, Turkey

*Address all correspondence to: yusuf.tutar@sbu.edu.tr; ytutar@outlook.com

References

[1] D. Patterson, "Molecular genetic analysis of Down syndrome," Hum. Genet., vol. 126, no. 1, pp. 195-214, 2009.

[2] T. F. Williams and A. J. Dalton, "Dementia and aging adults with intellectual disabilities: A handbook," Dement. Aging Adults with Intellect. Disabil. A Handb., pp. 1-488, 2014.

[3] C. M. Clarke and J. H. Edwards, "21-Trisomy / Normal," pp. 1028-1030, 1961.

[4] A. Kuliev, Z. Zlatopolsky, I. Kirillova, J. Spivakova, and J. Cieslak Janzen, "Meiosis errors in over 20,000 oocytes studied in the practice of preimplantation aneuploidy testing," Reprod. Biomed. Online, vol. 22, no. 1, pp. 2-8, 2011.

[5] M. Hattori, A. Fujiyama, and Y. Sakaki, "The DNA sequence of human chromosome 21," Tanpakushitsu Kakusan Koso., vol. 46, no. 16 Suppl, pp. 2254-2261, 2001.

[6] A. Letourneau and S. E. Antonarakis, "Genomic determinants in the phenotypic variability of Down syndrome," Prog. Brain Res., vol. 197, pp. 15-28, 2012.

[7] F. I. M. Craik and R. S. Lockhart, "Levels of Processing and Zinchenko's Approach to Memory Research," J. Russ. East Eur. Psychol., vol. 46, no. 6, pp. 52-60, 2008.

[8] O. Tunstall-Pedoe et al., "Abnormalities in the myeloid progenitor compartment in Down syndrome fetal liver precede acquisition of GATA1 mutations," Blood, vol. 112, no. 12, pp. 4507-4511, 2008.

[9] J. R. Korenberg et al., "Down syndrome phenotypes: The consequences of chromosomal imbalance," Proc. Natl. Acad. Sci. U. S. A., vol. 91, no. 11, pp. 4997-5001, 1994.

[10] M. Rachidi and C. Lopes, "Mental retardation in Down syndrome: From gene dosage imbalance to molecular and cellular mechanisms," Neurosci. Res., vol. 59, no. 4, pp. 349-369, 2007.

[11] K. J.O. et al., "The genetic architecture of Down syndrome phenotypes revealed by high-resolution analysis of human segmental trisomies," Proc. Natl. Acad. Sci. U. S. A., vol. 106, no. 29, pp. 12031-12036, 2009.

[12] L. E. Olson, J. T. Richtsmeier, J. Leszl, and R. H. Reeves, "A chromosome 21 critical region does not cause specific down syndrome phenotypes," Science (80-.)., vol. 306, no. 5696, pp. 687-690, 2004.

[13] J. Salvador, M. Arigita, E. Carreras, A. Lladonosa, and A. Borrell, "Evolution of prenatal detection of neural tube defects in the pregnant population of the city of Barcelona from 1992 to 2006," Prenat. Diagn., vol. 31, no. 12, pp. 1184-1188, 2011.

[14] K. Kerkel et al., "Altered DNA methylation in leukocytes with trisomy 21," PLoS Genet., vol. 6, no. 11, 2010.

[15] N. C. Lonberg and J. Nielsen, "Letters to the Editors Sere evskij-Turner's Syndrome or Turner's Syndrome," vol. 364, pp. 363-364, 1977.

[16] M. Fukami, A. Seki, and T. Ogata, "SHOX Haploinsufficiency as a Cause of Syndromic and Nonsyndromic Short Stature," Mol. Syndromol., vol. 7, no. 1, pp. 3-11, 2016.

[17] C. Trolle et al., "Widespread DNA hypomethylation and differential gene expression in Turner syndrome," Sci. Rep., vol. 6, 2016.

[18] S. N. Rajpathak, S. K. Vellarikkal, A. Patowary, V. Scaria, S. Sivasubbu, and D. D. Deobagkar, "Human 45,X fibroblast transcriptome reveals distinct differentially expressed genes including long noncoding RNAs potentially associated with the pathophysiology of turner syndrome," PLoS One, vol. 9, no. 6, 2014.

[19] J. Rovet, "Turner syndrome: A review of genetic and hormonal influences on neuropsychological functioning," Child Neuropsychol., vol. 10, no. 4, pp. 262-279, 2004.

[20] C. H. Gravholt, S. Juul, R. W. Naeraa, and J. Hansen, "Morbidity in Turner syndrome," J. Clin. Epidemiol., vol. 51, no. 2, pp. 147-158, 1998.

[21] F. Haverkamp et al., "Growth retardation in Turner syndrome: Aneuploidy, rather than specific gene loss, may explain growth failure," J. Clin. Endocrinol. Metab., vol. 84, no. 12, pp. 4578-4582, 1999.

[22] A. R. Zinn and J. L. Ross, "Molecular analysis of genes on Xp controlling Turner syndrome and premature ovarian failure (POF)," Semin. Reprod. Med., vol. 19, no. 2, pp. 141-146, 2001.

[23] C. A. Boucher, C. A. Sargent, T. Ogata, and N. A. Affara, "Breakpoint analysis of Turner patients with partial Xp deletions: Implications for the lymphoedema gene location," J. Med. Genet., vol. 38, no. 9, pp. 591-598, 2001.

[24] D. Hanahan and R. A. Weinberg, "The hallmarks of cancer," Cell, vol. 100, no. 1, pp. 57-70, 2000.

[25] G. SI, G. FR, and K. M, "Immunity, Inflammation and Cancer," Cell, vol. 140, pp. 883-899, 2010.

[26] R. Todd and D. T. Wong, "Oncogenes.," Anticancer Res., vol. 19, no. 6A, pp. 4729-46, 1999.

[27] M. Negrini, M. Ferracin, S. Sabbioni, and C. M. Croce, "MicroRNAs in human cancer: From research to therapy," J. Cell Sci., vol. 120, no. 11, pp. 1833-1840, 2007.

[28] A. Esquela-Kerscher and F. J. Slack, "Oncomirs - MicroRNAs with a role in cancer," Nat. Rev. Cancer, vol. 6, no. 4, pp. 259-269, 2006.

[29] J. Mendelsohn, P. M. Howley, M. A. Israel, J. W. Gray, and C. B. Thompson, "The Molecular Basis of Cancer," Mol. Basis Cancer, 2008.

[30] D. L. Burkhart and J. Sage, "Cellular mechanisms of tumour suppression by the retinoblastoma gene," Nat. Rev. Cancer, vol. 8, no. 9, pp. 671-682, 2008.

[31] S. Masri and P. Sassone-Corsi, "The emerging link between cancer, metabolism, and circadian rhythms," Nat. Med., vol. 24, no. 12, pp. 1795-1803, 2018.

[32] R. G. McKinnell, R. E. Parchment, A. O. Perantoni, G. B. Pierce, and I. Damjanov, The Biological Basis of Cancer. Cambridge: Cambridge University Press, 2006.

[33] J. T. Buijs and G. van der Pluijm, "Osteotropic cancers: From primary tumor to bone," Cancer Lett., vol. 273, no. 2, pp. 177-193, Jan. 2009.

[34] M. A. Nieto, R. Y. Y. J. Huang, R. A. A. Jackson, and J. P. P. Thiery, "Emt: 2016," Cell, vol. 166, no. 1, pp. 21-45, 2016.

[35] I. Yalim-Camci et al., "ETS1 is coexpressed with ZEB2 and mediates ZEB2-induced epithelial-mesenchymal transition in human tumors," Mol. Carcinog., vol. 58, no. 6, pp. 1068-1081, 2019.

[36] W. H. Koppenol, P. L. Bounds, and C. V. Dang, "Otto Warburg's contributions to current concepts of

cancer metabolism," Nat. Rev. Cancer, vol. 11, no. 5, pp. 325-337, 2011.

[37] R. B. Hamanaka and N. S. Chandel, "Targeting glucose metabolism for cancer therapy," J. Exp. Med., vol. 209, no. 2, pp. 211-215, 2012.

[38] A. M. Hosios et al., "Amino Acids Rather than Glucose Account for the Majority of Cell Mass in Proliferating Mammalian Cells," Dev. Cell, vol. 36, no. 5, pp. 540-549, 2016.

[39] C. M. Metallo et al., "Reductive glutamine metabolism by IDH1 mediates lipogenesis under hypoxia," Nature, vol. 481, no. 7381, pp. 380-384, 2012.

[40] P. J. Masiar and E. Medekova, "The role of serine and glutamine in the metabolism of malignant bone tumors and their significance in the diagnosis and prognosis of bone tumors," Neoplasma, vol. 35, no. 2, pp. 197-206, 1988.

[41] S. Pavlides et al., "The reverse Warburg effect: Aerobic glycolysis in cancer associated fibroblasts and the tumor stroma," Cell Cycle, vol. 8, no. 23, pp. 3984-4001, 2009.

[42] L. Hui and Y. Chen, "Tumor microenvironment: Sanctuary of the devil," Cancer Lett., vol. 368, no. 1, pp. 7-13, 2015.

[43] P. Sanità et al., "Tumor-stroma metabolic relationship based on lactate shuttle can sustain prostate cancer progression," BMC Cancer, vol. 14, no. 1, 2014.

[44] G. L. Semenza, "Tumor metabolism: Cancer cells give and take lactate," J. Clin. Invest., vol. 118, no. 12, pp. 3835-3837, 2008.

[45] J. L. Yecies and B. D. Manning, "Chewing the Fat on Tumor Cell Metabolism," Cell, vol. 140, no. 1, pp. 28-30, 2010.

[46] S. Zha et al., "Peroxisomal branched chain fatty acid β-oxidation pathway is upregulated in prostate cancer," Prostate, vol. 63, no. 4, pp. 316-323, 2005.

[47] I. Samudio et al., "Pharmacologic inhibition of fatty acid oxidation sensitizes human leukemia cells to apoptosis induction," J. Clin. Invest., vol. 120, no. 1, pp. 142-156, 2010.

[48] P. Caro et al., "Metabolic Signatures Uncover Distinct Targets in Molecular Subsets of Diffuse Large B Cell Lymphoma," Cancer Cell, vol. 22, no. 4, pp. 547-560, 2012.

[49] P. W. Szlosarek, S. J. Lee, and P. J. Pollard, "Rewiring mitochondrial pyruvate metabolism: Switching off the light in cancer cells?," Mol. Cell, vol. 56, no. 3, pp. 343-344, 2014.

[50] M. J. Holness and M. C. Sugden, "Regulation of pyruvate dehydrogenase complex activity by reversible phosphorylation," Biochem. Soc. Trans., vol. 31, no. 6, pp. 1143-1151, 2003.

[51] D. Mishra and D. Banerjee, "Lactate dehydrogenases as metabolic links between tumor and stroma in the tumor microenvironment," Cancers (Basel)., vol. 11, no. 6, 2019.

[52] D. M. Hockenbery, "Targeting mitochondria for cancer therapy," Environ. Mol. Mutagen., vol. 51, no. 5, pp. 476-489, May 2010.

[53] M. P. Murphy and R. A. J. Smith, "Targeting Antioxidants to Mitochondria by Conjugation to Lipophilic Cations," Annu. Rev. Pharmacol. Toxicol., vol. 47, no. 1, pp. 629-656, 2007.

[54] National Brain Tumor Society (NBTS), "The Essential Guide to Brain Tumors," 2012.

[55] M. C. Mabray, R. F. Barajas, and S. Cha, “Modern Brain Tumor Imaging,” Brain Tumor Res. Treat., vol. 3, no. 1, p. 8, 2015.

[56] H. M.E., M. A., L. W.L., and S. R., “Brain tumors: Molecular biology and targeted therapies,” Ann. Oncol., vol. 17, no. SUPPL. 10, pp. x191–x197, 2006.

[57] E. Lee, R. L. Yong, P. Paddison, and J. Zhu, “Comparison of glioblastoma (GBM) molecular classification methods,” Semin. Cancer Biol., vol. 53, pp. 201-211, 2018.

[58] H. Yan et al., “IDH1 and IDH2 mutations in gliomas,” N. Engl. J. Med., vol. 360, no. 8, pp. 765-773, Feb. 2009.

[59] B. H. Diplas et al., “The genomic landscape of TERT promoter wildtype-IDH wildtype glioblastoma,” Nat. Commun., vol. 9, no. 1, p. 2087, Dec. 2018.

[60] D. W. Parsons et al., “An integrated genomic analysis of human glioblastoma multiforme,” Science (80-.)., vol. 321, no. 5897, pp. 1807-1812, 2008.

[61] R. B. Jenkins et al., “A t(1;19)(q10;p10) mediates the combined deletions of 1p and 19q and predicts a better prognosis of patients with oligodendroglioma,” Cancer Res., vol. 66, no. 20, pp. 9852-9861, 2006.

[62] T. Rice et al., “Inherited variant on chromosome 11q23 increases susceptibility to IDH-mutated but not IDH-normal gliomas regardless of grade or histology,” Neuro. Oncol., vol. 15, no. 5, pp. 535-541, 2013.

[63] M. N. Bainbridge et al., “Germline Mutations in Shelterin Complex Genes Are Associated With Familial Glioma,” JNCI J. Natl. Cancer Inst., vol. 107, no. 1, p. c.30, Jan. 2015.

[64] W. Chen and C. Qin, “General hallmarks of microRNAs in brain evolution and development,” RNA Biol., vol. 12, no. 7, pp. 701-708, 2015.

[65] R. E. Andersen and D. A. Lim, “Forging our understanding of lncRNAs in the brain,” Cell Tissue Res., vol. 371, no. 1, pp. 55-71, 2018.

[66] M. Hanan, H. Soreq, and S. Kadener, “CircRNAs in the brain,” RNA Biol., vol. 14, no. 8, pp. 1028-1034, 2017.

[67] C. H. Yang et al., “MicroRNA-21 promotes glioblastoma tumorigenesis by down-regulating insulin-like growth factor-binding protein-3 (IGFBP3),” J. Biol. Chem., vol. 289, no. 36, pp. 25079-25087, 2014.

[68] G. Gabriely et al., “MicroRNA 21 Promotes Glioma Invasion by Targeting Matrix Metalloproteinase Regulators,” Mol. Cell. Biol., vol. 28, no. 17, pp. 5369-5380, 2008.

[69] Silber J. et al., “miR-124 and miR-137 inhibit proliferation of glioblastoma multiforme cells and induce differentiation of brain tumor stem cells,” Bmc Med., vol. 6, no. 14, 2008.

[70] Y. Yan, Z. Xu, Z. Li, L. Sun, and Z. Gong, “An insight into the increasing role of LncRNAs in the pathogenesis of gliomas,” Front. Mol. Neurosci., vol. 10, 2017.

[71] X. Q. Zhang and G. K. K. Leung, “Long non-coding RNAs in glioma: Functional roles and clinical perspectives,” Neurochem. Int., vol. 77, pp. 78-85, 2014.

[72] Z. J. et al., “Differential Expression of Circular RNAs in Glioblastoma Multiforme and Its Correlation with Prognosis,” Transl. Oncol., vol. 10, no. 2, pp. 271-279, 2017.

[73] L. Bolha and D. Glavač, “Circular RNA FBXW7: Implication in glioma tumorigenesis,” Transl. Cancer Res., vol. 7, pp. S521–S524, 2018.

[74] D. Barbagallo et al., "CircSMARCA5 inhibits migration of glioblastoma multiforme cells by regulating a molecular axis involving splicing factors SRSF1/SRSF3/PTB," Int. J. Mol. Sci., vol. 19, no. 2, 2018.

[75] R. Shi et al., "Exosomal levels of miRNA-21 from cerebrospinal fluids associated with poor prognosis and tumor recurrence of glioma patients," Oncotarget, vol. 6, no. 29, pp. 26971-26981, 2015.

[76] Q. Cai, A. Zhu, and L. Gong, "Exosomes of glioma cells deliver miR-148a to promote proliferation and metastasis of glioblastoma via targeting CADM1," Bull. Cancer, vol. 105, no. 7-8, pp. 643-651, 2018.

[77] H. L. Lang et al., "Glioma cells promote angiogenesis through the release of exosomes containing long non-coding RNA POU3F3," Eur. Rev. Med. Pharmacol. Sci., vol. 21, no. 5, pp. 959-972, 2017.

[78] H. L. Lang et al., "Glioma cells enhance angiogenesis and inhibit endothelial cell apoptosis through the release of exosomes that contain long non-coding RNA CCAT2," Oncol. Rep., vol. 38, no. 2, pp. 785-798, 2017.

[79] M. Goedert, "Alzheimer's and Parkinson's diseases: The prion concept in relation to assembled Aβ, tau, and α-synuclein," Science (80-.)., vol. 349, no. 6248, 2015.

[80] S. B. Prusiner, "Novel proteinaceous infectious particles cause scrapie," Science (80-.)., vol. 216, no. 4542, pp. 136-144, 1982.

[81] M. Jucker and L. C. Walker, "Self-propagation of pathogenic protein aggregates in neurodegenerative diseases," Nature, vol. 501, no. 7465, pp. 45-51, 2013.

[82] M. Goedert, B. Falcon, F. Clavaguera, and M. Tolnay, "Prion-like mechanisms in the pathogenesis of tauopathies and synucleinopathies," Curr. Neurol. Neurosci. Rep., vol. 14, no. 11, pp. 1-11, 2014.

[83] A. Goate et al., "Segregation of a missense mutation in the amyloid precursor protein gene with familial Alzheimer's disease," Nature, vol. 349, no. 6311, pp. 704-706, 1991.

[84] P. Poorkaj et al., "Tau is a candidate gene for chromosome 17 frontotemporal dementia," Ann. Neurol., vol. 43, no. 6, pp. 815-825, 1998.

[85] M. Hutton et al., "Association of missense and 5'-splice-site mutations in tau with the inherited dementia FTDP-17," Nature, vol. 393, no. 6686, pp. 702-704, 1998.

[86] M. G. Spillantini, J. R. Murrell, M. Goedert, M. R. Farlow, A. Klug, and B. Ghetti, "Mutation in the tau gene in familial multiple system tauopathy with presenile dementia," Proc. Natl. Acad. Sci. U. S. A., vol. 95, no. 13, pp. 7737-7741, 1998.

[87] P. M.H. et al., "Mutation in the alpha-synuclein gene identified in families with Parkinson's disease.," Science (80-.)., vol. 276, no. 5321, pp. 2045-2047, 1997.

[88] M. Goedert, M. G. Spillantini, R. Jakes, D. Rutherford, and R. A. Crowther, "Multiple isoforms of human microtubule-associated protein tau: sequences and localization in neurofibrillary tangles of Alzheimer's disease," Neuron, vol. 3, no. 4, pp. 519-526, 1989.

[89] C. F. et al., "Brain homogenates from human tauopathies induce tau inclusions in mouse brain," Proc. Natl. Acad. Sci. U. S. A., vol. 110, no. 23, pp. 9535-9540, 2013.

[90] D. W. Sanders et al., "Distinct tau prion strains propagate in cells and mice and define different tauopathies," Neuron, vol. 82, no. 6, pp. 1271-1288, 2014.

[91] B. Falcon et al., "Conformation determines the seeding potencies of native and recombinant Tau aggregates," J. Biol. Chem., vol. 290, no. 2, pp. 1049-1065, 2015.

[92] S. Boluda, M. Iba, B. Zhang, K. M. Raible, V. M. Y. Lee, and J. Q. Trojanowski, "Differential induction and spread of tau pathology in young PS19 tau transgenic mice following intracerebral injections of pathological tau from Alzheimer's disease or corticobasal degeneration brains," Acta Neuropathol., vol. 129, no. 2, pp. 221-237, 2015.

[93] R. A. Crowther and M. Goedert, "Abnormal tau-containing filaments in neurodegenerative diseases," J. Struct. Biol., vol. 130, no. 2-3, pp. 271-279, 2000.

[94] J. Kang et al., "The precursor of Alzheimer's disease amyloid A4 protein resembles a cell-surface receptor," Nature, vol. 325, no. 6106, pp. 733-736, 1987.

[95] C. L. Masters and D. J. Selkoe, "Biochemistry of amyloid β-protein and amyloid deposits in Alzheimer disease," Cold Spring Harb. Perspect. Med., vol. 2, no. 6, 2012.

[96] P. Lu et al., "Three-dimensional structure of human γ-secretase," Nature, vol. 512, no. 7513, pp. 166-170, 2014.

[97] T. Xie et al., "Crystal structure of the γ-secretase component nicastrin," Proc. Natl. Acad. Sci. U. S. A., vol. 111, no. 37, pp. 13349-13354, 2014.

[98] H. Acx et al., "Signature amyloid β profiles are produced by different γ-secretase complexes," J. Biol. Chem., vol. 289, no. 7, pp. 4346-4355, 2014.

[99] P. J. Barnes, "Similarities and differences in inflammatory mechanisms of asthma and COPD," Breathe, vol. 7, no. 3, pp. 229-238, 2011.

[100] S. Y. A. Rafael Lozano, Mohsen Naghavi, Kyle Foreman, Stephen Lim, Kenji Shibuya, Victor Aboyans*, Jerry Abraham*, Timothy Adair*, Rakesh Aggarwal* et al., "Global and regional mortality from 235 causes of death for 20 age groups in 1990 and 2010: a systematic analysis for the Global Burden of Disease Study 2010," Lancet, 2012.

[101] W. I. De Boer, V. K. T. Alagappan, and H. S. Sharma, "Molecular mechanisms in chronic obstructive pulmonary disease: Potential targets for therapy," Cell Biochem. Biophys., vol. 47, no. 1, pp. 131-147, 2007.

[102] B. P.J., "Alveolar macrophages as orchestrators of COPD," COPD, vol. 1, no. 1, pp. 59-70, 2004.

[103] P. J. Barnes, S. D. Shapiro, and R. A. Pauwels, "Chronic obstructive pulmonary disease: Molecular and cellular mechanisms," Eur. Respir. J., vol. 22, no. 4, pp. 672-688, 2003.

[104] K. Tomita et al., "Attenuated production of intracellular IL-10 and IL-12 in monocytes from patients with severe asthma," Clin. Immunol., vol. 102, no. 3, pp. 258-266, 2002.

[105] V. M. Keatings, P. D. Collins, D. M. Scott, and P. J. Barnes, "Differences in Interleukin-8 and Tumor Necrosis Facfor-α in Induced Sputum from Patients with Chronic Obstructive Pulmonary Disease or Asthma," Am. J. Respir. Crit. Care Med., vol. 153, no. 2, pp. 530-534, 1996.

[106] S. L. Traves, S. V. Culpitt, R. E. K. Russell, P. J. Barnes, and L. E. Donnelly, "Increased levels of the chemokines GROα and MCP-1 in sputum samples from patients with COPD," Thorax, vol. 57, no. 7, pp. 590-595, 2002.

[107] F. Bazzoni, M. A. Cassatella, F. Rossi, M. Ceska, B. Dewald, and M. Baggiolini, "Phagocytosing neutrophils produce and release high amounts of the neutrophil-activating peptide 1/ interleukin 8," J. Exp. Med., vol. 173, no. 3, pp. 771-774, 1991.

[108] G. R. Hellermann, S. B. Nagy, X. Kong, R. F. Lockey, and S. S. Mohapatra, "Mechanism of cigarette smoke condensate-induced acute inflammatory response in human bronchial epithelial cells," Respir. Res., vol. 3, 2002.

[109] K. B. Adler and Y. Li, "Airway epithelium and mucus: Intracellular signaling pathways for gene expression and secretion," Am. J. Respir. Cell Mol. Biol., vol. 25, no. 4, pp. 397-400, 2001.

[110] C. Pilette, Y. Ouadrhiri, V. Godding, J. P. Vaerman, and Y. Sibille, "Lung mucosal immunity: Immunoglobulin-A revisited," Eur. Respir. J., vol. 18, no. 3, pp. 571-588, 2001.

[111] S. Baraldo, K. L. Oliani, G. Turato, R. Zuin, and M. Saetta, "The Role of Lymphocytes in the Pathogenesis of Asthma and COPD," Curr. Med. Chem., vol. 14, no. 21, pp. 2250-2256, 2007.

[112] B. Mehrad and T. J. Standiford, "Role of cytokines in pulmonary antimicrobial host defense," Immunol. Res., vol. 20, no. 1, pp. 15-27, 1999.

[113] C. A. Janeway, P. Travers, M. Walport, and E. Al, "Principles of innate and adaptive immunity," Immunobiol. Immune Syst. Heal. Dis. 5th Ed., pp. 1-9, 2001.

[114] P. Bonniaud et al., "Smad3 Null Mice Develop Airspace Enlargement and Are Resistant to TGF-β-Mediated Pulmonary Fibrosis," J. Immunol., vol. 173, no. 3, pp. 2099-2108, 2004.

[115] W. I. De Boer et al., "Transforming growth factor β1 and recruitment of macrophages and mast cells in airways in chronic obstructive pulmonary disease," Am. J. Respir. Crit. Care Med., vol. 158, no. 6, pp. 1951-1957, 1998.

[116] M. Mohammadi, S. K. Olsen, and O. A. Ibrahimi, "Structural basis for fibroblast growth factor receptor activation," Cytokine Growth Factor Rev., vol. 16, no. 2 SPEC. ISS., pp. 107-137, 2005.

[117] M. Hoshino, Y. Nakamura, and Q. A. Hamid, "Gene expression of vascular endothelial growth factor and its receptors and angiogenesis in bronchial asthma," J. Allergy Clin. Immunol., vol. 107, no. 6, pp. 1034-1038, 2001.

[118] A. R. Kranenburg, W. I. De Boer, V. K. T. Alagappan, P. J. Sterk, and H. S. Sharma, "Enhanced bronchial expression of vascular endothelial growth factor and receptors (Flk-1 and Flt-1) in patients with chronic obstructive pulmonary disease," Thorax, vol. 60, no. 2, pp. 106-113, 2005.

[119] W. I. De Boer, "Cytokines and therapy in COPD: A promising combination?," Chest, vol. 121, no. 5 SUPPL., pp. 209S-218S, 2002.

[120] P. J. Barnes, "The cytokine network in asthma and chronic obstructive pulmonary disease," J. Clin. Invest., vol. 118, no. 11, pp. 3546-3556, 2008.

[121] P. J. Barnes, "Cellular and molecular mechanisms of asthma and COPD," Clin. Sci., vol. 131, no. 13, pp. 1541-1558, 2017.

[122] B. Lauby-Secretan, C. Scoccianti, D. Loomis, Y. Grosse, F. Bianchini, and K. Straif, "Body fatness and cancer

- Viewpoint of the IARC working group," N. Engl. J. Med., vol. 375, no. 8, pp. 794-798, Aug. 2016.

[123] F. Johnson, L. Cooke, H. Croker, and J. Wardle, "Changing perceptions of weight in Great Britain: Comparison of two population surveys," Bmj, vol. 337, no. 7664, pp. 270-272, 2008.

[124] J. Sulc, T. W. Winkler, I. M. Heid, and Z. Kutalik, "Heterogeneity in Obesity: Genetic Basis and Metabolic Consequences," Curr. Diab. Rep., vol. 20, no. 1, 2020.

[125] D. Albuquerque, E. Stice, R. Rodríguez-López, L. Manco, and C. Nóbrega, "Current review of genetics of human obesity: from molecular mechanisms to an evolutionary perspective," Mol. Genet. Genomics, vol. 290, no. 4, pp. 1191-1221, 2015.

[126] J. H. Yu and M. S. Kim, "Molecular mechanisms of appetite regulation," Diabetes Metab. J., vol. 36, no. 6, pp. 391-398, 2012.

[127] N. Sáinz, J. Barrenetxe, M. J. Moreno-Aliaga, and J. A. Martínez, "Leptin resistance and diet-induced obesity: Central and peripheral actions of leptin," Metabolism., vol. 64, no. 1, pp. 35-46, 2015.

[128] C. M. Steppan, J. Wang, E. L. Whiteman, M. J. Birnbaum, and M. A. Lazar, "Activation of SOCS-3 by Resistin," Mol. Cell. Biol., vol. 25, no. 4, pp. 1569-1575, 2005.

[129] S. Huether and K. McCance, Pathophysiology: The Biologic Basis for Disease in Adults and Children, vol. 13, no. 6. 2020.

[130] T. Sato, T. Ida, Y. Nakamura, Y. Shiimura, K. Kangawa, and M. Kojima, "Physiological roles of ghrelin on obesity," Obes. Res. Clin. Pract., vol. 8, no. 5, pp. e405–e413, 2014.

[131] A. Whang, R. Nagpal, and H. Yadav, "Bi-directional drug-microbiome interactions of anti-diabetics," EBioMedicine, vol. 39, pp. 591-602, 2019.

[132] "Pathophysiology of Obesity-Induced Health Complications," Pathophysiol. Obesity-Induced Heal. Complicat., 2020.

[133] N. Patel, C. Huang, and A. Klip, "Cellular location of insulin-triggered signals and implications for glucose uptake," Pflugers Arch. Eur. J. Physiol., vol. 451, no. 4, pp. 499-510, 2006.

[134] R. T. Atawia, K. L. Bunch, H. A. Toque, R. B. Caldwell, and R. W. Caldwell, "Mechanisms of obesity-induced metabolic and vascular dysfunctions," Front. Biosci. - Landmark, vol. 24, no. 5, pp. 890-934, 2019.

[135] G. Drews, P. Krippeit-Drews, and M. Duïfer, "Oxidative stress and beta-cell dysfunction," Pflugers Arch. Eur. J. Physiol., vol. 460, no. 4, pp. 703-718, Sep. 2010.

[136] S. P. Hunger and C. G. Mullighan, "Acute Lymphoblastic Leukemia in Children," N. Engl. J. Med., vol. 373, no. 16, pp. 1541-1552, Oct. 2015.

[137] S. Paul, H. Kantarjian, and E. J. Jabbour, "Adult Acute Lymphoblastic Leukemia," Mayo Clin. Proc., vol. 91, no. 11, pp. 1645-1666, 2016.

[138] D. G. Gilliland and M. S. Tallman, "Focus on acute leukemias," Cancer Cell, vol. 1, no. 5, pp. 417-420, 2002.

[139] E. J. Yeoh et al., "Classification, subtype discovery, and prediction of outcome in pediatric acute lymphoblastic leukemia by gene expression profiling," Cancer Cell, vol. 1, no. 2, pp. 133-143, 2002.

[140] S. A. Armstrong et al., "FLT3 mutations in childhood acute

lymphoblastic leukemia," Blood, vol. 103, no. 9, pp. 3544-3546, 2004.

[141] B. J. Druker et al., "Efficacy and safety of a specific inhibitor of the BCR-ABL tyrosine kinase in chronic myeloid leukemia," N. Engl. J. Med., vol. 344, no. 14, pp. 1031-1037, Apr. 2001.

[142] B. J. Druker, "Imatinib as a paradigm of targeted therapies," Adv. Cancer Res., vol. 91, pp. 1-30, 2004.

[143] N. Chiorazzi, K. R. Rai, and M. Ferrarini, "Chronic Lymphocytic Leukemia," N. Engl. J. Med., vol. 352, no. 8, pp. 804-815, Feb. 2005.

[144] D. Bhojwani and C.-H. Pui, "Relapsed childhood acute lymphoblastic leukaemia," Lancet Oncol., vol. 14, no. 6, pp. e205–e217, May 2013.

[145] J. H. Park et al., "Long-term follow-up of CD19 CAR therapy in acute lymphoblastic leukemia," N. Engl. J. Med., vol. 378, no. 5, pp. 449-459, 2018.

[146] C. H. June and M. Sadelain, "Chimeric antigen receptor therapy," N. Engl. J. Med., vol. 379, no. 1, pp. 64-73, 2018.

[147] A. Martyniszyn, A. C. Krahl, M. C. André, A. A. Hombach, and H. Abken, "CD20-CD19 Bispecific CAR T Cells for the Treatment of B-Cell Malignancies," Hum. Gene Ther., vol. 28, no. 12, pp. 1147-1157, 2017.

[148] B. Plenum et al., "Origin of HIV-1 in the chimpanzee *Pan troglodytes troglodytes*," Nature, vol. 397, no. February, pp. 436-441, 1999.

[149] W. Li et al., "Bats are natural reservoirs of SARS-like coronaviruses," Science (80-.)., vol. 310, no. 5748, pp. 676-679, 2005.

[150] E. I. Azhar et al., "Evidence for camel-to-human transmission of MERS coronavirus," N. Engl. J. Med., vol. 370, no. 26, pp. 2499-2505, 2014.

[151] P. Pradhan et al., "Uncanny similarity of unique inserts in the 2019-nCoV spike protein to HIV-1 gp120 and Gag," bioRxiv, p. 2020.01.30.927871, 2020.

[152] X. C., L. X., L. S., S. Y., G. S.-J., and G. F., "HIV-1 did not contribute to the 2019-nCoV genome," Emerg. Microbes Infect., vol. 9, no. 1, pp. 378-381, 2020.

[153] WHO., "WHO. Coronavirus Disease 2019 (COVID-19): Situation Report – 105.," WHO. Coronavirus Dis. 2019 Situat. Rep. – 105., p. 18, 2020.

[154] K. Pyrc et al., "Mosaic Structure of Human Coronavirus NL63, One Thousand Years of Evolution," J. Mol. Biol., vol. 364, no. 5, pp. 964-973, 2006.

[155] D. W. E., V. D. N., F. D., and M. V.J., "SARS and MERS: Recent insights into emerging coronaviruses," Nat. Rev. Microbiol., vol. 14, no. 8, pp. 523-534, 2016.

[156] "Coronaviridae - Figures - Positive Sense RNA Viruses - Positive Sense RNA Viruses (2011)," Int. Comm. Taxon. Viruses.

[157] J. S. Mani et al., "Natural product-derived phytochemicals as potential agents against coronaviruses: A review," Virus Res., vol. 284, 2020.

[158] A. Wu et al., "Genome Composition and Divergence of the Novel Coronavirus (2019-nCoV) Originating in China," Cell Host Microbe, vol. 27, no. 3, pp. 325-328, 2020.

[159] P. Zhou et al., "A pneumonia outbreak associated with a new coronavirus of probable bat origin," Nature, vol. 579, no. 7798, pp. 270-273, 2020.

[160] M. Hoffmann et al., "SARS-CoV-2 Cell Entry Depends on ACE2 and TMPRSS2 and Is Blocked by a Clinically Proven Protease Inhibitor," Cell, vol. 181, no. 2, pp. 271-280.e8, 2020.

[161] K. G. Andersen, A. Rambaut, W. I. Lipkin, E. C. Holmes, and R. F. Garry, "The proximal origin of SARS-CoV-2," Nat. Med., vol. 26, no. 4, pp. 450-452, 2020.

[162] T. Adhanom Ghebreyesus, "WHO Director-General's opening remarks at the media briefing on COVID-19," World Heal. Organ., no. March, p. 4, 2020.

[163] Z. Wu and J. M. McGoogan, "Characteristics of and Important Lessons from the Coronavirus Disease 2019 (COVID-19) Outbreak in China: Summary of a Report of 72314 Cases from the Chinese Center for Disease Control and Prevention," JAMA - J. Am. Med. Assoc., vol. 323, no. 13, pp. 1239-1242, 2020.

[164] S. A. Southern and C. S. Herrington, "Molecular events in uterine cervical cancer," Sex. Transm. Infect., vol. 74, no. 2, pp. 101-109, 1998.

[165] E.-K. Yim and J.-S. Park, "The Role of HPV E6 and E7 Oncoproteins in HPV-associated Cervical Carcinogenesis," Cancer Res. Treat., vol. 37, no. 6, p. 319, 2005.

[166] M. Julia Gargano, PhD; Elissa Meites, MD, MPH; Meg Watson, MPH; Elizabeth Unger, MD, PhD; Lauri Markowitz, Human Papillomavirus. .

[167] NCI, "National Cancer Institute. Human Papillomavirus (HPV) Vaccine Fact Sheet," 2015. [Online]. Available: http://www.cancer.gov/about-cancer/causes-prevention/risk/infectious-agents/hpv-vaccine-fact-sheet.

Chapter 2

Molecular Medicines for Parasitic Diseases

Bhawana Singh

Abstract

Being the cause for significant amount of morbidities and mortalities, parasitic diseases remain the major challenge for the healthcare community due to the limitations associated with the current chemotherapeutics. Drug discovery/invention can be achieved by collaborative efforts of biotechnologists and pharmacists for identifying potential candidates and successfully turn them into medicine for improving the healthcare system. Although molecular medicine for disease intervention is still in its infancy, however, significant research works and successful trials in short span of time have made it broadly accepted among the scientific community. This chapter identifies different molecular medicine approaches for dealing with parasites that have been coming up on the horizon with the new technological advances in bioinformatics and in the field of *omics*. With the better understanding of the genomics, molecular medicine field has not only raised hopes to deal with parasitic infections but also accelerated the development of personalized medicine. This will provide a targeted approach for identifying the druggable targets and their pathophysiological importance for disease intervention.

Keywords: CRISPR/Cas9 system, monoclonal antibody, immune checkpoint inhibitors, nanomedicine

1. Introduction

Parasitic diseases remain the threat to global healthcare sector, with considerable mortalities and morbidities associated with these diseases. Combating parasitic infection relies mostly on conventional chemotherapeutic approaches; however, an exponential rise in the number of recrudescent cases, lack of vaccines and toxicities issues associated with chemotherapies emphasized the need for the research to develop alternative strategies. It is noteworthy that emergence of drug resistance is not new; microbes have been evolving since ages, by knocking out one or the genes. In context of emerging drug resistance, World Health Organization (WHO) has warned for the upcoming "post-antibiotic era", therefore, molecular medicine has surged. Molecular medicine is the application of gene and/or DNA based information for therapeutic purpose. It involves the study of molecular mechanisms, identification of erroneous genetic and/or molecular pathways and development of molecular intervention with the aim to improve disease management.

This chapter provides an insight into how the anomalies in molecular pathways can be targeted leading to discovery of potential candidates for development of clinical medicine and innovative therapies to improve disease management strategies.

2. Evolution of molecular medicine

The field of molecular medicine evolved over a period of time since the discovery of DNA (in 1953) and recombinant DNA technology. Another major breakthrough in 1975, when it was discovered that DNA can be read base by base through the sequencing technique. Later, in 1985, it was known that DNA can be amplified with PCR, and this was major achievement in the field of molecular diagnostics. This journey gained pace with the advent of automated DNA sequencing in 1987 that served as the background for the human genome project (HGP) in 1990. The journey of HGP started the era of modern molecular medicine with the first successful gene therapy. In 1995, the success of unveiling the DNA sequence from the first model organism (*Hemophilus influenzae*) triggered the endeavor towards the completion of HGP. The completion of HGP (in 2000) and the free access to the human genome sequences provided the ground for the advent of omics era or post-genomic era (or functional genomics) [1].

This led to the use of increasing number of analytical platforms for DNA sequencing termed as the next generation sequencing platforms. Further, metagenomics approaches—omics and/or shot-gun approaches paved the way for the third-generation sequencing, that aimed to reduce the sequencing costs. These advances gained momentum with the computational approaches where synthetic biology has remarkably facilitated the DNA based analysis as well as the development of models for drug testing.

In order to deal with the limitation of the existing chemotherapeutic approaches there remains an urgent need for the conversion of biomedical knowledge into clinical application. Molecular medicine provides the opportunity to fill the gap between the basic research and the clinical application for the diagnosis, prevention and treatment of diseases. It involves the combinatorial application of pharmacology, biomedical and omics technologies for understanding and improving the molecular basis of the disease pathogenesis that will serve in designing disease intervention strategies. Development of molecular drug is a complex process that involves multidisciplinary effort including high throughput screening, chemical synthesis, modification, omics technologies, data mining, structure-based drug designing, phenotypic screening, target and lead identification and validation, etc. The development of molecular medicines involves following steps—first, the identification of target, potential tractability of target (i.e. identifying targets that are more druggable than others, depending upon their chemistry), establish genetic association of target with disease pathophysiology (some targets required for drug action may not necessarily associate with disease genetics) and validation of target (by establishing association of target with the disease development/persistence). Validation of target usually involves different molecular approaches to understand the role of target gene or protein in diseases pathophysiology. Overall, it is an interdisciplinary branch where recent technical advances have served as the milestone in gaining insight into the phenomenon of disease pathogenesis and development of innovative therapeutic measures.

Parasitic diseases are amongst the common infections in humans caused by protozoan and helminthic parasites. The causative agents, parasites, are diverse ranging from single celled protozoan to worms that be seen with naked eyes. Till the end of nineteenth century, parasitologists were mainly focused on understanding their life cycle; however, the concept took turn when some parasites were found to be associated with several human diseases that led to significant morbidity and mortality. Parasitic diseases are cosmopolitan, that may affect any part of world however, mostly the diseases are common in tropical countries, but tourism and migration can transmit them outside their geographical boundaries. The signs and symptoms of disease may not be obvious, and it may vary from mild abdominal pain to chronic

Diseases	Causative agent (pathogen)	Transmitting agent (vector)	Manifestation	Treatment options
Protozoan parasites				
Leishmaniasis (visceral, cutaneous and mucocutaneous)	*Leishmania* species	Sandfly (*Phlebotomus* & *Lutzomyia* species)	Fever, anemia, splenomegaly, lymphadenopathy; cutaneous forms manifests as skin lesions and ulcers	Liposomal amphotericin B, miltefosine, antimonials; fluconazole, itraconazole
Malaria	*Plasmodium* species	Female mosquito (*Anopheles* species)	Headache, fever, paroxysm, joint pain, anemia, jaundice; neurological symptoms in severe cases	Chloroquine, mefloquine, doxycycline
Chagas disease (American trypanosomiasis)	*Trypanosoma cruzi*	Kissing bugs (Triatominae)	Fever, malaise, enlargement (liver, spleen, lymph nodes), sometimes skin nodules (chagoma); chronic stages affects the brain, heart and digestive system	Benznidazole, nifurtimox
Human African Trypanosomiasis	*Trypanosoma brucei*	Tsetse fly (*Glossina* species)	First stage-intermittent fever, headache, swelling of lymph nodes, joint pain; second stage involves neurological symptoms	Pentamidine, suramin, fexinidazole, nifurtimox, eflornithine
Toxoplasmosis	*Toxoplasma gondii*	Oral route; transmitted by ingestion of parasite oocyst	Headache, fever, fatigue, muscle ache; skin manifestation includes erythema and roseola	Pyrimethamine, sulfadiazine, clindamycin, spiramycin
Trichomoniasis	*Trichomonas vaginalis*	Genital contacts	Pain, itchiness/burning in genitourinary organs, urethritis, prostatitis (in males) while frothy, foul-smelling discharge, vaginitis (in females)	Metronidazole
Giardiasis (beaver fever)	*Giardia* species	Feco-oral transmission by ingestion of cysts	Chronic diarrhea, abdominal cramps, nausea and vomiting	Nitroimdazole, quinacrine, furazolidone, paromomycin
Cryptosporidiosis	*Cryptosporidium* species	Oral transmission by consumption of contaminated water, undercooked food	Diarrhea, abdominal cramps, low-grade fever (in intestinal cryptosporidiosis); inflammation of nasal mucosa, cough, shortness of breath, hypoxemia(respiratory cryptosporidiosis)	Electrolyte replacement by rehydration therapy, nitazoxanide, azithromycin, paromomycin
Amoebiasis	*Entamoeba histolytica*	Feco-oral route	Diarrhea, severe abdominal pain	Amebicidals (metronidazole, tinidazole) and cysticidal agents (iodoquinol)

Diseases	Causative agent (pathogen)	Transmitting agent (vector)	Manifestation	Treatment options
Helminthic diseases				
Roundworm infection (in murine)	*Nippostrongylus braziliensis*	Skin penetration	Emphysema, loss of alveolar septa, lung hemorrhage	Tetramisole
Ascariasis (Roundworm infection, in human)	*Ascaris lumbricoides*	Feco-oral route	Fever, cough, weight loss, abdominal discomfort, intestinal ulcer accompanied with eosinophilia	Albendazole, mebendazole
Fasciolosis	*Fasciola hepatica*	Oral route, consumption of contaminated food	Acute phase marked by fever, nausea, skin rashes, abdominal pain; chronic phase manifests as jaundice, anemia and intermittent pain	Bromofenofos, triclabendazole, bithionol
Taeniasis	*Taenia* species	Consumption of undercooked pork or beef	Mild (abdominal pain and nausea) to no symptoms	Praziquantel, albendazole, niclosamide, mepacrine
Onchocerciasis (sub-cutaneous filariasis)	*Onchocerca* species	Blackfly (*Simulium* species)	Itchiness and bumps and depigmentation in skin to blindness	Ivermectin, moxidectin
Filariasis (lymphatic and serous cavity)	*Wuchereria bancrofti* and *Brugia* species	Blackflies and mosquitoes	Edema with skin thickening and underlying tissues	Diethylcarbamazine citrate (DEC)
Neural angiostrongyliasis (eosinophilic meningitis)	*Angiostrongylus cantonensis*	Oral route; upon ingestion larvae in undercooked prawn, snails, slugs, frogs	Headache, fever, malaise, nausea, neck stiffness, varying degree of neurological dysfunctions	No specific treatment, supportive care helps reduce the severity of symptoms
Schistosomiasis	*Schistosoma mansonii*	Contact with fresh water contaminated with parasites (released from fresh water snails)	Abdominal pain, diarrhea, fever, cough, bloody stool and/or blood in the urine	Praziquantel, oxamniquine, metrifonate, artesunate, mefloquine
Trichinosis	*Trichinella spiralis*	Consumption of undercooked pork	Nausea, vomiting, fever, diarrhea, facial swelling	Mebendazole, albendazole

Table 1.
Some parasitic diseases, their symptoms and treatment options.

hepatomegaly and eventually death. Some parasitic infections are easily treated while others are not. In the light of the lack of vaccine for parasitic infection, proper prophylactic measures (proper hygiene, prevention of contaminated food, water, preventing consumption of undercooked food, use of bednets, insecticide spraying to prevent vector borne diseases, etc.) and active disease surveillance remains the key for disease elimination. Unfortunately, poor disease management strategies have made parasitic infections a global healthcare challenge. In this article it's only possible to cover some important parasites (**Table 1**), for which research on molecular medicines are underway.

3. Molecular medicinal strategies and parasitic diseases

Parasitic infections (protozoan and helminthic infections) affect more than a quarter world population and cause chronic illness primarily in developing countries of world. These diseases affect the quality of life and treatment costs possess economic burden on families leading to viscous circle of poverty.

Molecular medicine is a broad field that includes insight into the molecular aspect of diseases. Recombinant DNA and cloning technologies are the conventional tools for studying the disease associated molecular profiles. Recent technical advances have paved the way for utilization of several molecular strategies for treating infectious diseases. Molecular medicine aims to understand the molecular basis of disease pathogenesis and allows the utilization of the information in designing specific diagnostic, therapeutic and prophylactic options. Mainly molecular medicine relies on two strategies—targeting genome and targeting signaling pathways, as targeted approach of disease management. Thus, it aims to improve the human health through the understanding of mechanism in human diseases.

3.1 Targeting genome

Apart from conventional approach of gene therapy (replacement of defective gene by exogenous DNA and editing mutated gene), recent technical advances have opened the arena for other strategies of manipulating the gene expression. Gene editing methods have gained limelight that involves the intrinsic molecular repair processes within the cell. The process of break repair in the DNA involves the homology-directed repair (HDR) and/or non-homologous end joining (NHEJ). The key step in gene-editing tool involves the precise introduction of double strand breaks. This process involves the use of engineered meganucleases, zinc-finger nucleases (ZFNs), transcription activator-like effector nucleases (TALENs) and the recent CRISPR/Cas system [2]. Further, short antisense oligonucleotides potentially serve as tools for abrogating the transcription of target gene. As compared to other genome editing methods CRISPR/Cas system using guide RNA has shown immense potential for future of molecular medicine.

3.1.1 Engineered meganucleases

Although there remains plethora of meganucleases to choose from, however, most commonly used meganucleases include the ZFNs that have DNA binding zinc finger protein domain and nuclease domain. Cys_2-His_2 zinc finger domain is amongst the most abundant types of DNA binding motifs in eukaryotes [3, 4]. The ZFNs work by binding to the DNA and cleaving it, which then undergoes repair by either homologous recombination or error-prone NHEJ [5]. Site-specific cleavage is induced by manipulating the ZFN complex to recognize two sequences that are on either side of target site. Upon identification, cleavage of genome is induced by restriction enzyme (FokI), thus generating double stranded breaks in genome that can be used for editing the region.

TALEN has been introduced as an alternative to ZFNs. These are similar to ZFNs in using restriction enzyme that incorporates with the DNA binding domain, but are of different origin. Similar to ZFNs, these protein structures lead to the double stranded breaks in DNA for genome editing [6]. Unfortunately, there are no evidences for the use of the aforementioned meganucleases for the development of molecular medicine for parasitic diseases.

3.1.2 RNA-guided engineered nucleases (CRISPR-Cas9 system)

After the discovery of clustered regularly interspaced palindromic repeats (CRISPR) (in 1987) as a part of bacterial immune system against invading viruses. This strategy has potential application in editing human chromosome with great accuracy. It is RNA guided gene editing tool that uses Cas9 endonuclease for generating double-stranded breaks at loci of interest, which are then repaired via. HDR (using a template) or NHEJ or error-prone microhomology-mediated end joining (MMEJ) [7]. Thus, leading to mutation (insertion, deletion or substitution) with no or minimal damage to host genome. Since the sequencing of the parasite genome, CRISPR/Cas9 genome editing tool accelerated the molecular research in parasitology.

Genome editing in malarial parasite (*P. falciparum* and *P. yoelii*) has provided the ground for development of molecular medicine [8, 9]. CRISPR system of genome editing has played crucial role in understanding the drug resistance and pathogen survival thus, genome editing of the parasite genome holds promises to trigger host immune responses while preventing disease pathology. There are several studies for CRISPR/Cas9 analyses in *T. gondii* however, the most remarkable one include the genome-wide screening that identified the genes involved in infection process [10, 11]. This has greatly accelerated the research to understand the parasite metabolic needs for survival and virulence, conversely, shedding light on dealing with drug resistance mechanisms. Similarly, CRISPR/Cas9 system for *T. cruzi* and *T. brucei* has facilitated functional studies of drug targets and/or vaccine candidates [12, 13]. Genetic manipulation has always remained arduous for *Leishmania* however, CRISPR/Cas9 system has proven efficacy for rapid genome editing and understanding gene functions with therapeutic implication [14, 15]. Similarly, genome editing for *T. vaginalis* has been recently introduced with potential *in vivo* toxicity issues which has been dealt by using nucleofusion based transfection [16, 17]. Large-scale functional genomic screening cannot rely on conventional CRISPR/Cas9 approach thus, CRISPRi and CRISPRa approaches have gained significant attention for generating knock-in/knock-down libraries.

Genome editing using CRISPR/Cas9 system in *Schistosoma mansoni* eggs reduced the infection induced granulomas. Similarly, CRISPR/Cas9 mediated deletion of granulin gene from liver fluke (*O. viverrini*) significantly improved the disease symptoms [18]. This is just the start of the use of CRISPR/Cas9 system in parasitic diseases, it has broader potential in designing molecular medicine for disease intervention.

3.1.3 RNA interference (RNAi)

RNA interference is the approach of inhibiting the gene expression or translation by insertion of double-stranded RNA into the cells and/or organism that mediates targeted degradation of its homologous RNA. It can be done *via*. Short interfering RNA (siRNAs), micro RNA (miRNA) and piwi-interacting (piRNA). It mediates gene silencing by forming RNA-induced silencing complex (RISC) that eventually degrades target mRNA. This unique ability of silencing target gene holds hopes for controlling parasitic infections.

T. brucei was the first protozoan parasite where RNAi based targeting of β-tubulin gene, changed parasite morphology [19]. Conversely, *T. cruzi* [20], *L. donovani* [21] and *L. major* [22] lack the essential protein (Ago-1) for suppressing the gene expression. RNAi mediated targeting of cathepsin B reduced the disease progression [23]. RNAi mediated targeting of topoisomerases and farnesyl pyrophosphate synthase have proven efficacy of RNAi based molecular medicine for disease intervention [24, 25]. Later, in 2011, RNAi target sequencing (RIT) identified several potential targets for genome-scale functional analyses which could potentially therapeutic targets [26]. RNA aptamers (synthetic RNA and DNA molecules) binds the target ligands (RNA/DNA) with high-specificity, and have been developed as pharmaceutically active compounds against *T. brucei* [27].

Malarial parasites lack the conventional RNAi pathway however, antisense oligodeoxynucleotides treatment (against parasite topoisomerase) has shown to significantly reduce the parasite multiplication [28]. Further, topoisomerase targeting antisense nanoparticles and chitosan-based nanoformulation have also been used to inhibit *P. falciparum* growth [29, 30]. Recently, synthetic siRNA targeting the β-actinin and cysteine protease served as potential molecular target for *T. vaginalis* infection [31]. Although still scrappy, better understanding of RNAi pathway in protozoan parasites is likely to revolutionize the molecular medicine due to its genome homeostatic potential.

RNAi based silencing of key genes involved in regulating the parasite survival and development have been potential candidates for therapeutics. Several miRNA have been known to regulate the nematode development and survival in the host microenvironment due to their immunoregulatory potential. These have also been crucial players of host-parasite interaction and have been used as diagnostic marker of infection. *Nippostrongylus brasiliensis* (rat parasite) was the first nematode where RNAi was reported [32]. Much evidences for RNAi based knock-down studies have been seen in *Schistosoma* [33, 34], *Brugia* [35], *Trichinella spiralis* [36], *Ascaris suum* [37], *Angiostrongylus cantonensis* [38], *Taenia saginata* [39], *Echinococcus* [40], *H. contortus* [41] and *Onchocerca volvulus* [42]. Unfortunately, RNAi has not achieved the expected success in parasitic nematodes (schistosomes being an exception) [43]. This could be attributed to the lack of several key components of RNAi pathway [44]. Thus, targeted therapy with RNAi based approach (especially miRNA) is still in its infancy, in context of helminthic infections, that needs orchestrated support from the investors as well as the scientific community in order to stand alone as potential candidate for development of molecular medicine.

3.2 Targeting cells and signaling pathways

This area of molecular medicine remains the hottest area of research in the field of parasitic diseases after the World Health Organization (WHO) warning about the risk of post-antibiotic era. The search for novel therapeutic strategies intends to enhance pathogen killing by targeting regulatory molecules/pathways. Better understanding of disease immunobiology and cellular signaling will provide momentum to the identification of the pathways of therapeutic importance. This area of research towards the development of molecular medicine involves the use of genetically engineered antibodies, recombinant proteins, small molecules to alter signaling pathways, targeting the immunometabolic pathways, inflammasomes, etc.

3.2.1 Immunotherapeutic approach

Immunotherapy is use of biological substances (antigen/antibody, immunomodulators administration) to regulate host immune system in order to fulfill prophylactic and/or therapeutic purpose. Immunotherapy aims to trigger the immune power by directly (antigen based or active immunotherapy) or indirectly (antibody based or passive immunotherapy) [45, 46]. This section describes various immunotherapeutic strategies of molecular medicine that have been reported for the parasitic diseases.

3.2.1.1 Recombinant proteins/cytokine therapy

Cytokines are the small molecular weight, chemical messengers that regulates the immune responses in autocrine and paracrine manner. There is plethora of evidences for the involvement of cytokines in determining the pathophysiological consequences. Recombinant protein (cytokine) based therapy aims to trigger T-cell immune responses and induces parasite clearance.

In *T. cruzi* infection, TGF-β (transforming growth factor-β) has been implicated to yield pathological consequences however, treatment with TGF-β receptor kinase, SB-431542, has shown to restrict the entrance of parasite in the cardiomyocytes and disease associated cardiomyopathy [47, 48]. Additionally, cytokine combination therapy with recombinant IFN-γ and TNF-α has anti-parasitic potential [49]. In context of leishmaniasis, Murray et al. first proved the significance of targeting the cytokine, they showed that monoclonal antibody-based treatment targeting the IL-10 receptor (anti-IL-10 receptor) instigated parasite clearance by inducing NO (nitric oxide) production [50]. Likewise, combination of recombinant IFN-γ therapy with conventional chemotherapy yielded promising results in controlling the disease pathology [51]. Not much has been reported about the cytokine-based therapy in other protozoan diseases.

Conversely, in helminthic infection, MAb (monoclonal antibody) based blocking of IL-4 and IL-10 has shown disease improvement by reducing parasitic burden and inducing TH1 immune responses [52]. Likewise, IL-4 based MAb therapy, in schistosomiasis, has shown to inhibit granuloma formation and hepatic fibrosis [53]. Similar findings of marked reduction in granuloma and hepatic fibrosis were reported upon treatment with *Schistosoma* eggs along with recombinant IL-12 treatment [54]. Exogenous IL-25 based therapy has shown to potentially modulate intestinal functions by regulating IL-13 mediated STAT6 signaling in order to favor protective immune responses in intestinal nematode infection by *N. brasiliensis* [55]. Conversely, exogenous treatment with IL-13 and IL-25 triggered ILCs (innate lymphoid cells) responses and conferred protection against helminthic infections [56]. In schistosomiasis, IL-13 inhibitor, sIL-13Ralpha2-Fc has proved therapeutic benefit by preventing tissue fibrosis due to T_H2 dominated inflammatory responses [49] .

The significance of exogenous cytokine therapy has also been underlined in trichiasis, where IL-33 is known to induce thymic stromal lymphopoietin that generates polarized TH2 responses to confer protection against intestinal nematodes [57]. While, IL-25 treatment instigated TH2 responses and restricted infection induced gastrointestinal inflammation [58], MAb based blockade of IL-10 ameliorated disease pathology. There are evidences for the IL-27 mediated suppression of T-cell proliferation thus IL-27 receptor (WSX-1) knock down improved the mucosal immunity [59]. The use of immune triggering cytokines (IFN-γ, IL-12, GM-CSF) and/or blocking immunoregulatory cytokines that possesses pathological consequences holds hopes for the development of molecular medicine. Thus, therapeutic potential of cytokine therapy can be exploited alone and/or in combination with conventional chemotherapy opening up the avenues for improving treatment outcomes.

3.2.1.2 Immune checkpoint therapy

Immune checkpoint molecules are involved in regulating the T-cell activation and functions. The expression of these molecules is enhanced during chronic infections as a result of immune subversion, thus, therapeutically targeting these molecules has shown promising results in cancer and infectious diseases vaccines [60, 61]. Indeed, T-cell dysfunctionality or exhaustion is the key for impaired T-cell responses during chronic infections; exhaustion is marked by loss of IL-2 production, reduced cytotoxicity, impaired production of pro-inflammatory mediators and reduced proliferative ability. The expression of multiple immune checkpoint molecules (PD-1, CTLA-4, LAG-3, Tim-3, TIGIT) remains the hallmark feature of exhausted cells; elevated expressions of these molecules are accompanied with progressive loss of T-cell functionality [62]. Immune checkpoint inhibitors have been novel strategy of reinvigorating the immune cell functions by abrogating the signaling by the immune checkpoint (or co-inhibitory molecules).

A number of immune checkpoint molecules have been reported in leishmaniasis including—LAG-3, Tim-3, CTLA-4, PD-1, etc. that negatively regulates T-cell functionality [63–65]. MAb based blockade of PD-1 and LAG-3 in malaria triggered pro-inflammatory cytokine responses and relieved T-cell inhibition [66]. Likewise, therapeutically targeting LAG-3 and PD-L1 restored CD4+ T-cells functions, restored follicular helper T-cells, plasma cells eventually cleared the blood stage of *Plasmodium* [67].

Unfortunately, this strategy of immune checkpoint therapy has been in its nascent stage for parasitic infections, and has yet not been used for HAT, Chagas disease, gastrointestinal protozoans as well as helminthic infections.

3.2.1.3 Immune cells and stem cell-based therapy

Immune cell manipulation offers another fascinating approach of molecular medicine to fight with parasitic diseases, when other treatment options fail to provide protective immunity [68, 69]. Direct transfer of immune cells has been holding great promises for conferring protection against protozoan, bacterial and viral infections [70]. Adoptive T-cell transfer therapy using tumor-infiltrating lymphocytes is the best example to clinical success of cellular therapy [71].

DC (dendritic cell) based vaccination approach using parasite peptide (KMP-11) elicited TH1 responses, reduced parasite load and induced lymphocyte proliferation in leishmaniasis infection [72]. Similarly, vaccination with DC along with histone H1 elicited pro-inflammatory responses (IFN-γ and IL-12), reduced the IL-10 and IL-4 producing cells and induced polarized TH1 responses [73]. Atypical progenitor cells (IL-7R+ c-kit+ cells) from malaria infected mice are potent fighters against infection, while transplantation of these cells had similar effects in disease recovery [74].

After the success of direct administration of MSCs (mesenchymal stromal cells) and antigen specific T-cells stem cell therapy has recently budded in the field of infectious diseases. MSCs have been shown to be equally important in conferring resistance against *P. berghei* infection, by suppressing IL-10, reducing the regulatory T-cells population and inducing the production of IL-12 [75, 76]. Likewise, autologous transplantation of MSCs and myoblasts has shown to significantly reduce the ventricular dysfunctions [77].

Transplantation of bone marrow mononuclear cells has marked effect on improving the inflammation and fibrosis in Chagas disease [78, 79]. Also, bone marrow transplantation holds promises for improving the quality of life in congestive heart failure due to Chagas disease [80, 81]. Adoptive immunotherapy in toxoplasmosis, by transferring CD8+ T-cells restricted parasite de-encystation; however, it failed to revert the T-cells exhaustion attributing to the short-lives of exhausted cells [82]. Further, MSCs therapy in toxoplasmosis has not been successful however, when used in combination with the spiramycin, pyrimethamine and folinic acid provided therapeutic benefits. Similarly, for coccidiosis, using adoptive transfer strategy, intraepithelial lymphocytes (IELs) and CD4+ T-cells from interferon gamma knock out (*Cryptosporidium parvum*-infected) mice has shown to provide protection against infection in naïve mice [83]. Likewise, adoptive transfer of sporozoites pulsed-DCs upon co-culture with CD4+ and CD8+ T-cells reduced parasite burden [84].

In helminthic diseases, MSC based therapy have been proven to be efficacious for reducing *Schistosoma japonicum* induced liver injury by using MSCs culture supernatant which inhibited macrophage activation by egg antigen. Macrophages primed with *N. brasiliensis* have been shown to clear the parasitic burden by neutrophil mediated mechanism of macrophage polarization [85] in strongyloidiasis. Filarial infections are associated with increased expression of Foxp3 expressing regulatory T-cells that impairs the CD4+ T-cell immunity. Regulatory T-cells targeted intervention using antibodies against CD25, glucocorticoid-induced TNF receptor family-related gene (GITR), provided cure for filarial infection [86]. In schistosomiasis, basophil depletion strategy has been shown to successfully ameliorate disease pathology and granulomatous lesions [87]. Similarly, *in vivo* DCs depletion has been an efficacious strategy to boost antigen specific T-cells expansion [88]. Antigen pulsed immune cell therapeutics has been extended to *F. hepatica* infection. DCs pulsed with parasite induces T_H1 responses and has been a viable vaccination option that protects against disease associated hepatic damage [89]. Similarly, transfer of *Hymenolepis diminuta* pulsed bone marrow derived DCs cells ameliorated colitis pathology by IL-4 signaling [90]. Therefore, cell based therapeutic strategy serves as potential molecular medicinal approach for parasitic infections.

3.2.1.4 Immunomodulators

Immunomodulators are small molecular inhibitors of signaling pathways that serve as molecular medicine for disease intervention. Imatinib, an Abl/Arg tyrosine kinase inhibitor, induces cytoskeleton remodeling to facilitate leishmanial parasite phagocytosis in the macrophages and reduces disease associated lesions [91]. Another signaling pathway inhibitor, AS-605240 (PI3K gamma inhibitor) has shown to be as efficacious as sodium stibogluconate (SSG) in the treating of *L. mexicana* infection [92]. Similarly, another PI3K inhibitor CAL-101 and IC87114 are known to effectively reduce parasitic burden by reducing the B-cells and regulatory T-cells populations [93, 94]. Another tyrosine kinase inhibitor, ibrutinib has been shown to treat leishmaniasis by triggering T_H1-polarized IFN-γ production [95]. Tellurium based immunomodulator (AS101) has shown to effectively revert t-cell anergy and promote NO production while inhibiting IL-10 signaling in *L. donovani* infection. In Chagas disease, inhibitors of GPCRs provide protection against the disease by preventing the parasite entry and infection [96]. Parasite derived thromboxane A2 signaling induces apoptosis, vasoconstriction and disease associated cardiomyopathy thus use of SQ29548, thromboxane A2 receptor antagonist abrogates the *T. cruzi* infection [97]. Conversely, platelet activating factor and leukotriene B4 induces NO production and effectively controls the parasite [98, 99].

Further, β-adrenergic receptor blockade along with carvedilol has been an effective strategy to improve clinical symptom of Chagas cardiomyopathy [100].

Tyrosine kinase inhibitors (lapatinib) have proven their efficacies in controlling Human African Trypanosomiasis (HAT) pathogenesis by blocking parasite endocytosis [101]. Furthermore, PI3Kγ/mTOR signaling inhibitors as NVP-BEZ235 restricts the *T. brucei* infection [102]. Lectin based therapy using parasite galactose-N-acetyl-D-galactosamine inhibitable lectin (Gallectin) instigates IL-12 production from DCs, T-cell proliferation and IFN-γ production [103].

Rosiglitazone, peroxisome proliferator-activator receptor gamma (PPARγ) agonist, is known to enhance phagocytic clearance of parasitized erythrocytes and reduce parasitic burden in malaria by inhibiting the mitogen-activated protein kinase (MAPK) and NF-κB signaling [104].

In helminthic infection (Strongyloidiasis), anakinra (IL-1β receptor antagonist) potentially improved innate cytokine responses (IL-33 and IL-25) eventually causing parasite expulsion [105]. Therefore, small molecular have shown potential therapeutic benefits in parasitic infection, here is just the tip of huge iceberg, research is underway to explore other molecules.

3.3 Nano-medicinal approach

The application of nanomaterials in the field of medicine for diagnosis and treatment received considerable attention in recent decades for parasitic diseases. The diagnostic potential of nanomaterials has been seen in malaria [106, 107], toxoplasmosis [108], cryptosporiodiosis [109], amebiasis [110] and leishmaniasis [111, 112].

Considering the nanoparticles as treatment option for parasitic diseases, these particles have proven efficacy in targeting the infected macrophages for treatment of VL [113]. Silver alone or in combination with chitosan nanoparticles exhibited anti-toxoplasma effects by exacerbating serum IFN-γ levels and lowering the parasitic burden [114]. Spiramycin loaded chitosan nanoparticles have shown to effectively treat toxoplasmosis [115]. In giardiasis, combination nanotherapy with silver, chitosan and curcumin nanoparticles have been shown to effectively clear the parasites from intestine and stool without any adverse effects [116]. Chitosan as nanosuspension has also shown lethal effects on *Cryptosporidium* oocysts [117]. Similarly, silver nanoparticles have also been shown to effectively reduced oocyst burden by triggering IFN-γ, without any adverse events as seen with standard therapeutic options [118].

The biodegradability and non-immunogenic properties of nanoparticles have made them suitable as delivery agents for drugs and vaccines. Nanoformulation of recombinant *P. falciparum* protein (Pfs25H) served as transmission blocking vaccine for malaria, by abrogating the parasite infectivity to mosquitoes. Similarly, polymeric vaccine using polymer poly(lactide-co-glycoside) acid (PLGA) nanoparticles with malaria antigen, VMP001, and immunostimulatory monophosphoryl A (MPL-A) triggered antigen-specific immune responses against *P. vivax* [119]. Furthermore, iron oxide nanoparticle conjugated with recombinant merozoite surface protein 1 (rMSP1) were efficiently engulfed by macrophages and DCs, that eventually triggered the pro-inflammatory responses [120]. In VL, conjugation of quercetin with gold nanoparticle [121], doxorubicin along with chitosan [122], amphotericin B as chitosan nanocapsule [123] and mannose-chitosan based nanoformulation of rifampicin served as effective delivery system for VL management [124]. Chitosan/poly (vinyl alcohol) based microspheres has also shown to abrogate the *Cryptosporidium* sporozoites attachment to the enterocytes thus served as potential oral chemotherapy for *Cryptosporidium* infection [125].

For helminthic infections, chitosan based albendazole formulation skewed the T-cell responses to T_H1 type and reduced the parasitic burden, which led to parasite clearance in echinococcosis [126, 127] as well as in toxocariasis [128]. Similarly, silver assembled on fungal (*Trichoderma harzianum*) cell wall in the form of nanoformulation improved the anti-fascioliasis potential of triclabendazole [129]. Liposomal nanoformulations (nanoparticles and nanocapsules) have been widely used for enhancing the efficacies and bioavailability of oral drugs for disease intervention. These formulations have gained significance as nanocarriers in helminthic infection due to their ability to diffuse through the intestinal mucosal layers. In schistosomiasis, liposome encapsulated praziquantel has shown significant reductions in parasitic burdens and hepatic granulomas due to increased affinity for parasite phospholipids [130]. Liposome based nanocapsules of praziquantel (PZQ-LNCs) improved the drug efficacy and ameliorated disease pathology [131]. Further, liposomal nanocapsules of miltefosine exerted potential schistosomal effects by ameliorating hepatic histology (reducing the granuloma size, number and inflammation) in single dose [132].

Nanoformulation has also been used for vaccine development and as adjuvants, self-assembling protein nanoparticles (SAPN) have shown to trigger protective antibodies and long-lived memory responses to confer sterile protection against malarial parasites (*P. berghei* and *P. falciparum*) [133]. SAPNs have also been used for delivering the epitopes to induce CD4+ and CD8+ T-cell responses against *Toxoplasma gondii* [134]. Archaea based nanoformulations (archaeosomes) have been used as adjuvant as a part of prophylactic vaccine against *T. cruzi*, instigated humoral as well as cell-mediated immune responses (T_H1 responses) leading to marked reduction in parasitic burdens [135]. Cationic solid lipid nanoparticles have been successfully used as adjuvant as part of prime-boost strategy to reduce the parasitic burdens during VL. The vaccination triggered IFN-γ production, NO production and high levels of immunoglobulins (IgG1 and IgG2a) [136]. Therefore, nanoparticles served as viable, safe and effective vaccine platform as well as development of molecular medicine for cost effective vaccine delivery.

4. Conclusion

In this world where cost of developing medicine for parasitic infections remain the greatest challenge, drug developers are embracing molecular medicine approach that promises to deal with the parasitic infections and improves the chances of successful treatment. Molecular medicine has revolutionized the field of drug discovery/development however, there are significant hurdles in turning the promise into reality. Perhaps, gradually but it is shaping the future of medicine with the help of molecular platforms, better bioinformatics services and better pharmacogenomic analyses has greatly facilitated the scientific community and the stakeholders to come on common platform to fight against the parasitic diseases.

DOI: http://dx.doi.org/10.5772/intechopen.91956

Author details

Bhawana Singh
Department of Medicine, Institute of Medical Sciences, Banaras Hindu University, Varanasi, India

*Address all correspondence to: bhavanasonali9@gmail.com

References

[1] Gannon F. Molecular medicine: Trendy title or new reality? EMBO Reports. 2003;**4**(8):733

[2] Porteus MH. Towards a new era in medicine: Therapeutic genome editing. Genome Biology. 2015;**16**:286

[3] Menoret S et al. Generation of Rag1-knockout immunodeficient rats and mice using engineered meganucleases. The FASEB Journal. 2013;**27**(2):703-711

[4] Gaj T, Gersbach CA, Barbas CF 3rd. ZFN, TALEN, and CRISPR/Cas-based methods for genome engineering. Trends in Biotechnology. 2013;**31**(7):397-405

[5] Carlson DF, Fahrenkrug SC, Hackett PB. Targeting DNA with fingers and TALENs. Molecular Therapy—Nucleic Acids. 2012;**1**:e3

[6] Bogdanove AJ, Voytas DF. TAL effectors: Customizable proteins for DNA targeting. Science. 2011;**333**(6051):1843-1846

[7] Karimian A et al. CRISPR/Cas9 technology as a potent molecular tool for gene therapy. Journal of Cellular Physiology. 2019;**234**(8):12267-12277

[8] Wagner JC et al. Efficient CRISPR-Cas9-mediated genome editing in *Plasmodium falciparum*. Nature Methods. 2014;**11**(9):915-918

[9] Ghorbal M et al. Genome editing in the human malaria parasite *Plasmodium falciparum* using the CRISPR-Cas9 system. Nature Biotechnology. 2014;**32**(8):819-821

[10] Sidik SM et al. A genome-wide CRISPR screen in toxoplasma identifies essential Apicomplexan genes. Cell. 2016;**166**(6):1423-1435 e12

[11] Sidik SM, Huet D, Lourido S. CRISPR-Cas9-based genome-wide screening of *Toxoplasma gondii*. Nature Protocols. 2018;**13**(1):307-323

[12] Chiurillo MA et al. Different roles of mitochondrial calcium uniporter complex subunits in growth and infectivity of *Trypanosoma cruzi*. mBio. 2017;**8**(3). pii: e00574-17

[13] Lander N et al. CRISPR/Cas9-mediated endogenous C-terminal tagging of *Trypanosoma cruzi* genes reveals the Acidocalcisome localization of the inositol 1,4,5-trisphosphate receptor. The Journal of Biological Chemistry. 2016;**291**(49):25505-25515

[14] Soares Medeiros LC et al. Rapid, selection-free, high-efficiency genome editing in protozoan parasites using CRISPR-Cas9 ribonucleoproteins. mBio. 2017;**8**(6). pii: e01788-17

[15] Beneke T et al. A CRISPR Cas9 high-throughput genome editing toolkit for kinetoplastids. Royal Society Open Science. 2017;**4**(5):170095

[16] Peng D et al. CRISPR-Cas9-mediated single-gene and gene family disruption in *Trypanosoma cruzi*. mBio. 2014;**6**(1):e02097-e02014

[17] Janssen BD et al. CRISPR/Cas9-mediated gene modification and gene knock out in the human-infective parasite *Trichomonas vaginalis*. Scientific Reports. 2018;**8**(1):270

[18] Arunsan P et al. Programmed knockout mutation of liver fluke granulin attenuates virulence of infection-induced hepatobiliary morbidity. eLife. 2019;**8**:e41463

[19] Ngo H et al. Double-stranded RNA induces mRNA degradation in *Trypanosoma brucei*. Proceedings of the National Academy of Sciences of the United States of America. 1998;**95**(25):14687-14692

[20] DaRocha WD et al. Tests of cytoplasmic RNA interference (RNAi) and construction of a tetracycline-inducible T7 promoter system in *Trypanosoma cruzi*. Molecular and Biochemical Parasitology. 2004;**133**(2): 175-186

[21] Zhang WW, Matlashewski G. Analysis of antisense and double stranded RNA downregulation of A2 protein expression in *Leishmania donovani*. Molecular and Biochemical Parasitology. 2000;**107**(2):315-319

[22] Robinson KA, Beverley SM. Improvements in transfection efficiency and tests of RNA interference (RNAi) approaches in the protozoan parasite Leishmania. Molecular and Biochemical Parasitology. 2003;**128**(2):217-228

[23] Abdulla MH et al. RNA interference of *Trypanosoma brucei* cathepsin B and L affects disease progression in a mouse model. PLoS Neglected Tropical Diseases. 2008;**2**(9):e298

[24] Prestrud P, Krogsrud J, Gjertz I. The occurrence of rabies in the Svalbard Islands of Norway. Journal of Wildlife Diseases. 1992;**28**(1):57-63

[25] Montalvetti A et al. Farnesyl pyrophosphate synthase is an essential enzyme in *Trypanosoma brucei*. In vitro RNA interference and in vivo inhibition studies. The Journal of Biological Chemistry. 2003;**278**(19):17075-17083

[26] Alsford S et al. High-throughput phenotyping using parallel sequencing of RNA interference targets in the African trypanosome. Genome Research. 2011;**21**(6):915-924

[27] Goringer HU et al. RNA aptamers as potential pharmaceuticals against infections with African trypanosomes. Handbook of Experimental Pharmacology. 2006;**173**:375-393

[28] Noonpakdee W et al. Inhibition of plasmodium falciparum proliferation in vitro by antisense oligodeoxynucleotides against malarial topoisomerase II. Biochemical and Biophysical Research Communications. 2003;**302**(4):659-664

[29] Foger F et al. Inhibition of malarial topoisomerase II in *Plasmodium falciparum* by antisense nanoparticles. International Journal of Pharmaceutics. 2006;**319**(1-2):139-146

[30] Attasart P et al. Inhibition of *Plasmodium falciparum* proliferation in vitro by double-stranded RNA nanoparticle against malaria topoisomerase II. Experimental Parasitology. 2016;**164**:84-90

[31] Ravaee R et al. Synthetic siRNAs effectively target cystein protease 12 and alpha-actinin transcripts in *Trichomonas vaginalis*. Experimental Parasitology. 2015;**157**:30-34

[32] Hussein AS, Kichenin K, Selkirk ME. Suppression of secreted acetylcholinesterase expression in *Nippostrongylus brasiliensis* by RNA interference. Molecular and Biochemical Parasitology. 2002;**122**(1):91-94

[33] Tchoubrieva EB et al. Vector-based RNA interference of cathepsin B1 in *Schistosoma mansoni*. Cellular and Molecular Life Sciences. 2010;**67**(21): 3739-3748

[34] Guidi A et al. Application of RNAi to genomic drug target validation in Schistosomes. PLoS Neglected Tropical Diseases. 2015;**9**(5):e0003801

[35] Aboobaker AA, Blaxter ML. Use of RNA interference to investigate gene function in the human filarial nematode parasite *Brugia malayi*. Molecular and Biochemical Parasitology. 2003;**129**(1): 41-51

[36] Chen MX et al. Identification and characterization of microRNAs in *Trichinella spiralis* by comparison

with *Brugia malayi* and *Caenorhabditis elegans*. Parasitology Research. 2011;**109**(3):553-558

[37] Wang J et al. Deep small RNA sequencing from the nematode Ascaris reveals conservation, functional diversification, and novel developmental profiles. Genome Research. 2011;**21**(9):1462-1477

[38] Chen MX et al. *Angiostrongylus cantonensis*: Identification and characterization of microRNAs in male and female adults. Experimental Parasitology. 2011;**128**(2):116-120

[39] Ai L et al. Characterization of microRNAs in *Taenia saginata* of zoonotic significance by Solexa deep sequencing and bioinformatics analysis. Parasitology Research. 2012;**110**(6):2373-2378

[40] Cucher M et al. High-throughput characterization of Echinococcus spp. metacestode miRNomes. International Journal for Parasitology. 2015;**45**(4):253-267

[41] Winter AD et al. Diversity in parasitic nematode genomes: The microRNAs of *Brugia pahangi* and *Haemonchus contortus* are largely novel. BMC Genomics. 2012;**13**:4

[42] Lustigman S et al. RNA interference targeting cathepsin L and Z-like cysteine proteases of *Onchocerca volvulus* confirmed their essential function during L3 molting. Molecular and Biochemical Parasitology. 2004;**138**(2):165-170

[43] Knox DP et al. RNA interference in parasitic nematodes of animals: A reality check? Trends in Parasitology. 2007;**23**(3):105-107

[44] Viney ME, Thompson FJ. Two hypotheses to explain why RNA interference does not work in animal parasitic nematodes. International Journal for Parasitology. 2008;**38**(1):43-47

[45] Hsueh EC, Morton DL. Antigen-based immunotherapy of melanoma: Canvaxin therapeutic polyvalent cancer vaccine. Seminars in Cancer Biology. 2003;**13**(6):401-407

[46] Morsink LM, Walter RB. Novel monoclonal antibody-based therapies for acute myeloid leukemia. Best Practice & Research. Clinical Haematology. 2019;**32**(2):116-126

[47] Waghabi MC et al. SB-431542, a transforming growth factor beta inhibitor, impairs *Trypanosoma cruzi* infection in cardiomyocytes and parasite cycle completion. Antimicrobial Agents and Chemotherapy. 2007;**51**(8):2905-2910

[48] Waghabi MC et al. Pharmacological inhibition of transforming growth factor beta signaling decreases infection and prevents heart damage in acute Chagas' disease. Antimicrobial Agents and Chemotherapy. 2009;**53**(11): 4694-4701

[49] Munoz-Fernandez MA, Fernandez MA, Fresno M. Synergism between tumor necrosis factor-alpha and interferon-gamma on macrophage activation for the killing of intracellular *Trypanosoma cruzi* through a nitric oxide-dependent mechanism. European Journal of Immunology. 1992;**22**(2):301-307

[50] Murray HW et al. Determinants of response to interleukin-10 receptor blockade immunotherapy in experimental visceral leishmaniasis. The Journal of Infectious Diseases. 2003;**188**(3):458-464

[51] Badaro R et al. Treatment of visceral leishmaniasis with pentavalent antimony and interferon gamma. The New England Journal of Medicine. 1990;**322**(1):16-21

[52] Macedo MS et al. Immunomodulation induced by *Ascaris suum* extract in mice: Effect of anti-interleukin-4 and anti-interleukin-10 antibodies. Scandinavian Journal of Immunology. 1998;**47**(1):10-18

[53] Cheever AW et al. Anti-IL-4 treatment of *Schistosoma mansoni*-infected mice inhibits development of T cells and non-B, non-T cells expressing Th2 cytokines while decreasing egg-induced hepatic fibrosis. Journal of Immunology. 1994;**153**(2):753-759

[54] Wynn TA et al. An IL-12-based vaccination method for preventing fibrosis induced by schistosome infection. Nature. 1995;**376**(6541):594-596

[55] Zhao A et al. Critical role of IL-25 in nematode infection-induced alterations in intestinal function. Journal of Immunology. 2010;**185**(11):6921-6929

[56] Huang Y et al. IL-25-responsive, lineage-negative KLRG1(hi) cells are multipotential 'inflammatory' type 2 innate lymphoid cells. Nature Immunology. 2015;**16**(2):161-169

[57] Humphreys NE et al. IL-33, a potent inducer of adaptive immunity to intestinal nematodes. Journal of Immunology. 2008;**180**(4):2443-2449

[58] Owyang AM et al. Interleukin 25 regulates type 2 cytokine-dependent immunity and limits chronic inflammation in the gastrointestinal tract. The Journal of Experimental Medicine. 2006;**203**(4):843-849

[59] Artis D et al. The IL-27 receptor (WSX-1) is an inhibitor of innate and adaptive elements of type 2 immunity. Journal of Immunology. 2004;**173**(9):5626-5634

[60] Pauken KE, Wherry EJ. Overcoming T cell exhaustion in infection and cancer. Trends in Immunology. 2015; **36**(4):265-276

[61] Butt AQ, Mills KH. Immuno-suppressive networks and checkpoints controlling antitumor immunity and their blockade in the development of cancer immunotherapeutics and vaccines. Oncogene. 2014;**33**(38):4623-4631

[62] Blackburn SD et al. Coregulation of CD8+ T cell exhaustion by multiple inhibitory receptors during chronic viral infection. Nature Immunology. 2009;**10**(1):29-37

[63] Singh B et al. A molecular signature for CD8(+) T cells from visceral leishmaniasis patients. Parasite Immunology. 2019;**41**(11):e12669

[64] Esch KJ et al. Programmed death 1-mediated T cell exhaustion during visceral leishmaniasis impairs phagocyte function. Journal of Immunology. 2013;**191**(11):5542-5550

[65] Murphy ML et al. B7-2 blockade enhances T cell responses to *Leishmania donovani*. Journal of Immunology. 1997;**159**(9):4460-4466

[66] Doe HT et al. Expression of PD-1/LAG-3 and cytokine production by CD4(+) T cells during infection with Plasmodium parasites. Microbiology and Immunology. 2016;**60**(2):121-131

[67] Butler NS et al. Therapeutic blockade of PD-L1 and LAG-3 rapidly clears established blood-stage Plasmodium infection. Nature Immunology. 2011;**13**(2):188-195

[68] Fajardo-Moser M, Berzel S, Moll H. Mechanisms of dendritic cell-based vaccination against infection. International Journal of Medical Microbiology. 2008;**298**(1-2):11-20

[69] Delamarre L, Mellman I. Harnessing dendritic cells for immunotherapy. Seminars in Immunology. 2011;**23**(1):2-11

[70] Steinman RM. Dendritic cells in vivo: A key target for a new vaccine science. Immunity. 2008;**29**(3):319-324

[71] Rosenberg SA et al. Durable complete responses in heavily pretreated patients with metastatic melanoma using T-cell transfer immunotherapy. Clinical Cancer Research. 2011;**17**(13):4550-4557

[72] Agallou M, Margaroni M, Karagouni E. Cellular vaccination with bone marrow-derived dendritic cells pulsed with a peptide of *Leishmania infantum* KMP-11 and CpG oligonucleotides induces protection in a murine model of visceral leishmaniasis. Vaccine. 2011;**29**(31):5053-5064

[73] Agallou M et al. Vaccination with Leishmania histone H1-pulsed dendritic cells confers protection in murine visceral leishmaniasis. Vaccine. 2012;**30**(34):5086-5093

[74] Belyaev NN et al. Induction of an IL7-R(+)c-Kit(hi) myelolymphoid progenitor critically dependent on IFN-gamma signaling during acute malaria. Nature Immunology. 2010;**11**(6):477-485

[75] Asami M et al. Susceptibility of multipotent haemopoietic stem cell deficient W/Wv mice to *Plasmodium berghei*-infection. Immunology and Cell Biology. 1991;**69**(**Pt 5**):355-360

[76] Thakur RS et al. Mesenchymal stem cells play an important role in host protective immune responses against malaria by modulating regulatory T cells. European Journal of Immunology. 2013;**43**(8):2070-2077

[77] Guarita-Souza LC et al. Simultaneous autologous transplantation of cocultured mesenchymal stem cells and skeletal myoblasts improves ventricular function in a murine model of Chagas disease. Circulation. 2006;**114**(1 Suppl):I120-I124

[78] Soares MB et al. Transplanted bone marrow cells repair heart tissue and reduce myocarditis in chronic chagasic mice. The American Journal of Pathology. 2004;**164**(2):441-447

[79] Topalis P et al. Anatomical ontologies of mosquitoes and ticks, and their web browsers in VectorBase. Insect Molecular Biology. 2008;**17**(1):87-89

[80] Vilas-Boas F et al. Bone marrow cell transplantation in Chagas' disease heart failure: Report of the first human experience. Arquivos Brasileiros de Cardiologia. 2011;**96**(4):325-331

[81] Vilas-Boas F et al. Early results of bone marrow cell transplantation to the myocardium of patients with heart failure due to Chagas disease. Arquivos Brasileiros de Cardiologia. 2006;**87**(2):159-166

[82] Bhadra R, Cobb DA, Khan IA. Donor CD8+ T cells prevent *Toxoplasma gondii* de-encystation but fail to rescue the exhausted endogenous CD8+ T cell population. Infection and Immunity. 2013;**81**(9):3414-3425

[83] Tessema TS, Dauber E, Petry F. Adoptive transfer of protective immunity from *Cryptosporidium parvum*-infected interferon-gamma and interleukin-12-deficient mice to naive recipients. Vaccine. 2009;**27**(47):6575-6581

[84] Bedi B, McNair NN, Mead JR. Dendritic cells play a role in host susceptibility to *Cryptosporidium parvum* infection. Immunology Letters. 2014;**158**(1-2):42-51

[85] Chen F et al. Neutrophils prime a long-lived effector macrophage phenotype that mediates accelerated helminth expulsion. Nature Immunology. 2014;**15**(10):938-946

[86] Taylor MD et al. Removal of regulatory T cell activity reverses hyporesponsiveness and leads to filarial parasite clearance in vivo. Journal of Immunology. 2005;**174**(8):4924-4933

[87] Anyan WK et al. Basophil depletion downregulates *Schistosoma mansoni* egg-induced granuloma formation. Parasitology International. 2013;**62**(6):508-513

[88] Lundie RJ et al. A central role for hepatic conventional dendritic cells

in supporting Th2 responses during helminth infection. Immunology and Cell Biology. 2016;**94**(4):400-410

[89] Falcon CR et al. Adoptive transfer of dendritic cells pulsed with *Fasciola hepatica* antigens and lipopolysaccharides confers protection against fasciolosis in mice. The Journal of Infectious Diseases. 2012;**205**(3):506-514

[90] Matisz CE et al. Suppression of colitis by adoptive transfer of helminth antigen-treated dendritic cells requires interleukin-4 receptor-alpha signaling. Scientific Reports. 2017;7:40631

[91] Wetzel DM, McMahon-Pratt D, Koleske AJ. The Abl and Arg kinases mediate distinct modes of phagocytosis and are required for maximal Leishmania infection. Molecular and Cellular Biology. 2012;**32**(15):3176-3186

[92] Cummings HE et al. Critical role for phosphoinositide 3-kinase gamma in parasite invasion and disease progression of cutaneous leishmaniasis. Proceedings of the National Academy of Sciences of the United States of America. 2012;**109**(4):1251-1256

[93] Khadem F et al. Pharmacological inhibition of p110delta subunit of PI3K confers protection against experimental leishmaniasis. The Journal of Antimicrobial Chemotherapy. 2017;**72**(2):467-477

[94] Vishwakarma P et al. Ammonium trichloro [1,2-ethanediolato-O,O′]-tellurate cures experimental visceral leishmaniasis by redox modulation of Leishmania donovani trypanothione reductase and inhibiting host integrin linked PI3K/Akt pathway. Cellular and Molecular Life Sciences. 2018;**75**(3):563-588

[95] Dubovsky JA et al. Ibrutinib is an irreversible molecular inhibitor of ITK driving a Th1-selective pressure in T lymphocytes. Blood. 2013;**122**(15):2539-2549

[96] Croxford JL et al. Effects of cannabinoid treatment on Chagas disease pathogenesis: Balancing inhibition of parasite invasion and immunosuppression. Cellular Microbiology. 2005;**7**(11):1592-1602

[97] Silva JF et al. Mechanisms of vascular dysfunction in acute phase of *Trypanosoma cruzi* infection in mice. Vascular Pharmacology. 2016;**82**:73-81

[98] Talvani A et al. Leukotriene B(4) induces nitric oxide synthesis in *Trypanosoma cruzi*-infected murine macrophages and mediates resistance to infection. Infection and Immunity. 2002;**70**(8):4247-4253

[99] Aliberti JC et al. Platelet-activating factor induces nitric oxide synthesis in *Trypanosoma cruzi*-infected macrophages and mediates resistance to parasite infection in mice. Infection and Immunity. 1999;**67**(6):2810-2814

[100] Botoni FA et al. A randomized trial of carvedilol after renin-angiotensin system inhibition in chronic Chagas cardiomyopathy. American Heart Journal. 2007;**153**(4):544 e1-544 e8

[101] Woodring JL et al. Evaluation of aromatic 6-substituted Thienopyrimidines as scaffolds against parasites that cause Trypanosomiasis, Leishmaniasis, and Malaria. MedChemComm. 2015;**6**(2):339-346

[102] Diaz-Gonzalez R et al. The susceptibility of trypanosomatid pathogens to PI3/mTOR kinase inhibitors affords a new opportunity for drug repurposing. PLoS Neglected Tropical Diseases. 2011;**5**(8):e1297

[103] Ivory CP, Chadee K. Activation of dendritic cells by the Gal-lectin of *Entamoeba histolytica* drives Th1 responses in vitro and in vivo. European Journal of Immunology. 2007;**37**(2):385-394

[104] Serghides L et al. Rosiglitazone modulates the innate immune

response to *Plasmodium falciparum* infection and improves outcome in experimental cerebral malaria. The Journal of Infectious Diseases. 2009;**199**(10):1536-1545

[105] Zaiss MM et al. IL-1beta suppresses innate IL-25 and IL-33 production and maintains helminth chronicity. PLoS Pathogens. 2013;**9**(8):e1003531

[106] Guirgis BS et al. Gold nanoparticle-based fluorescence immunoassay for malaria antigen detection. Analytical and Bioanalytical Chemistry. 2012;**402**(3):1019-1027

[107] Thiramanas R et al. Sensitivity and specificity of PS/AA-modified nanoparticles used in malaria detection. Microbial Biotechnology. 2013;**6**(4):406-413

[108] Wang H et al. A piezoelectric immunoagglutination assay for *Toxoplasma gondii* antibodies using gold nanoparticles. Biosensors & Bioelectronics. 2004;**19**(7):701-709

[109] Weigum SE et al. Amplification-free detection of *Cryptosporidium parvum* nucleic acids with the use of DNA/RNA-directed gold nanoparticle assemblies. The Journal of Parasitology. 2013;**99**(5):923-926

[110] Hemadi A et al. Bioconjugated fluorescent silica nanoparticles for the rapid detection of *Entamoeba histolytica*. Acta Tropica. 2015;**145**:26-30

[111] Andreadou M et al. A novel non-amplification assay for the detection of Leishmania spp. in clinical samples using gold nanoparticles. Journal of Microbiological Methods. 2014;**96**:56-61

[112] de la Escosura-Muniz A et al. Magnetic bead/gold nanoparticle double-labeled primers for electrochemical detection of isothermal amplified Leishmania DNA. Small. 2016;**12**(2):205-213

[113] Kunjachan S et al. Physicochemical and biological aspects of macrophage-mediated drug targeting in anti-microbial therapy. Fundamental & Clinical Pharmacology. 2012;**26**(1):63-71

[114] Gaafar MR et al. Chitosan and silver nanoparticles: Promising anti-toxoplasma agents. Experimental Parasitology. 2014;**143**:30-38

[115] Hagras NA et al. Successful treatment of acute experimental toxoplasmosis by spiramycin-loaded chitosan nanoparticles. Experimental Parasitology. 2019;**204**:107717

[116] Said DE, Elsamad LM, Gohar YM. Validity of silver, chitosan, and curcumin nanoparticles as anti-Giardia agents. Parasitology Research. 2012;**111**(2):545-554

[117] Ahmed SA, El-Mahallawy HS, Karanis P. Inhibitory activity of chitosan nanoparticles against *Cryptosporidium parvum* oocysts. Parasitology Research. 2019;**118**(7):2053-2063

[118] Gaafar MR et al. Silver nanoparticles as a therapeutic agent in experimental cyclosporiasis. Experimental Parasitology. 2019;**207**:107772

[119] Moon JJ et al. Antigen-displaying lipid-enveloped PLGA nanoparticles as delivery agents for a *Plasmodium vivax* malaria vaccine. PLoS One. 2012;**7**(2): e31472

[120] Pusic K et al. Iron oxide nanoparticles as a clinically acceptable delivery platform for a recombinant blood-stage human malaria vaccine. The FASEB Journal. 2013;**27**(3):1153-1166

[121] Das S et al. One pot synthesis of gold nanoparticles and application in chemotherapy of wild and resistant type visceral leishmaniasis. Colloids and Surfaces. B, Biointerfaces. 2013;**107**:27-34

[122] Kunjachan S et al. Chitosan-based macrophage-mediated drug targeting

for the treatment of experimental visceral leishmaniasis. Journal of Microencapsulation. 2011;**28**(4):301-310

[123] Asthana S et al. Immunoadjuvant chemotherapy of visceral leishmaniasis in hamsters using amphotericin B-encapsulated nanoemulsion template-based chitosan nanocapsules. Antimicrobial Agents and Chemotherapy. 2013;**57**(4):1714-1722

[124] Chaubey P, Mishra B. Mannose-conjugated chitosan nanoparticles loaded with rifampicin for the treatment of visceral leishmaniasis. Carbohydrate Polymers. 2014;**101**:1101-1108

[125] Luzardo Alvarez A et al. In vitro evaluation of the suppressive effect of chitosan/poly(vinyl alcohol) microspheres on attachment of *C. parvum* to enterocytic cells. European Journal of Pharmaceutical Sciences. 2012;**47**(1):215-227

[126] Abulaihaiti M et al. Efficacy of albendazole-chitosan microsphere-based treatment for alveolar Echinococcosis in mice. PLoS Neglected Tropical Diseases. 2015;**9**(9):e0003950

[127] Liang W et al. Efficacy of albendazole chitosan microspheres against *Echinococcus granulosus* infection in mice. Zhongguo Ji Sheng Chong Xue Yu Ji Sheng Chong Bing Za Zhi. 2014;**32**(3):188-192

[128] Barrera MG et al. In vivo evaluation of albendazole microspheres for the treatment of *Toxocara canis* larva migrans. European Journal of Pharmaceutics and Biopharmaceutics. 2010;**75**(3):451-454

[129] Gherbawy YA et al. The anti-fasciolasis properties of silver nanoparticles produced by *Trichoderma harzianum* and their improvement of the anti-fasciolasis drug triclabendazole. International Journal of Molecular Sciences. 2013;**14**(11):21887-21898

[130] Frezza TF et al. Liposomal-praziquantel: Efficacy against *Schistosoma mansoni* in a preclinical assay. Acta Tropica. 2013;**128**(1):70-75

[131] Amara RO et al. Praziquantel-lipid nanocapsules: An oral nanotherapeutic with potential *Schistosoma mansoni* tegumental targeting. International Journal of Nanomedicine. 2018;**13**: 4493-4505

[132] El-Moslemany RM et al. Miltefosine lipid nanocapsules: Intersection of drug repurposing and nanotechnology for single dose oral treatment of pre-patent *Schistosomiasis mansoni*. Acta Tropica. 2016;**159**:142-148

[133] Kaba SA et al. Protective antibody and CD8+ T-cell responses to the *Plasmodium falciparum* circumsporozoite protein induced by a nanoparticle vaccine. PLoS One. 2012;**7**(10):e48304

[134] El Bissati K et al. Effectiveness of a novel immunogenic nanoparticle platform for Toxoplasma peptide vaccine in HLA transgenic mice. Vaccine. 2014;**32**(26):3243-3248

[135] Higa LH et al. Archaeosomes display immunoadjuvant potential for a vaccine against Chagas disease. Human Vaccines & Immunotherapeutics. 2013;**9**(2):409-412

[136] Saljoughian N et al. Development of novel prime-boost strategies based on a tri-gene fusion recombinant L. tarentolae vaccine against experimental murine visceral leishmaniasis. PLOS Neglected Tropical Diseases. 2013;**7**(4):e2174

Section 2

Genes to Personalized Medicine and Molecular Therapie

Chapter 3

New Perspectives in Personalization of Therapy for Hematological Cancers

Małgorzata Rogalińska

Abstract

A progress in treatment of hematological cancers was achieved. Unfortunately, some youngsters, because of rare genetic alterations that are not easy to detect, as well as heavily pretreated old patients, because of coexisting diseases that lead to changes in patient metabolism, do not respond to therapy. Moreover, sometimes familiar diversities and alterations on genetic or epigenetic level that could be transferred on diversities in metabolism or cell signaling might be a reason why patients do not respond to therapy. Interestingly, for older patients a resistance to therapy could also occur as a reason of drug cross-reactivity. For designing of effective anticancer therapy for patient with chronic lymphocytic leukemia before drug administration, patient's leukemic cell response to anticancer drug(s) should be checked. Moreover, for patient response to treatment, also drugs prescribed previously by other medical doctors or even patients' diet could be important for achieving therapeutic success of therapy. Therefore it is important to choose the effective drugs before their administration to patient that will improve treatment efficacy and exclude resistance to therapy. It must be stated that the special attention for personalized therapy tests should be focused on patients previously resistant to therapy, more sensitive to drugs or heavily pretreated.

Keywords: personalization of therapy, resistance to treatment, anticancer drugs

1. Introduction

Several studies around the world are focus on molecular aspects related with developing of cancer. It seems to be not easy, because of high complexity of carcinogenesis and a difference between patients in disease progressing based on genetic, epigenetic or even environmental alteration. It is possible that in our bodies expression of proteins or external factors regulate hormone expression. Moreover, hormones could affect cell signal transduction and metabolism. It looks like we have some logical plan that coordinates gene expression, but because of potential involvement of many factors and familiar, sometimes even personal, predispositions for particular type of disease, diagnostic is not easy. The personal differences in disease progression activity and response to treatment reveal that even now cancers are the leading cause of death. The best way to avoid carcinogenesis is a health prophylactic since childhood. It is more likely that cancer or other diseases related with some disturbances in metabolism, except genetically related

 IntechOpen

documented cases, will develop in the group of overweight people with metabolic or hormonal disturbances and without physical exercises. For good health condition since childhood, we need to supplement probiotic bacteria to have bacterial flora in intestines that could cooperate somehow and save people against most infections and inflammation [1]. Moreover, it is very important what we consume. Food processing should be ecological, without unhealthy chemical additives [2, 3]. It must be underlined that health prophylactic might decrease the risk of getting ill or even save us from many diseases, including cancers. Proper screening tests that are able to find health problems in not advanced phase of disease are very important for prophylactic. It is extremely important to discover disease in early stage of development so we can effectively help patient to cure the disease, achieving success. It is always better and also cheaper to prevent than to cure diseases.

Before we had enough knowledge to cure successive cancers, the most effective in the war against cancers seems to be a prophylactic. The prophylactic tests should be designed for each person individually based on personal or genetic predispositions, work-related conditions, weight, or diet. Prophylactic test program should be organized by the Ministry of Health and paid from money directed to health service from our taxes.

The suitable prophylactic for professions, and increasing knowledge about disease development, could enlarge human life and decrease number of cases of cardiovascular diseases (e.g. stroke or heart attack). Therefore, we must remember that the special diet and physical exercises are able to regulate our hormone level, metabolism, and cell signaling leading to homeostasis [4, 5]. The disturbances in homeostasis could accompany the development of many diseases, including cancers.

There are several different types of lymphoproliferative disorders, characterized by disturbances in cell cycle and/or signal transduction that lead to fast proliferation of cancer cells (acute form) [6]. The other chronic type of neoplasm is caused, for example, by abrogation in apoptosis induction leading to accumulation of leukemic cells in peripheral blood. It was previously reported that in patient blood a quiescent and cycling cells were found that could be a problem in diagnostics and treatment [7–9].

Chronic lymphocytic leukemia (CLL), except bone marrow transplantation, for some patients is incurable. CLL usually occurs in older individuals but in youngsters could transform into a more aggressive form with fast developing disease [8].

Interestingly, a high heterogeneity in disease development, the characteristic accumulation in patient blood of mainly resting B lymphocytes, was observed. Leukemic cells accumulate in patient peripheral blood, because of inhibition in induction of apoptosis.

Several factors, even patient diet, could affect disease development and transformation into active form. It could lead to disturbances in cell cycle leading to increased cancer cell proliferation index. It could also induce changes in cell sensitivity to drug(s) [10]. The results of experiments directed toward personalization of therapy for CLL patients revealed that it is important to analyze before drug(s) administration if drug(s) will be active for this patient curing [10–14]. Moreover, during leukemic cell incubation with drugs, we are able to check also patients' cell sensitivity to in vitro incubation conditions. If in control untreated cells, cell viability decreases similarly like in treated ones, it is an indication that patient might need a reduction in drug dose in vivo [15]. Moreover, we need more knowledge on this topic to be able precisely to transform drug doses obtained in patient's blood into in vitro conditions. It must be underlined that for some patients more sensitive to drug(s) than others using above tests in vitro we are able to choose the proper drug(s) dose to optimize drug(s) doses administration in vivo. For patients responding to treatment in nonstandard way and for patients more sensitive than others to drugs, a personalized therapy test could be a chance to choose effective treatment for curing to avoid drug resistance, patient fatigue or sometimes also secondary cancers. Moreover, the ineffective treatment might reduce patients' life longevity. Therefore it is very important to check before administration if drug will be active to patient or in the case of resistance to search for other potentially effective drug.

The special value of personalized therapy tests is presented in **Figure 1**. The representative combined results obtained for CLL patient by tests such as cell viability (flow cytometry; Vybrant Apoptosis Assay), analyses of thermal profiles of nuclei (differential scanning calorimetry) and PARP expression/proteolytic cleavage (Western blot) for patient confirm the value for such test in choosing effective therapy for CLL patient (**Figure 1**). The representative results for CLL patient confirm that leukemic cells were more sensitive to the combination of cladribine and cyclophosphamide/mafosfamide than the combination of fludarabine and cyclophosphamide/mafosfamide. For this patient adding rituximab does not change anything in cells' reactivity to drugs (compare CM and Rit20CM results). The combination of cladribine and cyclophosphamide/mafosfamide will be more effective for this patient curing than the combination including fludarabine. Moreover, the addition of monoclonal antibody to CM combination did not change anything when we analyze all results obtained for patient.

In **Figure 2** there is an explanation why we should analyze each patient results separately. It must be stated that in the median results of cell viability presented in **Figure 2** (Section A), there are also results of both patients presented in Sections B (better responder to CM than FM) and C (resistant to therapy). The median results of cell viability for patients B and C could be misleading and suggest that both patients should be administered with fludarabine and cyclophosphamide. For both patients (see **Figure 2B** and **C**) fludarabine will not be an optimal drug for curing.

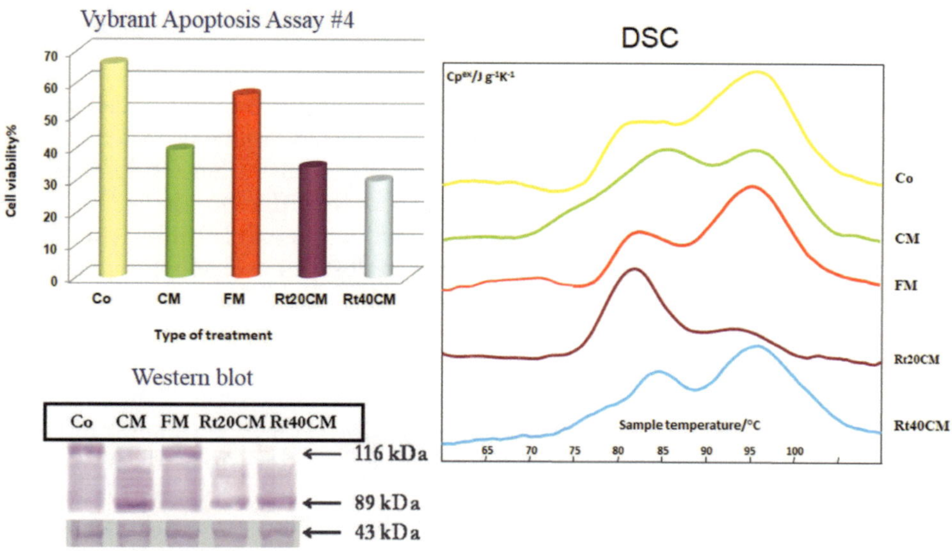

Figure 1.
Personalized therapy for CLL patient. Results of cell sensitivity with anticancer agents. Cell viability of chronic lymphocytic leukemia cells incubated for 48 h without Co and with anticancer drugs; Co, controlled untreated CLL cells; CM, cladribine + mafosfamide; FM, fludarabine + mafosfamide; RtCM (20 or 40 μM), rituximab + CM. Differences in thermal profiles were analyzed by differential scanning calorimetry (DSC). Analysis of protein expression related to apoptosis (PARP cleavage; 89 kDa) or actin (43 kDa) was studied by Western blot.

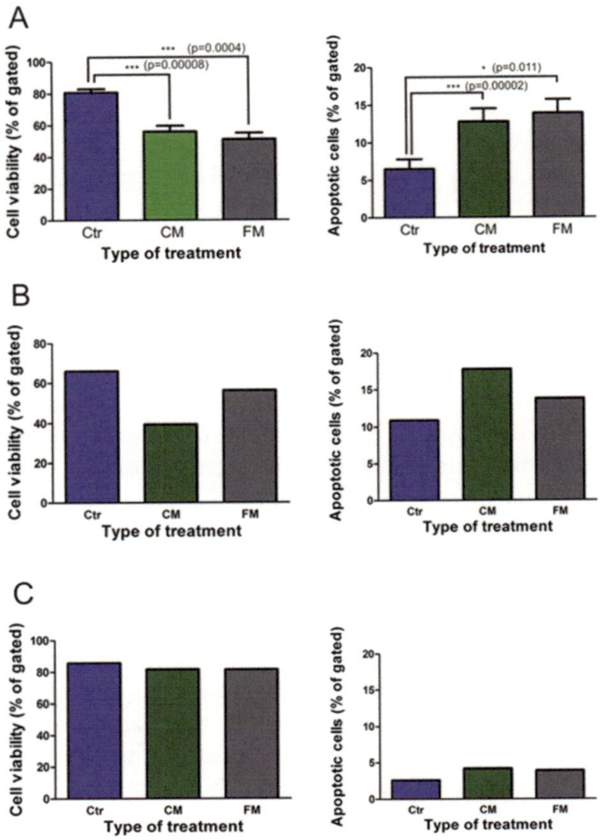

Figure 2.
Cell viability of chronic lymphocytic leukemia cells incubated for 48 h without Ctr and with anticancer drugs; CM, cladribine + mafosfamide; FM, fludarabine + mafosfamide; ***A****, median value of cell viability;* ***B****, results obtained for cells of CLL patient (better responded to CM than to FM);* ***C****, results obtained for cells of CLL patient resistant to treatment.*

Using above tests we can also monitor the differences in drug sensitivity during disease development (**Figure 3**) [10]. As presented in **Figure 3** results of cell sensitivity to anticancer agents could change during disease development. In active form of disease (year 2013), a higher leukocytosis than 18 months earlier results (year 2011) was noticed. For the same patient, we can observe differences in leukemic cell sensitivity to the same anticancer agents, i.e., combinations of cladribine + mafosfamide (cyclophosphamide), CM; fludarabine + mafosfamide (cyclophosphamide), FM; rituximab + CM (RCM); kinetin riboside (RK), that confirm the usefulness of personalized therapy tests also in monitoring of disease development and the changes in drug sensitivity [10].

Results of cell viability of chronic lymphocytic leukemia cells incubated for 48 h (24, 48 h) without Ctr and with anticancer drugs; CM, cladribine + mafosfamide; FM, fludarabine + mafosfamide; RCM, rituximab + CM; Rit, rituximab; RK, kinetin riboside [10].

The existing data confirm that in the development of CLL, some disturbances in cell signaling [16], apoptosis inhibition, or changes on epigenetic level [17–20] are observed. Moreover, the results of studies confirm that there are several molecules generated from encoded sequences of genes, characterized as miRNA that could affect gene expression, mainly by silencing. It could also be involved in regulation of protein synthesis important for cell cycle.

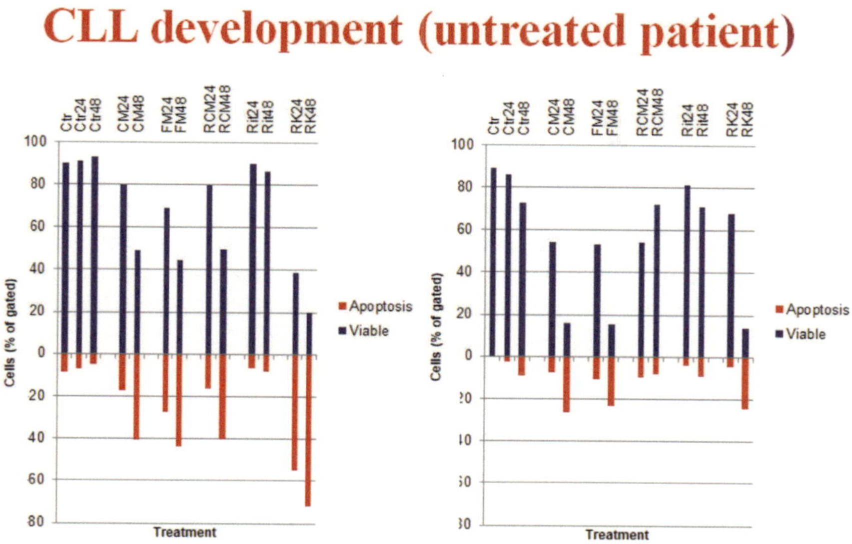

Figure 3.
Differences in drug sensitivity during disease development for the same CLL patient (results from year 2011 and 2013).

The background of chemoresistance includes one or more of the following mechanisms: induction of DNA repair, silencing of gene expression, some alterations in metabolism or in drug target structure, modifications in cell membrane or microenvironment composition, elevated expression of drug efflux pumps, and inhibition of apoptosis [21–24].

Everything is very complex, and on the one hand familiar diversities could affect cell signaling and metabolism; on the other hand also environmental factors could be important for final reaction of our cells and bodies to drugs, even human diet.

At the moment it is better to analyze the total effect of drug activity on leukemic cells before drug administration to CLL patient, preventing resistance to treatment.

Diagnostics for CLL are still based on the analysis of expression of characteristic clusters of differentiation (CD) as well as the presence of cytogenetic alterations (chromosomal aberrations) [25–27].

The currently used drugs in hematological clinics for CLL treatment are usually directed toward inhibition of Bcl-2 gene expression (venotoclax), inhibition of pathways related with signal transduction, for example, involved in inhibition of competitive binding of ATP to Bruton kinase (ibrutinib), or inhibition of PI3K signaling (idelalisib) [27–31]. Both kinases are involved in B-cell receptor signaling.

Venotoclax (VEN, ABT-199) is a selective inhibitor of antiapoptotic protein Bcl-2 expression. It is a BH3-mimetic molecule targeting BCL-2. VEN binds to BCL-2 and could activate BIM and induce apoptosis signaling. VEN demonstrates an activity in patients with poor prognostic, 17p-deleted chronic lymphocytic leukemia (CLL) [28]. VEN shows clinical activity on many hematological malignancies, lymphomas, acute myeloid leukemia, and early T-cell precursor ALL.

Ibrutinib directly works as an inhibitor of Bruton tyrosine kinase (BTK). Interestingly, there is crosstalk between Bruton tyrosine kinase signaling and bioenergetic stress responses. In primary chronic lymphocytic leukemia cells, a pharmacological interference between mitochondrial ATP synthesis and glucose metabolism could affect BTK activity. Moreover, ibrutinib could induce bioenergetic stress responses [32] that might affect for its resistance. Therefore ibrutinib activity could be regulated by glucose level, and patients with hyperglycemia might be resistant to ibrutinib treatment in TP53 deficient chronic lymphocytic leukemia (CLL) lymphocytes [28].

Idelalisib is an inhibitor of the delta isoform of the phosphatidylinositol 3-kinase (PI3K). Drug could be active on cell proliferation, survival, or even induction of apoptosis. Moreover the strong heterogeneity of CLL feature and involvement in PI3K signaling could be a reason of differences between patients in clinical development of CLL and diversities in response to therapy. Idelalisib could induce several possible side effects, including hepatotoxicity, diarrhea, colitis, pneumonitis, or intestinal perforation. A special importance for personalize therapy is a chance to avoid resistance to treatment and reduce the development of secondary cancer (melanoma, head and neck, prostate, breast, or lung) [16].

Drugs usually for some patients lead to disease remission that could last for many years. It is also possible that for the group of patients, drugs could be ineffective and cause resistance to therapy [31]. For CLL, drugs based on higher generations of monoclonal antibodies could usually cause cytotoxicity in B-cells and fast reductions in the number of B lymphocytes from peripheral blood, decreasing patient's immunological strength. To increase drug activity, the combined therapy based on few drugs could in theory increase patients' response to therapy. Based on our experience with leukemic cell incubations with anticancer drug(s), sometimes it does work this way; for other patients, for example, the addition of second drug will not change cell response to anticancer agents (**Figure 1**). It could prove that sometimes one drug will be enough instead of combined therapy that will not be more effective, will cause patient's weakness, and will not improve the final effect of treatment. For the group of patients, who do not react at standard way to anticancer drugs or are resistant to treatment, choosing the optimal way of treatment for patient seems to be very important for his curing.

There are several molecules, for example, generated from encoded sequences of genes (pre-mRNA), characterized as miRNA, that could affect gene expression, mainly by their silencing, and could decrease or block protein expression. Because of a high complexity of metabolic reactions and several metabolic pathways included inside the cells that could be activated by drugs, hormonal regulation of human body metabolism and several different factors, previously taken medicaments or even diet, could affect patient's response to anticancer treatment [19, 21, 23, 32, 33]. Several potential targets for anticancer agents met in the human body are a reason of drug's side effect. Moreover, some familiar or personal diversities could also change patient reactivity to drugs. Drug reactivity could also be affected by environmental factors or even patient's diet.

At the moment it is better to analyze the total effect of drug activity on leukemic cells before drug administration to patient to avoid potential resistance to treatment.

2. Conclusion

The best way to prevent diseases is a prophylactic. The well-balanced healthy diet, physical exercises, supplementation of probiotic bacteria, or screening tests showing our health condition are the best way to prevent diseases and increase life expectancy. We have to start thinking about our health since childhood, and several wrong decisions could shorten our life. Because of a high complexity in cells and human body function and not enough knowledge related to disease etiology, currently it is better to analyze in vitro the apoptosis induction potential of leukemic cells incubated for 48 h with anticancer drugs before drug administration to CLL patient to exclude resistance to treatment. The resistance to treatment is usually confirmed in CLL cells incubated for 48 h with anticancer drug(s).

While, after 24 h of cell incubation in vitro with anticancer drug(s), the necessity of dose modification usually for lower values in the case of CLL patients' more sensitive cells to drug(s) was noticed. It must be underlined that sometimes the addition of drug (rituximab) as presented in **Figure 1** does not change anything in CLL cell reactivity to drugs (CM and Rit20CM).

Acknowledgements

The author would like to thank Emeritus Professor Zofia M. Kilianska and Professor Henryk Piekarski from University of Lodz and Professor Tadeusz Robak (Department of Hematology, Medical University of Lodz), as well as Professor J. Wesierska-Gadek from Medical University of Vienna (Austria) for help and valuable advices in studies.

Author details

Małgorzata Rogalińska
Faculty of Biology and Environmental Protection, Department of Cytobiochemistry, University of Lodz, Lodz, Poland

*Address all correspondence to: malgorzata.rogalinska@biol.uni.lodz.pl; gosiar@wp.pl

References

[1] Reid G. The development of probiotics for women's health. Canadian Journal of Microbiology. 2017;**63**(4):269-277

[2] Singh RK, Chang HW, Yan D, Lee KM, Ucmak D, Wong K, et al. Influence of diet on the gut microbiome and implications for human health. Journal of Translational Medicine. 2017;**15**(1):73

[3] Shafei A, Ramzy MM, Hegazy AI, Husseny AK, El-Hadary UG, Taha MM, et al. The molecular mechanisms of action of the endocrine disrupting chemical bisphenol A in the development of cancer. Gene. 2018;**647**:235-243

[4] Liu J. Irisin as an exercise-stimulated hormone binding crosstalk between organs. European Review for Medical and Pharmacological Sciences. 2015;**19**(2):316-321

[5] Ha MS, Son WM. Combined exercise is a modality for improving insulin resistance and aging-related hormone biomarkers in elderly Korean women. Experimental Gerontology. 2018;**114**:13-18

[6] Dohner H, Weisdorf DJ, Bloomfield CD. Acute myeloid leukemia. The New England Journal of Medicine;**373**(12):1136-1152

[7] Klein U, Dalla-Favera R. Germinal centres: Role in B-cell physiology and malignancy. Nature Reviews. Immunology. 2008;**8**(1):22-33

[8] Hallek M. Chronic lymphocytic leukemia: 2020 update on diagnosis, risk stratification and treatment. American Journal of Hematology. 2020;**94**:1266-1287

[9] Robak T, Stilgenbauer S, Tedeschi A. Front-line treatment of CLL in the era of novel agents. Cancer Treatment Reviews. 2017;**53**:70-78

[10] Rogalińska M, Góralski P, Błoński JZ, Robak P, Barciszewski J, Koceva-Chyła A, et al. Personalized therapy tests for the monitoring of chronic lymphocytic leukemia development. Oncology Letters. 2017;**13**(4):2079-2084

[11] Rogalińska M, Błoński JZ, Góralski P, Wawrzyniak E, Hartman M, Rogalska A, et al. Relationship between in vitro drug sensitivity and clinical response of patients to treatment in chronic lymphocytic leukemia. International Journal of Oncology. 2015;**46**:1259-1267

[12] Rogalińska M, Kiliańska ZM. Personalized therapy versus targeted therapy, differences in the meaning. Global Journal for Research Analysis. 2015;**4**(1):5-8

[13] Rogalińska M, Franiak-Pietryga I, et al. Toward personalized therapy for chronic lymphocytic leukemia: DSC and cDNA microarray assessment of two cases. Cancer Biology & Therapy. 2014;**14**(1):1-7

[14] Góralski P, Rogalińska M, Błoński JZ, Pytel E, Robak T, Kiliańska ZM, et al. The differences in thermal profiles between normal and leukemic cells exposed to anticancer drug evaluated by differential scanning calorimetry. Journal of Thermal Analysis and Calorimetry. 2014;**118**:1339-1344

[15] Kubczak M, Szustka A, Błoński JZ, Gucký T, Misiewicz M, Krystof V, et al. Dose and drug changes in chronic lymphocytic leukemia cell response in vitro: A comparison of standard therapy regimens with two novel cyclin-dependent kinase inhibitors. Molecular Medicine Reports. 2019;**19**(5):3593-3603

[16] Wu M, Akinleye A, Zhu X. Novel agents for chronic lymphocytic leukemia. Journal of Hematology & Oncology. 2013;**6**:36

[17] Tari K, Shamsi Z, Reza Ghafari H, Atashi A, Shahjahani M, Abroun S. The role of the genetic abnormalities, epigenetic and microRNA in the prognosis of chronic lymphocytic leukemia. Experimental Oncology. 2018;**40**:261-267

[18] Martín-Subero JI, López-Otín C, Campo E. Genetic and epigenetic basis of chronic lymphocytic leukemia. Current Opinion in Hematology. 2013;**20**(4):362-368

[19] Bayraktar R, Van Roosbroeck K, Calin GA. Cell-to-cell communication: MicroRNAs as hormones. Molecular Oncology. 2017;**11**(12):1673-1686

[20] Shah MY, Ferrajoli A, Sood AK, Lopez-Berestein G, Calin GA. MicroRNA therapeutics in cancer—An emerging concept. eBioMedicine. 2016;**12**:34-42

[21] Qu Y, Dou B, Tan H, Feng Y, Wang N, Wang D. Tumor microenvironment-driven non-cell autonomous resistance to antineoplastic treatment. Molecular Cancer. 2019;**18**:69

[22] Si W, Shen J, Zheng H, Fan W. The role and mechanisms of action of microRNAs un cancer drug resistance. Clinical Epigenetics. 2019;**11**:25

[23] Galicia-Vázquez G, Aloyz R. Metabolic rewiring beyond Warburg in chronic lymphocytic leukemia: How much do we actually know? Critical Reviews in Oncology/Hematology. 2019;**134**:65-70

[24] Filip AA, Grenda A, Popek S, Koczkodaj D, Michalak-Wojnowska M, Budzyński M, et al. Expression of circulating miRNAs associated with lymphocyte differentiation and activation in CLL-another piece in the puzzle. Annals of Hematology. 2017;**96**(1):33-50

[25] Rodrigues CA, Goncalves MV, Ikoma MRV, et al. Diagnosis and treatment of chronic lymphocytic leukemia: Recommendations from the Brazilian Group of chronic lymphocytic leukemia. Revista Brasileira de Hematologia e Hemoterapia. 2016;**38**(4):346-357

[26] Wawrzyniak E, Haus O. In: Robak T, Warzocha K, editors. Znaczenie badań cytogenetycznych w hematologii. Wyd. Via Medica: Hematologia; 2016

[27] Montserrat E, Bauman T, Delgado J. Present and future of personalized medicine in CLL. Best Practice & Research. Clinical Haematology. 2016;**29**(1):100-110

[28] Seyfried F, Demir S, Hörl RL, et al. Prediction of venetoclax activity in precursor B-ALL by functional assessment of apoptosis signaling. Cell Death & Disease. 2019;**e 10**:571

[29] Choudhary G, Al-Harbi S, Mazumder S, et al. MCL-1 and BCL-xL-dependent resistance to the BCL-2 inhibitor ABT-199 can be overcome by preventing PI3K/AKT/mTOR activation in lymphoid malignancies. Cell Death & Disease. 2015;**6**:e1593

[30] Burger JA, Tedeschi A, Barr PM. Ibrutinib as initial therapy for patients with chronic lymphocytic leukemia. The New England Journal of Medicine. 2015;**373**:2425-2437

[31] Furman RR, Sharman JP, Coutre SE, et al. Idelalisib and rituximab in relapsed chronic lymphocytic leukemia. The New England Journal of Medicine. 2014;**370**:997-1007

[32] Sharif-Askari B, Doyon D, Paliouras M, et al. Bruton's tyrosine kinase is at the crossroads of metabolic adaptation in primary malignant

human lymphocytes. Scientific Reports. 2019;**9**:11069

[33] Rogalińska M. The role of mitochondria in cancer induction, progression and changes in metabolism. Mini Reviews in Medicinal Chemistry. 2016;**16**(7):524-530

Chapter 4

Genetic Risk Factors and Lysosomal Function in Parkinson Disease

Marcella Vieira Barroso Montenegro,
Carlos Eduardo de Melo Amaral
and Luiz Carlos Santana da Silva

Abstract

Parkinson disease is a complex disease that has multiple genetic and environmental factors. To achieve the early diagnosis and to be able to modify the disease progression, efforts are being made to identify individuals at risk. About 20 year ago, an evidence of major prevalence of Parkinsonism in patients with Gaucher Disease reported by studies worldwide led to the putative involvement of the *GBA* gene. Nowadays, the link from a rare disease with a common disease is well known and it is confirmed that mutations in the *GBA* gene are the most important genetic risk factor. Apart from rare mutations, genetic association studied appointed common variants in genes well associated with familial cases as *LRRK2* and *SNCA* may also contribute to the increased risk for sporadic cases. Other common variants in the *MAPT* gene were also reported. At least, genetic studies have been observed an excessive burden of relevant variants in genes with lysosomal function. Thus, a synergistic action of variants in genes that codifies proteins involved with the lysosome may be a mean of modulating the risk. In this chapter, we review the most robust genetic risk factor and the relevance of lysosomal function for Parkinson disease.

Keywords: Parkinson, GBA, risk factor, lysosome, GWAS

1. Introduction

Parkinson's disease (PD) is the second most common progressive neurodegenerative disease in humans and it is characterized by motor symptoms as muscular rigidity, resting tremor, bradykinesia, and postural instability and also by non-motor symptoms (hyposmia, constipation, depression, dementia, and postural hypotension, among others). These symptoms result primarily from the progressive loss of the dopaminergic neurons from the pars compacta of the mesencephalic substantia nigra and subsequent depletion of the dopamine neurotransmitter in the striatum, a central component of the basal ganglia that is responsible for the instigation and coordination of movements (**Figure 1**). The definitive diagnosis of PD is difficult being only confirmed with the presence of Lewy bodies, proteinaceous intracytoplasmic inclusion, in the reminiscent neurons of substantia nigra pars compacta and other regions in the brain postmortem analysis [1].

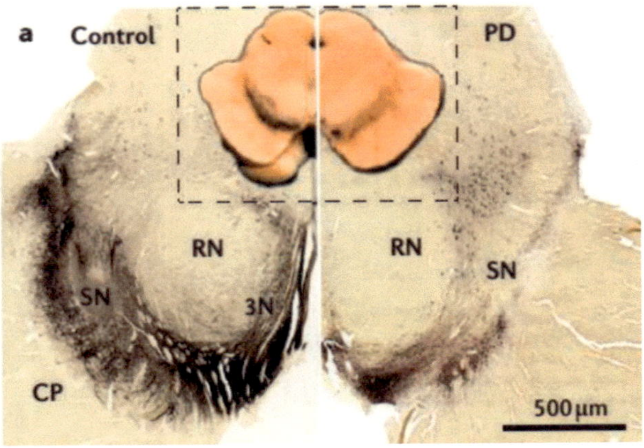

Figure 1.
Depigmentation of the substantia nigra (SN) (right panel) compared with control (left panel). Adapted from Ref. [1].

The etiology is not well understand, but PD is considered a complex disease, which counts with multiple genetic and environment factors. The most common is the sporadic PD for which the onset generally is late, after 60 years old. There is a rare form, the familial PD or monogenic PD (~10% of the cases), for which the disease is caused by mutations in a single gene and may present not only a late onset but also an earlier onset (below 45 years old) in some cases. Although less frequent, the study of monogenic forms of PD and their associated genes helps to understand the molecular basis of disease pathogenesis [1, 2].

Segregation studies of mutations in *SNCA* gene in large families with PD cases led to the discovery of the main protein involved in the disease pathogenesis, the α-synuclein. Shortly afterwards, postmortem studies in patients' brains revealed that this protein is the major component of Lewy bodies, in both sporadic and familial PD patients, reinforcing its important role in the development of PD [2–4]. Be it for genetic, environmental or both factors, the fact is that patients' brains do not have the soluble monomeric form of α-synuclein, which is easily degraded by lysosomal function, but the insoluble oligomeric forms [5, 6].

Nowadays, efforts have been directed to identify the individuals at risk of manifesting PD through clinical, genetic and biochemical markers in order to diagnose early and perhaps be possible to modify the progression of disease. For this purpose, genetic variations with the potential to alter the risk for PD have been widely researched. Both disease-causing variants and risk variants in genes associated with PD vary in frequency depending on ethnic background. Certain genetic variants may be a risk factor in an Asian population, but may not be statically significant in a European population, for example. The most robust and consistently replicated results are appointed to variants in the genes *LRRK2, MAPT, SNCA* and *GBA,* the last being the major genetic risk factor highlighting the importance of lysosomal pathway in the pathogenesis of PD [1–8].

2. Genetic risk factors

More than 20 years ago, Parkinson disease was understood as a disease caused by environmental factors only. It was from genetic analyzes in cases of familial PD that it was discovered that the genetic factor is also important and may even cause certain disease forms. Thus, we have monogenic PD, which can present a pattern of inheritance defied as autosomal dominant or autosomal recessive. In 1997, the discovery of mutations in the *SNCA* gene as the cause of PD in certain families also helped scientists to better understand the etiopathology of this complex disease through the association between the duplication and triplication of the *SNCA* gene with altered α-synuclein protein expression and the disease progression. Since then, diverse other genes were associated with mutations that cause PD, among them the genes *LRRK2* and *VPS35,* that along with *SNCA* are altered in autosomal dominant cases, and *PINK1*, *PARKIN*, *DJ-1* that are altered in autosomal recessive forms [3, 8].

However, the genetics of PD are not simply composed of variants that cause the disease. More recently, the focus has been on genetic variants that do not lead to PD alone but increase the risk of developing the disease. Among the genetic risk factors associated with sporadic PD, rare high-impact variants and common low-impact variants have been identified by candidate gene studies and genome-wide association studies (GWAS). The complexity of the PD genetic increases even more due to several risk variants for PD that are heterogeneous and dependent on the genetic background of each population. Genetic variants can be associated with PD in some populations, but not in others [8, 9].

Two largest GWAS studies in 2014 and 2017 identified in total 28 independent PD-associated risk loci, mainly in *SNCA*, *LRRK2*, *MAPT* and *GBA*. Genetic risk factors are present in several genes involved in metabolic pathways that may be directly related to α-synuclein metabolism or involved in processes that affect cellular homeostasis [10, 11].

2.1 SNCA

It is worthy to emphasize the fact that genes that carry rare casual mutations of monogenic PD observed in previous family studies are not excluded of the possibility to also carry common variants that confer risk for developing PD. This is the case of *LRRK2* and *SNCA*.

So far, five point mutations (A53T, A30P and E46K) and two copy number variation (duplication and triplication) in the gene *SNCA* are well known to cause autosomal dominant PD indistinguishable of sporadic PD, or an early-onset PD if the triplication of the gene is present [12]. Recently, single nucleotide polymorphisms (SNP) in *SCNA* were reported in non-coding regions, suggesting that those variants play a role in the regulation of the genetic expression through modifications post-transcriptional as interacting with microRNA or altering alternative splicing mechanism [7].

In 1999, the association between REP1, a complex polymorphic microsatellite repeat in the promoter region, and PD was pointed out by [13]. Seven years later, Maraganore [14] confirmed this association with a larger meta-analysis study using more than 5000 samples from 11 sites. Further, functional analysis studies provided evidence that the length of alleles affects the protein expression: the 261 bp-long risk allele is associated with an upregulation of α-synuclein expression mimicking *SNCA* locus multiplication, whereas the 259 bp-long protective variant shows reduced gene expression [15].

In 2009, Simón-Sánchez et al. [16] used GWAS in a great sample and identified additional signals of association with PD from intro 4 to after the 3′ UTR. One year later, Mata et al. [17] showed possible association between rs356219 in the 3′ UTR region and α-synuclein plasma levels. To definitely ascertain which variants in this region alter the risk for PD, more studies are necessary in large and genetically diverse samples.

2.2 LRRK2

In the region of chromosome 12 is localized the *LRRK2* gene where several genetic variants have been found; however, segregation in families with monogenic PD and case-control studies demonstrated that only seven point variants (R1441G, R1441C, R1441H, Y1699C, G2019S, I2020T and N1437H) have enough evidence to be defined as cause of PD. This gene encodes a protein of the same name composed of domains with kinase activity, GTPase and several domains of interaction with other proteins, suggesting that its function changes depending on which proteins form complexes, the type of cells and the stage of development. Mutations in *LRRK2* gene are the most common cause of PD familial cases. The mutation G2019S is the most prevalent worldwide, and it is present in 4% of familial PD and is associated with an indistinguishable phenotype from the clinical manifestations of sporadic PD [12–18].

Besides the prevalence in rare monogenic PD, this mutation can also confer risk in the sporadic PD, being found in 1% of the cases. G2019S has a penetrance variable, and its carrier's risk to develop PD depends on age and ethnic background. The age-related risk has been estimated to be 28% at age 59, 51% at 69, and 74% at 79 years. The frequency is higher in North African, Middle Eastern and Ashkenazi Jewish PD patients [18, 19].

G2019S is frequent in most populations worldwide, but it is very rare in the Asian population where it accounts for less than 1% of *LRRK2* mutations. In contrast, most common genetic variants SNPs G2385R and R1628P are more frequent in Asian populations than in Caucasian populations. Those SNPs are associated with an increased risk of 2.2 fold and 1.84 fold to develop PD, respectively [20, 21]. Lately, regions close to *LRRK2* have been appointed by GWAS as increasing by 1.2 fold the risk for PD. This fact alerts that the regulation of the gene expression is important to develop this disease [8].

Those works reinforce the idea that genes can carry both rare disease-causing variants and common variants that increase the risk for PD, as seen in *SNCA* and *LRRK2*. Additionally, common variants present in those genes enhance the importance of their proteins' role in the disease and implicate that there is a common neurodegenerative process between sporadic and familial PD.

2.3 MAPT

The gene *MAPT* is frequently associated with other neurodegenerative diseases as Alzheimer disease and frontotemporal dementia (FDT). *MAPT* encodes for the microtubule-associated protein tau, whose role is to regulate microtubule dynamics and assemble microtubules into parallel arrays within axons, essential for normal axonal transport in neurons. Polymorphisms in this gene have been found to be an indisputable risk factor of the synucleinopathy. The H1 and H2 haplotypes represent two distinct clades of subhaplotypes ensued from an inversion of ~900 kb on chromosome 17q21, spanning the entire *MAPT* coding region, and are tagged, among others, by genotypes at two SNPs: rs9468 and rs1800547 [4–8].

The H1 haplotype and its subhaplotype H1c have been significantly associated with an increased risk for a number of neurodegenerative diseases. Several studies proposed the most common H1 haplotype as susceptibility factor for PD with an odds ratio of 1.5. Recent studies that investigated the association between H1 and specific PD clinical manifestation also observed the higher prevalence of H1 in patients with cognitive defects, as dementia and H1 homozygous PD patients showed an increased risk to manifest non-tremor dominant subtype, which is a worse clinical prognosis [22, 23].

The underlying biological mechanisms that link the *MAPT* locus (and tau protein) to neurodegeneration are not yet adequately characterized. Through the functional characterization of variants in the *MAPT* gene, some theories of the tau protein effect in PD involve increased tau expression; altered gene splicing promoting aggregation; and altered 4/3 repeated transcript ratio. The emerging concept of H1 pathogenicity points to the role of each tau isoforms expressed rather than the overall number of transcripts.

According to this model, the H1 haplotype is associated with an underexpression of a protective isoform and an overexpression of the detrimental variant, which lead to a subtle neuronal dysfunction that accumulates over the years and induces or accelerates cellular degeneration [22–24]. However this locus harbors many genes and the extended linkage disequilibrium means that the tau protein may be not the cause of neurodegeneration and its DNA sequence is just close to the casual locus. Thus, while *MAPT* is a candidate, we cannot be certain that this is the true biological mediator of risk [7–16].

Diverse studies identified *MAPT* locus variants as a risk factor for PD, but it may not be true to any population. In the Caucasian population, there was this association, while it was absent in the Japanese population. This observation has potential implications for the analysis of complex traits across populations such as genetic heterogeneity, particularly at minor risk loci, highlighting the power of comparing GWAS across different populations [9–16].

Despite having a modest effect (less than 30% of the change in risk), these common variants can have a considerable impact when combined. Results from a 2015 study revealed that patients at an early age of onset of symptoms had a higher polygenic combination of risk variants than patients with a late onset. This demonstrates the possible effect of the synergistic value of the changes caused by these variants to modulate the PD clinic, such as the age of onset of symptoms [12].

3. GBA: the principal genetic risk factor for Parkinson disease

The *GBA* gene was initially described in association with a rare lysosomal storage disease (LSD) called Gaucher disease (GD). When mutated in homozygosis, depending on the mutation present, the resulting enzyme is malformed or even no enzyme is synthesized leading to enzyme glucocerebrosidase (GCase) partial or total deficiency and glucosylceramide (GlcCer) accumulation. The symptoms are multisystemic, with the brain, spleen, liver and bone marrow being the main organs affected. The presence and intensity of those symptoms differ between the three types of GD (GD1, GD2 and GD3). The heterozygous individuals do not present any clinical manifestation; however, in the last years, this perspective has changed [25, 26].

Further a number of studies have recorded the occurrence of parkinsonian manifestations in patients with GD and their relatives [27, 28]. In ref. [29] was showed that *GBA* mutations homozygous individuals have 21.4 fold increased risk to develop PD with probability of 9–12% to manifest motor symptoms before 80 years old. Despite being low, this risk is considerably higher than in the same age group in general population, 3%. The *GBA* and PD association was confirmed in the Jewish Ashkenazi, which showed a prevalence of *GBA* mutations in heterozygosis and homozygosis individuals in the PD population that by far outweighs the reported prevalence of mutations in other susceptibility genes for PD, as *Parkin* and *SNCA* [30].

Researchers worldwide have attempted to validate the same association in populations from many different genetic backgrounds [31–41]. In 2009, an international and multicenter study with a great sample of approximately 5000 PD patients and equal number of controls provided the definitive proof found for this association with an odds ratio greater than five (OR 5.3) and showed that mutations N370S and L444P are the most frequent in this gene. In other words, *GBA* mutation genes were recognized as the major genetic risk factor for PD until now [42].

In addition to alter the risk to manifest the disease, the presence of *GBA* mutations has also the potential to modify PD phenotype such as age of onset. The modulatory effects best described in the literature investigated the association with age of onset and declined cognitive. The association to other symptoms and patients survival rate has been not yet approached in more detail.

Whether in heterozygosis or in homozygosis individuals (GD patients), the age of onset of symptoms apparently occurs earlier than in PD patients without mutations, usually between the fourth and sixth decade of life [28–43]. In relation to symptoms is noticeable a cognitive decline earlier in PD patients with *GBA* mutations (PD-GBA) [26–45]. Dementia is one of the clinical manifestations that most affects the patient's quality of life and it is more frequent in GBA mutation carriers than in non-carriers. Longitudinal studies have shown that PD-GBA patients have a risk three times higher than patients without GBA mutations to present dementia [26, 44, 46]. Neuroimaging exams support this association by showing more expansive synucleinopathy in the neocortical and subcortical areas of PD-GBA patients, increasing the risk to dementia, psychosis and postural hypotension [46].

A few studies have evaluated the survival rate, if there is a greater risk of death in PD-GBA patients than in those without any mutations. A 2014 study found lower survival for the carrier group, but had a weak statistical value [47]. However, in 2016, a study with the largest sample number ever described replicated the same result with powerful statistical significance reinforcing this conclusion. It was defined in this study that there is a twice greater risk of mortality among PD-GBA patients. One explanation may be the increased presence of non-responsive levodopa motor impairments such as dysphagia and non-motor impairments such as orthostatic hypotension in the group of PD-GBA. There was no difference in disease duration compared to non-carriers, but patients were significantly younger at the time of death [46].

3.1 Genotype-phenotype correlations

Researchers have also observed different *GBA* mutations having a different impact in the clinical manifestations. Mutations generally associated with defined neuropathic forms of GD (GD type 2 and 3), such as L444P, are classified as severe mutations, while others associated with GD type 1, such as N370S, are classified as mild mutations [26–48].

A meta-analysis study included populations from North, Central and South America, Western and Eastern Europe, North Africa, Asia and Ashkenazi Jews, and its results showed a clear and significant differentiated effect comparing mild and severe mutations on the risk of developing PD and the age of onset of symptoms not only in Ashkenazi populations, but also worldwide. Severe mutations such as L444P confer a three to four times increased risk for its carriers to develop PD and are associated with the onset of symptoms 5 years earlier than mild mutations. The average age found for severe mutations was 53.1 (±11.2), whereas the average age for mild mutations was 58.1 (±10.6) [26].

The type of mutation was also relevant in modulating the cognitive impairments of PD patients. Ref. [46] observed that severe mutations conferred a higher risk of dementia for its carriers. The risk was three times greater compared to patients with mild mutations and five times greater when compared to the risk for PD without

GBA mutations. Another longitudinal study with a similar sample number corroborated with the increased risk of dementia for patients with severe mutations versus non-carriers [44]. With regard to other symptoms, motor impairments appear to be similar between patients with mild mutations and non-carriers, while those with severe mutations appear to be more aggravated and seem to have a higher frequency of non-motor symptoms such as psychosis, apathy and postural hypotension [46].

Patients' survival does not seem to differ when comparing the types of mutations with each other. However, when compared separately with non-carriers, mild mutations do not differ statistically from non-carriers, while mortality was shown to be greater for carriers of severe mutations than in non-carriers [46].

Due to the discovery and increasing number of proofs supporting the great influence of *GBA* mutations in PD, some authors consider the possibility of reclassifying them from risk factors for agents causing autosomal dominant PD [43, 49].

4. GBA-associated PD in different populations

Given the multifactorial etiology of PD, the different environment and ethnicity of a population may impact in the different results seen among the papers that investigated the frequency of *GBA* mutations in PD patients. Other possible causes of this variation can be the use of different techniques and methodologies.

The highest frequencies of mutations of the *GBA* gene have been found in PD patients of Ashkenazi Jewish ancestry, with rates of 13.7–31.3% in comparison with 4.5–6.2% in control groups [26–28]. The frequencies recorded in PD patients in non-Jewish populations representing other populations, such as Italians, Caucasian Americans, Greeks, Brazilians, British and Taiwanese, are invariably much lower—3.5% to 12.0%—while controls from the same populations range from 0% to 5.3% [31–41]. Previously, in North Africa, a study found no association between PD and mutations of the *GBA* gene; however, a more recent African study data suggested a risk association between mutations in the *GBA* gene and PD [37]. The lowest rate recorded to date was 2.3% in Norwegian PD patients, compared with 1.7% in the control [49].

The genetic background can also impact the frequency even within the same country. In Brazil, four studies evaluated the association between GBA and PD, with variances in frequencies depending on the region (**Table 1**). The North region had twice as many cases of PD patients with GBA mutations (7.4%) compared to the frequencies of the South and Southeast regions (3.5%) with a similar sample number. The fact may be explained by the different genetic composition of the North region, which, despite also has a European origin, has a higher Amerindian ancestry than the Southern Brazil, which is almost exclusively from European ancestry [31–50].

Greek and Italian studies have found significant differences comparing PD patients and controls from urban and rural areas, and from the North and South regions, respectively. In the Greek study, the frequency of *GBA* mutations between PD patients and controls was statically significant. However, when the cohorts were analyzed separately, there was a difference of frequencies. The difference between PD patients and controls was statistically significant only in the case of the patients of cohort A that is originated from Thessaly, a mainly rural area ($p = 0.021$, OR 4.2, 95% CI = 1.14–15.54) and not in the case of cohort B patients, the majority of which were residents and/or originated from the greater area of Athens, an urban environment ($p = 0.113$, OR 2.5, 95% CI = 0.77–8.42) [34].

In the Italian study, there was a lower frequency of mutations in PD patients (11/395, 2.8%) and in controls (1/483, 0.2%) from the Southern region, and the most common mutation was p.L444P. Conversely, in the Northern region, the most

Studies	Population studied	PD inclusion criteria	Method	Mutation analyzed	Patients mutation frequency	Control mutation frequency	Age of onset	*GBA* mutated PD and familiar history (FH)
Spitz et al. (2007)	65 PD patients and 267 control subjects from Southeastern Brazil	Early onset (<55 years).	PCR-RFLP, restriction endonucleases and electrophoresis	N370S and L444P	2/65 (**3%**); L444P 2/2 (100%); N370S 0/2 (0%)	0/267	Patient 1 at 46 yr old and patient 2 at 42 yr old	The two patients had FH, no statistical test was used.
Socal et al. (2008)	62 PD patients from Southern Brazil	All patients diagnosed were included.	PCR-RFLP, restriction endonucleases	N370S, L444P and IVS2þ1	2/62 (**3.5%**); L444P 1/2 (50%); N370S 1/2 (50%)	Not informed	Patients with mutation 37 ± 4 yr Patients without mutation 41.4 ± 10.8 yr	Not informed.
De Carvalho et al. (2012)	347 PD patients and 341 control subjects from Southeastern, Midwestern and Northern Brazil	All patients diagnosed were included.	Direct sequencing	N370S and L444P	13/347 (**3.7%**); L444P 8/13 (62%); N370S 5/13 (38%)	0/341	Patients with mutation 49.9 ± 11.3 yr Patients without mutation 52.5 ± 13.3 yr	Those with FH and those without FH did not present statistical significance.
Amaral et al. (2018)	81 PD patients and 81 control subjects from Northern Brazil	All patients diagnosed were included.	Amplification of the exon 8–exon 11, PCR-RFLP for N370S and L444P, restriction endonucleases and direct sequencing of N370S and L444P	N370S and L444P	6/81 (**7.4%**); L444P 3/6 (50%); N370S 3/6 (50%)	0/81	Patients with mutation 49.6 ± 17.4 yr Patients without 55.1 ± 11.6 yr	From the 6 patients, 2 had FH. No statistical test was used.

Bold valor are percentage.

Table 1.
GBA mutation among PD patients in different Brazilian regions.

frequent genetic defect found was p.N370S and the frequency of mutations in PD was 4.5% and 0.63% in controls. Therefore, the difference may be due to a particular frequency of *GBA* mutations in regions of Italy or to the sample size [36].

Although the frequency of *GBA* mutations in populations of PD patients has been well characterized worldwide, few data are available on the inverse relationship, that is, the risk of healthy heterozygous for *GBA* mutations in developing PD, since it is not known for sure the degree of influence that this genetic alteration has on the onset of the disease.

Anheim M et al. [43] published in 2012 an estimate of the penetration of PD in healthy heterozygous people for *GBA* mutations and reached a value of 7.6%, 13.7%, 21.4% and 29.7% for 50, 60, 70 and 80 years, respectively, based on a dominance model. However, in the same year, [51] found a lower value: 5% for 60 years and 15% for 80 years of age. Such difference is perhaps due to additional genetic factors or environmental factors, a fact that emphasizes the possibility of variance of the risk of developing PD according to the genetic background of the population. Families that have *GBA* mutations segregation through generations are a group at risk for developing PD and should be monitored for a possible early diagnosis to have better chances in modifying the disease.

5. Pathogenic mechanisms in PD

α-Synuclein is a key protein in the neuropathogenesis of PD, involved in several pathogenic processes. The physiological function of α-synuclein is not well understood, but studies show that it is normally located in presynaptic terminals where it binds to lipids and plays the role of regulating in more than one step the traffic of synaptic vesicles to be released. As cited above, the insoluble forms (oligomers and fibrils) of this protein accumulate and compound the Lewy bodies found in most PD patients and also contribute to neuronal cell death [5].

The reason behind this accumulation can be due to increased synthesis or decreased degradation (**Figure 2**). Mutations, as the triplications of the *SNCA* gene, can enhance the production of α-synuclein, while the interaction between the oligomers and fibrils formed with other mutant proteins can result in the deficiency of certain metabolic pathways and contribute to slowing down α-synuclein proteolysis. On the other hand, the initial deficiency of certain metabolic pathway caused by mutations in genes, advanced age or environmental factors can also be the trigger to accumulate α-synuclein resulting in the insoluble forms. This last theory has been

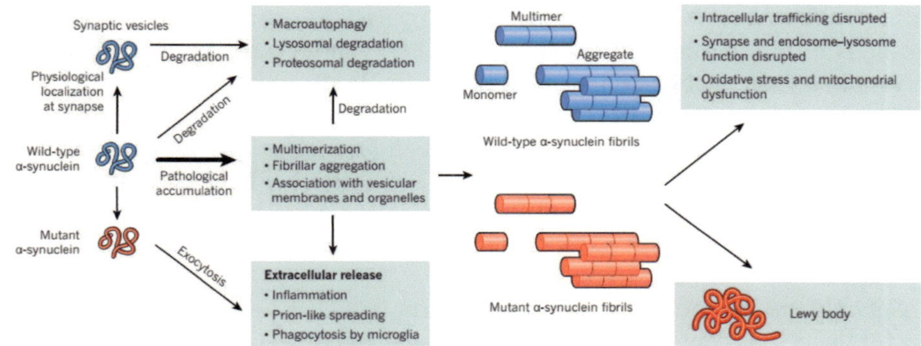

Figure 2.
The proposed physiological and PD-associated pathological functions of α-synuclein in neurons. Adapted from Ref. [6].

reinforced by the confirmed association of diverse genes involved in autophagy, endocytosis and lysosomal pathways as the *GBA* and *LRRK2* gene [1–6].

5.1 Lysosomal function-related genes and PD

The endosome-lysosome traffic processes, autophagy and lysosomal degradation, are essential functions for cell homeostasis, especially for neurons. The differentiated neurons have to maintain their homeostasis during the aging through degradation pathways since they do not divide in the same way as other eukaryotic cells. Moreover, cellular and animal models have also shown that the process of lysosome-autophagy and ubiquitin-proteasome has its activity reduced with natural aging. It may cause the accumulation of proteins whose homeostasis depends on those processes, such as α-synuclein. Indeed, the stimulation of degradation by macroautophagy through drugs proved to decrease intracellular levels of α-synuclein in experimental models [1–6].

Reciprocally, the accumulation of α-synuclein in the substantia nigra in experimental models leads to a reduction in lysosomal enzymes such as GCase, cathepsin B, β-galactosidase and hexosaminidase causing the inhibition of macroautophagy and ubiquitin-proteasome processes as a consequence enzyme transport to the lysosome interruption through dysfunction of vesicles and endosomes. The result is a vicious cycle where α-synuclein degradation mechanisms are inefficient resulting in the protein accumulation and it reinforces the inhibition of degradation activity [5–52].

Both GCase deficiency and the accumulation of its substrate (GlcCer) have been described to be associated with neurodegeneration (**Figure 3**). Feany M et al. [53] suggested that the connection of the α-synuclein to lipidic membranes would protect this protein from inadequate and clumped folding. Mutations of the *GBA* gene would alter the lipid composition of the membrane, which would favor a build-up of α-synuclein in the cytosol and subsequently in the Lewy bodies. Knockdown *GBA* in neuronal cells or in mouse models impairs α-synuclein clearance, whereas increasing glucocerebrosidase activity has the opposite effect, perhaps giving support to the loss-of-function theory in which the reduced or absent lysosomal enzyme is the trigger to α-synuclein accumulation [54].

Even excluding *GBA*, there was evidence for a burden damaging alleles in association with PD. In 2017, Ref. [55] performed a large study to examine the overlap between genes responsible for LSD and PD. More than half of PD cases in their cohort harbors one or more putative damaging variants among the 54 LSD genes. Specially, risk alleles in the genes *SMPD1* (Niemann-Pick type A/B), *GALC* (Krabbe disease), *SLC17A5* (Salla disease), *ASAH1* (Farber lipogranulomatosis) and *CTSD* (neuronal ceroid lipofuscinosis) have been candidate genes well replicated in different studies. *SMPD1* and *ASAH1,* along with *GBA*, participate in ceramide metabolism, and this fact can be evidence of the ceramide-associated process being relevant in a scenery of lysosomal dysfunction in PD [10–55].

The genes appointed as risk factor for PD to date explain only a fraction of PD heritability, suggesting the involvement of additional loci. Besides, the fact that *GBA* is the major genetic risk factor for PD makes other LSD genes attractive candidate risk factors. The results of [55] suggest that many genes that encode lysosomal enzymes besides *GBA* likely contribute to susceptibility for PD in Caucasian population.

Not only the lysosomal function is important, but also the previous steps necessary for the vesicle content to reach this organelle. In [10], a GWAS meta-analysis study found that PD-associated signals were enriched for autophagy and lysosomal function. *SCARB2* encodes a membrane protein (LIMP-2) required for correct targeting of GCase enzyme to the lysosome. Independent large GWAS have replicated

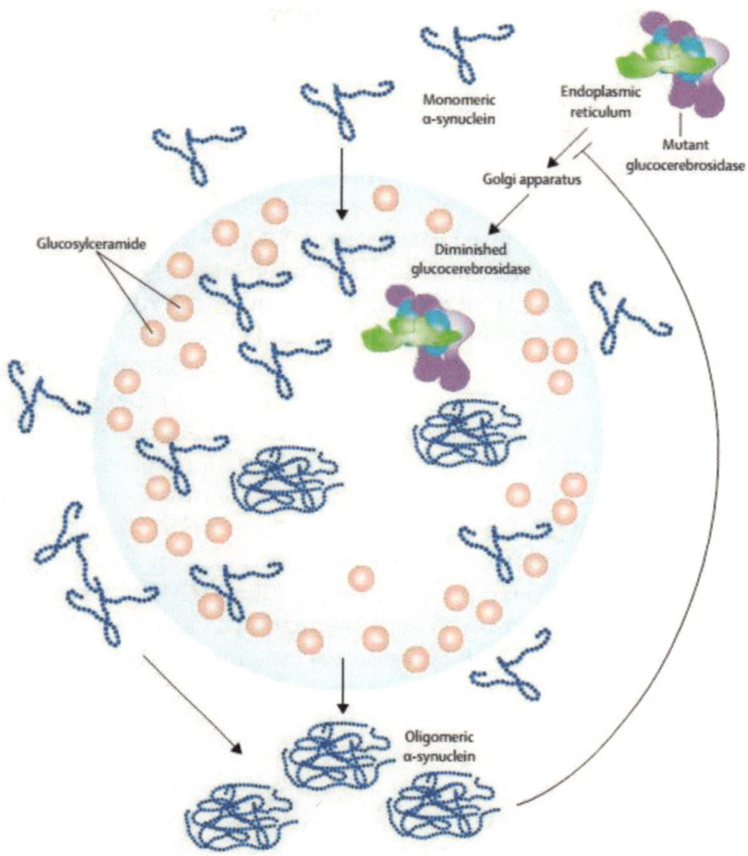

Figure 3.
The vicious cycle between the GCase and α-synuclein. Decreased glucocerebrosidase increases the lysosomal concentrations of glucosylceramide, which increases the formation of soluble α-synuclein oligomers. These oligomers also disrupt transport of newly synthesized glucocerebrosidase between the endoplasmic reticulum and Golgi apparatus, further compounding the problem. Adapted from reference [52].

common risk alleles in this gene. Functional analysis in cellular and animal model has shown that the reduction of LIMP-2 impairs the clearance of α-synuclein [55]. Those data reinforce that both the malfunction and the absence of the GCase, through mutations or impairment in the pathway, can result in α-synuclein accumulation.

The protein LRRK2 is complex and can work together with diverse proteins in different pathways, but for PD, the most relevant seems to be its endosome-to-lysosome trafficking function. Mutations in the kinase domain of the LRRK2 protein, such as the most common G2019S, compromise the traffic of the endosomal content to the lysosome through accentuated phosphorylation resulting in the dysregulation of proteins of the Rab family, responsible to target vesicles to the correct organelle membranes, including the lysosome [6–18].

In support of vesicular trafficking to lysosome impairment in PD, in 2009, two GWAS collaborative studies examining Caucasian and Asian subjects revealed significant risk alleles in *PARK16* locus for PD. This locus is a large linkage disequilibrium block that includes a Rab protein member of a subfamily that is implicated in vesicular transport to lysosomes and to lysosome-like organelles, the Rab-7 L1 (also known as RAB29) [9–16].

Mutations in the *VPS35* gene are one of the causes for autosomal dominant PD. Its protein is also involved in trafficking to lysosomes as a member of the retromer complex, which has the role to regulate the delivery of the protein content within endosomes to organelles. Some of the proteins carried by this complex are cation-independent mannose-6-phosphate receptors, necessary for the transport of lysosomal enzymes to the lysosome. In the dysfunction of the retromer complex, the receptors are not returned to the Golgi complex, thus impairing the lysosomal function. In addition, mutations in *ATP13A2* are a rare cause of recessive juvenile-onset Parkinsonism and dementia and are associated to lysosomal dysfunction. This gene codifies a lysosomal P-type ATPase [1, 6].

Interestingly, potentiated retromer function might suppress the altered trafficking and toxicity that are associated with mutations in *LRRK2* or the overexpression of α-synuclein85, which suggests a potential therapeutic avenue. This fact emphasizes the possibility that different genes can interact with each other influencing the lysosomal function and as a consequence modifying the PD progression.

These common and rare risk alleles in *ATP13A1, RAB7L1, LRRK2* and *VPS35*, which support a model of partial loss-of-function variants in genes regulating lysosomal activity by cellular trafficking, result in an increased vulnerability to α-synuclein mechanisms in PD [55]. Ref. [10], the largest GWAS meta-analysis study, concluded that PD-associated signals were enriched for autophagy and lysosomal function. It replicated the results for *GBA* and *TMEM175* genes, which encode a potassium channel involved in the regulation of lysosome and identified three novel candidate genes, *CTSB* (a lysosomal cysteine protease), *ATP60A1* (an ATPase) and *GALC* (a lysosomal enzyme).

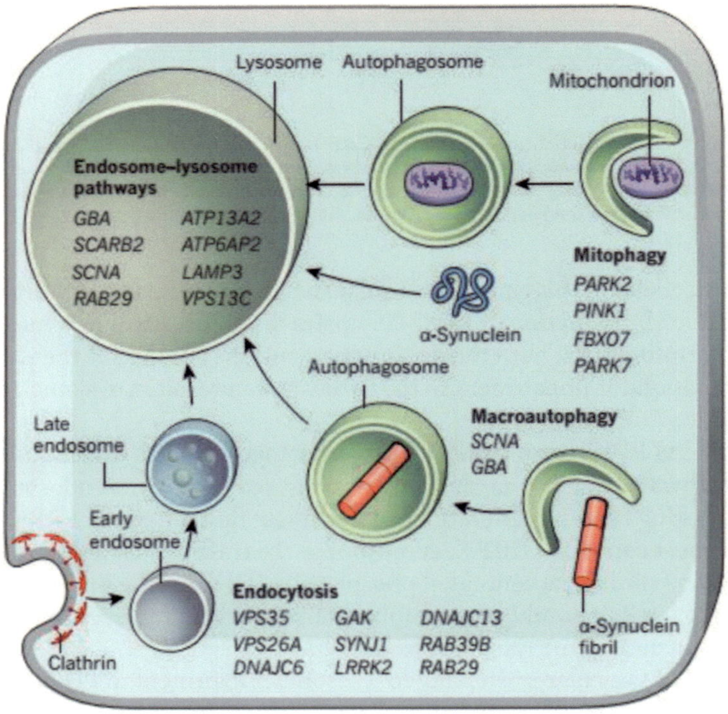

Figure 4.
Some of the PD-related genes associated with trafficking to the lysosome. Genes that encode intracellular trafficking components are associated with common sporadic and familial forms of PD, as well as related syndromes that share some of the clinical features of PD. Most of these genes are known to affect trafficking to the lysosome in the context of late endosome-to-lysosome pathways, clathrin-dependent endocytosis, macroautophagy or mitophagy. Wild-type α-synuclein (blue) can also enter lysosomes through chaperone-mediated autophagy. Adapted from Ref. [6].

Besides *GBA*, loss-of-function alleles are known as frequent PD risk factors, and some of those genes had the functional characterization made by analysis studies that showed knockout mice manifesting tremor phenotype with cerebral and cerebellar atrophy, thus corroborating with lysosome loss-of-function hypothesis to be involved with α-synuclein dysfunction and PD pathogenesis [10].

Therefore, advances in genetic and experimental model for PD have illuminated an important role for defects in intracellular transport pathways to lysosomes (**Figure 4**). The probability of discovering rare PD disease risk alleles at a single locus is low; however, if a set of lysosomal-related genes is investigated in conjunction, the chance of finding significant genetic variations is increased. Also, the candidate genes here appointed need further studies including even larger case–control studies and experiments in PD cellular or animal models.

6. Conclusion

Currently, genetic testing for PD is not a routine procedure, being restricted only to cases with a positive family history, with early onset or with the presence of specific atypical symptoms. In the future with the advance of genetic research, however, there is a possibility to use genetic variants to provide a perspective of the patient's clinical evolution. For this purpose, it is important to replicate risk variants for PD in large and genetically diverse samples due to the different results among populations. Genetic studies need to be a collaboration of the whole world to understand the genetics of a complex disease. In addition, candidate genes here appointed need further experiments in PD cellular or animal models understanding of the underlying pathology and molecular pathogenesis to provide perhaps the basis for the development of new therapies able to target mutated proteins that cause impairment in relevant pathways for PD as endosome trafficking, lysosome function and autophagy.

Acknowledgements

This study was performed with research grants from Instituto Nacional de Genética Médica e Populacional—INAGEMP (CNPq: 573993/2008-4), Fundação de Amparo à Pesquisa do Estado do Pará (FAPESPA) and Coordenação de Aperfeiçoamento de Pessoal de Nível Superior (CAPES) from Brazil.

Author details

Marcella Vieira Barroso Montenegro[1*], Carlos Eduardo de Melo Amaral[2]
and Luiz Carlos Santana da Silva[1]

1 Laboratory of Inborn Errors of Metabolism, Federal University of Pará (LEIM/UFPA), Belém, Brazil

2 Department of Molecular Biology, Center for Hemotherapy and Hematology of the Pará Foundation (HEMOPA), Belém, Brazil

*Address all correspondence to: marcella_montenegro3@hotmail.com

References

[1] Poewe W, Seppi K, Tanner C, Halliday G, Brundin P, Volkmann J, et al. Parkinson disease. Nature Reviews Disease Primers. 2017;**3**(1):1-21. DOI: 10.1038/nrdp.2017.13

[2] deSouza, Ruth-Mary, Schapira AH. Etiology and pathogenesis of Neurodegeneration. In: Schapira A, Wszolek Z, Dawson TM, Wood N, editors. 1st ed. 2017. pp. 46-52

[3] Polymeropoulos M. Mutation in the α-synuclein gene identified in families with Parkinson's disease. Science. 1997;**276**(5321):2045-2047. DOI: 10.1126/science.276.5321.2045

[4] Trotta L, Guella I, Soldà G, Sironi F, Tesei S, Canesi M, et al. SNCA and MAPT genes: Independent and joint effects in Parkinson disease in the Italian population. Parkinsonism & Related Disorders. 2012;**18**(3):257-262. DOI: 10.1016/j.parkreldis.2011.10.014

[5] Wong Y, Krainc D. α-Synuclein toxicity in neurodegeneration: Mechanism and therapeutic strategies. Nature Medicine. 2017;**23**(2):1-13. DOI: 10.1038/nm.4269

[6] Abeliovich A, Gitler A. Defects in trafficking bridge Parkinson's disease pathology and genetics. Nature. 2016;**539**(7628):207-216. DOI: 10.1038/nature20414

[7] Billingsley K, Bandres-Ciga S, Saez-Atienzar S, Singleton A. Genetic risk factors in Parkinson's disease. Cell and Tissue Research. 2018;**373**(1): 9-20. DOI: https://doi.org/10.1007/s00441-018-2817-y

[8] Kalinderi K, Bostantjopoulou S, Fidani L. The genetic background of Parkinson's disease: Current progress and future prospects. Acta Neurologica Scandinavica. 2016;**134**(5):314-326. DOI: 10.1111/ane.12563

[9] Satake W, Nakabayashi Y, Mizuta I, Hirota Y, Ito C, Kubo M, et al. Genome-wide association study identifies common variants at four loci as genetic risk factors for Parkinson's disease. Nature Genetics. 2009;**41**(12):1303-1307. DOI: 10.1038/ng.485

[10] Chang D, Nalls M, Hallgrímsdóttir I, Hunkapiller J, van der Brug M, Cai F, et al. A meta-analysis of genome-wide association studies identifies 17 new Parkinson's disease risk loci. Nature Genetics. 2017;**49**(10):1511-1516. DOI: 10.1038/ng.3955

[11] Nalls M, Pankratz N, Lill C, Do C, Hernandez D, Saad M, et al. Large-scale meta-analysis of genome-wide association data identifies six new risk loci for Parkinson's disease. Nature Genetics. 2014;**46**(9):989-993. DOI: 10.1038/ng.3043

[12] Ferreira M, Massano J. An updated review of Parkinson's disease genetics and clinicopathological correlations. Acta Neurologica Scandinavica. 2016;**135**(3):273-284. DOI: 10.1111/ane.12616

[13] Kruger R, Menezes Vieira-Saecker A, Kuhn W, Berg D, Muller T, Kohnl N, et al. Increased susceptibility to sporadic Parkinson's disease by a certain combined α-synuclein/apolipoprotein E genotype. Annals of Neurology. 1999;**45**(5):611-617

[14] Maraganore D. Collaborative analysis of α-synuclein gene promoter variability and Parkinson disease. Journal of the American Medical Association. 2006;**296**(6):661. DOI: 10.1001/jama.296.6.661

[15] Cronin K, Ge D, Manninger P, Linnertz C, Rossoshek A, Orrison B, et al. Expansion of the Parkinson disease-associated SNCA-Rep1 allele upregulates human α-synuclein in transgenic mouse brain. Human Molecular Genetics.

2009;**18**(17):3274-3285. DOI: 10.1093/hmg/ddp265

[16] Simón-Sánchez J, Schulte C, Bras J, Sharma M, Gibbs J, Berg D, et al. Genome-wide association study reveals genetic risk underlying Parkinson's disease. Nature Genetics. 2009;**41**(12):1308-1312. DOI: 10.1038/ng.487

[17] Mata I, Shi M, Agarwal P, Chung K, Edwards K, Factor S, et al. SNCA variant associated with Parkinson disease and plasma α-synuclein level. Archives of Neurology. 2010;**67**(11):1350-1356. DOI: 10.1001/archneurol.2010.279

[18] Hernandez D, Reed X, Singleton A. Genetics in Parkinson disease: Mendelian versus non-Mendelian inheritance. Journal of Neurochemistry. 2016;**139**:59-74. DOI: 10.1111/jnc.13593

[19] Healy D, Falchi M, O'Sullivan S, Bonifati V, Durr A, Bressman S, et al. Phenotype, genotype, and worldwide genetic penetrance of LRRK2-associated Parkinson's disease: A case-control study. The Lancet Neurology. 2008;**7**(7):583-590. DOI: 10.1016/s1474-4422(08)70117-0

[20] Farrer M, Stone J, Lin C, Dächsel J, Hulihan M, Haugarvoll K, et al. Lrrk2 G2385R is an ancestral risk factor for Parkinson's disease in Asia. Parkinsonism & Related Disorders. 2007;**13**(2):89-92. DOI: 10.1016/j.parkreldis.2006.12.001

[21] Ross O, Wu Y, Lee M, Funayama M, Chen M, Soto A, et al. Analysis of Lrrk2 R1628P as a risk factor for Parkinson's disease. Annals of Neurology. 2008;**64**(1):88-92. DOI: 10.1002/ana.21405

[22] Di Battista M, Pascale E, Purcaro C, Passarelli F, Passarelli E, Guglielmi R, et al. Clinical subtypes in Parkinson's disease: The impact of MAPT haplotypes. Journal of Neural Transmission. 2013;**121**(4):353-356. DOI: 10.1007/s00702-013-1117-7

[23] Williams-Gray C, Evans J, Goris A, Foltynie T, Ban M, Robbins T, et al. The distinct cognitive syndromes of Parkinson's disease: 5 year follow-up of the CamPaIGN cohort. Brain. 2009;**132**(11):2958-2969. DOI: 10.1093/brain/awp245

[24] Wade-Martins R. The MAPT locus—A genetic paradigm in disease susceptibility. Nature Reviews Neurology. 2012;**8**(9):477-478. DOI: 10.1038/nrneurol.2012.169

[25] Mistry P, Lopez G, Schiffmann R, Barton N, Weinreb N, Sidransky E. Gaucher disease: Progress and ongoing challenges. Molecular Genetics and Metabolism. 2017;**120**(1-2):8-21. DOI: 10.1016/j.ymgme.2016.11.006

[26] Gan-Or Z, Amshalom I, Kilarski L, Bar-Shira A, Gana-Weisz M, Mirelman A, et al. Differential effects of severe vs mild GBA mutations on Parkinson disease. Neurology. 2015;**84**(9):880-887. DOI: 10.1212/WNL.0000000000001315

[27] Bembi B, Zambito Marsala S, Sidransky E, Ciana G, Carrozzi M, Zorzon M, et al. Gaucher's disease with Parkinson's disease: Clinical and pathological aspects. Neurology. 2003;**61**(1):99-101. DOI: 10.1212/01.WNL.0000072482.70963.D7

[28] Alcalay R, Dinur T, Quinn T, Sakanaka K, Levy O, Waters C, et al. Comparison of Parkinson risk in Ashkenazi Jewish patients with Gaucher disease and GBA heterozygotes. JAMA Neurology. 2014;**71**(6):752. DOI: 10.1001/jamaneurol.2014.313

[29] Bultron G, Kacena K, Pearson D, Boxer M, Yang R, Sathe S, et al. The risk of Parkinson's disease in type 1 Gaucher disease. Journal of Inherited Metabolic

Disease. 2010;**33**(2):167-173. DOI: 10.1007/s10545-010-9055-0

[30] Aharon-Peretz J, Rosenbaum H, Gershoni-Baruch R. Mutations in the Glucocerebrosidase gene and Parkinson's disease in Ashkenazi Jews. New England Journal of Medicine. 2004;**351**(19):1972-1977. DOI: 10.1056/nejmoa033277

[31] Amaral C, Lopes P, Ferreira J, Alves E, Montenegro M, Costa E, et al. GBA mutations p.N370S and p.L444P are associated with Parkinson's disease in patients from northern Brazil. Arquivos de Neuro-Psiquiatria. 2019;**77**(2):73-79. DOI: 10.1590/0004-282x20190006

[32] Bras J, Paisan-Ruiz C, Guerreiro R, Ribeiro M, Morgadinho A, Januario C, et al. Complete screening for glucocerebrosidase mutations in Parkinson disease patients from Portugal. Neurobiology of Aging. 2009;**30**(9):1515-1517. DOI: 10.1016/j.neurobiolaging.2007.11.016

[33] Nichols W, Pankratz N, Marek D, Pauciulo M, Elsaesser V, Halter C, et al. Mutations in GBA are associated with familial Parkinson disease susceptibility and age at onset. Neurology. 2008;**72**(4):310-316. DOI: 10.1212/01.wnl.0000327823.81237.d1

[34] Moraitou M, Hadjigeorgiou G, Monopolis I, Dardiotis E, Bozi M, Vassilatis D, et al. β-Glucocerebrosidase gene mutations in two cohorts of Greek patients with sporadic Parkinson's disease. Molecular Genetics and Metabolism. 2011;**104**(1-2):149-152. DOI: 10.1016/j.ymgme.2011.06.015

[35] Winder-Rhodes S, Evans J, Ban M, Mason S, Williams-Gray C, Foltynie T, et al. Glucocerebrosidase mutations influence the natural history of Parkinson's disease in a community-based incident cohort. Brain. 2013;**136**(2):392-399. DOI: 10.1093/brain/aws318

[36] Asselta R, Rimoldi V, Siri C, Cilia R, Guella I, Tesei S, et al. Glucocerebrosidase Mutations in Primary Parkinsonism. Parkinsonism & Related Disorders. 2014;**20**(11):1215-1220. DOI: 10.1016/j.parkreldis.2014.09.003

[37] Lesage S, Condroyer C, Hecham N, Anheim M, Belarbi S, Lohman E, et al. Mutations in the glucocerebrosidase gene confer a risk for Parkinson disease in North Africa. Neurology. 2011;**76**(3):301-303. DOI: 10.1212/wnl.0b013e318207b01e

[38] Eblan M, Nguyen J, Ziegler S, Lwin A, Hanson M, Gallardo M, et al. Glucocerebrosidase mutations are also found in subjects with early-onset parkinsonism from Venezuela. Movement Disorders. 2006;**21**(2):282-283. DOI: 10.1002/mds.20766

[39] Noreau A, Rivière J, Diab S, Dion P, Panisset M, Soland V, et al. Glucocerebrosidase mutations in a French-Canadian Parkinson's disease cohort. Canadian Journal of Neurological Sciences/Journal Canadien des Sciences Neurologiques. 2011;**38**(5):772-773. DOI: https://doi.org/10.1017/S0317167100012300

[40] Mitsui J, Mizuta I, Toyoda A, Ashida R, Takahashi Y, Goto J, et al. Mutations for Gaucher disease confer high susceptibility to Parkinson disease. Archives of Neurology. 2009;**66**(5):571-576. DOI: 10.1001/archneurol.2009.72

[41] Mao X, Burgunder J, Zhang Z, An X, Zhang J, Yang Y, et al. Association between GBA L444P mutation and sporadic Parkinson's disease from mainland China. Neuroscience Letters. 2010;**469**(2):256-259. DOI: 10.1016/j.neulet.2009.12.007

[42] Sidransky E, Nalls M, Aasly J, Aharon-Peretz J, Annesi G, Barbosa E, et al. Multicenter analysis of glucocerebrosidase mutations in Parkinson's disease. New England Journal of Medicine.

2009;**361**(17):1651-1661. DOI: 10.1056/NEJMoa0901281

[43] Anheim M, Elbaz A, Lesage S, Durr A, Condroyer C, Viallet F, et al. Penetrance of Parkinson disease in glucocerebrosidase gene mutation carriers. Neurology. 2012;**78**(6):417-420. DOI: 10.1212/WNL.0b013e318245f476

[44] Liu G, Boot B, Locascio J, Jansen I, Winder-Rhodes S, Eberly S, et al. Specifically neuropathic Gaucher's mutations accelerate cognitive decline in Parkinson's. Annals of Neurology. 2016;**80**(5):674-685. DOI: 10.1002/ana.24781

[45] Beavan M, McNeill A, Proukakis C, Hughes D, Mehta A, Schapira A. Evolution of prodromal clinical markers of Parkinson disease in aGBAMutation–positive cohort. JAMA Neurology. 2015;**72**(2):201. DOI: 10.1001/jamaneurol.2014.2950

[46] Cilia R, Tunesi S, Marotta G, Cereda E, Siri C, Tesei S, et al. Survival and dementia inGBA-associated Parkinson's disease: The mutation matters. Annals of Neurology. 2016;**80**(5):662-673. DOI: 10.1002/ana.24777

[47] Brockmann K, Srulijes K, Pflederer S, Hauser A, Schulte C, Maetzler W, et al. GBA -associated Parkinson's disease: Reduced survival and more rapid progression in a prospective longitudinal study. Movement Disorders. 2014;**30**(3):407-411. DOI: 10.1002/mds.26071

[48] Thaler A, Bregman N, Gurevich T, Shiner T, Dror Y, Zmira O, et al. Parkinson's disease phenotype is influenced by the severity of the mutations in the GBA gene. Parkinsonism & Related Disorders. 2018;**55**:45-49. DOI: https://doi.org/10.1016/j.parkreldis.2018.05.009

[49] Toft M, Pielsticker L, Ross O, Aasly J, Farrer M. Glucocerebrosidase gene mutations and Parkinson disease in the Norwegian population. Neurology. 2006;**66**(3):415-417. DOI: 10.1212/01.wnl.0000196492.80676.7c

[50] Santos N, Ribeiro-Rodrigues E, Ribeiro-dos-Santos Â, Pereira R, Gusmão L, Amorim A, et al. Assessing individual interethnic admixture and population substructure using a 48-insertion-deletion (INSEL) ancestry-informative marker (AIM) panel. Human Mutation. 2010;**31**(2):184-190. DOI: 10.1002/humu.21159

[51] McNeill A, Duran R, Hughes D, Mehta A, Schapira A. A clinical and family history study of Parkinson's disease in heterozygous-glucocerebrosidasemutation carriers. Journal of Neurology, Neurosurgery & Psychiatry. 2012;**83**(8):853-854. DOI: 10.1136/jnnp-2012-302402

[52] Sidransky E, Lopez G. The link between the GBA gene and parkinsonism. The Lancet Neurology. 2012;**11**(11):986-998. DOI: https://doi.org/10.1016/S1474-4422(12)70190-4

[53] Feany M. New genetic insights into Parkinson's disease. New England Journal of Medicine. 2004;**351**(19):1937-1940. DOI: 10.1056/NEJMp048263

[54] Sardi S, Clarke J, Kinnecom C, Tamsett T, Li L, Stanek L, et al. CNS expression of glucocerebrosidase corrects α-synuclein pathology and memory in a mouse model of Gaucher-related synucleinopathy. Proceedings of the National Academy of Sciences. 2011;**108**(29):12101-12106. DOI: www.pnas.org/cgi/doi/10.1073/pnas.1108197108

[55] Robak L, Jansen I, van Rooij J, Uitterlinden A, Kraaij R, Jankovic J, et al. Excessive burden of lysosomal storage disorder gene variants in Parkinson's disease. Brain. 2017;**140**(12):3191-3203. DOI: 10.1093/brain/awx285

Chapter 5

Endogenous Retroelements in Cancer: Molecular Roles and Clinical Approach

Kang-Hoon Lee and Je-Yoel Cho

Abstract

Retroelements have been considered as "Junk" DNA although the encyclopedia of DNA elements (ENCODE) project has demonstrated that most of the genome is functional. Since the contribution of LINE1 (L1) and human endogenous retrovirus (HERV) has been suspected to cause human cancers, their regulations and putative molecular functions have been investigated in diverse types of cancer. Their diagnostic, prognostic, and therapeutic potentials have been incessantly proposed using cancer associated or specific properties, such as hypomethylation, increased transcripts, and reverse transcriptase, as well as cancer-associated antigens. This chapter presents the current knowledge on retroelements in various aspects during tumorigenesis and their clinical usage in many cancer studies.

Keywords: retrotransposons, repetitive elements, tumorigenesis, cancer, LINE, HERV, retroelement

1. Introduction

In recent decades, the development of genomic analysis technology has played an important role in the study and treatment of various diseases [1, 2]. However, these studies have been focused on genes that form proteins that account for about 1–2% of the entire genome, and the understanding of other parts remains relatively insufficient. A retroelement (RE), also called a retrotransposon, is a type I transposable element that replicates itself via RNA and reverse transcription and can be largely classified into two types based on the genome structure, including long terminal repeat sequences (LTRs). The intact endogenous retrovirus (ERVs) retains two LTRs at both ends of the genome, instead of long and short interspersed nuclear elements (LINE and SINE), which are non-LTR groups. LTRs compose ~8% of the human genome and most are known to be inactive due to accumulated mutations. Yet, interestingly, many are transcriptionally active [3]. The non-LTR groups can be divided again into autonomous LINEs and nonautonomous SINEs that need LINE's proteins [4]. The LINE1s (L1s), known as the only active REs, makes up ~17% of the human genome. Intact L1s retain ~6 kb of the genome, which encodes two proteins, ORF1 and ORF2, which are essential for replication and reverse transcription [5]. There are about 145 full-length, functional L1 elements in the human genome. On the other hand, SINEs, which are nonautonomous retroelements, have ~300 bp genomes without coding potential. Most SINEs are of the Alu type of which there are over one million copies in the human genome [6].

The association between REs and cancer has been suggested since 1950. As the presence of a viral-oncogene was unveiled and mouse mammary tumor virus (MMTV) became the accepted etiological agent of mammary tumors in mice, the possible carcinogenesis mechanism of ERV was also revealed, raising hope for overcoming cancer [7, 8]. Many studies have reported the association of RE expression with various cancer types, including breast cancer, melanoma, and kidney cancer [9]. However, the function of RE expression in cancer as a driver or passenger remains controversial [10, 11]. It is a chicken and egg situation, since the cancer-associated RE expression can cause malignant cell transformation and malignant cell transformation leads to global DNA hypomethylation, which in turn contributes to oncogenic RE expression [12–15]. In addition, the fact that most REs have lost their transposition activity due to accumulated mutations makes it difficult to evaluate the role of REs [16]. The RE sequences that occupies about half of the mammalian genome is known as "junk DNA," and, as the name suggests, little research has been done it [17]. However, in certain areas such as in the early embryogenesis process, degenerative disease, and cancer, the expression of REs have been studied relatively well [18, 19]. In particular, several studies have been conducted to reveal the relationship among the environmental stress, RE responses, and associated diseases [20, 21]. Although no direct relationship has been revealed yet, genome instability by activated RE is known to be the main mechanism linking RE with disease [22]. However, the transposition ratio of all the REs is about 0.02 germline events per generation [23], so it is too rare to explain their various roles.

In this chapter, we focus on the functional mechanisms of REs in various cancers from development to metastasis and from diagnosis to cancer therapy.

2. RE regulation in normal cells and abnormal reactivation and expansion in cancer

Fortunately, except for during the reprogramming process in early stage germ cells, most REs are strongly silenced by diverse epigenomic controls and their reactivation is molecularly inhibited [24, 25].

DNA methylation is a major epigenetic mechanism that contributes to retrotransposon silencing in both normal and cancer cells [26]. In early embryogenesis, a genome-wide DNA methylation is established by the DNA methyltransferase 3 (Dnmt3) and maintained by the methyltransferase1 (Dnmt1) [27]. Parental methylation pattern is genome-wide demethylated and methylated again at imprinted loci and REs by the Dnmt3, and these patterns are maintained by Dnmt1 in somatic cells [28–30]. Association between demethylation and RE expression was demonstrated in that the inactivation of DNMT3L, which is a non-catalytic homolog of DNMT3A/3B, causes the reactivation of L1 and IAP and leads to meiotic arrest as well as male sterility in male germ cells [31–33].

In cancer cells, a genome-wide DNA hypomethylation and the reactivation of REs that may result in the loss of chromosomal stability and imprinting patterns are well known [34]. Alteration of L1 methylation has been investigated in many types of cancers, including breast, colon, lung, ovarian, and prostate cancers [35–37]. Mostly, hypomethylation of the L1 promoter is associated with genome instability, aggressive histology, poor prognosis, and some metastasis [38]. Interestingly, some abnormal features, such as chromosome 8 abnormalities, are also associated with L1 hypomethylation [39]. In addition, due to their prevalent unmethylation in cancer samples, a moderate increase of Alu was also observed in cancer samples with a hypomethylated L1 promoter [40]. Similarly, hypomethylation of HERV has also been reported in various cancer cells [9, 12, 41–44]. Hypomethylation of its long terminal repeat (LTR) where the promoter is located is associated with its overexpression in cancer [45]. Numerous HERV family members were expressed in cancer cell lines and primary tumor tissues. In a head and neck cancer study, tumor-specific methylation changes were found in HERV-H, HERV-W, and HERV-K families [24, 46]. Similarly, the hypomethylated CpGs resulting in high expression of HERV-K, -W, and L1 was reported in ovarian cancer [47]. Moreover, the hypomethylation of REs has been observed in specific stages or subtypes of cancer, such as during ovarian cancer progression and in the basal subtype of invasive ductal carcinoma breast cancer [48, 49]. Remarkably, individual RE expressions associated with cancer such as HERV-K at 22q11.23 (H22q), HERV-H5, HERV-H48–1, and HERV-E4 are highlighted in various cancers [46, 50, 51]. Their transcripts or viral proteins have been detected in sera from bladder, breast, liver, lung, ovarian, and prostate cancer patients [11].

The last cellular epigenomic regulation mechanism for silencing RE expression is histone modification [52]. In normal spermatogonia, one of the repressive histone modification marks, histone 3 lysine 9 dimethylation (H3K9me2), causes transcriptional repression and is sufficient to maintain L1 silencing in the absence of DNA methylation. Thus, the loss of H3K9me2 combined with the absence of DNA methylation may be the cause of LINE1 activation [53]. On the other hand, in the study of the association of histone modification with RE expression in cancer, two repressive histone modifications, H3K9me3 and H3K27me3, were more enriched at H22q, HERVK17, and L1 sequences in PC3 than in LNCaP prostate cell lines, of which RE expression levels are high and low, respectively. By contrast, the active modification H3K4me3 was the most enriched in LNCaP at the H22q LTR [54].

The expressed RE transcripts can eventually be knocked down by the PIWI system [55]. Piwi-interacting RNA (piRNA) is a well-studied mechanism that contributes to the silencing of REs in many animal germline cells [56, 57]. The piRNA system is a ribonucleoprotein complex consisting of a piRNA, and a P-element-induced wimpy testis (PIWI) subfamily of Argonaut nucleases protein [58]. The piRNA recognizes RE sequences and the PIWI protein destroys the RE transcripts [58, 59]. The piRNA system silences RE expression both at the transcriptional and posttranscriptional levels by modifying repressive chromatin modifications and by cleaving RE transcripts, respectively [57, 60]. However, the role of piRNA in post-transcriptional regulation is not similar to that of miRNA via providing sequence specificity because most piRNA sequences are found not to be complementary to target gene transcripts, suggesting that piRNAs may be involved in epigenetic regulation rather than posttranscriptional regulation of mRNA [61]. The deficient of the piRNA pathway causes overexpression of REs, significantly compromised genome structure and, invariably, germ cell death and sterility [58]. The aberrant expression of piRNAs has been reported in the development of cancer including the proliferation, apoptosis, metastasis, and invasion of cancer cells [62]. Moreover, the high expression of PIWI proteins has been documented in many cancer types, including gastric cancer, liver cancer, intestinal cancer, breast cancer, nonsmall cell lung cancer, bladder cancer, ovarian cancer, and melanoma and is furthermore associated with the aggressiveness of sarcomas, gliomas, and leukemia [61, 63]. The roles of PIWI proteins have been investigated separately in cancer invasion, migration, proliferation, division, and survival [64]. PIWIL1 has been known to induce epithelial-mesenchymal transition and confer migration and invasion of endometrial cancer cells [65]. The association of PIWIL2 via increasing the expression of CDK2 and cyclin A in cancer cells is reported in glioma and nonsmall lung cancer (NSCLC) cells [66]. PIWIL3 promotes the cancer proliferation, migration, and invasion through the JAK2/STAT3 signal pathway [67]. PIWIL4 can promote cancer cell division, migration, and survival of breast cancer by activating TGF-β, MAPK/ERK, and FGF signaling pathways [68].

The apolipoprotein B mRNA editing catalytic polypeptide 3 (APOBEC3) proteins are cytidine deaminases of which family consists of seven family members (APOBEC3-A through -H) with diverse activities against a variety of retroviruses and endogenous REs, even though the activity of L1 suppression does not correlate either with antiviral activity against Vif-deficient HIV-1 and murine leukemia virus, or with patterns of subcellular localization [69, 70]. Thus, the inhibitory effect of APOBEC3 family members, specifically APOBEC3G on L1 transposition might not be due to deaminase activity, but due to novel mechanism(s) [70].

Besides APOBEC3G, MOV10, SAMHD1, and ZAP have all been identified to be able to inhibit L1 activity through diverse mechanisms [71]. MOV10 inhibits L1 mobility through interacting with L1 RNP resulting in L1 transcript degradation [72]. SAMHD1 inhibits the L1 RT activity [73]. ZAP also restricts L1 activity through the loss of L1 transcripts and ribonucleoprotein integrity [74].

Together, it will be a universal explanation for the various epigenomic modifications that are directly associated with both genome-wide RE silencing and reactivation that is much more commonly found in diverse human cancers as frequent as 4–100 de novo insertions per tumor.

3. Roles of RE expressed in cancers

The genomic instability caused by de novo insertions of REs that frequently occur in cancer is the major pathophysiological role accepted by the public [75, 76]. However, this is a very limited explanation of the universal functions of REs, because most REs lose their ability to mobilize [16]. Although some retain their coding potentials, these are silenced tightly by various mechanisms and at various levels, such as epigenomic mechanisms, transcription, and posttranscription [77]. Thus, a more in-depth understanding of RE function is mandatory.

3.1 The source of genome instability

De novo insertions of REs, despite their defective form, can both directly and indirectly affect surrounding human genome sequences [78]. Some of these events occur at high enough frequency to result in vast amounts of rearrangement of the host genome sequence [16]. This does not happen only via the mechanism of transposition activity followed by reintegration but also via the homologous recombination between dispersed REs, resulting in large structural variations (SVs) including duplications, inversions, and deletions [79]. REs are also the source of small SVs such as single-nucleotide variants (SNVs) and short indels, which are caused by template switching during repair of replication errors [16]. The SVs derived from reactivation and expansion of REs via either mobilization activity or homologous recombination have been frequently found in many cancers (~50%) [80, 81]. A high enrichment was reported especially in certain types of cancers, such as esophageal cancers, colon cancers, and squamous cell lung cancers (> 90%) [82]. Although this result indicated that somatic L1 insertions are very frequently found in certain cancers, it is known that a majority of RE somatic integrations are passenger mutations with little or no effect on cancer development [83].

Nevertheless, specific SV loci derived from somatic L1 insertions have also been identified as drivers in most cancer types, including colorectal, breast, lung, and liver cancers [84–88]. For example, disruption of the APC gene by the insertion of L1 in colon cancer has been well studied [89]. Additionally, a recent study identified driver SV by L1 insertion in liver cancer [90]. L1 integration in the intron of the ST18 gene disrupted a cis-regulatory repressor element, resulting in increased expression of the ST18 gene [84].

Several algorithms have also been developed for the sensitive and precise detection of SVs from the whole genome sequence (WGS) and whole exome sequence (WES) data published in large international consortia such as The International Cancer Genome Consortium (ICGC) and The Cancer Genome Atlas (TCGA), and driver SV events with remarkable functional consequences have been identified [82, 91]. The most SVs were generated by L1 (99%), followed by SINE VNTR Alu (SVA) and ERV [92]. Yet, few retrotranspositions of HERVs have been reported in human cancers [84, 93].

3.2 Epigenomic regulation and reactivation of REs in cancer

Since 1993 when the methylation status of L1 in cancer cells was first measured by Thayer et al., L1 hypomethylation has been reported in many types of human cancers, including prostate, ovarian, head and neck, lung, thyroid, and breast cancer [94, 95]. However, some controversial results showed no changes in L1 methylation levels of cancers including thyroid cancer, renal cancer, lymphoma, and leukemia [96]. This discrepancy may be due to differences in the tumor histological type, because association between L1 hypomethylation and clinical outcome has been demonstrated in melanoma patients. However, the mechanism of L1 hypomethylation effects on aggressive tumor behavior has not been fully investigated [49]. The most likely mechanism is the causing of DNA instability, which has been suspected as the main role of REs [92]. A DNA methyltransferase 1 (Dnmt1) mutation showed substantial genome-wide hypomethylation in all types of tissue and also known to be associated with aggressive T cell lymphomas [97, 98]. Notably, the mutation also showed a high frequency of chromosome 15 trisomy, which suggested that the DNA hypomethylation has a causal role in cancers by promoting genome instability [98]. Another possible mechanism is a dysregulation in transcription level, which activates proto-oncogenes and REs that affect tumor aggressiveness [99]. MicroRNAs, which are closely related to the development of human cancer, can be increased by global DNA hypomethylation, contributing to the acquisition of tumor aggressiveness [100]. In addition, it is possible that the L1 methylation state itself exerts a biological effect. It is known that L1 regulates the function of multiple genes by providing an alternative promoter and contributing to noncoding RNA expression [101, 102]. Therefore, further studies are needed to explain the mechanisms in which L1 hypomethylation affects tumor behavior.

3.3 REs, the origin of cancer associated non-coding transcripts

RNA sequencing using next-generation sequencing technology has provided a large amount of gene expression data in both normal and disease conditions, such as cancer [103]. Growing evidence suggests that REs in the intergenic regions of the human genome are sources of noncoding RNAs, including micro RNAs (miRNAs) and long noncoding RNAs (lncRNAs) [104]. Notably, about 30% of human lncRNAs originate from REs, specifically HERVs. In addition, about 80% of lncRNAs contain RE-originated sequences within or nearby their transcription start sites [105]. Importantly, a recent study has reported that many lncRNAs have a crucial role in a variety of fundamental cellular processes and diseases [106]. A recent study reported that a single-nucleotide polymorphism (SNP) in an L1-containing lncRNA sequence located in an intron of SLC7A2 leads to a decrease in its expression and results in a lethal encephalopathy phenotype [107]. Alu elements, which encode no functional proteins, are also frequently found at multiple locations in lncRNA sequences [108]. Recently, many studies have suggested that Alu sequence in lncRNAs can contribute to the function of lncRNAs. For example, Alu-mediated CDKN1A/p21 transcriptional regulator (APTR) negatively regulates p21 expression by recruiting polycomb repressive proteins to the p21 promoter. The Alu sequence is crucial to the localization of APTR on the p21 promoter that regulates cell growth and proliferation [109].

Despite the limited contribution of L1 and Alu to lncRNAs, a close association between HERVs and ncRNAs was reported by Kelley and Rinn [110]. Hundreds of ncRNAs originated from HERV-H. For example, the lncRNA ROR known to promote the progression of human cancers is one of the ncRNAs promoted by a HERV-H element [111]. Moreover, the lncRNA produced by HERV-K11 directly binds to polypyrimidine tract-binding protein-associated splicing factor (PSF), of which the function is to repress proto-oncogene transcription, reversing the PSF-mediated repression of proto-oncogene transcription and subsequently driving tumorigenesis [46, 112]. Other HERV-related lncRNAs with tumor-suppressive potential have also been identified in the intronic RNAs arising from ERV-9 [45]. It has been reported that its antisense RNA at 3′-untranslated regions was found to physically bind to key transcription factors for cell proliferation such as NF-Y, p53, and sp1. This means that the HERV-related lncRNAs may have a function as decoy targets or traps for the transcription factors resulting in the growth retardation of cancer cells [113].

Another role of RE transcripts related to human disease is to form a complex with the cytoplasmic cDNA of the reactivated RE transcripts to trigger the signal of the inflammatory pathway [23]; for example, RE-derived cytosolic DNA accumulated in Aicardi-Goutières syndrome (AGS) [114]. IFNB1 expression also has an anticorrelation with L1 retrotransposition in cancer cells [115]. Moreover, the study by Ishak et al. showed that mutation of the RB1 gene causes both genome-wide upregulation of L1 expression in somatic cells as well as increased susceptibility to leukemia [116]. Gasche et al. reported that the IL-6 treatment of a cancer cell line induced genome-wide L1 promoter hypomethylation [117]. Altogether, the evidence indicates that REs modify an important aspect of human tumorigenesis.

3.4 RE proteins associated with tumorigenesis

ORF1 and ORF2 in L1 and GAG, POL, and ENV in HERV are proteins encoded by REs that are essential to complete the replication cycle, whereas Alu's are RNA polymerase III-transcribed sequences without coding potential [118]. Most REs lose their coding potential due to accumulated mutations; however, it is well known that hundreds of L1 are still active to produce two essential proteins, ORF1 (p40, RNA binding protein) and ORF2 (p109, endonuclease and reverse transcriptase activities) [119, 120]. Additionally, although no infectious virus formed by HERVs is reported, multiple protein expressions and their functions have been studied in various HERV families [46]. Most comprehensive studies have reported on envelop proteins (ENV) and their pathogenic properties. The transcripts encoding capsid and protease (GAG) and reverse transcriptase with RNase H domain and integrase (POL) ORFs have been detected in many cells and tissues from both diseased and healthy individuals [121]. Remarkably, HERV-W encodes an ENV protein known as ERVWE1 (Syncytin1), which has been adopted by the human to functionally contribute in placenta biogenesis [122]. Similarly, Syncytin2 encoded by ERVFRD1 is known to have a key role in the implantation of human embryos [123]. Aberrant expression of HERV-W has been known to be associated with various human diseases including cancer [122, 124, 125].

In cancer, an increase in retroviral protein expression was generally detected. Overexpression of L1 ORF1 protein was detected from more than 90% of breast, ovarian, and pancreatic cancers followed by tubular gastrointestinal tract, lung, and prostate cancers (about 50%) [126, 127]. However, the high expression of L1 ORF1p expression is dependent on tumor origin, and it differs case by case even within a similar histological type of cancer. For example, L1 ORF1p is detected in lung adenocarcinoma at greatly varying levels (about 20% are very high, about 30% are moderate, and the rest are undetectable) [128]. Several antibodies targeting ORF2p have recently been produced, and thus, the overexpression of ORF2p was detected in many cancers. Although the functional effects of L1 proteins in human cancers remain unclear in most cancer contexts, this data suggests that L1 proteins are potential cancer biomarkers for the diagnosis of cancer development or the prognosis of clinical outcomes [126, 129]. On the other hand, the HERV-K ENV protein has been identified in various cancer tissues and several different mechanisms by which it associates with tumorigenesis have been proposed [130]. The melanocyte antigen HERV-K-MEL is expressed in about 85% of malignant melanocytes, whereas breast cancer, ovarian cancer, teratocarcinoma, sarcoma, and bladder cancer also express HERV-K ENV [131]. Other HERV families, HERV-E, and ERV3 have also been detected in more than 30% of ovarian cancer patients and are higher in patients with lymph-node-positive breast cancer [11, 132]. Moreover, some antibodies against HERV-K have been detected in serum samples with melanoma [133].

Despite HERVs being known to be incompetent in transposition, studies have shown that the protein-coding potentials can still promote neoplastic properties during tumorigenesis through diverse mechanisms [134]. The oncogenic role of HERV proteins is well investigated with NP9 and REC, which are accessory splice proteins of HERV-K [135]. The transcripts encoding these proteins are overexpressed in many tumors including breast cancers and both are known to interact with the promyelocytic leukemia zinc finger (PLZF) tumor suppressor, which is a transcriptional repressor and epigenetic modulator implicated in cancer. C-myc proto-oncogene is one of the major targets of PLZF. Interaction of NP9 and REC with PLZF abrogates the transcriptional repression of the c-Myc gene promoter, which results in c-Myc overproduction [136]. In addition, the abnormal cell-to-cell fusion activity of HERV-W ENV proteins has been shown to possibly contribute to tumor development and metastasis [130]. Further studies to characterize the expression and molecular functions of these HERV proteins in cancers are demanded.

4. Implementation of REs for cancer diagnosis and prognosis

4.1 Structural variations (SVs) associated with REs in cancer

Identification of somatic mutation hotspots associated with cancer is very important for functional analysis and diagnosis [137]. Several methods have been developed for the identification of somatic RE insertions in cancers (L1-seq, TIPseq, and ERVcaller), and many bioinformatics tools to discover somatic L1 insertions in silico using WGS or WES data have been developed [138, 139]. SVs via L1 insertion associated with cancer have been well investigated in a couple of genes, such as the APC gene that is considered to be a tumor suppressor of colorectal polyposis in colorectal cancer [89]. A potential suppressor of L1, TP53 mutation by L1 insertions, has been observed frequently in tumors. In addition, L1 insertional mutation of MOV10, which is a key L1 suppressor, decreased the expression of the MOV10 in tumors with high L1 insertions [140].

On the other hand, instead of cancer-associated SVs caused by RE insertion, genome variations that might be associated with HERVs or around gene expression in cancer have been identified. Chang et al. identified that four HERVs with mutation hotspots overlapped with exons of four human protein coding genes, which are TNN (HERV-9/LTR12), OR4K15 (HERV-IP10F/LTR10F), ZNF99 (HERV-W/HERV17/LTR17), and KIR2DL1 (MST/MaLR). They also evaluated the effect of each non-synonymous SNV on the survival of kidney cancer patients. Furthermore, they identified 788 HERVs harboring significantly increased the numbers of somatic single-nucleotide variations (SNVs) [141].

4.2 Global hypomethylation in cancer and identification of cancer associated RE methylation

Several studies have shown that global hypomethylation is very common in cancer [142]. The DNA methylation levels of L1 5′-untranslated region (UTR) in cancer have been extensively evaluated for potential use as an epigenomic marker for cancer diagnosis. The level of L1 hypomethylation increases in more advanced cancers; however, other types of REs, such as Alu and HERVs, have been lesser evaluated [143]. Since DNA methylation analysis has some benefits in handling tumor specimens, such as similar efficiency in fresh frozen and formalin-fixed paraffin-embedded tissue, many studies indeed have proposed DNA methylation as a diagnostic marker using fresh tumor biopsies or fixed tissue blocks [144]. Association between L1 hypomethylation and diagnostic and prognostic needs, such as tumor stage group, metastasis, the recurrence rate, and the survival rate, has been studied [145]. Also, L1 hypomethylation has been demonstrated to be a surrogate marker for predicting the response to cancer treatment [146]. Moreover, L1 hypomethylation is observed in very different types of specimen, including blood leukocyte DNA, serum, and oral rinse [147]. Hypomethylation of Alu was reported in several cancers, whereas hypomethylation of HERV-K and HERV-W genomes were found in urothelial cancer and ovarian cancer, respectively [47, 131, 148].

Classically, CpG methylation analyses have been performed in targeted sequence by discriminating between methylated and unmethylated DNA using bisulfite treatment followed by PCR amplification [149]. Although recent nanopore technology can separate between methylated and unmethylated DNA without any treatment, most analyses are usually based on methylation-specific PCR after bisulfite treatment (MSP) [150, 151]. Pyrosequencing-based analysis, specifically methylation-sensitive single-nucleotide-primer extension (MsSNuPE) and Methylight, is a promising method that can be used to reliably measure L1 methylation in paraffin-embedded cancer tissues with higher reproducibility [152]. Using this method, L1 hypomethylation has been tested in various human cancer patients, including gastric cancer, colon cancer, colorectal cancer, melanoma, and breast cancer, and its clinical implications have been suggested [153]. Recent studies have addressed that methylated L1 in circulating cell-free DNA (cfDNA) can be used as a potential prognostic and diagnostic target in cancers, and have promoted its potential as a minimally invasive screening technique. Lee et al. showed L1 hypomethylation in cfDNA of both human breast cancer and dog mammary tumor [154, 155].

Unfortunately, there are not many products in the marketplace that capitalize on the association between RE hypomethylation and diverse cancer types and features, even though many studies have provided evidence for it. Representatively, the only clinical test targeting methylation of L1 is used in the detection of bladder cancer in voided urine [156].

4.3 RE transcripts in cancer diagnosis

First of all, the quantitation of various HERV gene expressions was performed using a real-time PCR. The transcript expression of HERV-H, -K, -P, and -R ENV was significantly increased in the blood of lung cancer patients, and the level was generally much higher in the squamous cell carcinoma (SCC) subtype than the small-cell lung cancer (SCLC) subtype [157]. The level of HERV-K (HML-2) was found to be an independent prognostic factor for the overall survival rate of hepatocellular carcinoma patients [158]. The expression of HERV-H LTR-associating protein 2 (HHLA2) was significantly upregulated in bladder cancer, and it was suggested as a prognostic factor of tumor metastasis and poor survival of bladder cancer patients [159]. The elevated HERV-K (HML-2) was detected in both protein and transcripts level in the blood of breast cancer patients at an early stage and was further increased with developing metastasis. Thus, HERV-K (HML-2) expression will be one of a best candidate for the early detection of an increased risk for breast cancer in women [160]. The expression of HERV-E transcripts is observed in von Hippel-Lindau (VHL)-deficient renal carcinomas. Interestingly, the introduced VHL gene suppressed HERV-E expression in VHL-deficient carcinoma [11]. In addition, high blood levels of the ENV transcripts of various HERV types have been detected in breast cancer patients and that are decreased by treatment of adjuvant chemotherapy which means that alteration of blood HERV transcripts is a very good candidate for diagnosis and is a prognosis marker of breast cancer [132].

4.4 Detection of RE proteins in cancer specimens

A correlation between HERV protein expression and human cancer has been described [11]. HERV proteins, GAG, POL, and ENV, have been identified in cancer tissues, and several factors from environment and hormone response, such as UV radiation, inflammation, estrogen and smoking, have been proposed as a cause of HERV protein expression in various cancer tissues [161]. Remarkably, the envelop protein, ENV, of HERV-K has been identified in melanoma by immunohistochemistry [162]. In melanomas, the expression of HERV-K ENV is higher than that in benign lesions, especially in metastatic tumors. Moreover, it has also been found in other types of cancers, such as breast, ovarian, and bladder cancer. Antibodies targeting HERV-E, HERV-K (HML-2), and ERV3 have also been detected in more than 30% of ovarian cancer patients and are higher in patients with lymph-node-positive breast tumors. In addition, the presence of serum antibodies against HERV-K proteins has been suggested as a prognostic factor for poor survival of melanoma patients [11].

In L1 proteins, high levels of ORF1 protein was prevalent in certain cancers, including breast and ovarian cancer, whereas no or little expression was detected from other cancers such as renal, liver, and cervical cancer [36]. Rodic et al. and Ardeljan et al. separately detected ORF1 protein via IHC in ~90% of ovarian cancer and in ~90% of the breast cancer samples examined [127, 163]. Chen et al. reported that the ORF1 protein level is very high in ductal carcinoma in situ (DCIS) [164]. Moreover, the ORF1 level was the highest in high-grade ovarian carcinoma, but the expression of ORF1 in prostate cancer has not been fully confirmed [36]. Ardeljan et al. reported ORF1 positivity in ~41% of all prostate cancer tissue samples examined [163]. ORF1 levels could be clinically measured using CT scans on the blood of lung cancer patients. On the other hand, ORF2 has only been limitedly tested as a diagnostic marker for cancer when compared to ORF1 expression. However, since ORF2 encodes a reverse transcriptase that is heavily associated with L1 activity, similar to L1 hypomethylation, it may yet be a better diagnostic marker for L1-associated disease development. High expression of ORF2 in transitional colon mucosa but no expression in normal colon mucosa was detected via IHC. ORF2 was also detected in prostate intraepithelial neoplasia [36]. However, since the ORF2 expression has been reported to be much less than that of ORF1, there are challenges to measure it in clinic.

5. RE in cancer therapy

Aberration of RE activities in various aspects has been suggested as a potential target for cancer therapy [165]. Several studies have shown that inhibiting RT activity is a great therapeutic target for cancer. Sciamanna et al., 2005, uncovered that pharmacologic L1 inhibition by two reverse transcriptase inhibitors slows down the growth of malignant melanoma and prostatic cancer [166]. Carlini et al. similarly demonstrated the efficacy of reverse transcription inhibition of prostate cancer growth [167]. Furthermore, a clinical trial showed that Efavirenz, a non-nucleoside reverse transcriptase inhibitor (NNRTI), provides a therapeutic benefit by increasing the progression free survival in a high-stage castration-resistant prostate cancer cohort [168]. Recently, Efavirenz has been shown to suppress L1 activity and promote morphological differentiation in melanoma cells [169]. On the other hand, another class of RT inhibitor, the nucleoside reverse transcriptase inhibitor (NRTI), has also been shown to suppress L1 activity and induce anticancer activity in prostate cancer cell lines. Importantly, no significant effects were observed in normal cells [167]. Despite these successful findings, it is still unclear regarding the molecular function of RT inhibition in the gene expression regulation.

RNA interference (RNAi)-mediated downregulation of L1 generated identical effects to those observed with RT inhibitory drugs in human melanoma, which indicates that RT activity has a crucial role in L1 activity in human cancer [170]. Recently, a phase II human trial using Efavirenz on a cohort of metastatic patients with prostate cancer showed nonprogression when Efavirenz reached an optimal concentration in the blood [171]. Altogether, preclinical and clinical data provide evidence that RT inhibition is a potentially effective tool in a novel anticancer therapy against diverse human cancers with noncytotoxic effects on non-cancer cells [172].

Another approach regarding REs is an immunotherapy approach to target the pro-oncogenic effects of HERV ENV, which is possibly involved in tumor progression and in downstream metastatic spread, in a number of tissues. HERV ENVs exclusively upregulated in tumor tissues will be suitable targets to direct both passive and active immunotherapy against in cancer cells [130]. The antibodies recognizing the HERV ENVs has been developed, and currently, a monoclonal antibody against HERV-K (HML2) ENV successfully inhibits human breast cancer proliferation, with the activation of apoptosis [173]. On the other hand, various HERV-derived ENVs have been investigated as candidates of anticancer immunotherapy, either as tumor-associated or tumor-specific antigens in cancer cells [130]. ERVs were first used for antitumor immunization in the murine cancer models expressing ERV [9]. Similarly, in humans, protective immunity against the HERV-K MEL antigen in melanoma development has been investigated. This active immunotherapy is considered more advantageous with respect to passive immunization [130]. However, despite the antigenic similarity between HERV-K-MEL and yellow fever virus (YFV), no significant protective effects were shown in the 10 years post-anti-YFV vaccinations in the melanoma cohorts [174, 175]. HERV-H ENV (Xp22.3) is an another antigen significantly upregulated in a subset of gastrointestinal cancers. T cells that was sensitized to HERV-H ENV (Xp22.3) had lytic effects against colorectal cancer expressing the ENV. HERV-E ENV showed similar effects in renal carcinoma [130, 176].

In addition, demethylating drugs are commonly used as anticancer agents and are known to trigger RE reexpression [177]. Interestingly, DNA methyl transferase inhibitors are caused by immune attacks that increase the expression of HERV and thereby increase the viral dsRNA [178]. Accordingly, individual knocking down of MDA5, MAVS, or IRF7 inhibits the ability of DNA methyl transferase inhibitor to target colorectal cancers resulting in significantly reduced the anticancer activity [179]. Altogether, immunotherapy approaches targeting HERV ENV in a broad spectrum of cancers might be valuable for the expansion of target cancers and for use with other cancer therapies.

6. Conclusions

In this chapter, we reviewed and summarized the functions and regulatory mechanisms of retroelements in the development and progression of cancers, and further presented applications in the development of diagnosis and treatment targets using these characteristics (**Table 1**). We looked at the retrovirus as a functional genomic element that forms the genome, not as an ancient infected virus and its useless remnants. Reactivation of retroelements means that it affects various regulation processes of cells beyond not only controlling the functions of surrounding genes but also increasing the protein formed therefrom or its function, or prompting its reinsertion into a new position. Because of this, it is very important to analyze and understand retroelements' functions with regard to various target substances, for example, miRNA, transcription factors, epigenetic modifiers, and so on (**Figure 1**).

RE type	Cancer type	Experimental technique	References
L1	Colon, breast, lung, ovarian, prostate cancer	Bisulfite-pyrosequencing	[45]
		MCA/CpG island microarray	
L1	Intrahepatic cholangiocarcinoma	Bisulfite-pyrosequencing	[48]
L1	Prostate cancer	Southern blot analysis	[49]
Alu	Colon cancer	Next-generation sequencing of unmethylated Alu	[50]
HERV-K	Breast cancer	RT-PCR, northern blot, in situ hybridization	[51]
HERV-K	Breast cancer	TCGA RNA-seq, RPPA data anaylsis	[52]
HERV-K	Melanoma	IHC, immunoblotting	[53]
		Cell fusion-dependent colony formation assay	
HERV-K	Kidney cancer	RT-PCR, northern blot	[54]
HERV-K	Head and neck cancer	Microarray	[34]
LI	Ovarian cancer	Southern hybridization, RT-PCR	[57]
HERV-W	Ovarian cancer	Southern hybridization, RT-PCR	[57]
L1	Breast cancer	Absolute quantitative assessment of methylated alleles (AQAMA) PCR	[58]
HERV-K	Urothelial carcinoma	RT-PCT, bisulfite-pyrosequencing	[60]
L1	Urothelial carcinoma	RT-PCT, bisulfite-pyrosequencing	[60]
HERV-K	Pancreatic cancer	RT-PCR, IHC, IF, ELISA, female immunodeficient nude	[61]
HERV-K	Prostate cancer	RT-PCR, bisulfite-pyrosequencing, ChIP	[64]
LI	Colorectal, blood, brain, prostate, ovarian cancer	Tea (TE analyzer) from paired-end, whole-genome sequencing	[96]
L1	11 types of cancer	Whole genome, exome sequencing	[94]
L1	Lung, brain cancer	L1-seq	[97]
L1	Liver cancer	Retrotransposon capture sequencing (RC-seq)	[95]
L1	Colon cancer	Southern blot, isolation of the fragment containing the insertion	[98]

RE type	Cancer type	Experimental technique	References
L1	Liver cancer	RC-seq, whole genome sequencing	[99]
L1	Encephalopathy	DNA-seq, RT-PCR	[116]
Alu	Multiple cancer cell lines	RNA immunoprecipitation, RT-PCR	[118]
ERV-9	Multiple cancer cell lines	RT-PCR, western blot, RNA immunoprecipitation, xenograft models	[122]
L1	Multiple cancer cell lines	IF, LINE-1 activation assay, RT-PCR	[124]
L1	Leukemia	ChIP-seq, RNA-seq	[125]
L1	Oral cancer	Bisulfite-pyrosequencing	[126]
HERV-W	Testicular cancer	HERV GeneChip microarray, bisulfite sequencing PCR	[133]
HERV-W	Endometrial cancer	RT-PCR, DNA-seq, immunoblot	[134]
L1	Breast, ovarian, pancreatic, lung, prostate cancer	Immunohistochemistry	[136]
L1	Colon, prostate cancer	Immunoblot, IF, IHC	[138]
HERV	Breast cancer	RT-PCR	[141]
HERV-K	Teratocarcinoma	CRISPR/Cas9, immunoblot	[144]
HERV-K	Breast cancer	GST pull-down assay, Co-IP	[145]
L1	Gastrointestinal cancer	Tea (TE analyzer) from paired-end whole-genome sequencing, somatic SNV, indel call, RNA-seq for TCGA	[149]
HERV	Multiple cancer types	SNV, DNA functional elements analysis	[150]
L1	Liver cancer	Bisulfite pyrosequencing	[154]
L1	NSCLC	Methylation-specific real-time PCR assay	[155]
L1	Colon cancer	Bisulfite pyrosequencing	[162]
L1	Breast cancer	Bisulfite sequencing, MSRED, and RT-PCR	[163]
HERV	Lung cancer	RT-PCR	[166]
HERV-K	Liver cancer	RT-PCR	[167]
HERV-H	Multiple cancer types	Immunohistochemistry	[168]
HERV-K	Breast cancer	ELISA, RT-PCR	[169]
L1	Multiple cancer types	Immunohistochemistry	[172]
L1	Breast cancer	Western blot, IHC	[173]
L1	Melanoma, prostate cancer	IF, Western blot, xenograft model	[175]
L1	Prostate cancer	RT activity assay, RT-PCR	[176]
L1	Melanoma	IF, RT-PCR, western blot, xenograft model	[178]

Table 1.
RE expression in human cancers.

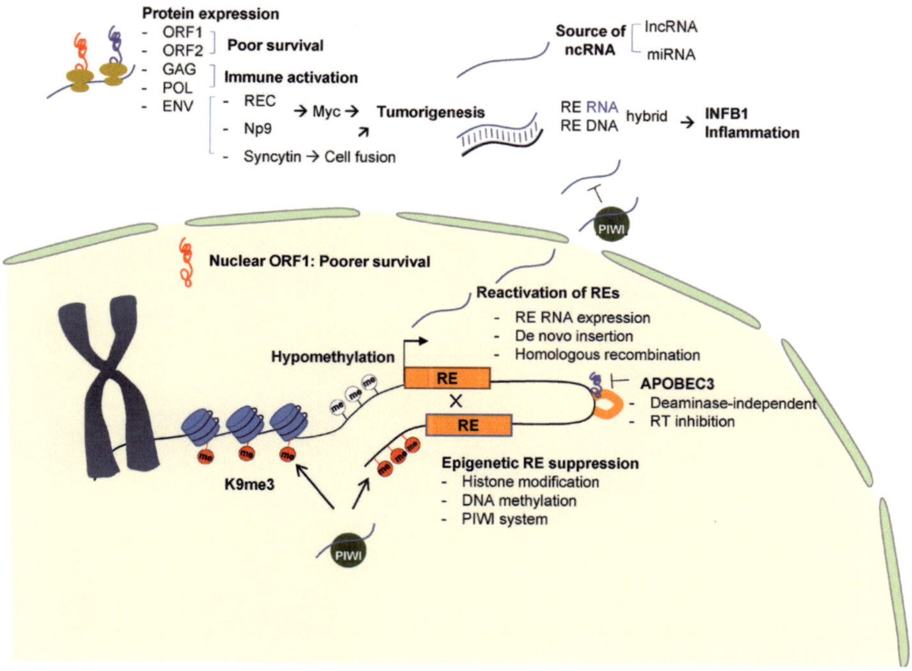

Figure 1.
Overall involvement of REs in cancer studies. RE expression was regulated by epigenomic controls such as histone modification and methylation. Reactivated RE by hypomethylation causes genome instability and the enrichment of cytoplasmic RE transcripts which may increase inflammatory signal. These may be involved in diverse biological process as a source of ncRNA including miRNAs. RE proteins are also involved in tumorigenesis process, and PIWI and APOBEC3 systems regulate RE activity in various ways.

Acknowledgements

This research was supported by the Bio & Medical Technology Development Program of the National Research Foundation (NRF), funded by the Ministry of Science and ICT (#2016M3A9B6026771) and by (NRF-2019R1I1A1A01060265) at least partially. J.Y.C. conceived and developed the entire study and revised the chapter, and K.H.L. mainly wrote the first draft. We thank Hyeon-Ji Hwang for data acquisition, and Johannes Schabort for English editing.

Conflict of interest

The authors declare no conflict of interest.

Author details

Kang-Hoon Lee and Je-Yoel Cho*
Department of Biochemistry, BK21 PLUS Program for Creative Veterinary Science Research and Research Institute for Veterinary Science, College of Veterinary Medicine, Seoul National University, Seoul, South Korea

*Address all correspondence to: jeycho@snu.ac.kr

References

[1] Collins FS et al. A vision for the future of genomics research. Nature. 2003;**422**(6934):835-847

[2] Hofker MH, Fu J, Wijmenga C. The genome revolution and its role in understanding complex diseases. Biochimica et Biophysica Acta. 2014;**1842**(10):1889-1895

[3] O'Donnell KA, Burns KH. Mobilizing diversity: Transposable element insertions in genetic variation and disease. Mobile DNA. 2010;**1**(1):21

[4] Cordaux R, Batzer MA. The impact of retrotransposons on human genome evolution. Nature Reviews. Genetics. 2009;**10**(10):691-703

[5] Beck CR et al. LINE-1 retrotransposition activity in human genomes. Cell. 2010;**141**(7):1159-1170

[6] Richardson SR et al. The influence of LINE-1 and SINE retrotransposons on mammalian genomes. Microbiology Spectrum. 2015;**3**(2) MDNA3-0061-2014

[7] Mason AL, Gilady SY, Mackey JR. Mouse mammary tumor virus in human breast cancer red herring or smoking gun? American Journal of Pathology. 2011;**179**(4):1588-1590

[8] Kassiotis G. Endogenous retroviruses and the development of cancer. Journal of Immunology. 2014;**192**(4):1343-1349

[9] Attermann AS et al. Human endogenous retroviruses and their implication for immunotherapeutics of cancer. Annals of Oncology. 2018;**29**(11):2183-2191

[10] Bannert N, Kurth R. Retroelements and the human genome: New perspectives on an old relation. Proceedings of the National Academy of Sciences of the United States of America. 2004;**101**(Suppl 2): 14572-14579

[11] Gonzalez-Cao M et al. Human endogenous retroviruses and cancer. Cancer Biology & Medicine. 2016;**13**(4):483-488

[12] Bannert N et al. HERVs new role in cancer: From accused perpetrators to cheerful protectors. Frontiers in Microbiology. 2018;**9**:178

[13] Yu HL, Zhao ZK, Zhu F. The role of human endogenous retroviral long terminal repeat sequences in human cancer (review). International Journal of Molecular Medicine. 2013;**32**(4):755-762

[14] Pfeifer GP. Defining driver DNA methylation changes in human cancer. International Journal of Molecular Sciences. 2018;**19**(4):1166

[15] Jansz N. DNA methylation dynamics at transposable elements in mammals. DNA Methylation. 2019;**63**(6):677-689

[16] Bourque G et al. Ten things you should know about transposable elements. Genome Biology. 2018;**19**:199

[17] Palazzo AF, Gregory TR. The case for junk DNA. PLoS Genetics. 2014;**10**(5):e1004351

[18] Tokuyama M et al. ERVmap analysis reveals genome-wide transcription of human endogenous retroviruses. Proceedings of the National Academy of Sciences of the United States of America. 2018;**115**(50):12565-12572

[19] Mita P, Boeke JD. How retrotransposons shape genome regulation. Current Opinion in Genetics & Development. 2016;**37**:90-100

[20] Casacuberta E, Gonzalez J. The impact of transposable elements in

environmental adaptation. Molecular Ecology. 2013;**22**(6):1503-1517

[21] Miousse IR et al. Response of transposable elements to environmental stressors. Mutation Research, Reviews in Mutation Research. 2015;**765**:19-39

[22] Jung YD et al. Retroelements: Molecular features and implications for disease. Genes & Genetic Systems. 2013;**88**(1):31-43

[23] Tam OH, Ostrow LW, Gale Hammell M. Diseases of the nervous system: Retrotransposon activity in neurodegenerative disease. Mobile DNA. 2019;**10**:32

[24] Szpakowski S et al. Loss of epigenetic silencing in tumors preferentially affects primate-specific retroelements. Gene. 2009;**448**(2):151-167

[25] Walter M et al. An epigenetic switch ensures transposon repression upon dynamic loss of DNA methylation in embryonic stem cells. eLife. 2016;**5**:e11418

[26] Li E, Zhang Y. DNA methylation in mammals. Cold Spring Harbor Perspectives in Biology. 2014;**6**(5):a019133

[27] Law JA, Jacobsen SE. Establishing, maintaining and modifying DNA methylation patterns in plants and animals. Nature Reviews. Genetics. 2010;**11**(3):204-220

[28] Adalsteinsson BT, Ferguson-Smith AC. Epigenetic control of the genome-lessons from genomic imprinting. Genes (Basel). 2014;**5**(3):635-655

[29] Leung D et al. Regulation of DNA methylation turnover at LTR retrotransposons and imprinted loci by the histone methyltransferase Setdb1. Proceedings of the National Academy of Sciences of the United States of America. 2014;**111**(18):6690-6695

[30] Jones PA, Liang GN. OPINION rethinking how DNA methylation patterns are maintained. Nature Reviews Genetics. 2009;**10**(11):805-811

[31] Rowe HM, Trono D. Dynamic control of endogenous retroviruses during development. Virology. 2011;**411**(2):273-287

[32] Zeng Y, Chen TP. DNA methylation reprogramming during mammalian development. Genes. 2019;**10**(4):257

[33] Zamudio N et al. DNA methylation restrains transposons from adopting a chromatin signature permissive for meiotic recombination. Genes & Development. 2015;**29**(12):1256-1270

[34] Costello JF, Plass C. Methylation matters. Journal of Medical Genetics. 2001;**38**(5):285-303

[35] Estecio MRH et al. LINE-1 hypomethylation in cancer is highly variable and inversely correlated with microsatellite instability. PLoS One. 2007;**2**(5):e399

[36] Lavasanifar A et al. Long interspersed nuclear element-1 mobilization as a target in cancer diagnostics, prognostics and therapeutics. Clinica Chimica Acta. 2019;**493**:52-62

[37] Cheung HH et al. DNA methylation of cancer genome. Birth Defects Research Part C-Embryo Today-Reviews. 2009;**87**(4):335-350

[38] Jeong S et al. Tumoral LINE-1 hypomethylation is associated with poor survival of patients with intrahepatic cholangiocarcinoma. BMC Cancer. 2017;**17**:588

[39] Schulz WA et al. Factor interaction analysis for chromosome 8 and DNA

methylation alterations highlights innate immune response suppression and cytoskeletal changes in prostate cancer. Molecular Cancer. 2007;**6**:14

[40] Jorda M et al. The epigenetic landscape of Alu repeats delineates the structural and functional genomic architecture of colon cancer cells. Genome Research. 2017;**27**(1):118-132

[41] Wang-Johanning F et al. Expression of human endogenous retrovirus k envelope transcripts in human breast cancer. Clinical Cancer Research. 2001;7(6):1553-1560

[42] Huang G et al. Human endogenous retroviral K element encodes fusogenic activity in melanoma cells. Journal of Carcinogenesis. 2013;**12**:5

[43] Cherkasova E et al. Detection of an immunogenic HERV-E envelope with selective expression in clear cell kidney cancer. Cancer Research. 2016;**76**(8):2177-2185

[44] Johanning GL et al. Expression of human endogenous retrovirus-K is strongly associated with the basal-like breast cancer phenotype. Scientific Reports. 2017;7:41960

[45] Babaian A, Mager DL. Endogenous retroviral promoter exaptation in human cancer. Mobile DNA. 2016;**7**:24

[46] Zhang M, Liang JQ, Zheng S. Expressional activation and functional roles of human endogenous retroviruses in cancers. Reviews in Medical Virology. 2019;**29**(2):e2025

[47] Menendez L, Benigno BB, McDonald JF. L1 and HERV-W retrotransposons are hypomethylated in human ovarian carcinomas. Molecular Cancer. 2004;**3**:12

[48] van Hoesel AQ et al. Hypomethylation of LINE-1 in primary tumor has poor prognosis in young breast cancer patients: A retrospective cohort study. Breast Cancer Research and Treatment. 2012;**134**(3):1103-1114

[49] Miousse IR, Koturbash I. The fine LINE: Methylation drawing the cancer landscape. BioMed Research International. 2015;**2015**:131547

[50] Kreimer U et al. HERV-K and LINE-1 DNA methylation and reexpression in urothelial carcinoma. Frontiers in Oncology. 2013;**3**:255

[51] Li M et al. Downregulation of human endogenous retrovirus type K (HERV-K) viral env RNA in pancreatic cancer cells decreases cell proliferation and tumor growth. Clinical Cancer Research. 2017;**23**(19):5892-5911

[52] Molaro A, Malik HS. Hide and seek: How chromatin-based pathways silence retroelements in the mammalian germline. Current Opinion in Genetics & Development. 2016;**37**:51-58

[53] Yang F, Wang PJ. Multiple LINEs of retrotransposon silencing mechanisms in the mammalian germline. Seminars in Cell & Developmental Biology. 2016;**59**:118-125

[54] Goering W, Ribarska T, Schulz WA. Selective changes of retroelement expression in human prostate cancer. Carcinogenesis. 2011;**32**(10):1484-1492

[55] Sytnikova YA et al. Transposable element dynamics and PIWI regulation impacts lncRNA and gene expression diversity in Drosophila ovarian cell cultures. Genome Research. 2014;**24**(12):1977-1990

[56] Ozata DM et al. PIWI-interacting RNAs: Small RNAs with big functions. Nature Reviews. Genetics. 2019;**20**(2):89-108

[57] Lim AK, Tao L, Kai T. piRNAs mediate posttranscriptional retroelement silencing and localization

to pi-bodies in the Drosophila germline. The Journal of Cell Biology. 2009;**186**(3):333-342

[58] Toth KF et al. The piRNA pathway guards the germline genome against transposable elements. Advances in Experimental Medicine and Biology. 2016;**886**:51-77

[59] Siomi MC et al. PIWI-interacting small RNAs: The vanguard of genome defence. Nature Reviews. Molecular Cell Biology. 2011;**12**(4):246-258

[60] Inoue K et al. Switching of dominant retrotransposon silencing strategies from posttranscriptional to transcriptional mechanisms during male germ-cell development in mice. PLoS Genetics. 2017;**13**(7):e1006926

[61] Cheng Y et al. Emerging roles of piRNAs in cancer: Challenges and prospects. Aging (Albany NY). 2019;**11**(21):9932-9946

[62] Yu Y, Xiao J, Hann SS. The emerging roles of PIWI-interacting RNA in human cancers. Cancer Management and Research. 2019;**11**:5895-5909

[63] Maleki Dana P, Mansournia MA, Mirhashemi SM. PIWI-interacting RNAs: New biomarkers for diagnosis and treatment of breast cancer. Cell & Bioscience. 2020;**10**:44

[64] Liu Y et al. The emerging role of the piRNA/piwi complex in cancer. Molecular Cancer. 2019;**18**(1):123

[65] Chen Z et al. Stem cell protein Piwil1 endowed endometrial cancer cells with stem-like properties via inducing epithelial-mesenchymal transition. BMC Cancer. 2015;**15**:811

[66] Qu X et al. PIWIL2 promotes progression of non-small cell lung cancer by inducing CDK2 and Cyclin A expression. Journal of Translational Medicine. 2015;**13**:301

[67] Jiang L et al. Downregulation of Piwil3 suppresses cell proliferation, migration and invasion in gastric cancer. Cancer Biomarkers. 2017;**20**(4):499-509

[68] Wang Z et al. The role of PIWIL4, an Argonaute family protein, in breast cancer. The Journal of Biological Chemistry. 2016;**291**(20):10646-10658

[69] Chiu YL, Greene WC. The APOBEC3 cytidine deaminases: An innate defensive network opposing exogenous retroviruses and endogenous retroelements. Annual Review of Immunology. 2008;**26**:317-353

[70] Kinomoto M et al. All APOBEC3 family proteins differentially inhibit LINE-1 retrotransposition. Nucleic Acids Research. 2007;**35**(9):2955-2964

[71] Liang W et al. APOBEC3DE inhibits LINE-1 Retrotransposition by interacting with ORF1p and influencing LINE reverse transcriptase activity. PLoS One. 2016;**11**(7):e0157220

[72] Choi J, Hwang SY, Ahn K. Interplay between RNASEH2 and MOV10 controls LINE-1 retrotransposition. Nucleic Acids Research. 2018;**46**(4):1912-1926

[73] Hu S et al. SAMHD1 inhibits LINE-1 retrotransposition by promoting stress granule formation. PLoS Genetics. 2015;**11**(7):e1005367

[74] Goodier JL et al. The broad-spectrum antiviral protein ZAP restricts human retrotransposition. PLoS Genetics. 2015;**11**(5):e1005252

[75] Kohnken R, Kodigepalli KM, Wu L. Regulation of deoxynucleotide metabolism in cancer: Novel mechanisms and therapeutic implications. Molecular Cancer. 2015;**14**:176

[76] Schneider AM et al. Roles of retrotransposons in benign and

malignant hematologic disease. Cell. 2009;**6**(2):121-145

[77] Crichton J et al. Defending the genome from the enemy within: Mechanisms of retrotransposon suppression in the mouse germline. Cellular and Molecular Life Sciences. 2014;**71**(9):1581-1605

[78] Huang CR, Burns KH, Boeke JD. Active transposition in genomes. Annual Review of Genetics. 2012;**46**:651-675

[79] Feschotte C, Pritham EJ. DNA transposons and the evolution of eukaryotic genomes. Annual Review of Genetics. 2007;**41**:331-368

[80] Belancio VP, Roy-Engel AM, Deininger PL. All y'all need to know 'bout retroelements in cancer. Seminars in Cancer Biology. 2010;**20**(4):200-210

[81] Solyom S, Kazazian HH Jr. Mobile elements in the human genome: Implications for disease. Genome Medicine. 2012;**4**(2):12

[82] Yi K, Ju YS. Patterns and mechanisms of structural variations in human cancer. Experimental & Molecular Medicine. 2018;**50**(8):98

[83] Erwin JA et al. L1-associated genomic regions are deleted in somatic cells of the healthy human brain. Nature Neuroscience. 2016;**19**(12):1583-1591

[84] Scott EC, Devine SE. The role of somatic L1 retrotransposition in human cancers. Viruses. 2017;**9**(6):131

[85] Helman E et al. Somatic retrotransposition in human cancer revealed by whole-genome and exome sequencing. Genome Research. 2014;**24**(7):1053-1063

[86] Shukla R et al. Endogenous retrotransposition activates oncogenic pathways in hepatocellular carcinoma. Cell. 2013;**153**(1):101-111

[87] Lee E et al. Landscape of somatic retrotransposition in human cancers. Science. 2012;**337**(6097):967-971

[88] Iskow RC et al. Natural mutagenesis of human genomes by endogenous retrotransposons. Cell. 2010;**141**(7):1253-1261

[89] Miki Y et al. Disruption of the APC gene by a retrotransposal insertion of L1 sequence in a colon cancer. Cancer Research. 1992;**52**(3):643-645

[90] Schauer SN et al. L1 retrotransposition is a common feature of mammalian hepatocarcinogenesis. Genome Research. 2018;**28**(5):639-653

[91] Nakagawa H, Fujita M. Whole genome sequencing analysis for cancer genomics and precision medicine. Cancer Science. 2018;**109**(3):513-522

[92] Hancks DC, Kazazian HH Jr. Roles for retrotransposon insertions in human disease. Mobile DNA. 2016;**7**:9

[93] Cakmak Guner B et al. Detection of HERV-K6 and HERV-K11 transpositions in the human genome. Biomedical Reports. 2018;**9**(1):53-59

[94] Thayer RE, Singer MF, Fanning TG. Undermethylation of specific LINE-1 sequences in human cells producing a LINE-1-encoded protein. Gene. 1993;**133**(2):273-277

[95] Baba Y et al. Long interspersed element-1 methylation level as a prognostic biomarker in gastrointestinal cancers. Digestion. 2018;**97**(1):26-30

[96] Piskareva O et al. The human L1 element: A potential biomarker in cancer prognosis, current status and future directions. Current Molecular Medicine. 2011;**11**(4):286-303

[97] Zhang W, Xu J. DNA methyltransferases and their roles in tumorigenesis. Biomarker Research. 2017;**5**:1

[98] Gaudet F et al. Induction of tumors in mice by genomic hypomethylation. Science. 2003;**300**(5618):489-492

[99] Lamprecht B, Bonifer C, Mathas S. Repeat-element driven activation of proto-oncogenes in human malignancies. Cell Cycle. 2010;**9**(21):4276-4281

[100] Veeck J, Esteller M. Breast cancer epigenetics: From DNA methylation to microRNAs. Journal of Mammary Gland Biology and Neoplasia. 2010;**15**(1):5-17

[101] Chishima T, Iwakiri J, Hamada M. Identification of transposable elements contributing to tissue-specific expression of long non-coding RNAs. Genes (Basel). 2018;**9**(1):23

[102] Tufarelli C, Cruickshanks HA, Meehan RR. LINE-1 activation and epigenetic silencing of suppressor genes in cancer: Causally related events? Mobile Genetic Elements. 2013;**3**(5):e26832

[103] Kukurba KR, Montgomery SB. RNA sequencing and analysis. Cold Spring Harbor Protocols. 2015;**2015**(11):951-969

[104] Zhang X et al. Non-coding RNAs and retroviruses. Retrovirology. 2018;**15**(1):20

[105] Kapusta A et al. Transposable elements are major contributors to the origin, diversification, and regulation of vertebrate long noncoding RNAs. PLoS Genetics. 2013;**9**(4):e1003470

[106] Sparber P et al. The role of long non-coding RNAs in the pathogenesis of hereditary diseases. BMC Medical Genomics. 2019;**12**(Suppl 2):42

[107] Cartault F et al. Mutation in a primate-conserved retrotransposon reveals a noncoding RNA as a mediator of infantile encephalopathy. Proceedings of the National Academy of Sciences of the United States of America. 2012;**109**(13):4980-4985

[108] Hadjiargyrou M, Delihas N. The intertwining of transposable elements and non-coding RNAs. International Journal of Molecular Sciences. 2013;**14**(7):13307-13328

[109] Negishi M et al. A new lncRNA, APTR, associates with and represses the CDKN1A/p21 promoter by recruiting polycomb proteins. PLoS One. 2014;**9**(4):e95216

[110] Kelley D, Rinn J. Transposable elements reveal a stem cell-specific class of long noncoding RNAs. Genome Biology. 2012;**13**(11):R107

[111] Pan Y et al. The emerging roles of long noncoding RNA ROR (lincRNA-ROR) and its possible mechanisms in human cancers. Cellular Physiology and Biochemistry. 2016;**40**(1-2):219-229

[112] Wang G et al. Regulation of proto-oncogene transcription, cell proliferation, and tumorigenesis in mice by PSF protein and a VL30 noncoding RNA. Proceedings of the National Academy of Sciences of the United States of America. 2009;**106**(39):16794-16798

[113] Xu L et al. A novel function of RNAs arising from the long terminal repeat of human endogenous retrovirus 9 in cell cycle arrest. Journal of Virology. 2013;**87**(1):25-36

[114] Stetson DB et al. Trex1 prevents cell-intrinsic initiation of autoimmunity. Cell. 2008;**134**(4):587-598

[115] Yu Q et al. Type I interferon controls propagation of long interspersed element-1. The Journal of Biological Chemistry. 2015;**290**(16):10191-10199

[116] Ishak CA et al. An RB-EZH2 complex mediates silencing of repetitive

DNA sequences. Molecular Cell. 2016;**64**(6):1074-1087

[117] Gasche JA et al. Interleukin-6 promotes tumorigenesis by altering DNA methylation in oral cancer cells. International Journal of Cancer. 2011;**129**(5):1053-1063

[118] Finnegan DJ. Retrotransposons. Current Biology. 2012;**22**(11):R432-R437

[119] Jiang F et al. Large-scale transcriptome analysis of retroelements in the migratory locust, *Locusta migratoria*. PLoS One. 2012;**7**(7):e40532

[120] Martin SL. The ORF1 protein encoded by LINE-1: Structure and function during L1 retrotransposition. Journal of Biomedicine & Biotechnology. 2006;**2006**(1):45621

[121] Garcia-Montojo M et al. Human endogenous retrovirus-K (HML-2): A comprehensive review. Critical Reviews in Microbiology. 2018;**44**(6):715-738

[122] Li F, Karlsson H. Expression and regulation of human endogenous retrovirus W elements. APMIS. 2016;**124**(1-2):52-66

[123] Soygur B, Sati L. The role of syncytins in human reproduction and reproductive organ cancers. Reproduction. 2016;**152**(5):R167-R178

[124] Gimenez J et al. Custom human endogenous retroviruses dedicated microarray identifies self-induced HERV-W family elements reactivated in testicular cancer upon methylation control. Nucleic Acids Research. 2010;**38**(7):2229-2246

[125] Strick R et al. Proliferation and cell-cell fusion of endometrial carcinoma are induced by the human endogenous retroviral Syncytin-1 and regulated by TGF-beta. Journal of Molecular Medicine (Berlin, Germany). 2007;**85**(1):23-38

[126] Burns KH. Transposable elements in cancer. Nature Reviews. Cancer. 2017;**17**(7):415-424

[127] Rodic N et al. Long interspersed element-1 protein expression is a hallmark of many human cancers. The American Journal of Pathology. 2014;**184**(5):1280-1286

[128] Sur D et al. Detection of the LINE-1 retrotransposon RNA-binding protein ORF1p in different anatomical regions of the human brain. Mobile DNA. 2017;**8**:17

[129] De Luca C et al. Enhanced expression of LINE-1-encoded ORF2 protein in early stages of colon and prostate transformation. Oncotarget. 2016;**7**(4):4048-4061

[130] Grandi N, Tramontano E. HERV envelope proteins: Physiological role and pathogenic potential in cancer and autoimmunity. Frontiers in Microbiology. 2018;**9**:462

[131] Cegolon L et al. Human endogenous retroviruses and cancer prevention: Evidence and prospects. BMC Cancer. 2013;**13**:4

[132] Rhyu DW et al. Expression of human endogenous retrovirus env genes in the blood of breast cancer patients. International Journal of Molecular Sciences. 2014;**15**(6):9173-9183

[133] Cherkasova E, Weisman Q, Childs RW. Endogenous retroviruses as targets for antitumor immunity in renal cell cancer and other tumors. Frontiers in Oncology. 2013;**3**:243

[134] Xue B, He L. An expanding universe of the non-coding genome in cancer biology. Carcinogenesis. 2014;**35**(6):1209-1216

[135] Chan SM et al. The HERV-K accessory protein Np9 controls viability

and migration of teratocarcinoma cells. PLoS One. 2019;**14**(2):e0212970

[136] Denne M et al. Physical and functional interactions of human endogenous retrovirus proteins Np9 and rec with the promyelocytic leukemia zinc finger protein. Journal of Virology. 2007;**81**(11):5607-5616

[137] Baeissa H et al. Identification and analysis of mutational hotspots in oncogenes and tumour suppressors. Oncotarget. 2017;**8**(13):21290-21304

[138] Steranka JP et al. Transposon insertion profiling by sequencing (TIPseq) for mapping LINE-1 insertions in the human genome. Mobile DNA. 2019;**10**:8

[139] Ewing AD. Transposable element detection from whole genome sequence data. Mobile DNA. 2015;**6**:24

[140] Jung H, Choi JK, Lee EA. Immune signatures correlate with L1 retrotransposition in gastrointestinal cancers. Genome Research. 2018;**28**(8):1136-1146

[141] Chang TC et al. Investigation of somatic single nucleotide variations in human endogenous retrovirus elements and their potential association with cancer. PLoS One. 2019;**14**(4):e0213770

[142] Ehrlich M. DNA methylation in cancer: Too much, but also too little. Oncogene. 2002;**21**(35):5400-5413

[143] Kitkumthorn N, Mutirangura A. Long interspersed nuclear element-1 hypomethylation in cancer: Biology and clinical applications. Clinical Epigenetics. 2011;**2**:315-330

[144] Locke WJ et al. DNA methylation cancer biomarkers: Translation to the clinic. Frontiers in Genetics. 2019;**10**:1150

[145] Miyata T et al. Prognostic value of LINE-1 methylation level in 321 patients with primary liver cancer including hepatocellular carcinoma and intrahepatic cholangiocarcinoma. Oncotarget. 2018;**9**(29):20795-20806

[146] Saito K et al. Long interspersed nuclear element 1 hypomethylation is a marker of poor prognosis in stage IA non-small cell lung cancer. Clinical Cancer Research. 2010;**16**(8):2418-2426

[147] Barchitta M et al. LINE-1 hypomethylation in blood and tissue samples as an epigenetic marker for cancer risk: A systematic review and meta-analysis. PLoS One. 2014;**9**(10):e109478

[148] Bakshi A et al. DNA methylation variation of human-specific Alu repeats. Epigenetics. 2016;**11**(2):163-173

[149] Leontiou CA et al. Bisulfite conversion of DNA: Performance comparison of different kits and methylation quantitation of epigenetic biomarkers that have the potential to be used in non-invasive prenatal testing. PLoS One. 2015;**10**(8):e0135058

[150] Kurdyukov S, Bullock M. DNA methylation analysis: Choosing the right method. Biology (Basel). 2016;**5**(1):3

[151] Shim J et al. Detection and quantification of methylation in DNA using solid-state Nanopores. Scientific Reports. 2013;**3**:1389

[152] Gonzalgo ML, Liang G. Methylation-sensitive single-nucleotide primer extension (Ms-SNuPE) for quantitative measurement of DNA methylation. Nature Protocols. 2007;**2**(8):1931-1936

[153] Irahara N et al. Precision of pyrosequencing assay to measure LINE-1 methylation in colon cancer, normal colonic mucosa, and peripheral blood cells. The Journal of Molecular Diagnostics. 2010;**12**(2):177-183

[154] Lee KH et al. Methylation of LINE-1 in cell-free DNA serves as a liquid biopsy biomarker for human breast cancers and dog mammary tumors. Scientific Reports. 2019;**9**(1):175

[155] Salvi S et al. Cell-free DNA as a diagnostic marker for cancer: Current insights. Oncotargets and Therapy. 2016;**9**:6549-6559

[156] Martinez VG et al. Epigenetics of bladder cancer: Where biomarkers and therapeutic targets meet. Frontiers in Genetics. 2019;**10**

[157] Zare M et al. Human endogenous retrovirus env genes: Potential blood biomarkers in lung cancer. Microbial Pathogenesis. 2018;**115**:189-193

[158] Ma WJ et al. Human endogenous retroviruses-K (HML-2) expression is correlated with prognosis and progress of hepatocellular carcinoma. BioMed Research International. 2016;**2016**:8201642

[159] Janakiram M et al. Expression, clinical significance, and receptor identification of the newest B7 family member HHLA2 protein. Clinical Cancer Research. 2015;**21**(10):2359-2366

[160] Wang-Johanning F et al. Human endogenous retrovirus type K antibodies and mRNA as serum biomarkers of early-stage breast cancer. International Journal of Cancer. 2014;**134**(3):587-595

[161] Downey RF et al. Human endogenous retrovirus K and cancer: Innocent bystander or tumorigenic accomplice? International Journal of Cancer. 2015;**137**(6):1249-1257

[162] Buscher K et al. Expression of human endogenous retrovirus K in melanomas and melanoma cell lines. Cancer Research. 2005;**65**(10):4172-4180

[163] Ardeljan D et al. The human long interspersed element-1 retrotransposon: An emerging biomarker of neoplasia. Clinical Chemistry. 2017;**63**(4):816-822

[164] Chen L et al. Prognostic value of LINE-1 retrotransposon expression and its subcellular localization in breast cancer. Breast Cancer Research and Treatment. 2012;**136**(1):129-142

[165] Anwar SL, Wulaningsih W, Lehmann U. Transposable elements in human cancer: Causes and consequences of deregulation. International Journal of Molecular Sciences. 2017;**18**(5):974

[166] Sciamanna I et al. Inhibition of endogenous reverse transcriptase antagonizes human tumor growth. Oncogene. 2005;**24**(24):3923-3931

[167] Carlini F et al. The reverse transcription inhibitor Abacavir shows anticancer activity in prostate cancer cell lines. PLoS One. 2010;**5**(12):e14221

[168] Hecht M et al. Efavirenz has the highest anti-proliferative effect of non-nucleoside reverse transcriptase inhibitors against pancreatic cancer cells. PLoS One. 2015;**10**(6):e0130277

[169] Oricchio E et al. Distinct roles for LINE-1 and HERV-K retroelements in cell proliferation, differentiation and tumor progression. Oncogene. 2007;**26**(29):4226-4233

[170] Sciamanna I, De Luca C, Spadafora C. The reverse transcriptase encoded by LINE-1 retrotransposons in the genesis, progression, and therapy of cancer. Frontiers in Chemistry. 2016;**4**:6

[171] Houede N et al. A phase II trial evaluating the efficacy and safety of efavirenz in metastatic castration-resistant prostate cancer. The Oncologist. 2014;**19**(12):1227-1228

[172] Sciamanna I et al. LINE-1-encoded reverse transcriptase as a target in

cancer therapy. Frontiers in Bioscience-Landmark. 2018;**23**:1360-1369

[173] Wang-Johanning F et al. Immunotherapeutic potential of anti-human endogenous retrovirus-K envelope protein antibodies in targeting breast tumors. Journal of the National Cancer Institute. 2012;**104**(3):189-210

[174] Hodges-Vazquez M et al. The yellow fever 17D vaccine and risk of malignant melanoma in the United States military. Vaccine. 2012;**30**(30):4476-4479

[175] Mastrangelo G et al. Does yellow fever 17D vaccine protect against melanoma? Vaccine. 2009;**27**(4):588-591

[176] Mullins CS, Linnebacher M. Endogenous retrovirus sequences as a novel class of tumor-specific antigens: An example of HERV-H env encoding strong CTL epitopes. Cancer Immunology, Immunotherapy. 2012;**61**(7):1093-1100

[177] Kong Y et al. Transposable element expression in tumors is associated with immune infiltration and increased antigenicity. Nature Communications. 2019;**10**:5228

[178] Grandi N, Tramontano E. Human endogenous retroviruses are ancient acquired elements still shaping innate immune responses. Frontiers in Immunology. 2018;**9**:2039

[179] Roulois D et al. DNA-demethylating agents target colorectal cancer cells by inducing viral mimicry by endogenous transcripts. Cell. 2015;**162**(5):961-973

Section 3

Genetics and Genomics in Clinical Practice

Chapter 6

Landscape Genetics: From Classic Molecular Markers to Genomics

Enéas Ricardo Konzen and Maria Imaculada Zucchi

Abstract

Landscape genetics combines population genetics and landscape ecology to understand processes that shape the distribution and organization of human, animal, or plant populations. This field of genetics emerged from the availability of several studies with classical molecular markers, such as isozymes, RAPD, AFLP, and microsatellites. Population genetic studies enabled the detection of population structure with those markers, but a more comprehensive analysis of natural populations was only possible with the development of statistical methods that combined both molecular data and environmental variables. Ultimately, the rapid development of sequencing technologies allowed studies at the genomic level, augmenting the resolution of association with environment factors. This chapter outlines basic concepts in landscape genetics, the main statistical methods used so far, and the perspectives of this field of knowledge into strategies for conservation of natural populations of plant and animal species. Moreover, we briefly describe the application of the field to understand historical human migration processes as well as how some diseases are spread throughout the world.

Keywords: molecular studies, environmental variables, population structure, genetic diversity, single nucleotide polymorphisms

1. Introduction

Population genetic studies deal with allele frequencies and processes that shape their variation within and among populations. Multiple studies have addressed genetic variation and their structure based on the screening of molecular markers such as allozymes (began with Lewontin and Hubby [1]), random amplified polymorphic DNA (RAPD) [2], amplified fragment length polymorphism (AFLP) [3], microsatellites or simple sequence repeats (SSR) [4], intersimple sequence repeats (ISSR) [5] and single nucleotide polymorphisms (SNP). The use of allozyme markers started up a series of population genetic studies, allowing relatively precise estimation of heterozygosity levels due to their codominance nature. Those markers were largely employed until the end of the 1990s. The development of techniques for screening directly at the level of DNA has accelerated the discovery of numberless markers in humans, animals, plants, fungi, and other organisms. RAPD, ISSR, and AFLP, in general, are more limited in describing genetic variation due to their dominance. In contrast, several SSR markers have been developed for studying a diverse set of species, enabling precise estimates of genetic diversity, gene flow, spatial genetic structure, paternity, linkage, and association mapping.

Ultimately, SNP markers have arisen as powerful markers for fine-scale genetic diversity, structure, and association mapping studies. The direct comparison among sequences of specific fragments generated by Sanger sequencing allowed the discovery of the first set of SNP. However, the revolution in sequencing technology of the last decade has provided numberless sequences for comparing individuals and deciphering population genetic mechanisms with high accuracy. The next-generation sequencing platforms generate millions of sequences that often result in thousands of SNP markers.

Nonetheless, the sole use of molecular data provides no definitive responses on evolutionary mechanisms operating in populations. An examination of the ecological factors, that drive the fate of individuals over generations or how current mechanisms impact in their adaptation or acclimation, is a much-needed task to better understand all species. Adequate statistical methods combining genetic and environmental variables are then necessary. Landscape genetics emerged as a field for the improvement of our understanding of the influence of geographical and environmental variables on the genetic structure of populations [6]. It diverges from the traditional basis of population genetics in the sense of more profound tests of the influence of landscape and environmental factors such as altitude, topography, and ground cover on population processes such as gene flow and population structure [7]. The rapid boost in genome-scale analyses also generated the terminology landscape genomics, as proposed by Joost et al. [8]. Landscape genomics differs from landscape genetics in the sense that it has become a powerful approach for scanning genes involved in complex adaptation mechanisms of species at populations and individual levels [9, 10].

This chapter is intended to provide brief concepts that cover the subject of landscape genetics and genomics. Furthermore, we outline potential applications of landscape genetic studies in the comprehension of adaptive traits of plants and animals and how such results may assist in the design of conservation strategies for endangered species. It is not our intent to provide an exhaustive panorama of landscape genetics studies so far, but rather contextualize concepts and applications with chosen case studies. Moreover, we briefly contextualize how landscape genetics is contributing in the comprehension of historical human migrations and the dispersion of human diseases.

2. Molecular markers and population structure studies

The most popular molecular markers employed in population genetic studies are SSR [4] and SNP. Simple sequence repeats are tandem repeated motifs with 1–6 bp [11] or up to 10 bp [12] with high frequency in genomes of all organisms. Plants commonly have AT-type repeats, whereas animals have the AC motif as the most common repeat unit [13]. High mutation rates are characteristics of microsatellite markers [12] providing markers with several alleles. SSR are codominant, hypervariable, and Mendelian inherited [14], which is implicated in high heterozygosity levels, increasing the discriminatory power among individuals and populations. Originally, SSR were developed from DNA libraries that required extensive laboratory work. Currently, however, the easiest way of discovering novel microsatellites if though direct sequencing of genomes and transcriptomes generated from NGS platforms [12]. With that available, SNP markers have actually been the most studied markers in recent years. SNP markers are the most abundant polymorphisms along plant and animal genomes. SNP consist on single base-pair changes present in the genome sequence that can occur as transitions or transversions, as nucleotide substitutions [15]. They can reach much higher density than all other types of markers in genomes. Next-generation sequencing can generate large amounts of sequence data, enabling the detection of thousands of SNP [16].

Microsatellites and SNP markers are powerful tools for population genetic analyses. They have been extensively employed in studies with humans as well as animal and plant models and non-model species. The codominance and multiallelic nature of microsatellites make them suitable for estimating variables such as heterozygosity, inbreeding, gene flow, outcrossing rates, differentiation among populations and population structure [17]. SNP markers are generally employed for determining population structure as well, but with much higher density of markers and therefore genomic coverage to explain such subdivision. A series of studies have used SNP to dissect complex traits with QTL mapping and genome-wide association studies (GWAS) [15].

3. The concepts of landscape genetics and landscape genomics

Landscape genetics is concerned with testing the effects of landscape features on gene flow and genetic population structure. In general, the first studies of landscape genetics involved an exploratory phase, by geographically widespread sampling of populations and analysis of the effects of various landscape variables [18]. Landscape features or variables consist of any biotic, climatic, soil, or other conditions that comprise the habitat of organisms [6]. The population structure means the organization of genetic variation as influenced by a combination of evolutionary forces such as recombination, mutation, drift, natural selection, and historic demographic processes [19]. This leads to the idea that a group of subpopulations that exchange migrants in an occasional fashion are part of metapopulations [6].

The current status of genomic technologies allows the discovery of thousands of SNP markers, which has increased the resolution power for studying the association of environmental variables with specific genomics regions, also with a much deeper understanding of evolutionary processes. Genotyping-by-sequencing has enabled the discovery of SNP markers even in non-model species, which may lack a reference genome so far [20, 21]. This is where the concept of landscape genomics comes forward. Landscape genomics focuses on detecting candidate genes under selection as putative signals of local adaptation. The design of a landscape genomics experiment involves replicated sampling of environmental factors that might be driving selection, augmenting the resolution for detection of candidate loci under selection [10].

4. A briefing on statistical approaches in landscape genetics

In a landscape genetics study, two steps of analyses are normally required. The first involves the analysis of patterns of genetic variation. Next, such patterns are correlated with landscape variables based on statistical methods [22]. To test for association of environmental variables with genetic data, one of the simplest and commonly used methods is the Mantel's test, originally developed for identifying time-space clustering of diseases [23]. The test uses permutations to address the significance of the linear correlation coefficient between two pair-wise similarity or dissimilarity matrices [22]. One of the simplest examples of its application in landscape genetics is to correlate the genetic distances between individuals with their geographic location [24].

The methods for determining association of genetic data with environmental variables can be broadly categorized into approaches that deal with (i) pair-wise landscape data and (ii) location-specific landscape data, as reviewed by Balkenhol et al. [22]. The development of methods in landscape genomics, however, expanded the range of tests for detecting loci under selection using genome scans, approaches for candidate gene discovery, QTL mapping and GWAS. Genome scans use two methods for detecting loci under selection, the differentiation outlier methods and the genetic-environmental association test, as reviewed by Storfer et al. [10]. Novel methods are continuously being developed, as more genomes are becoming sequenced or resequenced in populations.

5. Applications of landscape genetics

Several applications of landscape genetics or genomics can be described. We briefly account for case studies in plant and animal systems within this section. Moreover, a few examples of studies applied to humans are also given. In general, landscape genetics or genomics studies have provided association among geographic, abiotic, and biotic factors and genetic data provided by the screening of molecular markers in populations of diverse organisms. It has increased our power to detail inferences of movement and gene flow and potential adaptation to the landscape populations occur. However, studies for several organisms are still scarce or inexistent.

Cultivated crops such as maize, soybean, rice, and common bean were domesticated from wild progenitors which reflect their current adaptation to distinct environments. Landscape genomics studies have enabled a deeper understanding of processes shaping their distribution across multiple environments. Common bean (*Phaseolus vulgaris* L.) is an exceptional example of a widespread species original from America. Molecular data of wild germplasm identified two major gene pools, the Andean from Argentina to Colombia, and the Mesoamerican from Colombia to Mexico [25, 26]. A third smaller pool of wilds is also distinctive in a narrow area between Peru-Equador [27]. Microsatellites markers were broadly used to screen the genetic structure of wild and domesticated accessions of common bean (*Phaseolus vulgaris* L.), distinguishing from the broadest Andean and Mesoamerican gene pools to further subdivision within each one of them [25]. SNP markers from single fragments sequenced by Sanger also allowed an accurate distinction between Andean and Mesoamerican accessions, as well as their subdivisions [28]. The recognition of a parallel domestication event in each of the two major pools was also possible based on the detection of SNP markers in specific genomic regions of Andean and Mesoamerican genotypes [29]. Recent landscape genomics approaches enabled a more detailed description of the major events that determined the range expansion of *P. vulgaris* in America and how they were accompanied by environmental changes [26]. The climatic variability was also associated with differential drought adaptation and specific SNP markers were statistically related to root and shoot traits varying in a Mesoamerican panel of genotypes originated from regions with distinct precipitation regimes throughout the year [30].

Another application of landscape genomics concerns with the understanding of range expansion and ecological dominance of insect pests. The first step toward that is to know the population structure, gene flow and how natural selection is affecting adaptation. Zucchi et al. [31] described and addressed such problem by examining the population structure of *Piezodous guildiniis*, a soybean pest, in the United States and Brazil. A GBS-based set of SNP markers revealed genetic structure according to their geographic environment of origin. About 10% of loci were under positive selection, and their annotation revealed genes involved in genome reorganization, neuropeptides, and energy mobilization [31]. Addressing such problem is to assist future endeavors at managing pest spreading in cultivated crops.

Another equally important questions addressed by landscape genomics are the consequences of climate change and human intervention to natural populations of wilds plants and animals. *Euterpe edulis* Martius is a palm species native to the Atlantic Rain Forest in Brazil, known as heart-of-palm [32]. The species is the list of endangered species to extinction [33]. Several studies have addressed the genetic diversity and structure of natural populations of this palm (for a compilation see [34]). Soares et al. [35] studied the genetic diversity and structure of remnant fragments of *E. edulis* in Bahia state and related the data to landscape metrics such as composition and configuration and local variables including the logging activity as human disturbance variable. No evidence of spatial genetic structure was detected, but distinct genetic clusters could be identified, suggesting a reduction in gene flow between the fragments of this study [35]. Natural populations located in other regions of Brazil, such as in Sao Paulo state, revealed to have high genetic diversity, as shown from microsatellite markers. Adjacent populations that have been generated though germplasm collection for management and cultivation showed similar genetic diversity. Those genetic materials could be used for recovering overexploited populations [36].

Landscape genetics studies with wild animals have been focused in recognizing their patterns of moving across their habitats. On terrestrial lands, landscape genetics of animals has particular features in comparison to aquatic environments or even to terrestrial plants. Landscape patterns interfere with organism behavior, thereby affecting mating and dispersal and reflecting on population processes [37].

6. Landscape genetics and human populations and diseases

Genomic technologies have also enabled studies to uncover historical human migrations and the genetic structure and diversity of human populations. For example, a genome-wide study of Malaysian ethnic groups using a SNP array revealed that humans from the peninsular area of Malaysia had higher genetic diversity, which the authors associated with a contact zone for recent human migrations in the Asian continent [38]. Such an example suggests the association between the genetic structure of human populations with geographic variables. In fact, Peter et al. [39] show that genetic differentiation generally tends to increase over higher geographic distances; however, distortions in those patterns also frequently occur. The human population structure, then, seems to be quite dynamic.

Landscape genetics also has been employed in epidemiological studies of human diseases. Statistical methods can be used in the identification of hotspot areas of disease movement [40]. This will have important implications in designing strategies for spread containment. One challenge, however, has been the application of landscape genetics methods in vector-borne diseases, which was reviewed by Hemming-Schroeder [40]. A few studies have been dedicated to such goal with human diseases. One interesting example is the correlation found between the genetic structure of *Aedes mcintochi*, a major vector for Rift Valley fever in Kenya, and mean precipitation values [41].

In 2020, one of the major global health issues concerns the new COVID-19. Sequencing technologies coupled with landscape genomics approaches have the potential to identify dispersal patterns of the virus in order to contain its spreading. Landscape genetic approaches have the power of assisting the decision-making process.

7. Concluding remarks

Climate change and human interference are no longer to be neglected on natural ecosystems. Among several fields of study devoted to deciphering the impact of these processes, landscape genetics will provide a better comprehension of the interaction between organisms and their environment of origin. The boost in sequencing technologies is enabling the study of the most diverse range of organisms. In fact, the Earth BioGenome Project is intended to sequence, catalog, and characterize all eukaryotic diversity in the forthcoming decade [42]. With that information available, resequencing to the level of population and their association with landscape variables will provide information for designing appropriate strategies for the conservation of endangered forms of life as well as any other species. The resequencing of several human genomes will also enable a better comprehension of the human population structure throughout the world and how the landscape shapes its organization. This has been and will be continuing valuable information to comprehending the dispersion of human diseases as well.

Conflict of interest

The authors declare no conflict of interest.

Author details

Enéas Ricardo Konzen[1*] and Maria Imaculada Zucchi[2,3]

1 Interdisciplinary Department, Center of Limnological, Coastal and Marine Studies, Federal University of Rio Grande do Sul, Imbé, Rio Grande do Sul, Brazil

2 Secretary of Agriculture and Supply of São Paulo State, Piracicaba, São Paulo, Brazil

3 Institute of Biology, University of Campinas, Campinas, São Paulo, Brazil

*Address all correspondence to: erkonzen@gmail.com

References

[1] Lewontin RC, Hubby JL. A molecular approach to the study of genic heterozygosity in natural populations. II. Amount of variation and degree of heterozygosity in natural populations of *Drosophila pseudoobscura*. Genetics. 1966;**54**(2):595

[2] Williams JG, Kubelik AR, Livak KJ, Rafalski JA, Tingey SV. DNA polymorphisms amplified by arbitrary primers are useful as genetic markers. Nucleic Acids Research. 1990;**18**(22):6531-6535

[3] Vos P, Hogers R, Bleeker M, Reijans M, Lee TV, Hornes M, et al. AFLP: A new technique for DNA fingerprinting. Nucleic Acids Research. 1995;**23**:4407-4414

[4] Litt M, Luty JA. A hypervariable microsatellite revealed by in vitro amplification of a dinucleotide repeat within the cardiac muscle actin gene. American Journal of Human Genetics. 1989;**44**(3):397

[5] Lagercrantz U, Ellegren H, Kakanuga T. The abundance of various polymorphic microsatellite motifs differs between plants and vertebrates. Nucleic Acids Research. 1993;**21**:1111-1115

[6] Manel S, Schwartz MK, Luikart G, Taberlet P. Landscape genetics: Combining landscape ecology and population genetics. Trends in Ecology & Evolution. 2003;**18**(4):189-197

[7] Storfer A, Murphy MA, Evans JS, Goldberg CS, Robinson S, Spear SF, et al. Putting the 'landscape' in landscape genetics. Heredity. 2007;**98**(3):128

[8] Joost S, Bonin A, Bruford MW, Després L, Conord C, Erhardt G, et al. A spatial analysis method (SAM) to detect candidate loci for selection: Towards a landscape genomics approach to adaptation. Molecular Ecology. 2007;**16**(18):3955-3969

[9] Li Y, Zhang XX, Mao RL, Yang J, Miao CY, Li Z, et al. Ten years of landscape genomics: Challenges and opportunities. Frontiers in Plant Science. 2017;**8**:2136

[10] Storfer A, Patton A, Fraik AK. Navigating the interface between landscape genetics and landscape genomics. Frontiers in Genetics. 2018;**9**:68

[11] Kalia RK, Rai MK, Kalia S, Singh R, Dhawan AK. Microsatellite markers: An overview of the recent progress in plants. Euphytica. 2011;**177**(3):309-334

[12] Vieira MLC, Santini L, Diniz AL, Munhoz CDF. Microsatellite markers: What they mean and why they are so useful. Genetics and Molecular Biology. 2016;**39**(3):312-328

[13] Powell W, Morgante M, Andre C, Hanafey M, Vogel J, Tingey S, et al. The comparison of RFLP, RAPD, AFLP and SSR (microsatellite) markers for germplasm analysis. Molecular Breeding. 1996;**2**(3):225-238

[14] Abdul-Muneer PM. Application of microsatellite markers in conservation genetics and fisheries management: Recent advances in population structure analysis and conservation strategies. Genetics Research International. 2014;**2014**:1-11

[15] Nadeem MA, Nawaz MA, Shahid MQ, Doğan Y, Comertpay G, Yıldız M, et al. DNA molecular markers in plant breeding: Current status and recent advancements in genomic selection and genome editing. Biotechnology & Biotechnological Equipment. 2018;**32**(2):261-285

[16] Xia W, Luo T, Zhang W, Mason AS, Huang D, Huang X, et al. Development of high-density SNP markers and their application in evaluating genetic diversity and population structure in Elaeis guineensis. Frontiers in Plant Science. 2019;**10**:130

[17] Konzen ER. Towards conservation strategies for forest tree endangered species: The meaning of population genetic statistics. Advances in Forestry Science. 2014;**1**(1):45-51

[18] Storfer A, Murphy MA, Spear SF, Holderegger R, Waits LP. Landscape genetics: Where are we now? Molecular Ecology. 2010;**19**(17):3496-3514

[19] Andam CP, Challagundla L, Azarian T, Hanage WP, Robinson DA. Population structure of pathogenic bacteria. In: Genetics and Evolution of Infectious Diseases. Amsterdam: Elsevier; 2017

[20] Elshire RJ, Glaubitz JC, Sun Q, Poland JA, Kawamoto K, Buckler ES, et al. A robust, simple genotyping-by-sequencing (GBS) approach for high diversity species. PLoS One. 2011;**6**(5):e19379

[21] Poland JA, Brown PJ, Sorrells ME, Jannink JL. Development of high-density genetic maps for barley and wheat using a novel two-enzyme genotyping-by-sequencing approach. PLoS One. 2012;**7**(2):e32253

[22] Balkenhol N, Gugerli F, Cushman SA, Waits LP, Coulon A, Arntzen JW, et al. Identifying future research needs in landscape genetics: Where to from here? Landscape Ecology. 2009;**24**(4):455

[23] Mantel N. The detection of disease clustering and a generalized regression approach. Cancer Research. 1967;**27** (2 part 1):209-220

[24] Diniz-Filho JAF, Soares TN, Lima JS, Dobrovolski R, Landeiro VL, Telles MPDC, et al. Mantel test in population genetics. Genetics and Molecular Biology. 2013;**36**(4):475-485

[25] Kwak M, Gepts P. Structure of genetic diversity in the two major gene pools of common bean (*Phaseolus vulgaris* L., Fabaceae). Theoretical and Applied Genetics. 2009;**118**(5):979-992

[26] Ariani A, Mier B, Teran JC, Gepts P. Spatial and temporal scales of range expansion in wild *Phaseolus vulgaris*. Molecular Biology and Evolution. 2017;**35**(1):119-131

[27] Gepts P, Osborn TC, Rashka K, Bliss FA. Phaseolin-protein variability in wild forms and landraces of the common bean (*Phaseolus vulgaris*): Evidence for multiple centers of domestication. Economic Botany. 1986;**40**(4):451-468

[28] Bitocchi E, Nanni L, Bellucci E, Rossi M, Giardini A, Zeuli PS, et al. Mesoamerican origin of the common bean (*Phaseolus vulgaris* L.) is revealed by sequence data. Proceedings of the National Academy of Sciences. 2012;**109**(14):E788-E796

[29] Bitocchi E, Bellucci E, Giardini A, Rau D, Rodriguez M, Biagetti E, et al. Molecular analysis of the parallel domestication of the common bean (*Phaseolus vulgaris*) in Mesoamerica and the Andes. New Phytologist. 2013;**197**(1):300-313

[30] Teran JCBM, Konzen ER, Medina V, Palkovic A, Ariani A, Tsai SM, et al. Root and shoot variation in relation to potential intermittent drought adaptation of Mesoamerican wild common bean (*Phaseolus vulgaris* L.). Annals of Botany. 2019;**124**(6):917

[31] Zucchi MI, Cordeiro EM, Allen C, Novello M, Viana JPG, Brown PJ, et al. Patterns of genome-wide variation, population differentiation and SNP discovery of the red banded stink

bug (Piezodorus guildinii). Scientific Reports. 2019;**9**(1):1-11

[32] Reis MS, Guerra MP, Nodari RO, Ribeiro RJ, Reis A. Distribuição geográfica e situação atual das populações na área de ocorrência de Euterpe edulis Martius. Sellowia. 2000a;**49-52**:324-335

[33] Martinelli M, Moraes A. Livro Vermelho da Flora Do Brasil. Rio de Janeiro: Instituto de Pesquisas Jardim Botânico do Rio de Janeiro; 2013. p. 1100

[34] Konzen ER, Martins MP. Contrasting levels of genetic diversity among populations of the endangered tropical palm Euterpe edulis Martius. Cerne. 2017;**23**(1):31-42

[35] Soares LASS, Cazetta E, Santos LR, França DDS, Gaiotto FA. Anthropogenic disturbances eroding the genetic diversity of a threatened palm tree: A multi-scale approach. Frontiers in Genetics. 2019;**10**:1090

[36] Novello M, Viana JPG, Alves-Pereira A, de Aguiar Silvestre E, Nunes HF, Pinheiro JB, et al. Genetic conservation of a threatened Neotropical palm through community-management of fruits in agroforests and second-growth forests. Forest Ecology and Management. 2018;**407**:200-209

[37] Waits LP, Cushman SA, Spear SF. Applications of landscape genetics to connectivity research in terrestrial animals [chapter 12]. In: Balkenhol N, Cushman SA, Storfer AT, Waits LP, editors. Landscape Genetics: Concepts, Methods, Applications. 1st ed. West Sussex: John Wiley and Sons Ltd; 2016. pp. 199-219

[38] Deng L, Hoh BP, Lu D, Fu R, Phipps ME, Li S, et al. The population genomic landscape of human genetic structure, admixture history and local adaptation in peninsular Malaysia. Human Genetics. 2014;**133**(9):1169-1185

[39] Peter BM, Petkova D, Novembre J. Genetic landscapes reveal how human genetic diversity aligns with geography. Molecular Biology and Evolution. 2019;**37**(4):943-951

[40] Hemming-Schroeder E, Lo E, Salazar C, Puente S, Yan G. Landscape genetics: A toolbox for studying vector-borne diseases. Frontiers in Ecology and Evolution. 2018;**6**:21

[41] Campbell LP, Alexander AM. Landscape genetics of *Aedes mcintoshi* (Diptera: Culicidae), an important vector of rift valley fever virus in northeastern Kenya. Journal of Medical Entomology. 2017;**54**(5):1258-1265

[42] Lewin HA, Robinson GE, Kress WJ, Baker WJ, Coddington J, Crandall KA, et al. Earth BioGenome project: Sequencing life for the future of life. Proceedings of the National Academy of Sciences. 2018;**115**(17):4325-4333

Chapter 7

Clinical Validation of a Whole Exome Sequencing Pipeline

Debra O. Prosser, Indu Raja, Kelly Kolkiewicz, Antonio Milano and Donald Roy Love

Abstract

Establishing whole exome sequencing (WES) in an accredited clinical diagnostic space is challenging. The validation (as opposed to verification) of an approach that will lead to clinical reports requires adhering to international guidelines and recommendations and developing a robust analytical pipeline that can scale due to the increasing clinical demand for comprehensive gene screening. This chapter will present a step-wise approach to WES validation that any laboratory can follow. The focus will be on highlighting the pivotal technical issues that must be addressed in validating WES and the analytical tools and QC metrics that must be considered before implementing WES in a clinical environment.

Keywords: whole exome sequencing, next-generation sequencing, validation, bioinformatics, diagnostics

1. Introduction

The decision as to which type of genetic test should be implemented by a clinical laboratory is largely driven by the type of referrals received by the laboratory and the complexity of patients' clinical phenotypes. In the main, testing has advanced from single-gene to multi-gene panels in which next-generation sequencing (NGS) has offered the technical means of undertaking this approach at low cost and high throughput. However, with the increasing awareness of genetic heterogeneity combined with gene discovery, whole exome sequencing (WES) offers laboratories a more streamlined approach. By implementing a single wet-work pipeline of exome capture coupled with the ability to analyze a virtual gene panel or report on the whole exome, laboratories can perform NGS in a more efficient manner.

Since the inception of NGS over a decade ago, multiple recommendations and guidelines have been published for NGS [1–3]. Using these guidelines, the College of American Pathologists (CAP) and Association for Molecular Pathology (AMP) published their Practical Framework for Designing and Implementing NGS Tests for Inherited Disorders in 2019 [4], and this is available through the CAP website (https://www.cap.org/member-resources/precision-medicine/next-generation-sequencing-ngs-worksheets).

We adopted this framework to establish a diagnostic NGS service using whole exome sequencing as our capture procedure and analyzing virtual gene panels or WES for reporting purposes.

The framework provides guidance and editable worksheets for the five steps involved in test establishment and validation.

1. Test design: setup

2. Assay design and optimization

3. Test validation

4. Quality management

5. Bioinformatics and IT

Throughout the validation process, it is essential that the NGS workflow is informed by the real-world local environment in which clinical testing will be performed.

2. Test design: setup

In view of the diverse range of referrals made to the authors' genetics laboratory (serving the needs of a 400-bed women and children's hospital in the Middle East), a whole exome capture solution was chosen for library preparation. The principal motivation behind this determination was to achieve an efficient workflow that would allow appropriate batching coupled with a time-limited turnaround time (TAT) for all referrals.

The limited number of staff in the authors' laboratory demanded a WES workflow that could be easily automated, twinned with a data analysis package that would allow secure remote access with a strong databasing function. The whole exome solution capture by SOPHiA™ Genetics was chosen for library preparation. This platform allows for the analysis of WES, clinical exome sequencing (CES) and clinical gene panels, together with the identification of single-nucleotide variants (SNVs) and copy number variants (CNVs) using SOPHiA™ DDM software.

3. Assay design and optimization

The validation pipeline needs to be grounded from the beginning in terms of the requirements of the test, which must take into account the sample types the laboratory will receive and the parameters that need to be satisfied (see **Table 1**).

Routinely, whole blood samples collected in EDTA are received by the authors' laboratory for testing. Therefore, our validation focused only on genomic DNA extracted from whole blood using our standard methods. The baseline validation of the WES data required the inclusion of two HapMap gDNA samples: the NIST control (NA12878) and the commercial control (SG063) supplied by SOPHiA™ Genetics.

The WES capture by SOPHiA™ Genetics was used for library preparation following all the steps as set out by the automated WES 32 reaction protocol. For instrumentation, our validation was restricted to automated library preparation using the PE Sciclone® G3 NGS workstation and sequencing using the Illumina® HiSeq4000 platform.

A critical additional consideration was the need for copy number variant calls to be made. This required a minimum batch number of eight patients and high coverage requirements, which involved restricting the number of samples per Illumina® HiSeq4000 lane to one pool of eight patients.

Test requirements	Must have	Nice to have
WES		Y
CES	Y	
Clinical panels	Y	
CNV detection	Y	
Necessary sample throughput per month	16	32
How deeply does each position need to be covered for accurate variant calling (if known—otherwise address during test optimization)	>20x	>50x
DNA from whole blood collected in EDTA	Y	
DNA from external/commercial sources (limitations)	Y	
Required/expected TAT	3 months	2 months
Combine different tests (existing or planned) within a sequencing run	Y	

WES, whole exome sequencing; CES, clinical exome sequencing; CNV, copy number variant; TAT, turnaround time.

Table 1.
Test requirements and limitations.

Importantly, the naming of the sequence files (.bam,. FASTQ, etc.) should be considered during the early phase of test design and validation. File conventions that are used for the bioinformatic process may be limited in terms of the type of special characters and/or character length. Following recommendations in the CAP/AMP-Guidelines for Validating Next-Generation Sequencing Bioinformatics Pipelines [5], the identity of the sample must be preserved throughout all steps of the bioinformatic pipeline. These authors recommend the following four unique identifiers that should be applied to the sample file name:

i. Unique sample identifier

ii. Unique patient identifier

iii. Unique run identifier

iv. Laboratory location identifier

It is essential that the file naming convention that is decided upon for validation adheres to the above recommendations and can be universally implemented for all subsequent testing.

4. Test validation

Test validation mandates a need for accuracy, precision and stability. These assessments must be made in the context of expected clinical workloads and performance. For the authors' laboratory, the sample batch size was set at 16 samples per validation batch and a total of three validation runs performed over differing days with differing technologists.

Analytical performance was characterized by the assessment of precision, sensitivity and concordance of variant calls against previously validated data.

Inter-run and intra-run data were achieved by replicate analysis of two HapMap gDNAs, the NIST sample, NA12878, and the commercial control supplied by SOPHiA™ Genetics, SG063, as well as four well-characterized clinical samples previously reported by accredited laboratories. The remaining samples included a representative group of the clinical samples received by the authors' laboratory (see **Table 2**).

The complete NGS workflow should be included in the validation, from library preparation to bioinformatic analysis to report generation, which is highlighted below.

- Sample collection and DNA extraction. Genomic DNA is extracted and purified from blood samples using either the Gentra® PureGene® DNA Blood Mini Kit or the QIAsymphony® DSP DNA Midi kit (QIAGEN, Hilden, Germany). DNA quality is initially assessed by NanoDrop™ spectrophotometry.

  Genomic DNA preparation. The initial preparation of gDNA used in NGS library preparation is the most critical step in the NGS workflow, and the care and time taken here are key to successful library amplification and sequencing.

  High-quality gDNA can be by quantified using a Qubit™ fluorometer followed by sequential dilution with further quantification to the desired input concentration. It is essential to minimize pipetting gDNA volumes of less than 5 μl for dilution. In our study, gDNA is prepared to a working concentration of 40 ng/μl. After Qubit™ quantification, the integrity of the gDNA can be analyzed using an Agilent TapeStation 4200. Samples with a DNA integrity number (DIN) of greater than 7.5 can proceed to WES capture.

- Library preparation, targeted capture and sequencing. Whole exome sequencing was performed according to the SOPHiA™ Whole Exome Solution 32 Samples User Guide, in combination with the SOPHiA™ Library Preparation and Capture User Guide—automation with PerkinElmer Sciclone® G3 NGS workstation. Each validation run consists of 16 samples that are divided into 2 pools of 8 samples each, as shown in the validation grid in **Table 3**.

  The SOPHiA™ WES protocol for library construction subjects genomic DNA (200 ng) to enzymatic fragmentation, end repair and A-tailing. All these steps occur using a Sciclone® G3 NGS workstation. The adapter-ligated DNA is then amplified in a limited way via an eight-cycle PCR protocol.

  Post-amplification cleanup of the libraries is carried out using the Sciclone® G3 NGS workstation, and libraries are prepared for quantitation with a dilution factor of 4.

  Amplified libraries are analyzed using Qubit™ fluorometer and Agilent TapeStation 4200 to assess the quantity and quality of each individual library. Library DNA fragments should have a size distribution between 300 and 700 bp. Genomic DNA that has been fragmented, end repaired, A-tailed and adapter-ligated can then be considered library DNA, which is ready for pooling and then hybridization and capture. In the case of the SOPHiA™ WES protocol, eight samples are pooled (200 ng of each library) per capture.

  Prepared pools are hybridized for 4 h followed by post-capture amplification and cleanup on the Sciclone® G3 NGS workstation.

  Final library quantification is performed for each captured library pool using a Qubit™ fluorometer and Agilent TapeStation 4200. Subsequent pools are

Sample ID	Description	Purpose	Purpose (detail)	Specific variant/s of interest	Variant type	Measured metric
VAL-1	NA12878	Baseline validation	N/A	N/A	N/A	Intra-run variability Inter-run variability
VAL-2	SG063	Baseline validation	N/A	N/A	N/A	Intra-run variability Inter-run variability
VAL-3	Anonymized patient specimen	Baseline validation	Variant type	Ciliopathy gene panel CCDC39:c.2017G > T p.(Glu673*) CCDC39: Deletion of exons 14 to 20	SNV CNV	Inter-run variability Sensitivity
VAL-4	Anonymized patient specimen	Baseline validation	Variant type prevalent in gene	Single-gene analysis CFTR:c.1521_1523delCTT p.(Phe508del)	DEL	Inter-run variability Sensitivity
VAL-5	Anonymized patient specimen	Baseline validation	Variant type	Craniosynostosis gene panel CACNA1H:c.4318_4319delinsGC p.(Phe1440Ala)	DELINS	Inter-run variability Sensitivity
VAL-6	Anonymized patient specimen	Baseline validation	Variant type prevalent in gene	Tuberous sclerosis gene panel TSC2: Deletion of exons 2 to 16	CNV	Inter-run variability Sensitivity
VAL-7	Anonymized patient specimen	Gene-specific validation	Variant type	Arrhythmia cardiomyopathy gene panel SCN5A:c.4867C > T p.(Arg1623*)	SNV (stop)	Sensitivity
VAL-8	Anonymized patient specimen	Gene-specific validation	Variant type	Custom panel of 196 genes 200 genomic co-ordinates	SNV DEL/ DUP	Sensitivity
VAL-9	Anonymized patient specimen	Gene-specific validation	Variant type	Paroxysmal Dystonia gene panel Del 16p11.2 chr16:29,656,684-30,190,568	CNV	Sensitivity
VAL-10	Anonymized patient specimen	Gene-specific validation	Variant type	Leukodystrophy gene panel MLC1:c.908_918delinsGCA p.(Val303Glyfs*96)	DELINS	Sensitivity
VAL-11	Anonymized patient specimen	Gene-specific validation	Variant type	Epilepsy gene panel WWOX: Deletion of exons 1–5	CNV	Sensitivity
VAL-12	Anonymized patient specimen	Gene-specific validation	Variant range	Epilepsy gene panel	SNV DEL/ DUP	Sensitivity
VAL-13	Anonymized patient specimen	Gene-specific validation	Variant type	Single-gene analysis CFTR: deletion of exons 4–8	CNV	Sensitivity

Sample ID	Description	Purpose	Purpose (detail)	Specific variant/s of interest	Variant type	Measured metric
VAL-14	Anonymized patient specimen	Gene-specific validation	Variant range	Neuropathy gene panel	SNV DEL/ DUP	Sensitivity
VAL-15	Anonymized patient specimen	Gene-specific validation	Variant range	Cholestasis gene panel	SNV DEL/ DUP	Sensitivity
VAL-16	Anonymized patient specimen	Gene-specific validation	Variant type	Tuberous sclerosis gene panel (2 genes) TSC2:c.5238_5255del p.(His1746_Arg1751del)	DEL	Sensitivity
VAL-17	Anonymized patient specimen	Chromosomal CNV validation	Variant type	Molecular karyotype referral Dup 22q11.21 chr22:18,661,724-21,809,099	CNV	Sensitivity
VAL-18	Anonymized patient specimen	Gene-specific validation	Variant range	Primary ciliary dyskinesia gene panel DNAH5: Gain of exons 1 to 50 DNAH5:c.5503C > T p.(Gln1835*)	SNV CNV	Sensitivity
VAL-19	Anonymized patient specimen	Gene-specific validation (pseudogene)	Variant range	Inherited cancer gene panel CDKN2A:c.9_32dup p.(Ala4_Pro11dup)	SNV DEL	Sensitivity
VAL-20	Anonymized patient specimen	Gene-specific validation	Variant range	Custom panel of 196 genes 200 genomic coordinates	SNV DEL/ DUP	Blind analysis
VAL-21	Anonymized patient specimen	Chromosomal CNV validation	Variant type	Molecular karyotype referral Duplication at 16p13.11, deletion at 12p31 and duplication at Xp21.1	CNV	Sensitivity
VAL-22	Anonymized patient specimen	Gene-specific validation	Variant type prevalent in gene	Single-gene analysis DMD: duplication exons 45–62	CNV	Sensitivity
VAL-23	Anonymized patient specimen	Gene-specific validation	Variant type prevalent in gene	Dystrophinopathy gene panel DMD: deletion of exons 8–34	CNV	Sensitivity
VAL-24	Anonymized patient specimen	Gene-specific validation	Variant range	Custom panel of 196 genes 200 genomic co-ordinates	SNV DEL/ DUP	Sensitivity
VAL-25	Anonymized patient specimen	Gene-specific validation (pseudogene)	Pseudogene	Custom panel of nine genes	SNV DEL/ DUP	Sensitivity

Sample ID	Description	Purpose	Purpose (detail)	Specific variant/s of interest	Variant type	Measured metric
VAL-26	Anonymized patient specimen	Gene-specific validation	Variant type	Primary Immunodeficiency gene panel TBX1:c.1383_1421del p.(Ala464_Ala476del)	DEL	Sensitivity
VAL-27	Anonymized patient specimen	Gene-specific validation	Variant type	Dilated cardiomyopathy gene panel TTN:c.75984_75985insTACCA p.(Ala25329Tyrfs*32)	INS	Sensitivity
VAL-28	Anonymized patient specimen	Gene-specific validation	Variant type	Pediatric cancer gene panel SMARCB1:c.159_160delinsTATCTGGAGGCG (p.Leu54Ilefs*20)	DELINS	Sensitivity

DEL, deletion; INS, insertion; DUP, duplication; SNV, single-nucleotide variant; CNV, copy number variant.

Table 2.
Sample list.

		Run 001			Run 002			Run 003	
Pool A	**A**	VAL-1 NA12878	VAL-4	**A**	VAL-5	**VAL-13**	**A**	**VAL-21**	VAL-5
	B	**VAL-3**	VAL-10	**B**	VAL-2 SG-063	VAL-15	**B**	VAL-28	VAL-1 NA12878
	C	**VAL-11**	VAL-1 NA12878	**C**	**VAL-17**	VAL-2 SG-063	**C**	VAL-1 NA12878	VAL-24
	D	VAL-2 SG-063	VAL-12	**D**	VAL-16	VAL-19	**D**	**VAL-3**	VAL-25
Pool B	**E**	VAL-1 NA12878	**VAL-6**	**E**	VAL-2 SG-063	VAL-20	**E**	**VAL-22**	**VAL-6**
	F	VAL-7	VAL-8	**F**	**VAL-6**	**VAL-3**	**F**	**VAL-23**	VAL-2 SG-063
	G	VAL-2 SG-063	**VAL-9**	**G**	VAL-14	VAL-1 NA12878	**G**	VAL-4	VAL-27
	H	VAL-5	VAL-2 SG-063	**H**	**VAL-18**	VAL-4	**H**	VAL-1 NA12878	VAL-26

Copy number variant (CNV) samples are indicated in bold.

Table 3.
Validation grid.

diluted to 20 nM (in a total volume of 20 µl) and subjected to sequencing using an Illumina® HiSeq4000 Sequencing platform.

- Sequence analysis: performance metrics. Baseline performance metrics for the WES validation study must involve the analysis of well-characterized reference samples: the NIST sample (NA12878) and the SOPHiA™ Genetics control SG063. The sequence metrics for each sample in the run must be recorded and averages established using the reference samples. Samples must meet the sequencing metrics shown in **Table 4** in order to reach the threshold for clinical reporting.

  Analytical sensitivity and specificity must be calculated separately for each variant type (SNV, indel, CNV, etc.). Additional runs may be required to meet acceptable confidence intervals for less frequent variant types of insertions and deletions. For 95% confidence and 95% reliability, 59 variants of each type (and insertion/deletion range) should be analyzed [5]. The variant types that do not have strong confidence intervals must be listed in the test limitations of the clinical report until such time that the desired confidence levels have been achieved.

Selected sequencing metrics	Must have	Nice to have
Q30 score	>80	>85
Total number of reads per sample	>70 M	80–100 M
Percentage of mapped reads	>80%	>85%
Total percentage on-target reads	>90%	>95%
Coverage 10% quantile (at this depth, 90% target covered)	20x	50x

Table 4.
Sequencing metrics.

5. Quality management

The worksheets described by Santani et al. [4] set out very clear guidance for all quality aspects that need to be taken into consideration for the test to meet CAP requirements [4]. Through a validation study, the majority of a test's limitations will be discovered and can be recorded against the QC parameters. **Table 5** summarizes quality metrics that need to be addressed.

Section	Category	Criteria	Specific requirement Note that these may vary between tests and laboratories
Pre-analytical QC (per sample)	Specimen quality	Wrong specimen type	Whole blood
		Wrong type of tube	Purple top EDTA tube
		Insufficient quantity	≥0.5 ml
		Clotting (blood only)	No visible clots
		Insufficient labelling	Labelling contains name, DOB, barcode, date of collection
		Expired specimen	≤7 days since collection
		Expired collection tube	Collection tube not expired
	DNA quality and quantity	OD 260/280 ratio	>1.7
		Electrophoretic analysis	Shows intact high molecular weight DNA band
		Quantification	≥500 ng
		DNA integrity number (DIN)	>7.5
Analytical QC (per instrument run)	Instrument run QC	Cluster density	Not taken into account
		Base quality	Q30 ≥ 80
	Pipeline QC	Total reads passing filter	>280 M per lane
		% reads not assigned to any sample	<5%
	Control samples	Positive control	Expected variants found
Analytical QC (per sample)	Library preparation	Fragment size and distribution	>80% of fragments between 300 and 700 bp
		Pooled library concentration	>20 nM
	Sample de-multiplexing	% reads assigned to sample	8–12%
	Read alignment	% Reads aligned to target	>90%
		Distribution of coverage	>95% within 25–200×
		Coverage 10% quantile (at this depth 90% target covered at x)	>40×
		PCR duplicates	<20%
	Specimen identity	Accurate specimen identity, file names with 4 points of identification	All worksheets and transfers during bench work are witness checked for accurate specimen identification
	Data transfer Integrity	Data transfer to secure analysis platform	

Table 5.
Quality management.

	Considerations	Resources	Links
Gene selection	Clinical association	ClinGen	https://clinicalgenome.org/curation-activities/gene-disease-validity/ https://search.clinicalgenome.org/kb/gene-validity
		GeneReviews	https://www.ncbi.nlm.nih.gov/books/NBK1116/
Gene analysis	Appropriate transcripts	LRG RefSeq	https://www.lrg-sequence.org/ https://www.ncbi.nlm.nih.gov/refseq/rsg/
	Pseudogenes	Pseudogene. PanelApp – Genes and Entities	http://pseudogene.org/ https://panelapp.genomicsengland.co.uk/panels/entities/?tag=locus-type-pseudogene
	Evaluated homopolymeric regions	Ivády et al. [6]	DOI: 10.1186/s12864-018-4544-x
	Mutation spectrum—reported deep intronic and/or promoter region variants	PanelApp—Genes and Entities	https://panelapp.genomicsengland.co.uk/panels/entities/?
	CNV analysis	ClinVar	https://www.ncbi.nlm.nih.gov/clinvar/
		Decipher	https://decipher.sanger.ac.uk/
	Establish if critical variants are not covered by assay		
Virtual panel creation	Expert reviewed panels	PanelApp	https://panelapp.genomicsengland.co.uk/
		ClinGen	https://www.clinicalgenome.org/data-sharing/clinvar/
	Phenotype-driven	HPO	https://hpo.jax.org/app/

Table 6.
Considerations for gene selection, analysis and virtual panel creation.

6. Bioinformatics and IT

To assess accuracy, genetic variants must be compared against publicly available reference data obtained from 1000 Genomes Project.

Clinical association, gene validity and mutation spectrum are applied to the creation of virtual gene panels in order to aid variant interpretation and reporting. The considerations associated with constructing virtual gene panels and the analysis of variants are shown in **Table 6.**

7. Conclusions

The decision to implement WES in a clinical diagnostic environment is one that must take into account local context, which encompasses clinical complexity, staff resources, equipment resources and bioinformatic expertise. The decisions described here were made based on the above considerations with a view to establishing opportunity, the most important of which was to have a WES pipeline that could scale over time in terms of patients tested and with the potential to be a regional resource.

It should be stressed, however, that a WES pipeline is sandwiched by two critical elements: first, the need to focus on the quality and accurate quantitation of genomic DNA; which dictates the quality of everything that happens downstream, and second, to understand that the identification of DNA variants is technically demanding but the classification of those variants is not currently a fully automated process. The former can sometimes be overlooked, while the latter can be a daunting exercise. It is perhaps the subject of another book chapter to discuss the approaches to variant classification.

Conflicts of interest

The authors declare no conflicts of interest.

Thanks

The authors wish to thank Mr. Duncan Kay of Custom Science (NZ) for his generous suggestions regarding commercial providers for WES data analysis and Javier Botet of Sophia Genetics for his advice regarding quality management considerations.

Author details

Debra O. Prosser, Indu Raja, Kelly Kolkiewicz, Antonio Milano and Donald Roy Love*
Division of Pathology Genetics, Department of Pathology, Sidra Medicine, Doha, Qatar

*Address all correspondence to: dlove@sidra.org

References

[1] Rehm HL, Bale SJ, Bayrak-Toydemir P, Berg JS, Brown KK, Deignan JL, et al. ACMG clinical laboratory standards for next-generation sequencing. Genetics in Medicine. 2013;**15**(9):733-747. DOI: 10.1038/gim.2013.92

[2] Hegde M, Santani A, Mao R, Ferreira-Gonzalez A, Weck KE, Voelkerding KV. Development and validation of clinical whole-exome and whole-genome sequencing for detection of germline variants in inherited disease. Archives of Pathology & Laboratory Medicine. 2017;**141**:798-805. DOI: 10.5858/arpa.2016-0622-RA

[3] Matthijs G, Souche E, Alders M, Corveleyn A, Eck S, Feenstra I, et al. Guidelines for diagnostic next-generation sequencing. European Journal of Human Genetics. 2016;**24**:2-5. DOI: 10.1038/ejhg.2015.226

[4] Santani A, Simen BB, Briggs M, Lebo M, Merker JD, Nikiforova M, et al. Designing and implementing NGS tests for inherited disorders a practical framework with step-by-step guidance for clinical laboratories. The Journal of Molecular Diagnostics. 2019;**21**:369-374. DOI: 10.1016/j.jmoldx.2018.11.004

[5] Roy S, Coldren C, Karunamurthy A, Kip NS, Klee EW, Lincoln SE, et al. Standards and guidelines for validating next-generation sequencing bioinformatics pipelines a joint recommendation of the Association for Molecular Pathology and the College of American Pathologists. The Journal of Molecular Diagnostics. 2018;**20**(1):4-27. DOI: 10.1016/j.jmoldx.2017.11.003

[6] Ivády G, Madar L, Dzsudzsák E, Koczok K, Kappelmayer J, Krulisova V, et al. Analytical parameters and validation of homopolymer detection in a pyrosequencing-based next generation sequencing system. BioMed Central Genomics. 2018;**19**:158. DOI: 10.1186/s12864-018-4544-x

Chapter 8

Integrating Evolutionary Genetics to Medical Genomics: Evolutionary Approaches to Investigate Disease-Causing Variants

Ugur Sezerman, Tugce Bozkurt and Fatma Sadife Isleyen

Abstract

In recent years, next-generation sequencing (NGS) platforms that facilitate generation of a vast amount of genomic variation data have become widely used for diagnostic purposes in medicine. However, identifying the potential effects of the variations and their association with a particular disease phenotype is the main challenge in this field. Several strategies are used to discover the causative mutations among hundreds of variants of uncertain significance. Incorporating information from healthy population databases, other organisms' databases, and computational prediction tools are evolution-based strategies that give valuable insight to interpret the variant pathogenicity. In this chapter, we first provide an overview of NGS analysis workflow. Then, we review how evolutionary principles can be integrated into the prioritization schemes of analyzed variants. Finally, we present an example of a real-life case where the use of evolutionary genetics information facilitated the discovery of disease-causing variants in medical genomics.

Keywords: genomics, evolution, variant discovery

1. Introduction

NGS technologies can be integrated into medical diagnostics in several ways which vary in the number and type of sequenced regions. While targeted tests include sequencing particular disease-specific genes, sequencing all ~20,000 protein-coding genes by Whole-exome sequencing (WES) and entire genomes by Whole-genome Sequencing (WGS) are non-targeted approaches. These sequencing approaches are precise ways to detect genetic variation of a patient and in relation to a healthy population or healthy reference genome. However, sequencing-based diagnostic methods generate large amounts of genomic data. Approximately, 60,000–100,000 single nucleotide variations (SNV) and small insertions and deletions (indel) in each patient's personal genome can be detected on WES [1]. Translating these high numbers of genomic variants into useful clinical information is a crucial task. Although several methods have been introduced to help reduce the vast number of possible genes to clinically causative ones, this process still remains challenging.

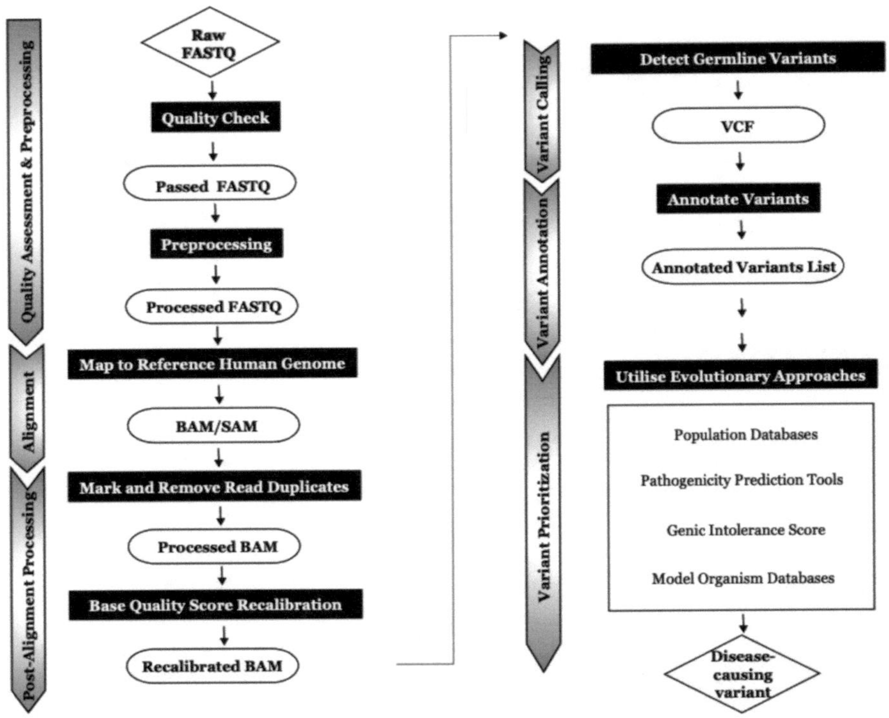

Figure 1.
A general workflow for WES data analysis. Six main steps, quality assessment & preprocessing, alignment, post-alignment processing, variant calling, variant annotation, and variant prioritization integrated with evolutionary approaches, are shown.

Disease-related genes show non-random distribution characteristics in the genome with the majority of them being already present in the eukaryotic ancestor [2]. Mendelian disease genes that underlie single-gene disorders tend to have a more ancient evolutionary origin [3]. Considering disease-related genes have evolved under the effect of natural selection like other genes, evolutionary approaches can provide powerful insight not only to understand human genetic diseases but also to detect genomic variants that cause them.

Here, we briefly describe the analysis workflow from raw data to genomic variants as the first step of the translation to the clinical outcome. We primarily focus on WES analysis because most variations that are responsible for Mendelian disorders disrupt protein-coding regions [4]. Then we give an insight into how evolutionary principles are integrated into the prioritization of detected variants. The framework of the chapter can be found in **Figure 1.**

2. From raw data to genomic variations

The common file format for the storage of data produced by sequencers is FASTQ [5]. FASTQ format stores both nucleotide sequence and its corresponding Phred quality scores [6, 7]. The Phred score related to the base-calling error probabilities indicates the quality of each nucleotide within a read. In a FASTQ file, each read is shown by four lines: The first line begins with a "@" and continues with a sequence identifier and an optional description. The second line consists of the raw sequence letters: A, T, G, C, and N (unknown). The third line starts with a "+"

character and can be followed by the same sequence identifier again. The "+" sign specifies the end of the sequence. The fourth line includes the quality scores for the sequence in the second line.

Here, we give an overview of the data analysis workflow from a FASTQ file to obtain annotated genomic variants.

2.1 Quality assessment and preprocessing

Although NGS platforms are capable of generating massively parallel sequences even in a single run, the quality of sequencing reads may not be perfect due to some reasons such as the failure in experimental processing and technical machine errors. The quality of raw FASTQ data should be assessed in the first step of the workflow since these errors affect downstream analysis.

A number of tools have been developed to evaluate raw FASTQ data. These tools generally take FASTQ files as input and generate summary statistics and graphs for a quick overview of the raw read quality. In addition to the most commonly used one FASTQC [8], developed by Simon Andrews at Babraham Institute, other tools are also available such as FQStat [9], Quack [10], SeqAssist [11], QC-Chain [12]. Based on the result of the quality check step, if there is a need, preprocessing is necessary before alignment.

The standard preprocessing step consists of trimming of low-quality bases and adapter sequence removal at the end of the reads. Adapter sequences can be ligated to 3′ and 5′ ends of reads depending on the used library preparation protocol during the sequencing. These adapter fragments should be removed correctly because of leading to either missed alignments or wrong genotyping in further downstream analyses. Many tools with different principles of implementation have been developed to perform preprocessing. Ktrim [13], PE-Trimmer [14], SeqPurge [15], AdapterRemoval [16], PEAT [17], Skewer [18], Trimmomatic [19], QcReads [20], AlienTrimmer [21], and Btrim [22] are tools can be used for adapter and quality trimming depending on the study design. In addition to these, some tools such as FastqCleaner [23], FastProNGS [24], EasyQC [25], fastp [26], TrimGalore, FASTX-Toolkit, afterQC, ClinQC, NGS QC Toolkit, PRINSEQ, fastQ_brew carry out both quality check and preprocessing functions.

2.2 Alignment of reads

After quality check and preprocessing of raw data, processed reads must be aligned to the reference genome. Both GRCh37 (hg19) and GRCh38 (hg38) are widely used as a reference for the human genome. Optimal alignment to reference sequences is not easy computational task and requires a fast and tolerant algorithm to obtain an imperfect alignment due to genomic variations. Several tools have been developed to align short reads. They mainly use the Burrows-Wheeler Transformation (BWT) algorithm, the Smith-Waterman (SW) dynamic programming algorithm or a combination of both of them. Bowtie2 [27] and BWA [28], which implement the BWT algorithm, are widely used for short reads alignment. Novoalign [29], MOSAIK [30], and SHRiMP2 [31] implement SW algorithm. For a comprehensive review of these methods and their differences, benchmark studies can be found in the literature [32, 33].

The output of the alignment step is the Sequence Alignment Map (SAM) file which contains mapped reads. BAM stands for Binary Alignment Map and is the binary version of a SAM file. Both BAM files and SAM files have the same information which include a header and an alignment section. The header section provides some information such as reference sequence, read group, sequencing platform details and applied process information to the reads. The alignment section includes the genomic position with relevant descriptive information of each sequence.

SAMtools [34] and Integrative Genomics Viewer (IGV) [35] are also commonly used programs to view BAM/SAM files for further confirmation analysis of detected variants.

2.3 Post-alignment processing

Processing of aligned reads is recommended to improve the quality of downstream variant calling analysis. The processing step generally consists of marking read duplicates and base quality score recalibration (BQSR) to minimize technical biases.

During the sequencing, a library of DNA fragments from a particular genomic region is prepared using PCR amplification to provide adequate DNA fragments for the sequencing process. Therefore, some amplified fragments could share the same sequence and the same corresponding alignment position leading to bias in variant detection. These duplicates should be removed to eliminate PCR-introduced bias. MarkDuplicates available in the Picard [36] and SAMtools [34] are widely-used tools to detect read duplicates based on their identical 5′ region and position on the genome.

In addition to marking duplicates, base quality is also an important factor for variant detection. As mentioned in the section "Quality check and preprocessing", each sequence read has a Phred quality score generated by the sequencing machine. However, the machine could generate systematically biased scores. On the contrary, BQSR patterns errors empirically to recalibrate the base quality scores using a machine learning approach. Thus, technical bias is significantly minimized. The key point in this process is to exclude known variants before BQSR since they are true genomic variations. So, they should not be considered as sequencing errors. The most widely used tool for recalibration of base qualities is BaseRecalibrator available in Genome Analysis Toolkit (GATK) [37].

2.4 Variant calling

After the post-alignment processing step, variant analysis can be started on an analysis-ready BAM file. In the variant calling step, the differences between the reference genome and genome of interest are calculated. Variants can be categorized as germline and somatic variants while dealing with variant calling. Germline variants are inherited variations present in the germ cells. Somatic variants are present only in somatic cells and can be specific to a tissue. In this chapter, we focus on the identification of germline SNV and indels. Several tools based on different algorithms have been developed to call germline short variants. Tools such as HaplotypeCaller available in GATK [38], SAMtools [34], FreeBayes [39], and Platypus [40] are based on Bayesian approaches. VarScan [41] relies on a heuristic approach to identify variants, while SNVer [42] uses a frequentist approach. The performance of different tools has been evaluated by recent studies [43–45], yet, these tools mostly generate an analysis-ready VCF (Variant Call Format) file. A VCF file is a text file that contains header lines and data lines. The header lines begin with "##" symbol. The first header line is always the VCF format version and continues with lines defining the name, length, value type, and description of each item in relevant fields of each data line.

2.5 Variant annotation and prioritization

After variants are detected, biologically important features such as gene symbols, genomic position, amino acid change, and consequences of variants add to a VCF file in the annotation step. In addition to the basic annotation, several tools can be used to integrate the annotations from countless sources including information of known variants with minor allele frequency (MAF) found in public databases and pathogenicity prediction of variants. There are numerous variant annotation tools that implement different methods and most widely used ones are AnnoVar [46], VEP [47], SnpEff [48], GEMINI [49], VarAFT [50], AnnTools [51], SVA [52], NGS-SNP [53]. These annotation tools enable to filtering and prioritizing potential disease-causing mutations. The prioritization of clinically causative mutation among a vast amount of annotated variations is the most challenging part of the analysis and is not a fully automatized. In the next section, we are going to discuss how evolutionary approaches can be used to prioritize genomic variants.

3. Utilizing evolutionary information in variant prioritization

We have described the process of obtaining annotated variations from raw FASTQ data. Experimentally evaluation of each variant at a genomic scale would be an impractical process, but evolutionary principles can provide us a valuable set of an experiment from nature. Integrating evolutionary approaches into the prioritization step have the potential to distinguish the variant responsible for a particular disease among all annotated variants. Indeed, the association between disease and evolution has been attributed to natural selection [54, 55]. During evolution, variations at highly conserved genomic regions are exposed to natural selection because of their negative impact on fitness that make these conserved genes intolerant to variations [56]. On the contrary, at the faster-evolving regions of the genome, many variations have been tolerated over evolutionary time and accumulate in the population with high MAF. However, there is a predisposition for Mendelian disease genes to be more intolerant than the other genes [57]. These genes are also more conserved across species allowing us to compare the phenotypes of different mutant genes on a multispecies level [58].

In this part, we discuss the role of evolutionary approaches in variant prioritization. The first prioritization method aims to filter variants using information from allele frequencies in population databases. Then we introduce several pathogenicity prediction tools to interpret the rest of the variants, especially the ones with uncertain significance. Following that, we describe the usage of gene intolerance information while making inference the variant pathogenicity. Finally, we list commonly used model organism databases that can be used for the comparison of mutant gene phenotypes in several species.

3.1 Population databases

During human evolution, present and novel variations have been evaluated in terms of their biological impact. Population databases record the outcomes of genetic variations providing an extensive catalog that include thousands of individuals' genomic variations to researchers. At the end of the 1990s, the establishment of dbSNP has led to record genotype-phenotype associations via variant databases [59]. Latterly, large-scale projects such as gnomAD and 1000 Genome Project Databases that actively collect genomic data from various populations have become available MAF at population level found in these databases is one of the primary guides to interpret that variant pathogenicity. Because causative variants related to most Mendelian disorders have deleterious effects on reproductive fitness. Generally, causative alleles are less likely to reside in these databases or are present with low frequencies. In any global population database, except for the well-known founder alleles, >5% MAF can be considered as benign [60]. Therefore, a subset of the total number of variants inside these databases can be used for variant filtration. This is often achieved according to three different approaches. The first approach, called discrete filtering, assumes that a disease-causing variant should not found in these databases [61, 62]. This approach can be useful for very rare Mendelian disorders, but it can be problematic in some cases. Excluding observed alleles, independent from their MAF, can lead to the elimination of truly pathogenic alleles found in the general population at low frequencies because of the increasing number of genomes in databases. Especially, elucidating autosomal recessive disorders are affected by this risk. The second approach, called 1%-approach, is based on allele frequency thresholds that change according to the inheritance model of variants. While the analysis of autosomal recessive variants MAF threshold can be set at 1%, MAF cutoff of 0.1% can be useful for autosomal dominant variants [62]. Alternatively, the third approach, called the quantile-based approach, employs frequency thresholds as in the previous method. However, the thresholds in the quantile-based method are variable and depend on disease prevalence, mode of inheritance, database size, and database characteristics [63].

Depending on the case, different approaches can be employed using population databases with different scopes and data collection. Here, we summarize the widely used population databases. 1000 Genome Project (1KGP) Database.

3.1.1 1000 Genome Project (1KGP) database

1KGP database provides a comprehensive set of human genetic variations from a diverse set of individuals of multiple populations. The database includes the reconstructed genomes of 2504 individuals from 26 populations obtained by combining low-coverage whole-genome sequencing, deep exome sequencing, and dense microarray genotyping. The database contains over 88 million variants, which consist of around 84.7 million SNPs, 3.6 million indels, and 60,000 structural variants [64, 65].

3.1.2 The Genome Aggregation Database (gnomAD)

gnomAD is an extensive collection of exome and genome sequencing data from several large-scale sequencing projects. The first release of gnomAD is also known as the Exome Aggregation Consortium (ExAC) dataset. gnomAD short variant v2 release contains 125,748 exomes, and 15,708 whole genomes mapped to the GRCh37/hg19 reference sequence. In contrast, the short variant v3 release contains 71,702 whole genomes, including most of the whole genomes from v2 release mapped to the GRCh38 reference sequence. Therefore, gnomAD v2 provides higher power for the analysis of the coding regions, while v3 offers a valuable resource for the analysis of non-coding regions. For the analysis of structural variants, gnomAD SV v2.1 data set grants access to a total of 10,847 genomes aligned against the GRCh37 reference sequence [66].

3.1.3 Database of short genetic variations (dbSNP) and the database of genomic structural variations (dbVar)

The National Center for Biotechnology Information (NCBI) maintains dbSNP and dbVar databases which together contain almost 2 billion submitted human variants. Although dbVar does not have a reference structural variant database since the current technology cannot detect the precise breakpoints in the genome, dbSNP presents the reference variants as rs identifiers. Other contents of the dataset include population frequency, geographic origin of the population, population-specific genotype and allele frequencies as well as population-specific heterozygosity estimates. Besides serving as a human population database, dbSNP and dbVar also contain a variety of organisms′ genomic variations that can be a valuable resource for evolutionary studies [67, 68].

3.1.4 ClinVar

ClinVar is a public database that archives genetic variances of any type and the interpretations of their clinical significance for reported conditions. Unlike dbSNP and dbVar that are also maintained by NCBI, ClinVar only focuses on the medically relevant variations. Although ClinVar reviews the submissions of variants for validation, the clinical significance of the variants is reported directly from submitters. ClinVar displays any conflict between the interpretations for the same variant from different submitters or the consensus. In the strict comparison approaches, the algorithm evaluates submissions for a variant to be pathogenic and likely pathogenic as conflicting. In the more relaxed approach, the variants can be categorized as pathogenic/likely pathogenic, benign/likely benign, or uncertain significance [69].

3.1.5 Database of chromosomal imbalance and phenotype in humans using Ensembl resources (DECIPHER)

DECIPHER provides a catalog of common copy-number changes in healthy populations as well as chromosome rearrangements of patients and their phenotype record submitted by clinical researchers upon informed consent [70]. Therefore, DECIPHER can serve as a valuable platform during variant prioritization. Users can check both the healthy population database and the previously submitted clinical records within DECIPHER to understand the effect of the variant of interests better and to identify novel and potentially pathogenic variants.

3.2 Pathogenicity prediction tools

Even population MAF-based filtering, individuals generally have many variants that are not present in databases. Most of these variants do not classify definitively as benign or pathogenic according to criteria proposed by some clinical guidelines such as the American College of Medical Genetics and Genomics (ACMG) [60]. These types of alterations termed variants of uncertain significance (VUS). Further filtering approaches must use to reduce the number of VUS. For this purpose, numerous pathogenicity prediction tools based on different principles have been developed to evaluate the variant effect. ACMG and the European Society of Human Genetics (ESHG) [71] guidelines also recommend these in-silico methods to interpret variant pathogenicity.

The first methods were proposed to predict computationally whether an amino acid substitution will disturb the protein function. These methods, now part of the PolyPhen algorithm [72], use physical properties of the mutational change along with a multispecies alignment as a basis to evaluate mutations. Many methods have been derived from this idea and are based on different principles. Evolutionary conservation is among the most useful features for such predictions. Some methods such as SIFT [73], PROVEAN [74] and PANTHER [75] rely on sequence conservation. For example, SIFT, as the most widely used algorithm, compares the alignments of related sequences by performing a PSI-BLAST search to check if the variant is tolerated in an evolutionary aspect. In addition to sequence conservation, another group of methods which take into account several features such as amino acid physicochemical properties, the context of variation position, protein structural features through machine learning algorithms are also available. CADD [76], MutationTaster2 [77], PolyPhen-2 [72], DANN [78] and VEST3 [79] are well-known examples of such tools.

The predicted impact of a variation obtained from different tools may not be the same. This problem led to researchers making efforts to develop meta predictors that combine the results from existing tools by using several approaches such as logistic regression, decision trees, random forests, and support vector machines to make their own decisions. MetaSVM and MetaLR [80], M-CAP [81] and REVEL [82] are well-known examples of meta-predictors.

Below, several useful tools are explained without a performance comparison. However, various benchmark studies that have extensively examined the accuracy of these tools can be found in the literature [83–85].

3.2.1 MutationTaster2

MutationTaster2, using a naive Bayes classifier, predicts the functional consequences of variants that are both in exonic and intronic regions by incorporating a scoring system for the evolutionary conservation around DNA variants. MutationTaster uses information from several variant databases, including 1KGP and ClinVar. The tool automatically predicts a variant as neutral if it is found more than four times in the homozygous state in these databases and as disease-causing if it is reported as pathogenic in ClinVar by listing the associated disease phenotypes [77].

3.2.2 Combined annotation-dependent depletion (CADD)

CADD combines 63 genomic features derived from evolutionary constraint, surrounding sequence context, and functional predictions to evaluate SNVs and short indels. The tool integrates all of these features into a single CADD score using a machine learning approach trained on a binary distinction between simulated variants and variants that have become fixed in human populations since the split between humans and chimpanzees. C scores correlate with pathogenicity of a variant and disease severity [76].

3.2.3 The Mendelian clinically applicable pathogenicity (M-CAP)

M-CAP uses a supervised learning classifier to interpret genomic variants and focus especially on coding mutations for Mendelian diseases. As a meta-predictor, it uses nine existing tools SIFT, PolyPhen-2, CADD, MutationTaster, MutationAssessor [86], FATHMM [87], LRT [88], MetaLR and MetaSVM. It also combines information of base-pair, amino acid, genomic region, and gene conservation from RVIS [89], PhyloP [90], PhastCons [91], SIPHY [92], GERP [93], PAM250 and BLOSUM62 [94]. Additionally, M-CAP establishes multiple-sequence alignments of 99 primate, mammalian, and vertebrate genomes to the human genome as a new feature [81].

3.2.4 PrimateAI

PrimateAI [95] is a deep neural network trained by a comprehensive dataset that includes around 380,000 common missense variants from humans and six non-human primate species. PrimateAI categorizes the common missense mutations from other primate species as non-pathogenic for humans. Thus, it enables the identification of the pathogenic variants. PrimateAI has previously shown 88% accuracy in disease-causing variant identification and allowed the discovery of 14 novel candidate genes related to intellectual disability. PrimateAI also incorporates protein structure information as it learns to predict the secondary structure and solvent accessibility from amino acid sequences. PrimateAI provides a score to the user in which a threshold of >0.8 is for likely pathogenic classification, <0.6 is for likely benign, and 0.6–0.8 is as intermediate in genes with dominant modes of inheritance, and a threshold of >0.7 is for likely pathogenic and <0.5 for likely benign in genes with recessive modes of inheritance.

3.3 Genic intolerance

Genic intolerance is a gene-level assessment that has a potential to prioritize genomic variants. It has been developed as a scoring system to calculate tolerance of genes to a functional genetic variation on a genome-wide scale and rank them using 6503 WES data available in the National Heart, Lung, and Blood Institute-NHLBI Exome Sequencing Project [89]. This system predicts the expected common functional variation in the gene and compares them to apparently neutral variation found in the gene. The deviation from this prediction is attributed to the intolerance score, namely the Residual Variation Intolerance Score (RVIS). While genes with a positive RVIS score have more common functional variation than expected, genes with negative RVIS scores have less. A negative RVIS score indicates that the gene is intolerant. The scoring system also shows that the genes that cause Mendelian diseases are significantly more intolerant to functional variation than genes that do not cause any known disease.

3.4 Model organism databases

The evolutionary conservation of many biological processes among species allows the usage of several different model organisms to study human diseases. Although not all the human genes are conserved in invertebrate models such as worms and fruit flies, vertebrate models such as zebrafish and mouse provide valuable resources to study such genes. When evaluating the function of a conserved gene in model organisms, it is critical to keep in mind that orthologous genes usually cause different phenotypes in different species, although the gene products have a similar molecular function. The model organism databases listed below provide the related information on the molecular function of query genes so that they serve as a valuable resource during the variant prioritization process.

3.4.1 Mouse genome informatics (MGI)

MGI is the primary database that integrates genetic, genomic, and biological data for the laboratory Mouse. Mouse Genome Database (MGD) and Mouse Gene Expression Database (GXD) are the two largest contributors to MGI, both serving as valuable resources for the studies of human disease. MGD provides curated phenotypes and functional annotations for mouse genes and alleles, while GXD contains mouse gene expression data with an emphasis on endogenous gene expression during mouse development [96, 97]. The Human-Mouse Disease Connection tool within MGI is another important feature that facilitates exploring gene-phenotype-disease relationships between human and mouse. By simply searching the list of human genes on MGI, the algorithm finds matching mouse genes and their homologs and displays the both human and mouse phenotypes associated with the genes of interest. MGI is updated once every week by adding new annotations from the literature.

3.4.2 International Mouse Phenotyping Consortium (IMPC)

IMPC aims to establish a comprehensive dataset of mouse genome and phenome by knocking out each gene individually and characterizing the physical and chemical changes, thus providing the foundations for the functional analysis of human genetic variation [98]. The project also aims to generate putative human pathogenic variants in both coding and non-coding regions of the mouse genome.

IMPC uses an algorithm that has been developed to detect phenotypic similarities between the mouse strains of IMPC and more than 7000 rare diseases. The algorithm evaluates a very diverse set of phenotyping parameters that comprise neurological, behavioral, metabolic, cardiovascular, pulmonary, reproductive, respiratory, sensory, musculoskeletal, and immunological parameters and provides a quantitative measure on how well a mouse model recapitulates disease features.

So far, over 3000 genes have already been cataloged and revealed models for 360 diseases, with 90% of the annotated phenotypes being novel [99]. By 2021, IMPC plans to analyze more than 9000 mouse genes to facilitate the prioritization and validation of variations obtained from clinical sequencing efforts.

3.4.3 Rat Genome Database (RGD)

RGD provides genetic, genomic, phenotypic, and disease-related data for the laboratory rat, *Rattus norvegicus*. Rats have been one of the most commonly used model organisms for human disease research. RGD catalogs the rat data and also serves as a comparative data analysis platform between species such as rat, mouse, and human by validating the orthologous relationships. The database currently contains more than 1300 rat strains with disease/phenotype annotations [100]. RGD contains several tools that facilitate the analysis of data in disease-related content. PhenoMiner is such a tool that standardizes the phenotype data obtained from different rat studies by using a variety of ontologies developed at RGD [101]. Users can select one of the Phenominer search categories that include rat strains, experimental conditions, clinical measurements, and measurement methods to begin their search. Then, the algorithm filters the data according to the selected conditions and displays the results.

3.4.4 FlyBase

FlyBase is the central resource for integrated Drosophila genetic and genomic data, including but not limited to sequence-level gene models, mutant phenotypes, mutant lesions and chromosome aberrations, as well as gene expression patterns [102]. The fruit fly—*Drosophila melanogaster*—is a member of the Drosophila family widely used as a model for human disease research.

FlyBase allows different approaches for data presentation to facilitate Drosophila translational research as the two main methods being the gene-centric and disease-centric ones. The Gene Report displays information on individual genes. The report also lists the mutant alleles of the gene and the expression pattern of the gene products. The Human Disease Model Report provides background information on a specific disease and presents summaries of the experimental data and results from previous fruit fly studies.

FlyBase also incorporates orthology prediction tools such as OrthoDB and DIOPT that have been developed to identify orthologs of fly genes in multiple organisms [103, 104]. Integrating the results of these tools to the Gene Reports provides users the identification of orthologs in up to 5000 species. The predicted orthologs serve as a valuable resource for the human disease gene variants prediction as FlyBase also indicates whether the human ortholog functionally complements the fly mutant upon transfer into the Drosophila genome.

3.4.5 WormBase

WormBase serves as the main database for genetic, genomic, and biological information on C.elegans and related nematodes. *C. elegans* is a widely used model for human disease variant research as over 40% of human genes have a C.elegans ortholog. WormBase catalogs the available mutant strains for each gene as well as related nematode studies. WS273 release of WormBase contains over 160,000 gene summaries for 10 nematode species. The gene summaries also include human ortholog diseases and phenotypes to aid the detection of human disease-causing variants [105].

3.4.6 Zebrafish Information Network (ZFin)

ZFIN is the main database that provides genetic, genomic, and phenotypic data from zebrafish studies [106]. Zebrafish—*Danio reriro*—is a model organism extensively used in biomedical research, especially for developmental and genomic studies. Powerful approaches are available to model human diseases using zebrafish. Genetic manipulation of zebrafish orthologs of human disease genes is a common strategy to model genetic disorders such as Duchenne muscular dystrophy [107] and Rett Syndrome [108]. Another strategy of disease modeling is generating transgenic zebrafish lines that express human genes. This approach allows testing the function of the potential disease-causative variant in disease pathology. For example, a transgenic zebrafish model confirmed the pathogenicity of two novel XPNPEP3 gene mutations predicted to be ciliopathy-causing in the clinic [109]. Users can easily search ZFIN to reach information on disease models, including the transgenic lines and mutant phenotypes related to their query.

4. Real-life case

4.1 Variation in the frizzled class receptor 6 (FZD6) protein found in individuals with the nail disorder

Nonsyndromic congenital nail disorder 1 (OMIM #1161050) is a condition affecting the fingernails and toenails characterized by extremely thick nails, onycholysis, hyponychia and claw-like appearance. Autosomal recessive mutations in the FZD6 gene (OMIM *603409) were found to be associated with this disorder [110]. FZD6 is a member of the highly conserved WNT receptors family crucial for developmental processes and differentiation. The study conducted on mice demonstrated that FZD6-mediated Wnt signaling has a regulatory role in the differentiation process of claw/nail formation [111].

In a previous study from our group, a Turkish family with three affected individuals reported. After performing WES on the index case, 96 de novo heterozygous, 421 homozygous, and 185 compound heterozygous variants were obtained from data analysis. Employing population MAF frequency filtering according to the mode of inheritance has decreased the number of variants to 19, 46, 3 for de novo heterozygous, homozygous, compound heterozygous variants respectively. Further prioritization approaches were applied by integrating pathogenicity prediction scores provided by PrimateAI and other tools, model organism phenotypes, and gene intolerance scores. Ultimately, the FZD6 gene was found to be the most prominent gene even though the gene does not have a high intolerance score. However, the potential functional impact of the mutation was supported by the examination of the evolutionary conservation of the disturbed amino acid region. The region was found to be evolutionarily conserved in other FZD6 orthologues including *Pan troglodytes*, *Macaca mulatta*, *Pongo abelii*, *Bos taurus*, *Canis lupus familiaris*, *Rattus norvegicus*, *Mus musculus*, *Xenopus laevis*. The index case had a homozygous 8 bp deletion on the FZD6 gene caused p.Gly559Aspfs*16. Additionally, this mutation has previously been reported in two other Turkish families. It is also reported that all three families have a common ancestor. In this study, the pathogenicity mechanism for this mutation in nail dysplasia is provided for the first time. The mutation causes a frameshift and creates a premature stop codon at position 16 of the new reading frame [112].

This case study demonstrated that the promising applications of evolutionary approaches assist the clinical diagnosis.

5. Conclusion

Associating genomic variants with diseases is a multistep process. The early steps of this process are highly automated through the usage of several bioinformatics tools. However, the final prioritization step, which is the most critical step, is not completely automated. It requires a comprehensive interpretation together with integrative approaches. In this chapter, we aimed to explain the potential of integrating evolutionary principles into variant prioritization toward clinical utility. This chapter provides sufficient basic information to understand the required bioinformatics tools, various databases with increasing sequence data from individuals as well as model organism research. Finally, we conclude that the pre-evaluation of individual variations with evolutionary approaches can help shorten the diagnostic odyssey, hence saving time and resources. This chapter aims to contribute to the integration of evolutionary genetics to medical genomics. Further studies that combine theoretical and analytical approaches are needed to improve the field of precision medicine via the use of evolutionary insight.

Conflict of interest

The authors declare no conflict of interest.

Author details

Ugur Sezerman*, Tugce Bozkurt and Fatma Sadife Isleyen
Graduate School of Health Sciences, Biostatistics and Bioinformatics Program, Acibadem Mehmet Ali Aydinlar University, Istanbul, Turkey

*Address all correspondence to: sezermanu@gmail.com

References

[1] Jamuar SS, Tan E-C. Clinical application of next-generation sequencing for Mendelian diseases. Human Genomics. 2015;**9**:10. DOI: 10.1186/s40246-015-0031-5

[2] Domazet-Loso T, Tautz D. An ancient evolutionary origin of genes associated with human genetic diseases. Molecular Biology and Evolution. 2008;**25**:2699-2707. DOI: 10.1093/molbev/msn214

[3] Cai JJ, Borenstein E, Chen R, Petrov DA. Similarly strong purifying selection acts on human disease genes of all evolutionary ages. Genome Biology and Evolution. 2009;**1**:131-144. DOI: 10.1093/gbe/evp013

[4] Stenson PD, Ball EV, Howells K, Phillips AD, Mort M, Cooper DN. The human gene mutation database: Providing a comprehensive central mutation database for molecular diagnostics and personalised genomics. Human Genomics. 2009;**4**:69. DOI: 10.1186/1479-7364-4-2-69

[5] Cock PJA, Fields CJ, Goto N, Heuer ML, Rice PM. The sanger FASTQ file format for sequences with quality scores, and the Solexa/Illumina FASTQ variants. Nucleic Acids Research. 2010;**38**:1767-1771. DOI: 10.1093/nar/gkp1137

[6] Ewing B, Hillier L, Wendl MC, Green P. Base-calling of automated sequencer traces using *Phred*. I. Accuracy assessment. Genome Research. 1998;**8**:175-185. DOI: 10.1101/gr.8.3.175

[7] Ewing B, Green P. Base-calling of automated sequencer traces using *Phred*. II. Error probabilities. Genome Research. 1998;**8**:186-194. DOI: 10.1101/gr.8.3.186

[8] Available from: https://www.bioinformatics.babraham.ac.uk/projects/fastqc/

[9] Chanumolu SK, Albahrani M, Otu HH. FQStat: A parallel architecture for very high-speed assessment of sequencing quality metrics. BMC Bioinformatics. 2019;**20**:424. DOI: 10.1186/s12859-019-3015-y

[10] Thrash A, Arick M, Peterson DG. Quack: A quality assurance tool for high throughput sequence data. Analytical Biochemistry. 2018;**548**:38-43. DOI: 10.1016/j.ab.2018.01.028

[11] Peng Y, Maxwell AS, Barker ND, Laird JG, Kennedy AJ, Wang N, et al. SeqAssist: A novel toolkit for preliminary analysis of next-generation sequencing data. BMC Bioinformatics. 2014;**15**:S10. DOI: 10.1186/1471-2105-15-S11-S10

[12] Zhou Q, Su X, Wang A, Xu J, Ning K. QC-chain: Fast and holistic quality control method for next-generation sequencing data. PLoS One. 2013;**8**:e60234. DOI: 10.1371/journal.pone.0060234

[13] Sun K. Ktrim: An extra-fast and accurate adapter- and quality-trimmer for sequencing data. Bioinformatics. 2020:btaa171. DOI: 10.1093/bioinformatics/btaa171

[14] Liao X, Li M, Zou Y, Wu F, Pan Y, Wang J. An efficient trimming algorithm based on multi-feature fusion scoring model for NGS data. IEEE/ACM Transactions on Computational Biology and Bioinformatics. 2019:1-1. DOI: 10.1109/TCBB.2019.2897558

[15] Sturm M, Schroeder C, Bauer P. SeqPurge: Highly-sensitive adapter trimming for paired-end NGS data. BMC Bioinformatics. 2016;**17**:208. DOI: 10.1186/s12859-016-1069-7

[16] Schubert M, Lindgreen S, Orlando L. AdapterRemoval v2: Rapid adapter trimming, identification,

and read merging. BMC Research Notes. 2016;**9**:88. DOI: 10.1186/s13104-016-1900-2

[17] Li Y-L, Weng J-C, Hsiao C-C, Chou M-T, Tseng C-W, Hung J-H. PEAT: An intelligent and efficient paired-end sequencing adapter trimming algorithm. BMC Bioinformatics. 2015;**16**:S2. DOI: 10.1186/1471-2105-16-S1-S2

[18] Jiang H, Lei R, Ding S-W, Zhu S. Skewer: A fast and accurate adapter trimmer for next-generation sequencing paired-end reads. BMC Bioinformatics. 2014;**15**:182. DOI: 10.1186/1471-2105-15-182

[19] Bolger AM, Lohse M, Usadel B. Trimmomatic: A flexible trimmer for Illumina sequence data. Bioinformatics. 2014;**30**:2114-2120. DOI: 10.1093/bioinformatics/btu170

[20] Ma Y, Xie H, Han X, Irwin DM, Zhang Y-P. QcReads: An adapter and quality trimming tool for next-generation sequencing reads. Journal of Genetics and Genomics. 2013;**40**:639-642. DOI: 10.1016/j.jgg.2013.11.001

[21] Criscuolo A, Brisse S. AlienTrimmer: A tool to quickly and accurately trim off multiple short contaminant sequences from high-throughput sequencing reads. Genomics. 2013;**102**:500-506. DOI: 10.1016/j.ygeno.2013.07.011

[22] Kong Y. Btrim: A fast, lightweight adapter and quality trimming program for next-generation sequencing technologies. Genomics. 2011;**98**:152-153. DOI: 10.1016/j.ygeno.2011.05.009

[23] Roser LG, Agüero F, Sánchez DO. FastqCleaner: An interactive bioconductor application for quality-control, filtering and trimming of FASTQ files. BMC Bioinformatics. 2019;**20**:361. DOI: 10.1186/s12859-019-2961-8

[24] Liu X, Yan Z, Wu C, Yang Y, Li X, Zhang G. FastProNGS: Fast preprocessing of next-generation sequencing reads. BMC Bioinformatics. 2019;**20**:345. DOI: 10.1186/s12859-019-2936-9

[25] Rangamaran VR, Uppili B, Gopal D, Ramalingam K. EasyQC: Tool with interactive user Interface for efficient next-generation sequencing data quality control. Journal of Computational Biology. 2018;**25**:1301-1311. DOI: 10.1089/cmb.2017.0186

[26] Chen S, Zhou Y, Chen Y, Gu J. Fastp: An ultra-fast all-in-one FASTQ preprocessor. Bioinformatics. 2018;**34**:i884-i890. DOI: 10.1093/bioinformatics/bty560

[27] Langmead B, Salzberg SL. Fast gapped-read alignment with bowtie 2. Nature Methods. 2012;**9**:357-359. DOI: 10.1038/nmeth.1923

[28] Li H, Durbin R. Fast and accurate short read alignment with burrows-wheeler transform. Bioinformatics. 2009;**25**:1754-1760. DOI: 10.1093/bioinformatics/btp324

[29] Available from: http://www.novocraft.com/products/novoalign/

[30] Lee W-P, Stromberg MP, Ward A, Stewart C, Garrison EP, Marth GT. MOSAIK: A hash-based algorithm for accurate next-generation sequencing short-read mapping. PLoS One. 2014;**9**:e90581. DOI: 10.1371/journal.pone.0090581

[31] David M, Dzamba M, Lister D, Ilie L, Brudno M. SHRiMP2: Sensitive yet practical short read mapping. Bioinformatics. 2011;**27**:1011-1012. DOI: 10.1093/bioinformatics/btr046

[32] Fonseca NA, Rung J, Brazma A, Marioni JC. Tools for mapping high-throughput sequencing data. Bioinformatics. 2012;**28**:3169-3177. DOI: 10.1093/bioinformatics/bts605

[33] Hatem A, Bozdag D, Toland AE, Çatalyürek ÜV. Benchmarking short sequence mapping tools. BMC Bioinformatics. 2013;**14**:184. DOI: 10.1186/1471-2105-14-184

[34] Li H, Handsaker B, Wysoker A, Fennell T, Ruan J, Homer N, et al. The sequence alignment/map format and SAMtools. Bioinformatics. 2009;**25**:2078-2079. DOI: 10.1093/bioinformatics/btp352

[35] Robinson JT, Thorvaldsdóttir H, Winckler W, Guttman M, Lander ES, Getz G, et al. Integrative genomics viewer. Nature Biotechnology. 2011;**29**:24-26. DOI: 10.1038/nbt.1754

[36] picard n.d. Available from: http://broadinstitute.github.io/picard/

[37] DePristo MA, Banks E, Poplin RE, Garimella KV, Maguire JR, Hartl C. A framework for variation discovery and genotyping using next-generation DNA sequencing data. Nature Genetics. 2011;**43**:491-498. DOI: 10.1038/ng.806

[38] Auwera GA, Carneiro MO, Hartl C, Poplin R, del Angel G, Levy-Moonshine A, et al. From FastQ data to high-confidence variant calls: The genome analysis toolkit best practices pipeline. Current Protocols in Bioinformatics. 2013;**43**. DOI: 10.1002/0471250953.bi1110s43

[39] Garrison E, Marth G. Haplotype-based variant detection from short-read sequencing. ArXiv:12073907 [q-Bio]; 2012

[40] Rimmer A, Phan H, Mathieson I, Iqbal Z, Twigg SRF, et al. Nature Genetics. 2014;**46**:912-918. DOI: 10.1038/ng.3036

[41] Koboldt DC, Chen K, Wylie T, Larson DE, McLellan MD, Mardis ER, et al. VarScan: Variant detection in massively parallel sequencing of individual and pooled samples. Bioinformatics. 2009;**25**:2283-2285. DOI: 10.1093/bioinformatics/btp373

[42] Wei Z, Wang W, Hu P, Lyon GJ, Hakonarson H. SNVer: A statistical tool for variant calling in analysis of pooled or individual next-generation sequencing data. Nucleic Acids Research. 2011;**39**:e132-e132. DOI: 10.1093/nar/gkr599

[43] Sandmann S, de Graaf AO, Karimi M, van der Reijden BA, Hellström-Lindberg E, Jansen JH, et al. Evaluating variant calling tools for non-matched next-generation sequencing data. Scientific Reports. 2017;**7**:43169. DOI: 10.1038/srep43169

[44] Chen J, Li X, Zhong H, Meng Y, Du H. Systematic comparison of germline variant calling pipelines cross multiple next-generation sequencers. Scientific Reports. 2019;**9**:9345. DOI: 10.1038/s41598-019-45835-3

[45] Kumaran M, Subramanian U, Devarajan B. Performance assessment of variant calling pipelines using human whole exome sequencing and simulated data. BMC Bioinformatics. 2019;**20**:342. DOI: 10.1186/s12859-019-2928-9

[46] Wang K, Li M, Hakonarson H. ANNOVAR: Functional annotation of genetic variants from high-throughput sequencing data. Nucleic Acids Research. 2010;**38**:e164-e164. DOI: 10.1093/nar/gkq603

[47] McLaren W, Gil L, Hunt SE, Riat HS, Ritchie GRS, Thormann A, et al. The Ensembl variant effect predictor. Genome Biology. 2016;**17**:122. DOI: 10.1186/s13059-016-0974-4

[48] Cingolani P, Platts A, Wang LL, Coon M, Nguyen T, Wang L, et al. A program for annotating and predicting the effects of single nucleotide

polymorphisms, SnpEff: SNPs in the genome of *Drosophila melanogaster* strain w^{1118}; iso-2; iso-3. Fly. 2012;**6**: 80-92. DOI: 10.4161/fly.19695

[49] Paila U, Chapman BA, Kirchner R, Quinlan AR. GEMINI: Integrative exploration of genetic variation and genome annotations. PLoS Computational Biology. 2013;**9**:e1003153. DOI: 10.1371/journal.pcbi.1003153

[50] Desvignes J-P, Bartoli M, Delague V, Krahn M, Miltgen M, Béroud C, et al. VarAFT: A variant annotation and filtration system for human next generation sequencing data. Nucleic Acids Research. 2018;**46**:W545-W553. DOI: 10.1093/nar/gky471

[51] Makarov V, O'Grady T, Cai G, Lihm J, Buxbaum JD, Yoon S. AnnTools: A comprehensive and versatile annotation toolkit for genomic variants. Bioinformatics. 2012;**28**:724-725. DOI: 10.1093/bioinformatics/bts032

[52] Ge D, Ruzzo EK, Shianna KV, He M, Pelak K, Heinzen EL, et al. SVA: Software for annotating and visualizing sequenced human genomes. Bioinformatics. 2011;**27**:1998-2000. DOI: 10.1093/bioinformatics/btr317

[53] Grant JR, Arantes AS, Liao X, Stothard P. In-depth annotation of SNPs arising from resequencing projects using NGS-SNP. Bioinformatics. 2011;**27**:2300-2301. DOI: 10.1093/bioinformatics/btr372

[54] Miller MP. Understanding human disease mutations through the use of interspecific genetic variation. Human Molecular Genetics. 2001;**10**:2319-2328. DOI: 10.1093/hmg/10.21.2319

[55] Thomas PD, Kejariwal A. Coding single-nucleotide polymorphisms associated with complex vs. Mendelian disease: Evolutionary evidence for differences in molecular effects. Proceedings of the National Academy of Sciences. 2004;**101**:15398-15403. DOI: 10.1073/pnas.0404380101

[56] Zhu Q, Ge D, Maia JM, Zhu M, Petrovski S, Dickson SP, et al. A genome-wide comparison of the functional properties of rare and common genetic variants in humans. The American Journal of Human Genetics. 2011;**88**:458-468. DOI: 10.1016/j.ajhg.2011.03.008

[57] Cooper DN, Kehrer-Sawatzki H. Exploring the potential relevance of human-specific genes to complex disease. Human Genomics. 2011;**5**:99. DOI: 10.1186/1479-7364-5-2-99

[58] Botstein D, Risch N. Discovering genotypes underlying human phenotypes: Past successes for Mendelian disease, future approaches for complex disease. Nature Genetics. 2003;**33**:228-237. DOI: 10.1038/ng1090

[59] Sherry ST, Ward M, Sirotkin K. dbSNP—Database for Single Nucleotide Polymorphisms and Other Classes of Minor Genetic Variation. n.d.:4

[60] Richards S, Aziz N, Bale S, Bick D, Das S, et al. Standards and guidelines for the interpretation of sequence variants: A joint consensus recommendation of the American College of Medical Genetics and Genomics and the Association for Molecular Pathology. Genet Med. 2015;**17**:405-423. DOI: 10.1038/gim.2015.30

[61] Stitziel NO, Kiezun A, Sunyaev S. Computational and statistical approaches to analyzing variants identified by exome sequencing. Genome Biology. 2011;**12**:227. DOI: 10.1186/gb-2011-12-9-227

[62] Bamshad MJ, Ng SB, Bigham AW, Tabor HK, Emond MJ, Nickerson DA, et al. Exome sequencing as a tool for

Mendelian disease gene discovery. Nature Reviews. Genetics. 2011;**12**: 745-755. DOI: 10.1038/nrg3031

[63] Broeckx BJG, Peelman L, Saunders JH, Deforce D, Clement L. Using variant databases for variant prioritization and to detect erroneous genotype-phenotype associations. BMC Bioinformatics. 2017;**18**:535. DOI: 10.1186/s12859-017-1951-y

[64] The 1000 Genomes Project Consortium. A global reference for human genetic variation. Nature. 2015;**526**:68-74. DOI: 10.1038/nature15393

[65] Sudmant PH, Rausch T, Gardner EJ, Handsaker RE, Abyzov A, et al. An integrated map of structural variation in 2,504 human genomes. Nature. 2015;**526**:75-81. DOI: 10.1038/nature15394

[66] Karczewski KJ, Francioli LC, Tiao G, Cummings BB, Alföldi J, Wang Q, et al. The mutational constraint spectrum quantified from variation in 141,456 humans. Genomics. 2019. DOI: 10.1101/531210

[67] Sherry ST. dbSNP: The NCBI database of genetic variation. Nucleic Acids Research. 2001;**29**:308-311. DOI: 10.1093/nar/29.1.308

[68] MacDonald JR, Ziman R, Yuen RKC, Feuk L, Scherer SW. The database of genomic variants: A curated collection of structural variation in the human genome. Nucl Acids Res. 2014;**42**:D986-D992. DOI: 10.1093/nar/gkt958

[69] Landrum MJ, Lee JM, Benson M, Brown G, Chao C, Chitipiralla S, et al. ClinVar: Public archive of interpretations of clinically relevant variants. Nucleic Acids Research. 2016;**44**:D862-D868. DOI: 10.1093/nar/gkv1222

[70] Firth HV, Richards SM, Bevan AP, Clayton S, Corpas M, Rajan D, et al. DECIPHER: Database of chromosomal imbalance and phenotype in humans using Ensembl resources. The American Journal of Human Genetics. 2009;**84**:524-533. DOI: 10.1016/j.ajhg.2009.03.010

[71] Matthijs G, Souche E, Alders M, Corveleyn A, Eck S, Feenstra I, et al. Guidelines for diagnostic next-generation sequencing. European Journal of Human Genetics. 2016;**24**:2-5. DOI: 10.1038/ejhg.2015.226

[72] Adzhubei IA, Schmidt S, Peshkin L, Ramensky VE, Gerasimova A, Bork P, et al. A method and server for predicting damaging missense mutations. Nature Methods. 2010;7:248-249. DOI: 10.1038/nmeth0410-248

[73] Ng PC. SIFT: Predicting amino acid changes that affect protein function. Nucleic Acids Research. 2003;**31**:3812-3814. DOI: 10.1093/nar/gkg509

[74] Choi Y, Sims GE, Murphy S, Miller JR, Chan AP. Predicting the functional effect of amino acid substitutions and Indels. PLoS One. 2012;7:e46688. DOI: 10.1371/journal.pone.0046688

[75] Thomas PD. PANTHER: A library of protein families and subfamilies indexed by function. Genome Research. 2003;**13**:2129-2141. DOI: 10.1101/gr.772403

[76] Kircher M, Witten DM, Jain P, O'Roak BJ, Cooper GM, Shendure J. A general framework for estimating the relative pathogenicity of human genetic variants. Nature Genetics. 2014;**46**:310-315. DOI: 10.1038/ng.2892

[77] Schwarz JM, Cooper DN, Schuelke M, Seelow D. MutationTaster2: Mutation prediction for the deep-sequencing age. Nature Methods.

2014;**11**:361-362. DOI: 10.1038/nmeth.2890

[78] Quang D, Chen Y, Xie X. DANN: A deep learning approach for annotating the pathogenicity of genetic variants. Bioinformatics. 2015;**31**:761-763. DOI: 10.1093/bioinformatics/btu703

[79] Carter H, Douville C, Stenson PD, Cooper DN, Karchin R. Identifying Mendelian disease genes with the variant effect scoring tool. BMC Genomics. 2013;**14**:S3. DOI: 10.1186/1471-2164-14-S3-S3

[80] Dong C, Wei P, Jian X, Gibbs R, Boerwinkle E, Wang K, et al. Comparison and integration of deleteriousness prediction methods for nonsynonymous SNVs in whole exome sequencing studies. Human Molecular Genetics. 2015;**24**:2125-2137. DOI: 10.1093/hmg/ddu733

[81] Jagadeesh KA, Wenger AM, Berger MJ, Guturu H, Stenson PD, Cooper DN, et al. M-CAP eliminates a majority of variants of uncertain significance in clinical exomes at high sensitivity. Nature Genetics. 2016;**48**:1581-1586. DOI: 10.1038/ng.3703

[82] Ioannidis NM, Rothstein JH, Pejaver V, Middha S, McDonnell SK, Baheti S, et al. REVEL: An ensemble method for predicting the pathogenicity of rare missense variants. The American Journal of Human Genetics. 2016;**99**:877-885. DOI: 10.1016/j.ajhg.2016.08.016

[83] Li J, Zhao T, Zhang Y, Zhang K, Shi L, Chen Y, et al. Performance evaluation of pathogenicity-computation methods for missense variants. Nucleic Acids Research. 2018;**46**:7793-7804. DOI: 10.1093/nar/gky678

[84] Schaafsma GCP, Vihinen M. Representativeness of variation benchmark datasets. BMC Bioinformatics. 2018;**19**:461. DOI: 10.1186/s12859-018-2478-6

[85] Niroula A, Vihinen M. How good are pathogenicity predictors in detecting benign variants? PLoS Computational Biology. 2019;**15**:e1006481. DOI: 10.1371/journal.pcbi.1006481

[86] Reva B, Antipin Y, Sander C. Predicting the functional impact of protein mutations: Application to cancer genomics. Nucleic Acids Research. 2011;**39**:e118-e118. DOI: 10.1093/nar/gkr407

[87] Shihab HA, Gough J, Cooper DN, Stenson PD, Barker GLA, Edwards KJ, et al. Predicting the functional, molecular, and phenotypic consequences of amino acid substitutions using hidden Markov models. Human Mutation. 2013;**34**:57-65. DOI: 10.1002/humu.22225

[88] Chun S, Fay JC. Identification of deleterious mutations within three human genomes. Genome Research. 2009;**19**:1553-1561. DOI: 10.1101/gr.092619.109

[89] Petrovski S, Wang Q, Heinzen EL, Allen AS, Goldstein DB. Genic intolerance to functional variation and the interpretation of personal genomes. PLoS Genetics. 2013;**9**:e1003709. DOI: 10.1371/journal.pgen.1003709

[90] Pollard KS, Hubisz MJ, Rosenbloom KR, Siepel A. Detection of nonneutral substitution rates on mammalian phylogenies. Genome Research. 2010;**20**:110-121. DOI: 10.1101/gr.097857.109

[91] Siepel A. Evolutionarily conserved elements in vertebrate, insect, worm, and yeast genomes. Genome Research. 2005;**15**:1034-1050. DOI: 10.1101/gr.3715005

[92] Garber M, Guttman M, Clamp M, Zody MC, Friedman N,

Xie X. Identifying novel constrained elements by exploiting biased substitution patterns. Bioinformatics. 2009;**25**:i54-i62. DOI: 10.1093/bioinformatics/btp190

[93] Davydov EV, Goode DL, Sirota M, Cooper GM, Sidow A, Batzoglou S. Identifying a high fraction of the human genome to be under selective constraint using GERP++. PLoS Computational Biology. 2010;**6**:e1001025. DOI: 10.1371/journal.pcbi.1001025

[94] Henikoff S, Henikoff JG. Amino acid substitution matrices from protein blocks. Proceedings of the National Academy of Sciences. 1992;**89**:10915-10919. DOI: 10.1073/pnas.89.22.10915

[95] Sundaram L, Gao H, Padigepati SR, McRae JF, Li Y, Kosmicki JA, et al. Predicting the clinical impact of human mutation with deep neural networks. Nature Genetics. 2018;**50**:1161-1170. DOI: 10.1038/s41588-018-0167-z

[96] Bult CJ, Blake JA, Smith CL, Kadin JA, Richardson JE, The Mouse Genome Database Group, et al. Mouse Genome Database (MGD) 2019. Nucleic Acids Research. 2019;**47**:D801-D806. DOI: 10.1093/nar/gky1056

[97] Smith CM, Hayamizu TF, Finger JH, Bello SM, McCright IJ, Xu J, et al. The mouse gene expression database (GXD): 2019 update. Nucleic Acids Research. 2019;**47**:D774-D779. DOI: 10.1093/nar/gky922

[98] The International Mouse Phenotyping Consortium, Dickinson ME, Flenniken AM, Ji X, Teboul L, Wong MD, et al. High-throughput discovery of novel developmental phenotypes. Nature. 2016;**537**:508-514. DOI: 10.1038/nature19356.

[99] The International Mouse Phenotyping Consortium, Meehan TF, Conte N, West DB, Jacobsen JO, Mason J, et al. Disease model discovery from 3,328 gene knockouts by the International Mouse Phenotyping Consortium. Nature Genetics. 2017;**49**:1231-1238. DOI: 10.1038/ng.3901.

[100] Smith JR, Hayman GT, Wang S-J, Laulederkind SJF, Hoffman MJ, Kaldunski ML, et al. The year of the rat: The rat genome database at 20: A multi-species knowledgebase and analysis platform. Nucleic Acids Research. 2019:gkz1041. DOI: 10.1093/nar/gkz1041

[101] Laulederkind SJF, Liu W, Smith JR, Hayman GT, Wang S-J, Nigam R, et al. PhenoMiner: Quantitative phenotype curation at the rat genome database. Database. 2013;**2013**:bat015. DOI: 10.1093/database/bat015

[102] Thurmond J, Goodman JL, Strelets VB, Attrill H, Gramates LS, Marygold SJ, et al. FlyBase 2.0: The next generation. Nucleic Acids Research. 2019;**47**:D759-D765. DOI: 10.1093/nar/gky1003

[103] Zdobnov EM, Tegenfeldt F, Kuznetsov D, Waterhouse RM, Simão FA, Ioannidis P, et al. OrthoDB v9.1: Cataloging evolutionary and functional annotations for animal, fungal, plant, archaeal, bacterial and viral orthologs. Nucleic Acids Research. 2017;**45**:D744-D749. DOI: 10.1093/nar/gkw1119

[104] Hu Y, Flockhart I, Vinayagam A, Bergwitz C, Berger B, Perrimon N, et al. An integrative approach to ortholog prediction for disease-focused and other functional studies. BMC Bioinformatics. 2011;**12**:357. DOI: 10.1186/1471-2105-12-357

[105] Harris TW, Arnaboldi V, Cain S, Chan J, Chen WJ, Cho J, et al. WormBase: A modern model organism information resource. Nucleic Acids Research. 2019:gkz920. DOI: 10.1093/nar/gkz920

[106] Ruzicka L, Howe DG, Ramachandran S, Toro S, Van Slyke CE, Bradford YM, et al. The Zebrafish information network: New support for non-coding genes, richer gene ontology annotations and the Alliance of genome resources. Nucleic Acids Research. 2019;**47**:D867-D873. DOI: 10.1093/nar/gky1090

[107] Berger J, Currie PD. Zebrafish models flex their muscles to shed light on muscular dystrophies. Disease Models & Mechanisms. 2012;**5**:726-732. DOI: 10.1242/dmm.010082

[108] Pietri T, Roman A-C, Guyon N, Romano SA, Washbourne P, Moens CB, et al. The first mecp2-null zebrafish model shows altered motor behaviors. Frontiers in Neural Circuits. 2013;**7**:1-10. DOI: 10.3389/fncir.2013.00118

[109] O'Toole JF, Liu Y, Davis EE, Westlake CJ, Attanasio M, Otto EA, et al. Individuals with mutations in XPNPEP3, which encodes a mitochondrial protein, develop a nephronophthisis-like nephropathy. The Journal of Clinical Investigation. 2010;**120**:791-802. DOI: 10.1172/JCI40076

[110] Fröjmark A-S, Schuster J, Sobol M, Entesarian M, Kilander MBC, Gabrikova D, et al. Mutations in frizzled 6 cause isolated autosomal-recessive nail dysplasia. The American Journal of Human Genetics. 2011;**88**:852-860. DOI: 10.1016/j.ajhg.2011.05.013

[111] Cui C-Y, Klar J, Georgii-Heming P, Fröjmark A-S, Baig SM, Schlessinger D, et al. Frizzled6 deficiency disrupts the differentiation process of nail development. Journal of Investigative Dermatology. 2013;**133**:1990-1997. DOI: 10.1038/jid.2013.84

[112] Saygi C, Alanay Y, Sezerman U, Yenenler A, Özören N. A possible founder mutation in FZD6 gene in a Turkish family with autosomal recessive nail dysplasia. BMC Medical Genetics. 2019;**20**:15. DOI: 10.1186/s12881-019-0746-6

COMPUTATIONAL FLOW MODELING FOR CHEMICAL REACTOR ENGINEERING

Process Systems Engineering Series
A series edited by George Stephanopoulos and John Perkins

Volume 1
Mathematical Modeling
Rutherford Aris

Volume 2
Data Processing and Reconciliation for Chemical Process Operations
José A Romagnoli & Mabel Cristina Sánchez

Volume 3
Linear Algebra and Linear Operators in Engineering
Ted H Davis & Kendall T Thomson

Volume 4
Process Modelling and Model Analysis
Katalin Hangos & Ian Cameron

Volume 5
Computational Flow Modeling for Chemical Reactor Engineering
Vivek V Ranade

COMPUTATIONAL FLOW MODELING FOR CHEMICAL REACTOR ENGINEERING

Vivek V. Ranade
Industrial Flow Modeling Group
Chemical Engineering Division
National Chemical Laboratory
Pune 411008, India

ACADEMIC PRESS
A Harcourt Science and Technology Company

San Diego San Francisco New York Boston London Sydney Tokyo

This book is printed on acid-free paper.

Academic Press
A Harcourt Science and Technology Company
525 B Street, Suite 1900, San Diego, California 92101-4495, USA
http://www.academicpress.com

Academic Press
Harcourt Place, 32 Jamestown Road, London NW1 7BY, UK
http://www.academicpress.com

ISBN 0-12-576960-1

Library of Congress Catalog Number: 2001090198
A catalogue record of this book is available from the British Library

Typeset by Newgen Imaging Systems (P) Ltd., Chennai, India
Printed and bound in Great Britain by Bookcraft, Bath, UK

02 03 04 05 06 07 BC 9 8 7 6 5 4 3 2 1

To Nanda & Vishakha

CONTENTS

7 Numerical Solution of Complex Flow Models

8 Computational Tools for Simulating Flow Processes

III CFM FOR CRE

9 Flow Modeling for Reactor Engineering

IV APPLICATIONS

10 Stirred Reactors

11 Bubble Column Reactors

12 Fluidized Bed Reactors

13 Fixed Bed and Other Types of Reactors

V EPILOGUE

14 Epilogue

PREFACE

Industrial Flow Modeling Group, *iFMg* at National Chemical Laboratory undertakes contract research and consultancy projects in the general area of reactor engineering. We use computational flow modeling to carry out these industrial projects. Computational flow modeling is a powerful tool for the design and analysis of industrial flow processes. Though it is routinely used as a design tool in aerospace engineering, chemical engineers have started exploiting the power of computational flow modeling only recently. Considering the central role played by reactors in chemical process industries, there is tremendous potential for applying computational flow-modeling tools to improve reactor engineering.

Through interactions with practicing engineers from industry, it has been realized that there is insufficient help available to harness state of the art computational flow modeling tools for complex, industrial reactor engineering applications. Many reactor engineers either consider that the flow complexities of industrial reactors are impossible to simulate, or expect miracles from off-the-shelf, commercial flow modeling tools. These two diverse views arise because of inadequate interactions between the flow modeling and industrial reactor engineering communities. It is essential to clearly understand the role of flow modeling in reactor engineering. It is necessary to relate the individual aspects of reactor engineering and computational flow modeling in a coherent and consistent way to realize the potential of computational flow modeling for reactor engineering research and practice. To assist practicing engineers in these aspects, workshops on 'computational flow modeling for chemical process industries' were started at the National Chemical Laboratory. The enthusiastic response to these workshops has encouraged me to write this book, which is an expanded and formalized presentation of workshop notes. I have tried to provide sufficient information to understand and to define the specific role of computational flow modeling for reactor engineering applications, to select appropriate tools and to apply these tools to link reactor hardware to reactor performance. The intended audience of the book is practicing chemical engineers working in industry as well as chemical engineering scientists and research students working in the area of reactor engineering. Some prior background in reactor engineering and numerical techniques is assumed.

The information in the book is organized to facilitate the central task of reactor engineer, that is, relating reactor hardware to reactor performance. Several steps to achieve such a task are discussed to clearly define the role of flow modeling in the overall reactor engineering activity. The necessity of using a hierarchy of modeling tools and establishing a clear relationship between the objectives of reactor engineering and the computational flow model is emphasized with the help of examples. The overall methodology of achieving the objectives of reactor engineering via computational flow modeling is discussed. Desirable characteristics and key issues in selecting appropriate computational fluid dynamics (CFD) codes are briefly discussed. A number of examples and case studies covering the four major reactor types used in chemical industries, namely, stirred reactors, bubble column reactors, fluidized bed reactors and fixed bed reactors are included. In view of the wide range of reactor types, however, it is impossible to cover all the reactor types and flows relevant to these reactor types. Emphasis on certain topics and the selection of examples is biased and is directly related to my own research and consulting experience. Some topics, like radiative heat transfer, laminar reactive flows are completely omitted. I have, however, made an attempt to evolve general guidelines, which will be useful for solving practical reactor engineering problems. Some comments on future trends in computational flow modeling and its use by the chemical engineering community are also included.

The material included in this book may be used in several ways and at various stages of flow modeling projects. It may be used as a basic resource for making appropriate decisions about investment in the application of CFD to reactor engineering. It may be used as a study material for an in-house course to facilitate the appreciation and application of computational flow modeling for reactor engineering. It may be used as a companion book while solving practical reactor engineering problems. I hope that this book will encourage chemical engineers to exploit the potential of computational flow modeling and will eventually lead to better reactor engineering.

This book is essentially the outcome of my last fifteen years of association with this subject. I have received a great deal of help from numerous persons over these years in formulating and revising my views on both computational flow modeling and chemical reactor engineering. I am particularly indebted to my teacher and mentor, Professor J.B. Joshi, who has been one of the leading practitioners of process fluid dynamics for three decades. There are not adequate words to express his contributions to this book. I was fortunate to have an opportunity to work with Dr R.V. Chaudhari and Dr R.A. Mashelkar at the National Chemical Laboratory. Both of them always extended their full support and encouragement in my every endeavor. Without their support, it would not have been possible to develop our industrial flow modeling activity, on which this book is based. I would like to acknowledge the support provided by Professor H.E.A. van den Akker of Delft University of Technology and by

Professors G.F. Versteeg and J.A.M. Kuipers of University of Twente, The Netherlands. My brief stay at Professor van den Akker's laboratory at Delft introduced me to different commercial CFD solvers and expanded my horizons. The idea of this book was formalized during my second visit to The Netherlands at University of Twente. I would also like to thank Dr Bharatan Patel of Fluent Inc. and Mr Paresh Patel of Fluent India for their support.

I am grateful to my associates and collaborators with whom I worked on different industrial projects. In particular, I owe much to Professor J.R. Bourne, Mr Vaibhav Deshpande, Ms S.M.S. Dommeti and Mr Yatin Tayalia. My students, especially Kapil Girotra, Ashwin Sunthankar, Ranjit Utikar, Aravind Rammohan, Sachin Muthian, Avinash Khopkar, Prashant Gunjal, Vivek Buwa and Shishir Sable have contributed to this book in different ways. This includes technical contributions either in a direct or indirect way, helping me to collect the required information and reading the draft manuscript. My father, Mr V.B. Ranade also has painstakingly read the entire manuscript and suggested several ways to enhance the clarity of presentation. The manuscript was improved wherever their suggestions were incorporated. Any remaining errors or shortcomings are, needless to say, the responsibility of the author. Finally, I wish to thank my wife, Nanda, for her patience, understanding and enthusiastic support, which carried me through this long and arduous writing process.

Vivek V. Ranade
December 2000
Pune

PART I
INTRODUCTION

1 REACTOR ENGINEERING AND FLOW MODELING

All industrial chemical processes are designed to transform cheap raw materials to high value products (usually via chemical reactions). A 'reactor', in which such chemical transformations take place, has to carry out several functions such as bringing reactants into intimate contact (to allow chemical reactions to occur), providing an appropriate environment (temperature and concentration fields, catalysts) for an adequate time and allowing for the removal of products. Chemical reactor engineering includes all the activities necessary to evolve the best possible hardware and operating protocol of the reactor to carry out the desired transformation of raw materials (or reactants) to value added products. A reactor engineer has to ensure that the reactor hardware and operating protocol satisfy various process demands without compromising safety, the environment and economics. To realize this, the reactor engineer has to establish a relationship between reactor hardware and operating protocols and various performance issues (Fig. 1.1).

Successful reactor engineering requires expertise from various fields including thermodynamics, chemistry, catalysis, reaction engineering, fluid dynamics, mixing and heat and mass transfer. The reactor engineer has to interact with chemists to understand the basic chemistry and peculiarities of the catalyst. Based on such an understanding and proposed performance targets, the reactor engineer has to abstract the information relevant to identifying the characteristics of the desired fluid dynamics of the reactor. The reactor engineer then has to conceive suitable reactor hardware and operating protocols to realize this desired fluid dynamics in practice. Thus, fluid

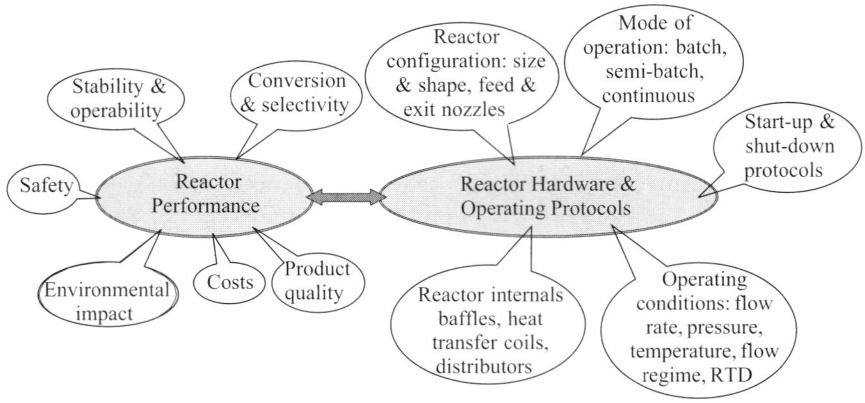

FIGURE 1.1 Chemical reactor engineering.

dynamics plays a pivotal role in establishing the relationship between reactor hardware and reactor performance.

To establish the relationship between reactor hardware and reactor performance, it is necessary to use a variety of different tools/models. Creative application of the best possible tools is required to evolve the best possible hardware configuration and operating protocol for the reactor under consideration. Various tools for modeling chemical kinetics and reactions are already well developed and routinely used in practice. This activity constitutes the major part of conventional chemical reaction engineering. Several excellent textbooks discussing these tools are available (for example, Aris, 1965; Levenspiel, 1972; Westerterp *et al.*, 1984; Naumann, 1987). Most models falling in this category make use of drastic simplifications when treating the reactor fluid dynamics. Indeed, sophisticated models and theories are available to predict the interaction between chemistry and transport processes such as mixing, heat and mass transfer. However, these models rarely attempt to rigorously relate transport properties with the reactor hardware and operating protocol. For a specific chemistry/catalyst, the reactor performance is a complex function of the underlying transport processes. These transport processes are, in turn, governed by the underlying fluid dynamics, and therefore by a variety of design and operating parameters of the process equipment. In conventional reaction engineering, experimental and semi-theoretical methods (like cold flow simulations or tracer studies) are used to relate fluid dynamics and mixing with reactor hardware and operating parameters. The information obtainable from these methods is usually described in an overall/global parametric form. This practice conceals detailed local information about turbulence and mixing, which may ultimately determine reactor performance. This approach essentially relies on prior experience and trial and error methods to evolve suitable reactor hardware. These tools, therefore, are increasingly perceived as being expensive and time consuming ways of developing better reactor technologies. It is necessary to adapt and develop better techniques and tools to relate reactor hardware with fluid dynamics and resultant transport processes.

Over the years, aerospace engineers, who are most concerned with the task of establishing the relationship between the hardware and resulting fluid dynamics, have developed and routinely use computational fluid dynamics. Computational fluid dynamics (CFD) is a body of knowledge and techniques used to solve mathematical models of fluid dynamics on digital computers. In recent years, chemical engineers have realized that, although establishing a relationship between reactor hardware and fluid dynamics is less central (compared to aerospace engineers) to their role, it is no less important. With the development of high performance computers and advances in numerical techniques and algorithms, chemical engineers have started exploiting the power of computational fluid dynamics tools. Considering the central role of reactors in chemical process industries, there is tremendous potential for applying these tools for better reactor engineering. If applied properly, computational flow modeling (CFM) may reduce development time, leading to reduced time to market, shorter payback time and better cash flow. It is, however, necessary to adapt CFD techniques and to develop a computational flow modeling approach to apply them to chemical reactor engineering. This book is written with the intention of assisting practicing engineers and researchers to develop such an approach. Individual aspects of chemical reactor engineering and computational flow modeling (CFM) are discussed and related in a coherent way to convey and clarify the potential of computational flow modeling for reactor engineering research and practice. The emphasis is not on providing a complete review but is on equipping the reader with adequate information and tips to undertake a complex flow-modeling project. The focus is on modeling fluid flows and developing tractable reactor engineering models. Numerical issues are dealt with in adequate detail to provide appreciation of the important aspects and to guide the development and incorporation of new models into available solvers. Readers interested in developing their own complete solvers may refer to specialized books on CFD (for example, Ferziger and Peric, 1995; Patankar, 1980).

The information in this book is organized to facilitate the central task of a reactor engineer, that is, relating reactor hardware to reactor performance. This chapter provides a brief introduction to the contents to be covered in detail in subsequent chapters. Here, the roles of flow modeling and computational flow modeling are discussed in the context of reactor engineering. Various aspects of chemical reaction and reactor engineering are discussed in Section 1.1 to clearly define the role of flow modeling in overall activity. Computational flow modeling, its advantages and limitations are discussed in Section 1.2. Introduction to the use of CFM for reactor engineering is given in Section 1.3. This chapter, as a whole, will be used to appreciate and identify the potential of CFM for reactor engineering.

The theoretical and numerical basis of computational flow modeling (CFM) is described in detail in Part II. The three major tasks involved in CFD, namely, mathematical modeling of fluid flows, numerical solution of model equations and computer implementation of numerical techniques are discussed. The discussion on mathematical modeling of fluid flows has been divided into four chapters (2 to 5). Basic governing equations (of mass, momentum and energy), ways of analysis and possible simplifications of these equations are discussed in Chapter 2. Formulation of different boundary conditions (inlet, outlet, walls, periodic/cyclic and so on) is also discussed. Most of the discussion is restricted to the modeling of Newtonian fluids (fluids exhibiting the linear dependence between strain rate and stress). In most cases, industrial reactors are operated under a turbulent flow regime. Introduction to turbulence and various approaches (direct numerical simulations or DNS, large eddy simulations or LES and Reynolds averaged Navier–Stokes equations or RANS simulations) to modeling turbulent flows are discussed in Chapter 3. Turbulence models based on the RANS approach are discussed in more detail, with special consideration to reactor engineering applications. For several industrial applications, multiphase reactors are used, which involves contacting more than one phase. Various approaches to modeling such multiphase flows are discussed in Chapter 4 with special emphasis on dispersed multiphase flows. The interactions between chemical reactions and fluid dynamics are discussed in Chapter 5.

Model equations governing flow processes relevant to reactor engineering applications are quite often complex, non-linear and coupled. More often than not, analytical solutions are not possible and numerical methods are required to obtain a solution to the model equations. The numerical methods relevant to solving model equations are discussed in Chapters 6 and 7. Chapter 6 covers use of the finite volume method to solve generic flow models. Various aspects of the finite volume method such as discretization schemes, grid arrangements, implementation of boundary conditions and algorithms for handling pressure–velocity coupling are discussed in detail. Applications of these methods to solve turbulent flows, multiphase flows and reactive flows are discussed in Chapter 7. Guidelines for making appropriate selection of the available techniques based on the objective at hand are discussed. Practical ways of estimating errors in numerical solutions of model equations are discussed. The methodology and the desired qualities of computational tools required to implement these numerical methods on a digital computer to solve model equations are discussed in Chapter 8.

Part III of the book discusses the overall methodology of using computational flow modeling for reactor engineering. The necessity of using a hierarchy of modeling tools and establishing a clear relationship between the objectives of reactor engineering and the computational flow model is illustrated with the help of examples. The importance of a physical understanding of the system for facilitating rational simplification of the problem, formulation of appropriate boundary conditions and identification of key issues is emphasized. The information discussed in Part I and Part II is used to evolve a systematic methodology for linking reactor hardware with reactor performance. The methodology is illustrated with the help of some practical examples.

Details of the application of computational flow modeling to different types of reactors are discussed in Part IV. A separate chapter is devoted to three major reactor types used in chemical industries, namely, stirred reactors, bubble column reactors and fluidized bed reactors. Applications to fixed bed reactors and other miscellaneous reactor types are briefly discussed in Chapter 13. Recent work on modeling the complex fluid dynamics in these reactors is critically reviewed. The modeling approaches and the flow results obtained therefrom are evaluated from the point of view of their application to reactor engineering. Limitations of the current state of knowledge in describing the complex underlying physics of some of the flows relevant to reactor engineering are discussed. Despite such limitations, suggestions are made for making the best use of these computational flow models for reactor engineering applications.

The Epilogue recapitulates the lessons learnt from our experience of applying computational flow modeling while addressing practical reactor engineering problems. The advantages of using CFM and the probable pit falls are re-emphasized. Some comments on future trends in computational flow modeling and its application by the chemical/reactor engineering community are included.

1.1. CHEMICAL REACTOR ENGINEERING (CRE)

Chemical reactor engineering activity is related to the engineering of chemical transformations. Chemical transformations or reactions can occur only if the reactant molecules are brought into molecular contact (mixed) under the appropriate environment (temperature and concentration fields, catalysts) for an adequate time. A process vessel which provides the necessary conditions to favor the desired reaction and allows for removal of products, is called a 'reactor'. A large variety of equipment

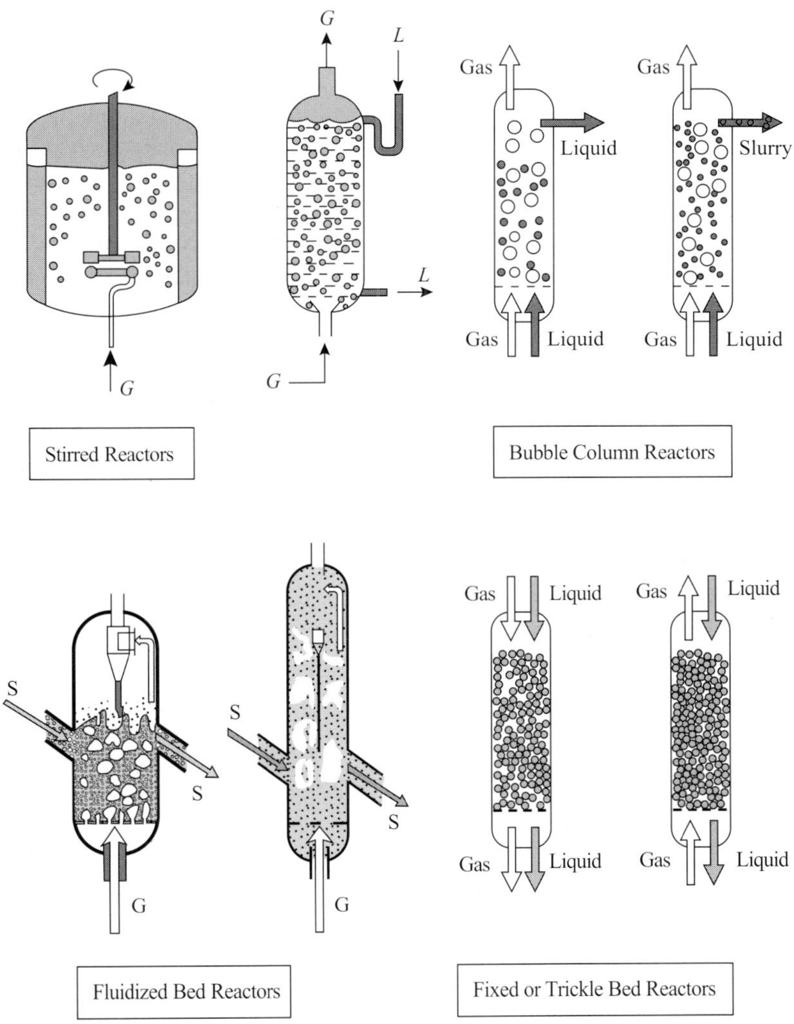

FIGURE 1.2 Commonly used reactor types.

is being used as reactors in practice. Some of the commonly used types of reactor are shown in Fig. 1.2. Although the reactors included in this figure show contacting of two phases (gas–liquid or gas–solid), similar equipment can also be used to carry out reactions involving a single phase (homogeneous reactions) or more than two phases. Several different versions of these four major reactor types are used in practice. By looking at these configurations, one can imagine the complexities of the underlying fluid dynamics in these equipments. A reactor engineer is faced with a host of questions when establishing a relationship between reactor hardware, operating protocol and reactor performance. In this section, some of these questions and the relevant tasks required of a reactor engineer are discussed briefly to bring out the role of flow modeling in the overall activity.

The major questions being faced by a reactor engineer can be grouped into three classes:

1. What chemical transformations are expected to occur?
2. How fast will these changes occur?
3. What is the best way to carry out these transformations?

The first question concerns thermodynamics and chemistry. Knowledge of chemistry and reaction mechanisms is helpful to identify the various possible chemical reactions. Thermodynamics provides models and tools to estimate free energies and heat of formations of chemical compounds from which the energetics of all the possible chemical reactions can be examined. These tools help a reactor engineer to identify thermodynamically more favorable operating conditions. The theories and modeling tools required to carry out these functions are fairly well developed and do not involve any consideration of actual reactor hardware and underlying fluid dynamics. These tools are, therefore, not discussed here. More information on these topics can be found in chemical engineering thermodynamics textbooks (for example, Smith and van Ness, 1959; Sandler, 1998). Thermodynamics provides tools to estimate physical properties (density, solubility, vapor pressure, heat capacity, conductivity, etc.) and the state of transforming species under operating conditions. This information is required for flow modeling. A brief discussion of these issues and the key references are given in Chapter 2.

The second question (estimating how fast the thermodynamically possible chemical transformations will occur) involves a knowledge of chemistry, reaction kinetics and various transport processes such as mixing, heat and mass transfer. Analysis of the transport processes and their interaction with chemical reactions can be quite difficult and is intimately connected to the underlying fluid dynamics. Such a combined analysis of chemical and physical processes constitutes the core of chemical reaction engineering. The overall framework of reaction engineering is briefly discussed here.

The first step in any reaction engineering analysis is formulating a mathematical framework to describe the rate (and mechanism) by which one chemical species is converted into another in the absence of any transport limitations (chemical kinetics). The rate is the mass, in moles of a species, transformed per unit time, while the mechanism is the sequence of individual chemical events, whose overall result produces the observed transformation. Though a knowledge of the mechanism is not necessary for reaction engineering, it is of great value in generalizing and systematizing the reaction kinetics. A knowledge of the rate of transformation, however, is essential for any reaction engineering activity. The rate of transforming one chemical species into another cannot be predicted with accuracy. It is a system specific quantity, which must be determined from experimental measurements. Recent advances in computational chemistry and molecular modeling have led to some successes in making *a priori* predictions of reaction kinetics (Senken, 1992; Dixon and Feller, 1999). However, in spite of such progress, most of the practical reaction engineering analysis will have to rely on experimental measurements of reaction kinetics (at least in the immediate to intermediate future).

Measuring the rate of chemical reactions in the laboratory is itself a specialized branch of science and engineering. The rate is formally defined as the change in moles of a component per unit time and per unit volume of reaction mixture. It is important that this rate is an intrinsic property of a given chemical system and is not a function of any physical process such as mixing or heat and mass transfer. Thus, the rate must be a local or point value referring to a differential volume of reaction mixture around that point. It is, therefore, essential to separate the effects of physical processes from the measured experimental data to extract information about the intrinsic reaction kinetics. It is a difficult task and has some parallels with the reactor engineering activity in reverse order (measurement of reactor performance–transport processes–fluid dynamics–intrinsic kinetics). More information about chemical kinetics and about laboratory reactors used to obtain intrinsic kinetics can be found in such textbooks as Smith (1970), Levenspiel (1972) and Doraiswamy and Sharma (1984). Assuming that such intrinsic rate data is available, chemical kineticists have developed a number of valuable generalizations to formulate rate expressions including those for catalytic reactions. Various textbooks cover aspects of chemical kinetics in detail (Smith, 1970; Levenspiel, 1972; Froment and Bischoff, 1984). Mathematical models (and corresponding model parameters) of intrinsic reaction kinetics will be assumed to be available to reactor engineers using this book.

Once the intrinsic kinetics is available, the production rate and composition of the products can be related, in principle, to the reactor volume, reactor configuration and mode of operation by solving mass, momentum and energy balances over the reactor. This is the central task of a reaction and reactor engineering activity. The difference between reaction engineering and reactor engineering lies in the treatment of momentum balances or in other words, of the underlying fluid dynamics. In reaction engineering, emphasis is given to reaction-related issues by making simplifications in the underlying fluid dynamics. In this way, it is possible to establish a relationship between the process design of a reactor and the performance of a reactor. Reactor engineering combines reaction engineering with the rigorous modeling of underlying fluid dynamics to establish a relationship between actual reactor hardware and its performance.

In order to understand these aspects, it may be useful to consider the operation of a single-phase reactor of arbitrary type. The microscopic mass balance of a reactant over an element of reactor volume (Fig. 1.3) can be written in the following general form applicable to any reactor type:

$$\begin{array}{l} \textit{accumulation of} \\ \textit{component } \phi \end{array} = \begin{array}{l} \textit{rate of change of} \\ \textit{component } \phi \textit{ due} \\ \textit{to convection} \end{array} + \begin{array}{l} \textit{rate of change of} \\ \textit{component } \phi \textit{ due} \\ \textit{to dispersion} \end{array} + \begin{array}{l} \textit{rate of change of} \\ \textit{component } \phi \textit{ due} \\ \textit{to reaction} \end{array} \qquad (1.1)$$

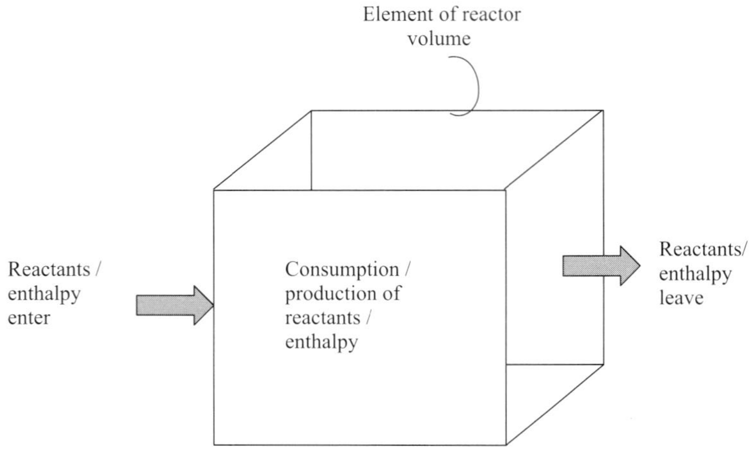

FIGURE 1.3 Conservation over element of reactor volume.

This general balance over an element of reactor volume can be represented mathematically as

$$\frac{\partial(\rho\phi)}{\partial t} + \frac{\partial(\rho U_i \phi)}{\partial x_i} = \frac{\partial}{\partial x_i}\left(\Gamma_\phi \frac{\partial \phi}{\partial x_i}\right) + S_\phi \qquad (1.2)$$

where ρ is the density of the fluid, ϕ is the concentration of any component, U_i is the local velocity in the x_i direction, Γ_ϕ is the effective diffusivity of ϕ and S_ϕ is a volumetric source term (rate of production of ϕ per unit volume) of ϕ. The terms appearing in Eq. (1.2) represent corresponding terms in Eq. (1.1). More complete and detailed mathematical formulation of general conservation-governing equations is discussed in Chapter 2 (and in references cited therein). It is important to remember that the source term, S_ϕ, will be equal to the rate based on intrinsic kinetics only if there is no physical resistance, i.e. there are no concentration or temperature gradients within the volume element under consideration. In non-isothermal operations, it is necessary to solve an energy balance equation along with the material balance equation. The form of the energy balance equation is similar to Eq. (1.2) with ϕ being an enthalpy content of the fluid. The material and energy balance equations are strongly coupled with each other since the source term of the energy balance equations depends on the rate of reaction. The material and energy balance equations are starting points for all reaction engineering analysis. Strictly speaking, it is necessary to know the velocity field at each point in the reactor in order to solve the material and energy balances discussed above. For any arbitrary reactor type, the velocity field can be predicted by solving corresponding momentum balance equations over the reactor. However, over the years, chemical reaction engineering analysis has made significant contributions by making judicious simplifications of these general equations to draw useful conclusions about the behavior of the reactor and to bring out the limiting behavior of reactors without solving the momentum balance equations.

The most fruitful and extensively used concept along these lines is the concept of an 'ideal' reactor. The simplest reactor, whose performance is governed by the so-called 'zero dimensional' equation is a 'completely mixed reactor'. The key assumption is that mixing in the reactor is complete, so that the properties of the

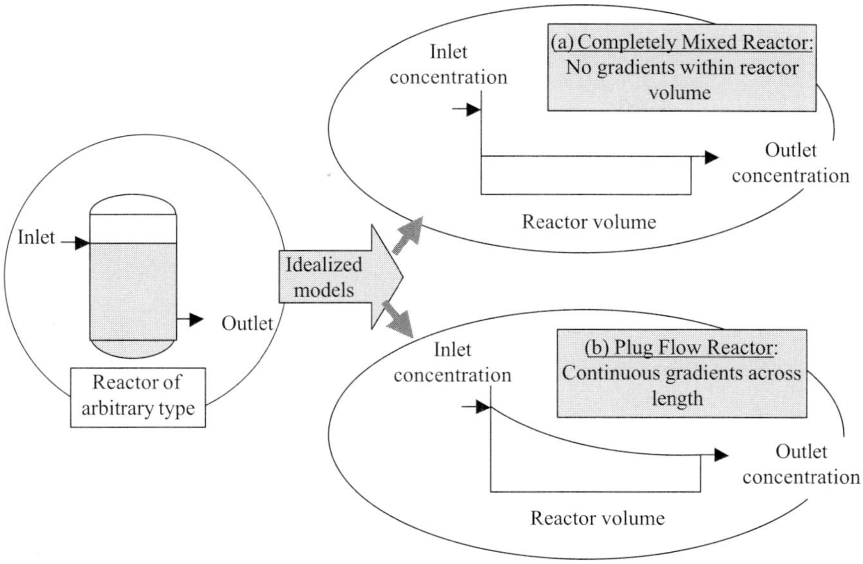

FIGURE 1.4 Ideal reactors.

reaction mixture are uniform in all parts of the reactor vessel and are, therefore, the same as those in the 'exit' stream (Fig. 1.4a). It means that mixing is much faster than the reaction and residence time based on net flow. It also means that the differential volume element chosen for the microscopic balance can cover the entire reactor. This greatly simplifies the governing equations and allows a reaction engineer to evaluate different modes of reactor operation (batch, semi-batch and continuous) and to understand the key features of the chemical system under investigation. An analysis based on a completely mixed reactor concept provides one of the limiting solutions for the performance expected from a practical reactor.

The other ideal reactor concept, known as a 'plug flow reactor' is based on a 'one dimensional' approximation of the material and energy balance equations. In an ideal plug flow reactor, unidirectional flow through the reactor is assumed (like flow through a tube). The velocity is assumed to be uniform over all the planes normal to the flow direction. In addition, it is assumed that no mixing takes place in the direction of flow and there are no gradients in the planes normal to the flow direction. These assumptions allow maximum variation of concentrations from reactor inlet to reactor outlet in contrast to the mixed reactor concept (Fig. 1.4b). Therefore, reaction engineering analysis of a reactor using this approximation provides a second limit on the performance expected from a practical reactor.

It may not be an exaggeration to say that carrying out the analysis of an industrial reactor using these concepts of ideal reactors is one of the most important tasks of a reactor engineer. Such an analysis results in a crucial understanding and useful information about the sensitivity of reactor performance to underlying mixing. It also helps to identify the characteristics of desirable mixing within the reactor. Such information can be very useful in optimizing reactor performance while carrying out multiple reactions and catalytic or autocatalytic reactions. In addition, ideal reactor concepts can be extensively used to understand the interaction between chemical and thermal processes. The simplifications in the underlying flow and mixing allow reactor

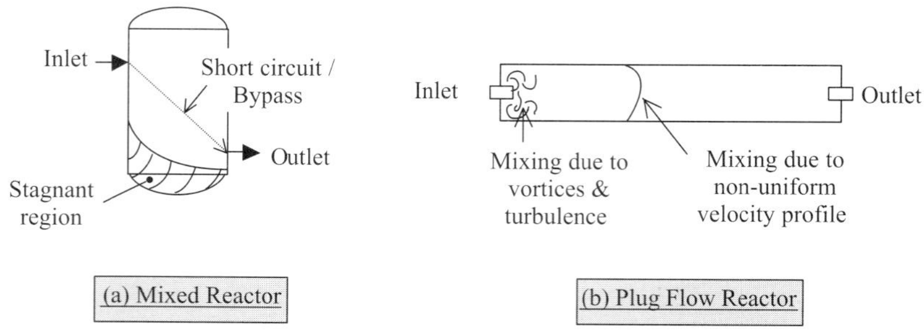

FIGURE 1.5 Deviations from ideal reactors.

engineers to carry out sophisticated operability and stability analysis of reactors (see reviews by Razon and Schmitz, 1987; Morbidelli and Carra, 1987). The concepts of ideal reactors have also been extensively used to understand the behavior of a variety of multiphase reactors, which are discussed a little later in this section.

After establishing such understanding and analysis of the reaction system using ideal reactor concepts, the next most important question facing the reactor engineer is to evaluate the consequences of the assumptions involved in the concepts of ideal reactors to estimate the behavior of an actual reactor. The mixing in an actual reactor may deviate significantly from that assumed for ideal reactors. This deviation can be caused by channeling of fluid, by recycling of fluid or by the formation of stagnant regions within the reactor (Fig. 1.5). If pockets of stagnant fluid exist within the reactor, conversion will approach the upper limit in these regions, but this fluid does not leave the reactor. The fed reactants will flow through the remaining volume of the reactor and, therefore, will have less time to react. The result will be an average conversion lower than that for the ideal reactor. A similar result may occur if there is a short-circuit and fluid by-passes through the reactor without mixing. Deviations from ideal plug flow behavior in the form of some mixing in the direction of flow (instead of no mixing) and incomplete mixing in the plane normal to the flow direction may also occur. Bypassing and short-circuiting may also occur in a plug flow reactor. If one knows the complete history of all the fluid elements (velocity and mixing) flowing through the reactor, it is possible to solve the differential material and energy balances to quantitatively estimate the influence of such non-ideal behavior. In the absence of such knowledge, reaction engineers have devised ingenious tools to quantify the effects of non-ideal behavior.

The residence time distribution (RTD) and state of mixedness are the two most important concepts used for such analysis. RTD, as the name suggests, indicates the spread of residence time experienced by different fluid elements while flowing through the reactor. The response data or measurements of the variation of reactor outlet concentration for the known change of inlet concentration can be used to estimate the RTD of a given reactor. For reactions following other than first-order kinetics, knowledge of RTD will not be sufficient to estimate the reactor performance. It is necessary to know the state of mixing between fluid elements of different ages flowing through the reactor. Here again, it may be noted that completely segregated (assuming no mixing between fluid elements of different ages) and completely mixed fluid elements constitute the two limiting solutions. Obtaining the RTD of an actual reactor and applying these two limiting assumptions to obtain the bounds on performance of the reactor is a practical method for a useful reaction engineering analysis.

Several sophisticated techniques and data analysis methodologies have been developed to measure the RTD of industrial reactors (see, for example, Shinnar, 1987). Various different types of models have been developed to interpret RTD data and to use it further to predict the influence of non-ideal behavior on reactor performance (Wen and Fan, 1975). Most of these models use ideal reactors as the building blocks (except the axial dispersion model). Combinations of these ideal reactors with or without by-pass and recycle are used to simulate observed RTD data. To select an appropriate model for a reactor, the actual flow pattern and its dependence on reactor hardware and operating protocol must be known. In the absence of detailed quantitative models to predict the flow patterns, selection of a model is often carried out based on a qualitative understanding of flow patterns and an analysis of observed RTD data. It must be remembered that more than one model may fit the observed RTD data. A general philosophy is to select the simplest model which adequately represents the physical phenomena occurring in the actual reactor.

A flow model representing the actual flow patterns and mixing within the reactor is necessary for realistic description of reactor behavior. Such a flow model can even be just a qualitative understanding to guide model development or can be a model with varying degrees of sophistication. For example, Van de Vusse (1962) proposed a model for simulating a stirred tank reactor based on intuitive understanding of flow generated by an impeller. He visualized the flow pattern within the stirred reactor in the form of three loops (Fig. 1.6a) and constructed a mixing model based on this visualization (Fig. 1.6b). Such a model can predict the influence of flow patterns within the reactor on reactor performance. In order to relate reactor configuration (for example, degree of baffling) and operating conditions (for example, impeller rotational speed) with reactor performance, it is necessary to establish a relationship between these hardware/operating parameters and model parameters. This can be accomplished by fitting model parameters to simulate the observed RTD experiments conducted with different reactor configurations. Results by Takamatsu and Sawada (1968) relating type of impeller, degree of baffling and impeller Reynolds number (rotational speed) are shown in Fig. 1.6c. Although these experimental findings do not provide any generalized correlations for stirred reactors, they were useful to indicate the general trends and, probably, were among the first attempts to directly connect the reactor hardware and operating conditions to reactor performance via a reactor model.

Several such models with increasing complexity were developed. Mann and his coworkers developed models based on 200 to 400 completely mixed zones or cells with finite exchange between neighboring reactors connected in such a way as to represent the actual flow generated by an impeller (Mann and Mavros, 1982; Wang and Mann, 1992). In these models (shown schematically in Fig. 1.7), they used experimental measurements of velocity data for prescribing flow through different zones. They were reasonably successful in simulating reactor performance for fast, mixing controlled reactions. However, an approach which relies either on RTD data and qualitative understanding of the flow patterns or on experimental measurements of flow, to establish the relationship between reactor hardware and a reactor model or reactor performance has obvious limitations for general application. The extent of non-ideality, and therefore model parameters, will change with the reactor scale and operating conditions. These studies have increasingly pointed out the need for more rigorous flow modeling of chemical reactors, even for single-phase flows.

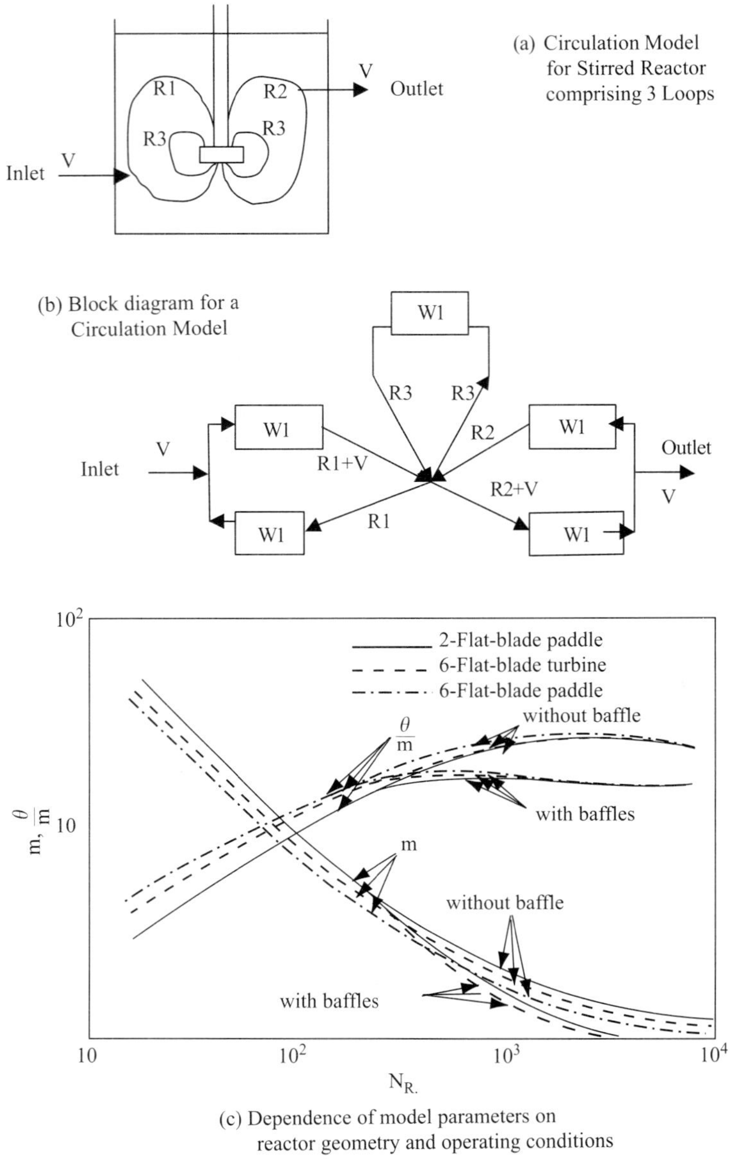

FIGURE 1.6 Flow model for stirred reactors (from Wen and Fan, 1975).

Discussions on flow modeling so far have been more or less restricted to single-phase reactors. However, in a broad range of application areas, multiple phases are involved in chemical reactions (see examples cited by Ramachandran and Choudhari, 1983; Doraiswamy and Sharma, 1984; Kunii and Levenspiel, 1991; Shah, 1991; Dudukovic *et al.*, 1999). Reactors carrying out such reactions are generically termed multiphase reactors. There are several types of multiphase reactors and several methods are available to classify these reactors. One of the simplest methods of

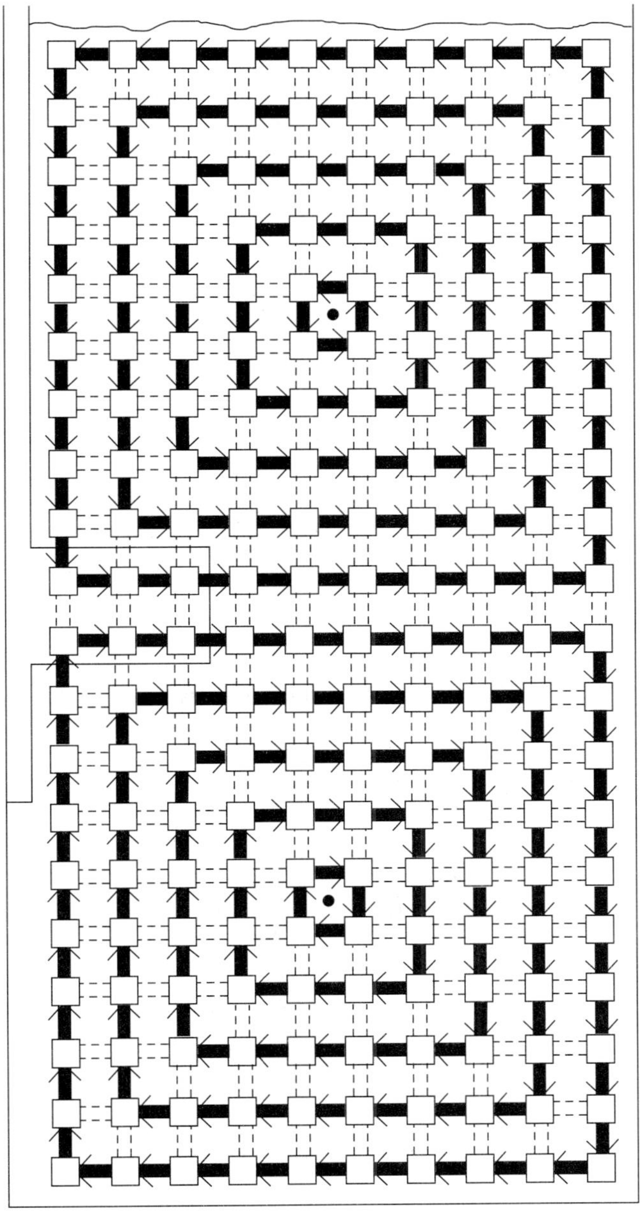

FIGURE 1.7 Network of zones model for stirred reactors: 2 x 10 x 10 network. Flow through different zones was specified using experimental measurements (from Mann and Mavros, 1982).

classification is based on the presence of phases, such as:

Gas–liquid reactors: Stirred reactors, bubble column reactors, packed columns, loop reactors.

Gas–liquid–solids reactors: Stirred slurry reactors, three-phase fluidized bed reactors (bubble column slurry reactors), packed bubble column reactors, trickle bed reactors, loop reactors.

Gas–solid reactors: Fluidized bed reactors, fixed bed reactors, moving bed reactors.

Some of these reactors are shown schematically in Fig. 1.2. The existence of multiple phases opens up a variety of choices in bringing these phases together to react. Questions like operability, and stability of the flow regime need to be answered. When reactants under operating conditions constitute more than one phase, the need to understand flows and quantitative predictions becomes even more crucial. Each of these reactors exhibits complex fluid dynamics and can be operated in a variety of flow regimes. For example, a gas–solid reactor can be operated in a variety of regimes ranging from a fixed bed reactor (where a bed of solid particles is stationary and gas flows through the voids between the solid particles) to a fast-fluidized bed reactor (where solid particles are transported by the gas phase). Bubble column reactors may be operated in a homogeneous regime (with more or less uniform bubbles and uniform gas volume fraction distribution within the reactor) or in a heterogeneous regime (with wide bubble size distribution and non-uniform gas volume fraction distribution within the column, which leads to significant internal re-circulation). Gas–liquid stirred reactors may also exhibit different flow regimes depending on the type, size and location of the impeller, gas flow rate and impeller speed. As an example, these flow regimes are illustrated schematically in Fig. 1.8. For very low impeller speeds, flow generated by rising gas bubbles dominates the flow generated by the impeller (Fig. 1.8a). In such cases, the gas phase behaves like a plug flow and the liquid phase may exhibit varying degrees of mixedness depending on relative time scales of mass transfer, reaction and mixing. For the other extreme, where flow is dominated by the impeller (Fig. 1.8e), gas bubbles follow liquid streamlines and are dispersed all over the reactor. In such a case, the gas phase behaves as if it is completely mixed. Thus, fluid dynamics and mixing in these multiphase reactors is determined by the operating flow regime. To select an appropriate reactor model, it is therefore essential to know the prevailing operating regime in the reactor (for the given hardware and operating conditions). Some generic multiphase flow regimes are shown in Fig. 1.9. It is not possible to discuss the intricacies of all of these reactors and their operating regimes here. More information may be obtained from the books cited above (and references cited therein) and from Chapters 10 to 13 of this book.

Apart from the flow regimes, several other issues control the performance of these multiphase reactors. For example, in a gas–liquid reactor, the rate of mass

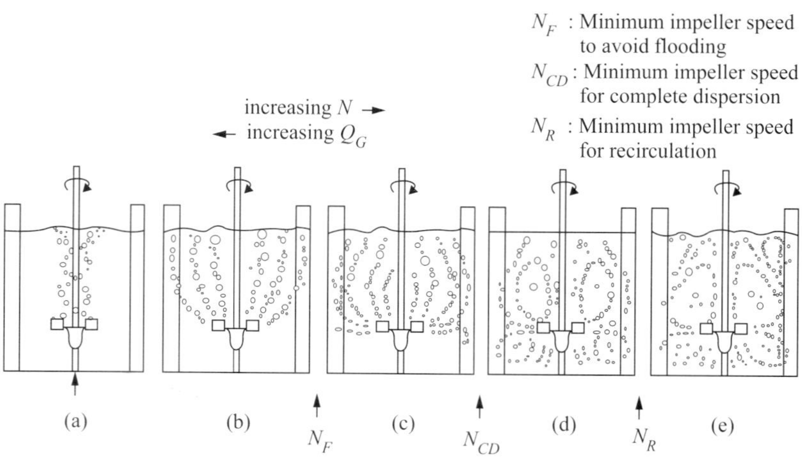

FIGURE 1.8 Flow regimes of gas–liquid stirred reactor (from Middleton, 1992).

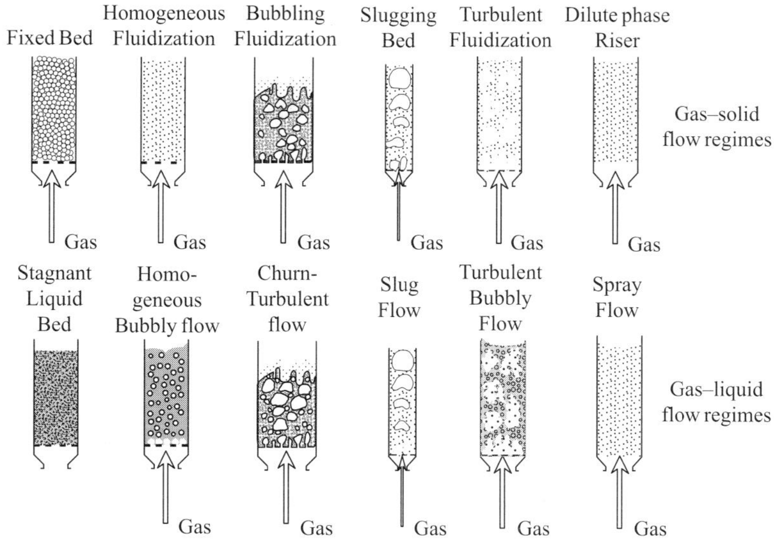

FIGURE 1.9 Some flow regimes of multiphase systems (from Krishna, 1994).

transfer from gas phase to liquid phase is determined by the mass transfer coefficient, interfacial area and concentration driving force for mass transfer. Each of these aspects is intimately related to the underlying fluid dynamics. Overall interfacial area and its distribution within the reactor is controlled by local gas volume fraction and local bubble size distribution. Local as well as global mean and turbulent flow fields control local bubble size. Local mass transfer coefficient is also dependent on local turbulence. Gas volume fraction and its distribution are also intimately related to overall fluid dynamics and interphase coupling of gas and liquid phases. One can imagine that the method of gas introduction (design of gas distributor, location, size and so on) can significantly affect the gas distribution and therefore the overall fluid dynamics of gas–liquid reactors. The flow field will also be very sensitive to reactor internals. This is not typical for gas–liquid reactors only but, in fact, is true for all multiphase reactors. For all multiphase reactors, hardware details and operating conditions have very significant impact on the resulting flow and therefore on the reactor performance. Even small-scale hardware details like the design of feed nozzles, gas distributors and baffles may have a dramatic influence on flow structure. The issues of scale-up and scale-down become much more complicated for multiphase reactors, because not all the relevant properties can be scaled proportionately. For example, in the case of gas–liquid–solid reactors, the relative dimensions of solid particles, gas bubbles and the reactor are bound to change with different reactor scales. Therefore, for reliable scale-up, interphase mass and heat transfer, which ultimately depends on microscopic fluid dynamics near the interface, overall flow patterns and mixing need to be analyzed at all the considered scales separately. An iterative methodology needs to be adopted to design most of these multiphase reactors. Without referring to any specific reactor type, the overall reactor engineering methodology for designing and validating an industrial reactor is shown in Fig. 1.10.

It is often necessary to carry out a small number of iterations over the sequence of steps shown in Fig. 1.10. Reaction engineering with idealized models is used to

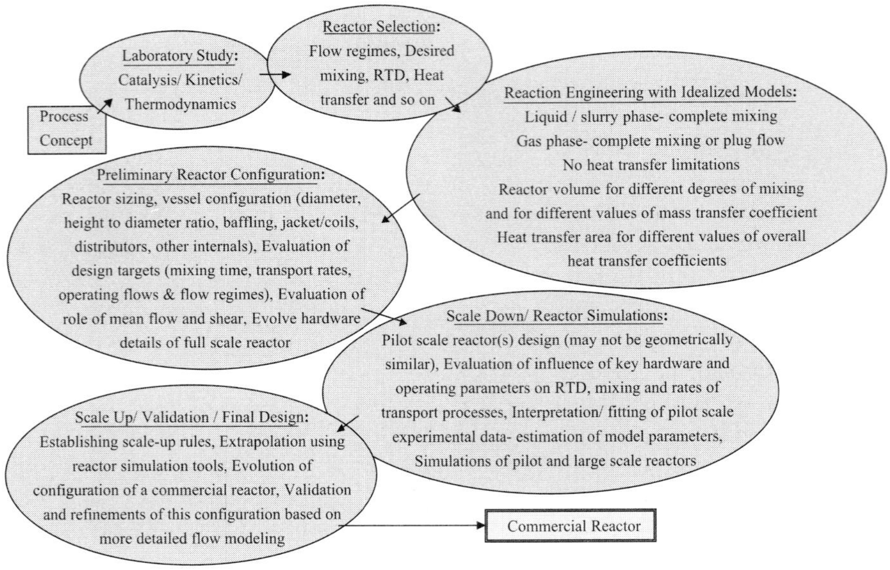

FIGURE 1.10 Methodology of reactor engineering.

understand the upper and lower bounds on performance and to identify important factors which control the performance. Studies using idealized models are also helpful in determining the desired performance targets for transport processes such as mixing, mass and heat transfer. Engineering creativity, experience and accumulated empirical information is generally used to evolve preliminary reactor configurations. Reactor simulation models are then developed to evaluate these different reactor configurations. Using a conventional methodology, a reactor engineer has to rely on experimental and semi-empirical tools to obtain a knowledge of fluid dynamics, which is essential when addressing many crucial design issues. Several reviews and books have been published which analyze published empirical correlations to estimate parameters necessary for the design and simulation of reactors (for example, see Shah, 1991: stirred reactors; Deckwer, 1991: bubble column reactors; Kunii and Levenspiel, 1991: fluidized bed reactors and so on). Wherever such available information is not adequate, experiments on pilot scale reactors are designed and carried out. The usefulness of pilot scale studies depends on how well these pilot reactors mimic the fluid dynamics and mixing in proposed large-scale reactors. For obvious reasons, such conventional design methods using empirical correlations have rather limited reliability. Uncertainty associated with extrapolation may be unacceptably high. Such methods are not able to relate details of reactor hardware with reactor performance. This non-capability narrows down the choice of reactor configurations. New ideas and new reactor configurations are often sidelined in favor of proven and conventional reactor types when there is an excessive reliance on empirical information and experiments.

To achieve and retain a competitive edge, it is becoming more and more important to address the third question 'what is the best way to carry out the desired transformation?' and to design the reactor hardware and operating protocols accordingly. To answer this question, it is necessary for a reactor engineer to establish accurately the relationship between reactor hardware and reactor performance. Computational flow modeling tools can make substantial contributions in establishing such a relationship.

CFM tools can accelerate the reactor engineering tasks shown in Fig. 1.10 with minimum experimentation on pilot scales and with enhanced confidence levels. Use of CFM for reactor engineering is briefly discussed in Section 1.3 and Parts III and IV of this book. Traditional methods of flow modeling, which rely either on experimental investigations or on making drastic simplifications of the flow problem to allow analytical solutions, are proving to be increasingly inadequate for this purpose. These methods have served us well to establish the reactor engineering profession, which has shaped the present chemical industry. However, to make further progress, it is essential to make creative use of the best possible tools available to reactor engineers. This is especially true for multiphase reactors. The ultimate wish of any reactor engineer is to know the complete history of all the fluid elements flowing through the reactor. This was considered hitherto not possible for most practical reactors. Recent advances in understanding the physics of flows, numerical techniques and digital computers can make tremendous contributions to realizing this ultimate wish by enabling simulations of complex flows in industrial equipment. Of course, there are still many unanswered questions and problems which need to be overcome to realize this dream. It is, however, important that reactor engineers are aware of the potential of these recent advances and are equipped to apply computational flow modeling tools creatively in their endeavors to develop innovative and better reactor hardware and operating protocols. The major features of these advances which are relevant to reactor engineering are discussed in the next section.

1.2. COMPUTATIONAL FLOW MODELING (CFM)

As mentioned in the previous section, the equations of fluid mechanics are analytically solvable for only a limited number of flows. Though known solutions are extremely useful in providing an understanding of the fluid dynamics, these rarely can be used for engineering analysis and design. Although many key ideas for the numerical solution of partial differential equations were established more than a century ago, these were of little use before the advent of digital computers. The revolution in the ability of computers to store the data and to perform algebraic operations has greatly accelerated the development of numerical techniques for the solution of equations of fluid mechanics. This has led to the birth of a specialized discipline called computational fluid dynamics (CFD). It takes little imagination to realize that rapid advances in computing power and CFD can make significant contributions to various engineering fields. Before we discuss applications to reactor engineering, various aspects of CFD and computational flow modeling (CFM) are introduced in this section.

CFD deals with the solution of fluid dynamic equations on digital computers and the related use of digital computers in fluid dynamic research. CFD requires relatively few restrictive assumptions and gives a complete description of the flow field for all variables. Quite complex configurations can be treated and the methods are relatively easy to apply. It can incorporate a variety of processes simultaneously. CFD simulations serve as a bridge between theory and reality. Simulations have the added advantage that diagnostic ‘probing’ of a computer simulation does not disturb the flow and normal operation! The detailed predicted flow field gives an accurate insight to the fluid behavior and can sometimes give information which cannot be obtained from experiments. CFD simulations may allow one to switch on and off various interactions included in the model to understand the relative contributions of each individual process, which is extremely difficult – if not impossible – to achieve in experiments. These simulations allow detailed analysis at an earlier stage in the design cycle, with less cost, with lower risk and in less time than experimental testing. It sounds almost too good to be true. Indeed, these advantages of CFD are conditional and may be realized only when the fluid dynamic equations are solved accurately, which is extremely difficult for most engineering flows of interest. It must be remembered that numerical simulations will always be approximate. There can be various reasons for differences between computed results and 'reality'. Errors are likely to arise from each part of the process used to generate numerical simulations:

- fluid dynamic equations;
- input data and boundary conditions;
- numerical methods and convergence;
- computational constraints;
- interpretation of results, and so on.

It is necessary to develop an appropriate methodology to harness the potential of CFD tools for engineering analysis and design despite some of the limitations. Computational flow modeling (CFM) includes such overall methodology and all the other activities required to use CFD to achieve the engineering objectives.

Computational flow modeling for reactor engineering requires broad-based expertise in process and reactor engineering and an in-depth understanding of various aspects of CFD, along with a generous dose of creativity. Activities involved in a typical computational flow-modeling project are shown in Fig. 1.11. The identification of objectives for flow modeling and the application of a validated CFD model to achieve the set objectives are discussed in the next section with specific reference to chemical reactor engineering. Other aspects of computational flow modeling are introduced in this section and are discussed in detail in Part II (Chapters 2 to 8) of this book.

After establishing the modeling goals, the starting point of any computational flow-modeling project is to develop a mathematical model (equations and boundary conditions) to describe the relevant flow phenomena. This involves a rigorous analysis of fluids and type of flow under consideration. The first step is the rheological characterization of fluids under consideration. For Newtonian fluids, the knowledge of fluid viscosity is sufficient to develop the governing fluid dynamic equations. For non-Newtonian and rheologically complex fluids, it may be necessary to characterize the behavior of the fluid by more than one parameter. In this book, scope is restricted to the analysis of Newtonian fluids. Once the viscosity is known, it is necessary to distinguish the type of flow to select or develop an appropriate flow model. Some of the types are as follows:

- compressible/incompressible;
- laminar/turbulent;
- steady/unsteady;
- isothermal/non-isothermal;
- passive/reactive;
- single phase/multiphase.

Each of these types will have special features. For example, unsteady flows may be either forced unsteady, like a flow generated by a rotating impeller, or inherently

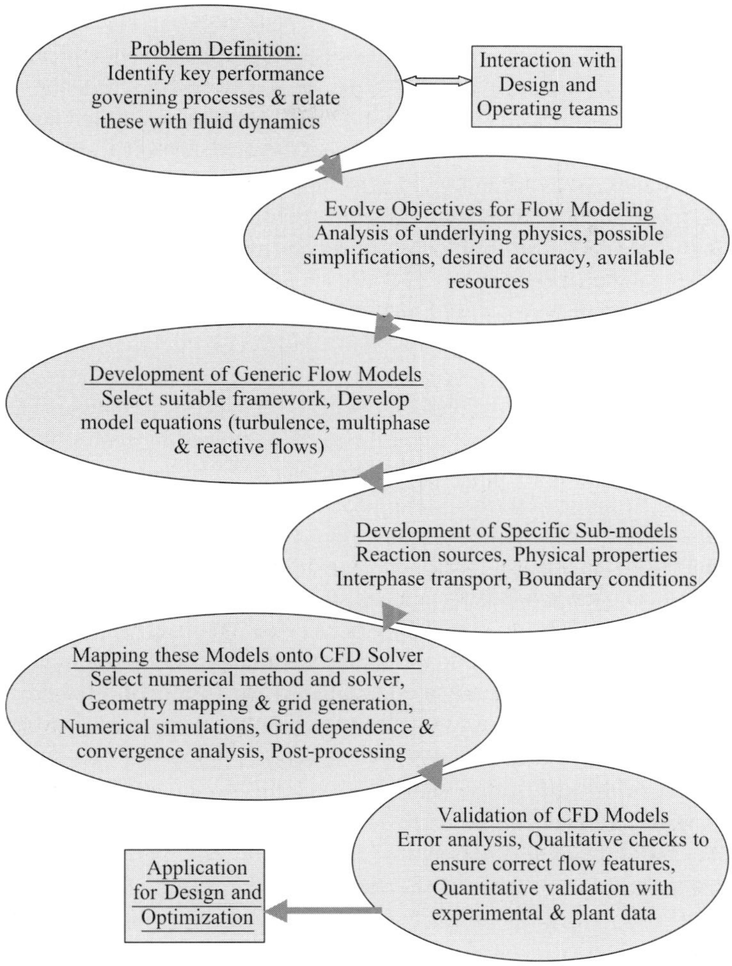

FIGURE 1.11 Typical flow modeling project.

unsteady, like vortex shedding behind a bluff body. Multiphase flows cover a very wide range of flows and have several sub-types depending on the nature of the phases (see for example, Fig. 1.9). For more details on multiphase reactors and commonly encountered flow regimes, refer to the discussion in Section 1.1.

Each of these different types of flows is governed by a set of equations having special features. It is essential to understand these features to select an appropriate numerical method for each of these types of equations. It must be remembered that the results of the CFD simulations can only be as good as the underlying mathematical model. Navier–Stokes equations rigorously represent the behavior of an incompressible Newtonian fluid as long as the continuum assumption is valid. As the complexity increases (such as turbulence or the existence of additional phases), the number of phenomena in a flow problem and the possible number of interactions between them increases at least quadratically. Each of these interactions needs to be represented and resolved numerically, which may put strain on (or may exceed) the available computational resources. One way to deal with the resolution limits and overall simulation costs is to isolate the expensive processes and to replace them with simplified phenomenological models. These phenomenologies are physically reasonable, approximate models. The parameters of such models are guesses, fits to experiments or calibrated from a more detailed but more restricted numerical model. Several phenomenological turbulence models are widely used in engineering analysis. It is essential to assess the underlying assumptions and limitations of such phenomenological models before they are used for a specific application. Similar or even more caution is necessary for multiphase flows and reactive turbulent flows. In many of these, even the underlying physics is not adequately understood and an engineer has to negotiate the challenges with inadequately validated phenomenological models. It must be remembered that if a phenomenological model is used to treat one of the controlling physical or fluid-dynamic processes in a simulation, the overall simulation is no more accurate than the phenomenology. It is necessary to evolve an appropriate methodology to use and to interpret the results obtained by such simulations.

Reactive flows have special problems over and above the complexities of underlying fluid dynamics. A reactor engineer wishes to know the history (path followed through the reactor and concentrations along the path) of all the fluid elements flowing through the reactor. This poses fundamental difficulties in modeling turbulent reactive flows. In a Eulerian approach (in which fluid motion and mixing is modeled using a stationary frame of reference), the location of a fluid element may be known exactly but its state (concentration) is not known accurately. In a Lagrangian approach (in which fluid motions and mixing is modeled using a frame of reference moving with the fluid particles), the state of the fluid element may be known accurately, however, its location is not known exactly. Several hybrid approaches have been used to find a way around this difficulty. Here again, similar to any phenomenological model, appropriate care needs to be taken when developing the model and interpreting its results. More detailed discussion of the modeling of fluid dynamics with special emphasis on turbulent flows, dispersed multiphase flows and reactive flows is given in Part II. Suggested references for developing model equations for other types of flows are also provided. Apart from the basic governing equations, it is necessary to develop specific sub-models for the system under consideration, such as models for variations of physical properties, interphase transport terms (momentum, heat and mass) and reaction sources.

After developing suitable governing equations, it is necessary to set the required boundary (and initial) conditions to solve these equations. This includes decisions about the extent of the solution domain. The process of isolating the system under consideration from its surrounding environment and specifying the outside influences in terms of boundary conditions may not be as straightforward as it sounds. In many cases, inappropriate decisions about the extent of the solution domain and the boundary conditions may give misleading results. Some examples of this are discussed in Chapter 2.

After finalizing the model equations and boundary conditions, the next task is to choose a suitable method to approximate the differential equations by a system of algebraic equations in terms of the variables at some discrete locations in space and time (called a discretization method). There are many such methods; the most important are finite difference (FD), finite volume (FV) and finite element (FE) methods. Other methods, such as spectral methods, boundary element methods or cellular automata are used, but these are generally restricted to special classes of problems. All methods yield the same solution if the grid (number of discrete locations used to represent the differential equations) is adequately fine. However, some methods are more suitable to particular classes of problems than others and the preference is often determined by ease of application, required computational resources and familiarity of the user.

Finite difference (FD) is probably the oldest method for the numerical solution of partial differential equations (PDEs). In this method, the solution domain is covered by a computational grid. At each grid point, the terms containing partial derivatives in the differential equation are approximated by expressions in terms of the variable values at grid nodes. This results in one algebraic equation per grid node, in which the variable value at that node and a certain number of neighboring nodes appear as unknowns. Taylor series expansions or polynomial fitting is used to obtain approximations for the first- and second-order derivatives. For simple geometry and structured grids (grid types are discussed later in this chapter and then in Part II), the FD method is very simple and effective. However, in finite difference methods, conservation is not enforced unless special care is taken. This is one of the major limitations of FD methods from the reactor engineering point of view. The restriction to simple geometry is also a significant disadvantage, since most industrial reactors have complex geometrical constructions.

In the finite element (FE) method, the solution domain is broken into discrete volumes or finite elements (generally unstructured; in 2D they are triangles or quadrilaterals and in 3D they are tetrahedra or hexahedra). The distinguishing feature of FE methods is that the equations are multiplied by a weight function before they are integrated over the entire domain. This approximation is then substituted into the weighted integral of the conservation law. By minimizing the residual, a set of non-linear algebraic equations is obtained. An important advantage of the FE method is its superior ability to deal with a solution domain having complex geometry. It is, however, difficult to develop computationally efficient solution methods for strongly coupled and non-linear equations using FE.

The finite volume (FV) method uses the integral form of the conservation equations as its starting point to ensure global conservation. The solution domain is again divided into number of computational cells (similar to FE). The differential equation is integrated over the volume of each computational cell to obtain the algebraic equations. Variable values are stored at the cell centers and interpolation is used to express variable values at cell faces in terms of the cell center values. Surface and volume integrals are approximated using suitable quadrature formulae. As a result, one obtains an algebraic equation per computational cell, in which a number of neighboring cell center values appear as unknowns. The FV methods can accommodate any type of grid and is, therefore, suitable for handling complex geometry. All terms that need to be approximated have physical meaning in the FV approach. Finite volume methods are, therefore, quite popular with engineers. The disadvantage, however, of FV methods is that higher than second-order approximations of gradient terms are difficult to implement, especially in 3D. Despite this, FV is the method of choice of many engineers and so it is, for this book. Detailed descriptions of various aspects of the FV method will be given in Part II (Chapters 6 and 7).

Having selected the numerical method, it is necessary to generate an appropriate grid, i.e. discrete representation of the solution domain and discrete locations at which variables are to be calculated. Two types of grids, namely structured and unstructured grids, are briefly discussed here. In a structured grid, there are families of grid lines

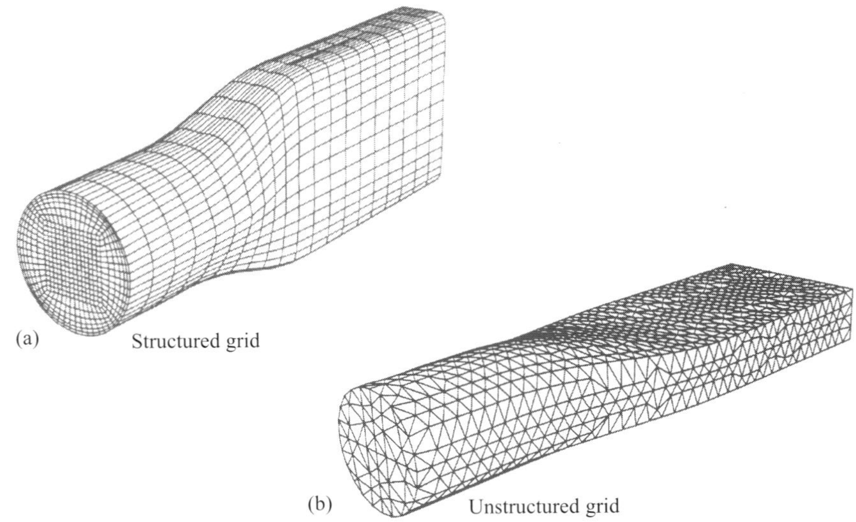

FIGURE 1.12 Examples of structured and unstructured grids.

following the constraint that grid lines of the same family do not cross each other and cross each member of the other families only once. The position of a grid point within the solution domain is, therefore, uniquely identified by a set of two (in 2D) or three (in 3D) indices. It is thus logically equivalent to a Cartesian grid. The properties of a structured grid can be exploited to develop very efficient solution techniques. One major disadvantage is the difficulty in controlling the grid distribution. In a structured grid, concentration of grid points in one region for more accuracy may unnecessarily lead to small spacing in other parts of the solution domain. A block-structured grid is used to eliminate or reduce this disadvantage. In a block-structured grid, the solution domain is divided into a number of blocks which may or may not overlap. Within each block, a structured grid is defined. This kind of grid is more flexible as it allows local (block-wise) grid refinement. For very complex geometry, unstructured grids, which can fit an arbitrary solution domain boundary, are used. In this case, there is no restriction on the shape of the control volume and the number of neighboring nodes. Triangles and quadrilaterals in 2D and tetrahedra or hexahedra in 3D are the most widely used grid shapes in practice. Examples of structured and unstructured grids are shown in Fig. 1.12. Unstructured grids can be refined locally and allow more control of the variation of aspect ratio, etc. The advantage of flexibility is often offset by the disadvantage of the irregularity of the data structure. The solvers for algebraic equation systems of unstructured grids are generally slower than those for structured grids. Methods of grid generation will not be covered in this book. Several excellent texts on grid generation are available (see for example, Thompson *et al.*, 1985; Arcilla *et al.*, 1991). Some discussion on assessing the quality of the generated grid and tips for rectifying observed deficiencies are given in Part II.

Following the choice of grid type, one has to select the approximations to be used in the discretization process. For the finite volume method, one has to select the methods of approximating surface and volume integrals. The choice of method of approximation influences the accuracy and computational costs. The number of nodes involved in approximation controls the memory requirements, speed of the code and difficulty in implementing the method in the computer program. More accurate approximation involves a larger computational molecule (more nodes) and gives fuller coefficient matrices. A judicious compromise between simplicity, ease of implementation, accuracy and computational efficiency has to be made. More discussion and details of choices with such a compromise in mind are given in Part II.

Discretization yields a large system of algebraic equations. The choice of solver depends on the type of flow, grid type and the size of the computational molecule (number of nodes appearing in each algebraic equation). A wide variety of solvers and accelerators are available; some of which are discussed in Part II. The set of algebraic equation is usually solved iteratively (so-called 'inner iterations'). The details of solvers of algebraic equations will not be discussed in this book. Interested readers may refer to specialized texts on these topics (for example, Press *et al.*, 1992; Fergizer and Peric, 1995). The 'outer iterations' involve repeating this process many times over to deal with the non-linearity and coupling among the model equations. Deciding when to stop the iterative process (convergence criterion) at each level is important, from both accuracy and efficiency points of view. These issues are also briefly discussed in Part II. Some tips for assessing the degree of overall convergence and tuning of solver parameters are also given.

Of course, before tuning the solver parameters, it is necessary to develop a computer program to implement the numerical techniques selected to solve the mathematical model. It takes an organized and dedicated effort to design an efficient and error-free computer program. After adequate testing, the program can be a valuable tool for engineers trying to understand and manipulate the complex fluid dynamics in industrial equipment. The steps in developing and testing the program are, therefore, of the utmost importance. It is difficult to discuss guidelines for the development of computer programs since this encompasses widely different issues. Patankar (1980) has listed some such suggestions in his book. In this book, it will be assumed that an error-free computer program, which takes care of grid generation and the solver part, is available to the reactor engineer. This assumption is not as unrealistic as it sounds, since there is an increasing tendency, especially in chemical process industries, to use commercially available CFD codes. This brief introduction and the discussion in Part II will allow chemical engineers to use such programs efficiently and effectively. The emphasis in this book is on discussions concerning the modeling of fluid flows relevant to chemical reactor engineers and on the usage of such tools to solve the model equations and reactor engineering problems.

The path of chemical reactor engineers, hoping to use CFD tools and programs to enhance the productivity of a reactor, is crowded by complex challenges offered by multiphase flows, turbulent flows, reactive flows, non-Newtonian flows and so on. Understanding CFD and having access to a CFD program is only part of the solution. It is necessary to appreciate various issues and make decisions about modeling strategies and the interpretation of results. It is necessary to devise an appropriate methodology to achieve reactor engineering objectives by creatively employing the best available knowledge and tools.

1.3. CFM FOR CRE

The Competitive edge of any reactor technology rests on how well the underlying flow processes are designed and operated. If the underlying flow processes are adequately studied and controlled, there is always scope for performance enhancement and for evolving innovative design solutions. There have been many instances in the past where innovative, clever analysis and engineering of flow processes have realized substantial enhancements even in so-called 'mature' technologies. One of the most striking examples of using a knowledge of fluid dynamics to substantially enhance the performance of a reactor is the development of the super-condensed mode of operation for the fluidized bed polymerization (of olefins) reactors. The capacity of such fluidized bed polyolefin reactors is constrained by the heat removal capacity of the reactor hardware and operating conditions. In the super-condensed mode of operation, a volatile liquid is injected into the fluidized bed to maximize the heat removal rates (via evaporation of the injected liquid). The realized increase in heat removal capacity obviously depends on a variety of parameters including location and method of liquid injection, distribution of the injected liquid, contact between liquid and suspended solid particles, and so on. In recent years, instead of injecting the gas and liquid mixture at the bottom of fluidized bed reactors, liquid is injected separately into the fluidized bed (Fig. 1.13). Detailed knowledge of complex multiphase fluid dynamics and mixing occurring in such complex equipment allows the correct selection of nozzle design and nozzle locations. Recent optimization efforts (Sinclair, 1995) based on rigorous experiments and modeling of multiphase fluid dynamics resulted in a substantial increase (by 50 to 100%) in the capacity of these polyolefin reactors (this means producing 50 000–100 000 tons per year of polyethylene more from the existing reactor)! Several such examples may be cited from the current process industry. Because of confidentiality issues, many of these examples may not be published in the open literature. Some of the examples are discussed in Chapter 9 to illustrate the methodology and more are discussed in Part IV of this book.

Performance enhancement of existing or new reactors may be realized in a variety of ways, such as:

(1) producing more from existing equipment;
(2) producing better quality products;
(3) reducing energy consumption;
(4) more safety of operations;
(5) reducing pollution, and so on.

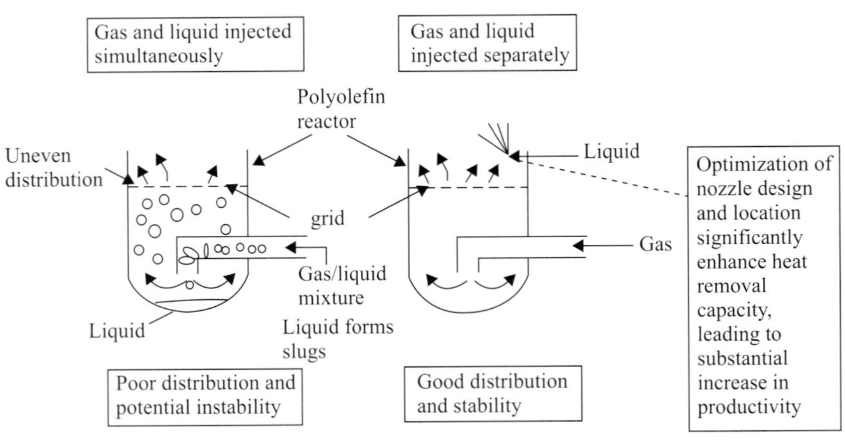

FIGURE 1.13 Super-condensed mode of olefin polymerization.

Realization of enhancement in any of the aspects mentioned above requires expertise from various fields ranging from chemistry and catalysis to reaction engineering, fluid dynamics, mixing and heat and mass transfer. For the given chemistry/ catalysts, the performance of industrial processes or equipment is a complex function of the underlying transport processes. These transport processes are in turn governed by the fluid dynamics and, therefore, by a number of design and operating parameters of the process equipment. Computational fluid dynamics has the potential to significantly enhance the power of reactor engineers to analyze, predict and manipulate the fluid dynamics of industrial reactors. It requires a broad-based knowledge of reactor engineering and computational fluid dynamics. A brief introduction to reaction and reactor engineering and computational fluid dynamics has been given in the previous sections. The essentials of harnessing the power of computational flow modeling to reactor engineering are briefly introduced here.

One of the most important steps in using CFM for reactor engineering is to clearly identify and define goals for modeling the flow. This appears to be quite obvious to everybody. Unfortunately, in practice, causes of many of the not so successful applications of CFM in reactor engineering can be traced to inadequate attention to this step. As emphasized repeatedly here, the performance of the reactor depends on a variety of complex issues and interactions among them. It is not always easy to understand and separate the role of flow modeling in the overall performance. The task of defining specific objectives of the flow model itself may involve several steps, some of which are discussed below.

Before defining the objectives of a flow model it is necessary to outline the performance objectives of the reactor in as much detail as possible. In both of these steps of outlining the objectives, it is useful to construct 'wish lists'. The first wish list should be about the overall performance of the reactor. This list may contain all the items by which reactor performance will be judged (some of this may be just qualitative). It is then necessary to re-examine such a list in light of the constraints posed by the given chemistry and catalysis of the system. A conventional reaction engineering model, which makes drastic simplifications of the underlying fluid dynamics, should be developed to understand the limiting behavior of the reactor. It is essential to carry out a detailed sensitivity analysis with respect to fluid dynamical issues using these performance models. This exercise often leads to identification of key processes governing the overall performance of the reactor. It is also often necessary to carry out simulations of the start-up and shutdown processes of continuous reactors in order to identify any specific requirements during those periods.

Identification of such key processes facilitates firming up the performance objectives for the reactor. These objectives in turn need to be related to the underlying fluid dynamics. This leads to the preparation of a second wish list about the flow and mixing characteristics of the reactor. After finalizing such a list, the reactor engineer has to visualize a reactor configuration (design and operating protocol) realizing as many items in the list as possible without violating the other constraints (economics, fabrication and so on). Here the role of flow modeling starts to become clearer. It must be pointed out here that though the steps discussed here appear sequential, it is often necessary to repeat the whole process to evolve an adequate understanding. During the process, interaction with design and operating teams is essential to capture the key issues.

The sensitivity analysis and wish list of underlying fluid dynamics allow one to quantitatively specify the objectives of the flow model. More often than not, reactor engineers are dealing with extremely complex phenomena in a complex geometry. It is, therefore, necessary to understand the limitations of the current knowledge of physics of flows and their implications on the predicted results. As a guideline, a chart, whose two axes correspond with the complexity in the flow physics and chemistry is shown in Fig. 1.14 (adapted from Boris, 1989). Two 'dimensions' of difficulty are considered in this figure: the complex physics of chemical kinetics and multiphase reactive flows along the horizontal axis and the geometry-related resolution-bound processes of fluid dynamics on the vertical axis. Each axis spans a range of difficulty from EASY to HARD. On the horizontal axis, an easy problem might involve single-phase laminar flow with simple, slow chemical reactions involving few species. A hard problem involves several reactions of dozens of species in turbulent, multiphase flows. These latter problems almost always need a phenomenological representation in a practical CFD model. Along the vertical axis, an easy problem might involve a one-dimensional flow simulation with simple geometry. A hard problem involves transient, three-dimensional flow simulation in a complex geometry exhibiting widely different spatial and temporal scales. As one can see from this figure, most of the 'CAN DO' region involves problems with either an easy physics component or an easy geometry component. The 'COULD DO' region is an extension of the 'CAN DO' region. If ample computational resources are available and the computations are directed at answering a few, specific questions, the 'COULD DO' region can be simulated. The outer regions of Fig. 1.14 involve problems with difficult physics and other computational aspects, so that detailed solution is considered impractical and phenomenology is invoked. Turbulent reactive flows (and multiphase flows) fall in this category. At this juncture, it is important to clearly understand the characteristics of the 'learning' versus 'simulation' model.

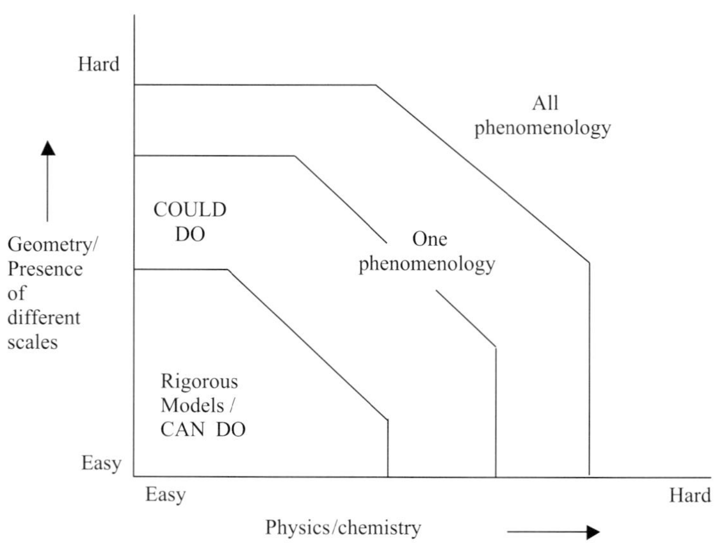

FIGURE 1.14 Interactions of fluid dynamics and chemistry (adapted from Boris, 1989).

It may be possible to develop a rigorous model of an idealized flow situation, which can be used as a 'learning' tool. For example, complex interactions between turbulence and chemical reactions can be simulated rigorously using the direct numerical simulation (DNS) approach. These simulations can provide a wealth of information about the interactions and can provide data which is very difficult to obtain from experiments. Therefore, although such simulations are restricted to low Reynolds number flows and simple geometry, these can lead to better understanding and insight into the development of better phenomenological models. The objectives when developing such a model, obviously, will be very different from those involved when simulating a reactive flow in an industrial reactor. The latter model has to relate the reactor hardware to the performance using the finite computational resources. Several such examples can be given, especially in multiphase flows, where the underlying physics is very complex. A clear understanding and visualization of the expected results and their proposed use is, therefore, essential for defining the objectives of the flow model.

After establishing the relationship between reactor performance and underlying flow as well as finalizing the objectives of the flow model, it is necessary to select an appropriate level of complexity of the flow model to meet these objectives. This includes not only the mathematical models of fluid flows but also various other aspects including the required degree of accuracy of predicted results and available resources. It is essential to give sufficient thought to the required degree of accuracy of the predictions of the flow model right at the first stage. The intended use of the results from the flow model dictates the required accuracy levels. The available time, expertise and computational facilities also need to be examined to define realistic goals. Thorough analysis of these issues will allow one to clearly define the goals of the flow model and in the process will also evolve a methodology for using the results from the flow model to achieve the performance objectives.

Various issues in the development of a flow model and its numerical simulation have been already discussed in the previous section. It will be useful to make a few comments on the validation of the simulated results and their use in reactor engineering. More details are discussed in Part III and Part IV. Even before validation, it is necessary to carry out a systematic error analysis of the generated computer simulations. The influence of numerical issues on the predicted results and errors in integral balances must be checked to ensure that they are within the acceptable tolerances. The simulated results must be examined and analyzed using the available post-processing tools. The results must be checked to verify whether the model has captured the major qualitative features of the flow such as shear layers and trailing vortices.

Whenever phenomenological models are used, further quantitative validation of simulated results is essential. Even if the objective of the flow model is to qualitatively screen possible alternative configurations, it is important to validate the simulations quantitatively to ensure that they have adequately captured the basic phenomena controlling the performance. In many cases, however, the data on flow fields generated in the industrial equipment is not available and is difficult to measure. Direct quantitative validation is not possible in such cases. The reactor engineer has to then assess the simulations based on indirect validations by comparing residence time distribution or mixing time, etc. It may often be necessary to independently validate various sub-models and the phenomenology incorporated in the overall flow model. Here again, emphasis should be on verifying whether the key processes are adequately simulated. Prior experience and engineering judgement should be used while interpreting simulation results, which are not grid independent.

Despite some of these limitations, computational flow modeling can prove to be a great help to the reactor engineer in realizing the 'wish lists'. The validated computational flow model can be used to evaluate new reactor concepts, designs and configurations. Again this is generally an iterative process. The reactor engineer has to 'dream up' configurations which are likely to satisfy the wish list. Detailed analysis of the simulations of a flow model will lead to identification of the most promising configuration among the investigated configurations, and to further ideas for evolving new reactor configurations. Though the major process improvements will, no doubt, stem from improved chemistry and catalysis, there is still tremendous scope for enhancing performance by harnessing computational flow modeling to reactor engineering. The following parts of the book discuss the basics of computational flow modeling and the overall methodology of using computational flow modeling for reactor engineering, illustrated with several case studies.

REFERENCES

Arcilla, A.S., Hauser, J., Eiseman, P.R. and Thompson, J.F. (1991), "Numerical Grid Generation in Computational Fluid Dynamics and Related Fields", North-Holland, Amsterdam.

Aris, R. (1965), "Introduction to the Analysis of Chemical Reactors", Prentice Hall, Englewood Cliff, NJ.

Boris, J.P. (1989), New directions in computational fluid dynamics, *Ann. Rev. Fluid Mech.*, **21**, 345–385.

Deckwer, W.D. (1991), "Bubble Column Reactors", Wiley, New York.

Dixon, D.A. and Feller, D. (1999), Computational chemistry and process design, *Chem. Eng. Sci.*, **54**, 1929–1939.

Doraiswamy, L.K. and Sharma, M.M. (1984), "Heterogeneous Reactions – Analysis Examples and Reactor Design", Vol. **2**, John Wiley & Sons, New York.

Dudukovic, M.P., Larachi, F. and Mills, P.L. (1999), Multiphase reactors – revisited, *Chem. Eng. Sci.*, **54**, 1975–1996.

Ferziger, J.H. and Peric, M. (1995), "Computational Methods for Fluid Dynamics", Springer Verlag, Berlin.

Froment, G.F. and Bischoff, K.B (1984), "Chemical Reactor Analysis and Design", John Wiley & Sons, New York.

Krishna, R. (1994), A systems approach to multiphase reactor selection, *Adv. Chem. Eng.*, **19**, 201–250.

Kunii, D. and Levenspiel, O. (1991), "Fluidization Engineering", John Wiley & Sons, New York.

Levenspiel O. (1972), "Chemical Reaction Engineering", 2nd edition, John Wiley & Sons, New York.

Mann, R. and Mavros, P. (1982) Proceedings of 4th European Conference in Mixing, p. 35.

Middleton, J.C. (1992), Gas–liquid dispersion and mixing, in "Mixing in the Process Industries", Butterworth-Heinemann, Woburn, MA.

Morbidelli, M. and Carra, S. (1987) Gas–Liquid Reactors, in "Chemical Reaction and Reactor Engineering", Vol. **26**, Marcel Dekker, New York.

Naumann, E.B. (1987), "Chemical Reactor Design", John Wiley and Sons, New York.

Patankar, S.V. (1980), "Numerical Heat Transfer and Fluid Flow", Hemisphere, Taylor & Francis Group, New York.

Press, W.H., Flannery, B.P., Teukolsky, S.A. and Velyerling, W.T. (1992), "Numerical Recipes – The Art of Scientific Computing (FORTRAN version)", Cambridge University Press, Cambridge.

Ramchandran, P.A. and Choudhari, R.V. (1983), "Three Phase Catalytic Reactors", Gordon and Breach, New York.

Razon, L.F. and Schmitz, R.A. (1987), Multiplicities and instabilities in chemically reacting systems – a review, *Chem. Eng. Sci.*, **42**(5), 1005–1047.

Sandler, S.I. (1998) "Chemical and Engineering Thermodynamics", 3rd edition, John Wiley & Sons, New York.

Senken, S.M. (1992), Detailed chemical kinetic modeling, *Adv. Chem. Eng.*, **18**, 95–196.

Shah, Y.T. (1991), Design parameters for mechanically agitated reactors, *Adv. Chem. Eng.*, **17**, 1–206.

Shinnar, R. (1987), Use of residence – and contact – time distribution in reactor design, in "Chemical Reaction and Reactor Engineering", Marcel Dekker, New York.

Sinclair, K.B. (1995), Third generation polyolefin technologies and their capabilities, Society of Plastics Engineers Polyolefins IXth International Conference, Texas USA.

Smith, J.M. (1970), "Chemical Engineering Kinetics", 2nd edition, McGraw Hill, New York.

Smith, J.M. and Van Ness, H.S. (1959), "An Introduction to Chemical Engineering Thermodynamics", 2nd edition, McGraw Hill, New York.

Takamatsu, T. and Sawada, T.J. (1968), *Jpn Assoc. Automatic Control Engrs*, **12**, 11.

Thompson, J.F., Warsi, Z.U.A. and Mastin, C.W. (1985), "Numerical Grid Generation", North-Holland, Amsterdam.

Van de Vusse, J.G. (1962), A new model for the stirred tank reactors, *Chem. Eng. Sci.*, **17**, 507.

Wang, Y.-D. and Mann, R. (1992), Partial segregation in stirred batch reactors, *Chem. Eng. Res. Des.*, **70A**, 282–290.

Wen, C.Y. and Fan L.T. (1975), "Models for flow systems and chemical reactors", Marcel Dekker, New York.

Westerterp, K.R., Van Swaaij, W.P.M. and Beenackers, A.A.C.M. (1984), "Chemical Reactor Design & Operation", 2nd edition, John Wiley & Sons, New York.

PART II
COMPUTATIONAL FLOW MODELING

2 MATHEMATICAL MODELING OF FLOW PROCESSES

A clear understanding and analysis of the role of flow processes in determining reactor performance leads to specific definitions of the objectives of the flow model. The next step is to develop a mathematical model for simulating flow processes occurring in the reactor, which will meet the defined objectives. Numerous types of chemical reactors, having different hardware configurations and modes of operation, are used in practice. More often than not, the flow processes occurring in these industrial reactors are turbulent and may involve more than one phase. It is, however, essential to understand the basics of mathematical modeling of single phase flow processes before one attempts to model complex flow processes occurring in industrial reactors. The scope of this chapter is restricted to discussing these basic aspects of mathematical modeling of single-phase flow processes. This chapter, thus, will form a basis for further discussions on the modeling of turbulent, multiphase and reactive flow processes (the following three chapters). This chapter is divided into three sections: governing equations, auxiliary equations and boundary conditions. A brief discussion and summary is provided at the end.

2.1. BASIC GOVERNING EQUATIONS

It is customary for chemical reactor engineers to start their analysis of flow processes occurring in a reactor with the formulation of species conservation equations along with the energy conservation equations. The reactor fluid dynamics is often simplified to avoid the need for solving momentum conservation equations. The model equations are often written in terms of molar concentrations of species and temperature. These equations are further simplified by assuming special conditions (such as mixing is much faster than reactions) to derive most of the commonly used reaction engineering models. As mentioned in Section 1.1, such simplifications have been extensively used to analyze the behavior of reactors. In order to further enhance our abilities to understand and control the flow processes occurring in reactors, it is necessary to provide a more rigorous treatment of momentum conservation and to consider mass, momentum and energy conservation equations simultaneously.

Any rigorous analysis of flow processes starts with the application of the universal laws of conservation of mass, momentum and energy. It may be of interest to point out that the conservation laws of momentum and energy may be derived from the homogeneity of space and time (Bird, 1998). It is very important to clearly identify and understand the implications of the underlying assumptions (both, explicit and implicit) when describing physical processes in mathematical equations. In this chapter, we will describe and discuss the basic governing equations based on these three laws for any continuous fluid. Without going into rigorous definition, an assumption of continuous fluid means that the 'mean free path' of the constituent molecules of the fluid is much smaller than the characteristic length scales of flow processes. For gases, the mean free path is of the order of 10^{-7} m and for liquids it is of the order of 10^{-10} m. Most flow processes which are of interest to reactor engineers can therefore be modeled using the continuous fluid approximation. Additional information about the governing equations may be found in Bird *et al.* (1960), Bird and Graham (1998) and Bird (1998). In addition to the basic governing equations developed from the universal laws, it is necessary to develop relevant constitutive equations and equations of state for the fluids under consideration to close the system of equations.

There are two approaches for deriving basic governing equations. In the Eulerian approach, an arbitrary control volume in a stationary reference frame is used to derive the basic governing equations. In an alternative, Lagrangian approach, equations are derived by considering a control volume (material volume) such that the velocity of the control volume surface always equals the local fluid velocity (Fig. 2.1). For single-phase flows, both the approaches give the same final form of the conservation equations (see Deen, 1998 for more discussion on different approaches to deriving conservation equations). These two approaches, however, offer different routes to simulate multiphase flow processes. Modeling multiphase flows and turbulent reactive flows based on these two approaches is discussed in Chapters 4 and 5 respectively. Basic governing equations for single-phase flow processes are discussed here.

2.1.1. Conservation of Mass

It is often suitable to write the mass conservation equations in terms of mass fractions of species rather than molar concentrations, especially for flow processes, where properties of the fluid may vary with composition and temperatures. The mass conservation equation for species k can therefore be written (in vector symbolism):

$$\frac{\partial}{\partial t}(\rho m_k) + \nabla \cdot (\rho U m_k) = -\nabla \cdot (j_k) + S_k \qquad (2.1)$$

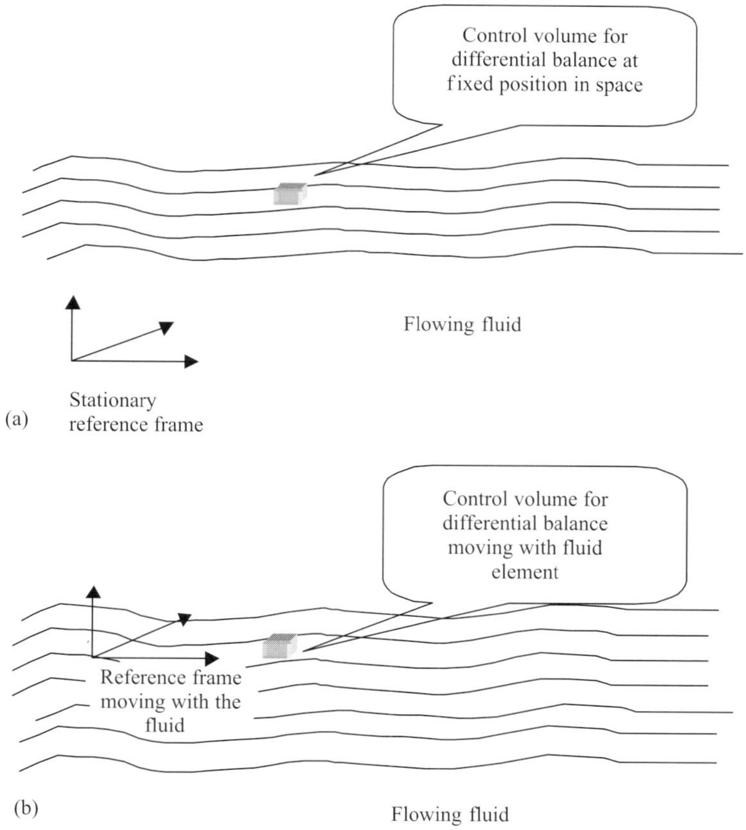

FIGURE 2.1 Two approaches to deriving governing equations. (a) Eulerian; (b) Lagrangian.

where t is time, ρ is fluid density, m_k is the mass fraction of species k and U is fluid velocity. The first term of the left-hand side of this equation represents accumulation of species k in a volume element and the second term represents change in species mass fraction due to convection. The first term of the right-hand side represents the change in species mass fraction due to the diffusive fluxes, j_k. S_k is the source of species k (net rate of production per unit volume). In principle, the volumetric source can be a rate of production or consumption due to chemical reactions or net exchange of species k with other phases, if present. For the non-reactive single-phase flows, source terms will be generally absent. Source term formulations for reactive flow processes will be discussed in Chapter 5. The velocity field may be known or may be obtained by solving momentum conservation equations (to be discussed later). It will be necessary to formulate equations for diffusive fluxes j_k in terms of species mass fractions in order to use these equations to determine the species concentration fields in the reactor.

In general, the diffusive mass flux is composed of diffusion due to concentration gradients (chemical potential gradients), diffusion due to thermal effects (Soret diffusion) and diffusion due to pressure and external forces. It is possible to include the full multicomponent model for concentration gradient driven diffusion (Taylor and Krishna, 1993; Bird, 1998). In most cases, in the absence of external forces, it is sufficient to use the following expression for diffusive flux:

$$J_k = -\rho D_{k\mathrm{m}} \nabla m_k - D_{k\mathrm{T}} \frac{\nabla T}{T} \tag{2.2}$$

where $D_{k\mathrm{m}}$ is the diffusion coefficient for species k in the mixture and $D_{k\mathrm{T}}$ is the thermal mass diffusion coefficient for species k. In many cases of interest to a reactor engineer, the contribution of thermal diffusion is very small compared to the diffusive flux due to concentration gradients. For modeling pressure-driven separation processes, it may be necessary to include the diffusive flux due to pressure (for more details, see Brodkey and Hershey, 1988; Bird, 1998). If only the most dominant term, the diffusion due to concentration gradient, is considered, the species conservation equations become

$$\frac{\partial}{\partial t}(\rho m_k) + \nabla \cdot (\rho U m_k) = \nabla \cdot (\rho D_{k\mathrm{m}} \nabla m_k) + S_k \tag{2.3}$$

The summation of species conservation equations of this form (written in terms of mass fractions) for all the species present in the continuous phase results in the overall mass conservation equations:

$$\frac{\partial}{\partial t}(\rho) + \nabla \cdot (\rho U) = \sum_k S_k \tag{2.4}$$

The terms appearing in this equation have similar significance to those of the individual species equations, that is, the first term represents accumulation, the second represents the contribution of convection and the third term represents the sum of volumetric sources of all the components. For single-phase flow processes, the summation of sources of all the components will be zero (since there cannot be net generation or destruction of mass).

The performance equations of ideal reactors, which are well known to any reactor engineer, are just the limiting cases of these general mass conservation equations. Possible simplifications of these equations are discussed later in the chapter after discussing all the governing equations and their dimensionless forms.

2.1.2. Conservation of Momentum

Application of the law of conservation of momentum yields a basic set of equations governing the motion of fluids, which are used to calculate velocity and pressure fields. Details of the derivation of momentum transport equations may be obtained from such textbooks as Bird *et al.* (1960), Brodkey and Hershey (1988) or Deen (1998). The governing equations can be written:

$$\frac{\partial}{\partial t}(\rho U) + \nabla \cdot (\rho U U) = -\nabla \cdot \pi + \rho g + F \tag{2.5}$$

In these equations, π is the molecular flux of momentum and g and F are gravitational acceleration and external body forces, respectively. The physical interpretation of the various terms appearing in these equations again follows similar lines: the first term is the rate of increase in momentum per unit volume; the second term represents change in momentum per unit volume, caused by convection; the fourth and fifth terms represent the gravitational force per unit volume and any other external force, if present, respectively. The third term represents molecular contributions, which include pressure and viscous force per unit volume and is given as

$$-\nabla \cdot \pi = -\nabla p + \nabla \cdot \tau \tag{2.6}$$

where p is pressure and τ is the viscous stress tensor. It may be noted that the second term of the right-hand side is not simple divergence because of the tensorial nature of τ.

In order to use these general momentum conservation equations to calculate the velocity field, it is necessary to express viscous stress terms in terms of the velocity field. The equations which relate the stress tensor to the motion of the continuous fluid are called constitutive equations or rheological equations of state. Although the governing momentum conservation equations are valid for all fluids, the constitutive equations, in general, vary from one fluid material to another and possibly also from one type of flow to another. Fluids, which follow Newton's law of viscosity (although it is referred to as a law, it is just an empirical proposition) are called Newtonian fluids. For such fluids, the viscous stress at a point is linearly dependent on the rates of strain (deformation) of the fluid. With this assumption, a general deformation law which relates stress tensor and velocity components can be written:

$$\tau_{ij} = \mu\left(\nabla U + \nabla U^{\mathrm{T}}\right) + \left(\kappa - \frac{2}{3}\mu\right)\delta_{ij}\left(\nabla \cdot U\right) \tag{2.7}$$

where δ_{ij} is the Kronecker delta ($\delta_{ij} = 1$ if $i = j$ and $\delta_{ij} = 0$ if $i \neq j$) function, μ is the coefficient of viscosity and κ is the coefficient of bulk viscosity. The superscript 'T' denotes the transpose of a tensor quantity. In general, it is believed that, except in the study of shock waves and in the absorption and attenuation of acoustic waves, it is convenient to ignore the coefficient of bulk viscosity. Substitution of Eq. (2.7) into Eq. (2.6) and Eq. (2.5) results in the complete momentum conservation equation. A special case of these momentum conservation equations for constant density and constant viscosity fluids is the famous Navier–Stokes equation, which provides the usual starting point for the analysis of flow processes (Bird *et al.*, 1960; Deen, 1998).

Any fluid, which does not obey Newton's law of viscosity, is called a non-Newtonian fluid. This class covers widely different materials/fluids, varying from those exhibiting slight deviation from Newtonian behavior to almost elastic solids. Fluids exhibiting slight deviations from Newtonian behavior, such as power law fluids (which exhibit a power law relationship between stress and strain) or Bingham plastic fluids (which require finite yield stress for flowing), can be readily modeled using the same framework. The molecular viscosity term appearing in Eq. (2.7) is replaced by an effective viscosity term, which may be a function of local stress and strain values. More complex behavior, e.g. viscoelastic behavior, requires a completely different framework to develop satisfactory constitutive equations. The subject of developing suitable constitutive equations for viscoelastic fluids, is extremely complex and outside the scope of this book. As stated earlier, the focus in this book is on simulating turbulent, multiphase and reactive flows. Detailed discussion about the rheology and motion of complex fluids can be found in Tanner (1985), Bird *et al.* (1987) (constitutive equations, models) and Crochet *et al.* (1984) (numerical simulation).

2.1.3. Conservation of Energy

Application of the law of conservation of energy can be used to derive transport equations for total energy. In order to derive an equation for internal energy, it is first necessary to derive a transport equation for mechanical energy, which can then be subtracted from the equation for total energy to obtain the governing equation for internal energy (Bird *et al.*, 1960; Bird, 1998). Without going into details, the equation for internal energy written in terms of static enthalpy is given below:

$$\frac{\partial}{\partial t}(\rho h) + \nabla \cdot (\rho U h) = -\nabla \cdot (q) + \frac{Dp}{Dt} - (\tau : \nabla U) - \nabla \cdot \left(\sum_k h_k j_k\right) + S_h \tag{2.8}$$

Here h is an enthalpy, which is defined as

$$h = \sum_k m_k h_k \quad \because \quad h_k = \int_{T_{\text{ref}}}^{T} C_{\text{p}k}\, dT \tag{2.9}$$

where T_{ref} is a reference temperature and $C_{\text{p}k}$ is the specific heat of species k, at constant pressure. q is a flux of enthalpy. The first and second terms of the energy conservation equation represent accumulation and change of enthalpy due to convection. The third term represents change in the enthalpy due to conduction. The fourth and fifth terms represent reversible and irreversible change in the enthalpy due to pressure and viscous dissipation, respectively. The sixth term accounts for changes in enthalpy due to diffusive mass fluxes and the final term is the volumetric source of enthalpy (due to say, chemical reactions). In the energy conservation equation, the flux of enthalpy, q can be written in terms of temperature gradient as

$$q = -k\nabla T \tag{2.10}$$

where k is thermal conductivity of the fluid.

The energy conservation equation is intimately linked to momentum conservation equations via the fourth and fifth terms. For most reacting systems, the contribution of energy released or absorbed by chemical reactions usually dominates the other terms originating from pressure and viscous effects. For highly viscous flows with low heats of reaction, it may be important to consider the viscous heating terms. An order of magnitude analysis is often used to examine the relative importance of different terms.

These equations have general applicability for any continuous medium and are valid for any co-ordinate system. Additional information about the formulations of basic governing equations can be found in Bird *et al.* (1960).

2.1.4. Analysis/Simplification of Governing Equations

A reactor engineer has to evaluate and analyze various terms appearing in the basic governing equations to explore the possibilities of simplifying them and tailoring them to suit the needs of the problem under consideration. It is often useful and instructive to re-write the governing equations in non-dimensional form by using characteristic reference scales (length, velocity, time, temperature and so on). The dimensionless form allows one to identify major factors governing the flow process. The choice of characteristic reference scales is obvious in simple flows (for example, average velocity, geometric length scale of the equipment). Use of such reference scales leads to a dimensionless form of governing equations containing some characteristic dimensionless numbers.

By examining these characteristic dimensionless numbers, it is possible to appreciate possible interactions of different processes (convection, diffusion, reaction and so on) and to simplify the governing equations accordingly. A typical dimensionless form of the governing equation can be written (for a general variable, ϕ):

$$\left(\frac{\rho_r\phi_r}{t_r}\right)\frac{\partial}{\partial t}(\rho\phi)+\left(\frac{\rho_r U_r\phi_r}{L_r}\right)\nabla\cdot(\rho U\phi)=\left(\frac{\Gamma_r\rho_r\phi_r}{L_r^2}\right)\nabla\cdot(j_\phi)+\left(\frac{\rho_r\phi_r}{t_r}\right)S_k \tag{2.11}$$

where the subscript 'r' indicates characteristic values (or reference values) used to make the governing equations dimensionless. Γ_r is the effective diffusion coefficient of variable ϕ. All the symbols appearing without this subscript denote dimensionless quantities. If the characteristic time scale, t_r is defined as the ratio of characteristic length (L_r) and velocity (U_r) scales, the dimensionless form of the equation can be rewritten:

$$\frac{\partial}{\partial t}(\rho\phi)+\nabla\cdot(\rho U\phi)=\left(\frac{\Gamma_r}{U_r L_r}\right)\nabla\cdot(j_\phi)+S_k \tag{2.12}$$

The dimensionless form of the equation contains one dimensionless parameter as a multiplier of the first term of the right-hand side and maybe some additional dimensionless parameters, which may appear within the dimensionless source term, S_k. Depending on the general variable, ϕ, the effective diffusion coefficient, Γ_r appearing in this dimensionless number will be different, leading to different dimensionless numbers. For the species mass fraction, momentum and enthalpy transport equations, the effective diffusion coefficient will be molecular diffusion coefficient, the kinematic viscosity of the fluid and the thermal diffusivity of the fluid respectively. The corresponding dimensionless numbers are, therefore, defined as follows.

Reynolds number, Re: may be interpreted as the ratio of the convective transport to the molecular transport of momentum or as the ratio of the inertial to viscous forces:

$$\mathrm{Re}=\frac{L_r U_r}{(\mu_r/\rho_r)} \tag{2.13}$$

Examination of the relevant dimensionless numbers, with reference to specific characteristics of the problem under consideration, is useful for simplifying the governing equations. For example, for very high speed flows, the reciprocal of the Reynolds number tends to zero and it may be reasonable to ignore viscous stress terms in the momentum conservation equations. Under these conditions, momentum conservation equations reduce to well-known Euler equations. Aerospace engineers have used this simplification extensively for simulating high speed flows around complex shaped objects. On the other hand, when the Reynolds number is small (that is, when flow velocity or the size of the equipment is very small or the fluid is very viscous), the convective or inertial terms in the Navier–Stokes equations can be neglected. This approximation leads to well-known creeping flow equations.

Peclet Number, Pe: dimensionless number appearing in enthalpy or species mass conservation equations (defined for heat transfer and mass transfer, respectively). It is interpreted again as the ratio of the convective transport to the molecular transport and is defined as

$$\mathrm{Pe}_{\mathrm{heat}} = \frac{L_r U_r}{\left(k_r/\rho C_{\mathrm{pr}}\right)} \quad \text{and} \quad \mathrm{Pe}_{\mathrm{mass}} = \frac{L_r U_r}{D_r} \tag{2.14}$$

If these Peclet numbers are divided by the Reynolds number, the resulting dimensionless numbers are called the Pradtl number, Pr and Schmidt number, Sc, respectively. The Prandtl number (Pr) is the ratio of momentum diffusivity and thermal diffusivity. The Schmidt number (Sc) is the ratio of momentum diffusivity and mass diffusivity. These five dimensionless numbers can convey very useful information about the relative contributions of convective and molecular transport and relative magnitudes of momentum, heat and mass transfer.

It must be noted that apart from these five dimensionless numbers, some additional dimensional parameters may appear in the dimensionless source terms. The source terms appearing in basic conservation equations are made dimensionless by dividing the reference source term, S_r defined as

$$S_r = \frac{\rho_r U_r \phi_r}{L_r} \tag{2.15}$$

The dimensionless source term essentially represents the ratio of generation to convection. For various generation terms, several additional dimensionless numbers may be defined. For example, if the generation of momentum due to gravitational forces is considered, a dimensionless number, called as the Froude number (Fr), is defined as the ratio of convection to gravitational factors. The dimensionless numbers discussed here along with other dimensionless numbers are listed in Table 2.1 together with their physical interpretation.

Apart from analyzing the relative contributions of various transport and generation mechanisms, the reactor engineer has to use basic engineering judgement to evolve suitable simplifications of the mathematical model. For example, when the flow under consideration has a predominant direction and the variation of geometry is gradual, it is possible to use so called 'boundary layer approximations'. In such cases, the flow is influenced mainly by what is happening upstream. Special, efficient methods have been developed to solve such specific simplified forms of the equations. Various possibilities for simplification, for example ignoring the variation of fluid properties such as density, viscosity, heat capacity etc., need to be evaluated by considering the possible implications on the application of the model. Compressibility effects may be neglected when the characteristic velocity of the fluid is much smaller than the speed of sound in that fluid.

The basic governing equations, written in a form suitable for any co-ordinate system, are useful for understanding the basic concepts and significance of various terms. It is, however, necessary to rewrite these equations, after considering the possible simplifications, for a specific co-ordinate system appropriate to the problem under consideration. Cartesian and cylindrical co-ordinate systems are the most commonly used systems for analyzing flow processes in simple geometry. The basic governing equations incorporating the relevant constitutive relationships (for Newtonian fluids)

TABLE 2.1 Dimensionless Numbers

Name	Symbol	Definition	Physical Significance
Reynolds number	Re	$\mathrm{Re} = \frac{\rho_r L_r V_r}{\mu_r}$	Ratio of inertial forces to viscous forces; Ratio of momentum transfer by convection and by molecular action of viscosity
Peclet number	Pe	$\mathrm{Pe} = \frac{\rho_r C_p L_r V_r}{k}$ or $\frac{L_r V}{D}$	Ratio of convective transport to molecular transport (of energy or mass)
Prandtl number	Pr	$\mathrm{Pr} = \frac{C_p \mu}{k}$	Ratio of momentum diffusivity to thermal diffusivity
Schmidt number	Sc	$\mathrm{Sc} = \frac{\mu}{\rho D}$	Ratio of momentum diffusivity to mass diffusivity
Nusselt number or Sherwood number	Nu or Sh	$\mathrm{Nu} = \frac{hL}{k}$ $\mathrm{Sh} = \frac{k_M L}{D}$	Ratio of total transfer to molecular transfer (of energy or mass)
Damkohler number	Da_1	$\frac{L K_n C_A^{n-1}}{U}$	Ratio of convective time scale to reaction time scale; ratio of convective transport to rate of generation due to chemical reaction
Damkohler number	Da_2	$\frac{L^2 K_n C_A^{n-1}}{D}$	Ratio of diffusion time scale to reaction time scale; ratio of diffusive transport to rate of generation due to chemical reaction
Stanton number	St	$\frac{h}{C_p \rho U}$ or $\frac{k_{L,\text{ave}}}{U_{z,\text{ave}}}$	Ratio of interface transport to bulk transport
Euler number	Eu	$\frac{p}{(\rho U^2)}$	Ratio of pressure forces to inertial forces
Froude number	Fr	$\frac{U^2}{(Lg)}$	Ratio of inertial forces to gravitational forces
Lewis number	Le	$\frac{k}{\rho C_p D}$	Ratio of thermal diffusivity to mass diffusivity
Weber number	We	$\frac{U^2 L \rho}{\sigma}$	Ratio of inertial to surface forces

For more discussion on dimensionless numbers relevant for flow process, see Bird *et al.* (1960) and Brodkey and Hershey (1988).

written in cylindrical co-ordinates are listed in Table 2.2. To model flow processes in complex process equipment, it may be necessary to use a more general co-ordinate system. It is possible to transform the equations listed in Table 2.2 into any such suitable co-ordinate systems. Anderson *et al.* (1984) listed governing equations applicable to any orthogonal curvilinear co-ordinates.

TABLE 2.2 Governing Equations in Cylindrical Co-ordinates

$$\frac{\partial(\rho\phi)}{\partial t}+\frac{1}{r}\frac{\partial}{\partial r}(\rho rU\phi)+\frac{1}{r}\frac{\partial}{\partial\theta}(\rho V\phi)+\frac{\partial}{\partial z}(\rho W\phi)$$
$$=\frac{1}{r}\frac{\partial}{\partial r}\left(\Gamma_\phi r\frac{\partial\phi}{\partial r}\right)+\frac{1}{r}\frac{\partial}{\partial\theta}\left(\frac{\Gamma_\phi}{r}\frac{\partial\phi}{\partial\theta}\right)+\frac{\partial}{\partial z}\left(\Gamma_\phi\frac{\partial\phi}{\partial z}\right)+S_\phi$$

ϕ	Γ_ϕ	S_ϕ
1 (continuity)	0	0
U (r momentum)	μ	$-\frac{\partial p}{\partial r}+\frac{1}{r}\frac{\partial}{\partial r}\left(\Gamma_\phi r\frac{\partial U}{\partial r}\right)+\frac{1}{r}\frac{\partial}{\partial\theta}\left(\Gamma_\phi r\frac{\partial(V/r)}{\partial r}\right)$ $+\frac{\partial}{\partial z}\left(\Gamma_\phi\frac{\partial W}{\partial r}\right)-\frac{2\Gamma_\phi}{r^2}\frac{\partial V}{\partial\theta}-\frac{2\Gamma_\phi U}{r^2}+\frac{\rho V^2}{r}$
V (θ momentum)	μ	$-\frac{1}{r}\frac{\partial p}{\partial\theta}+\frac{1}{r}\frac{\partial}{\partial r}\left(\Gamma_\phi\frac{\partial U}{\partial\theta}\right)+\frac{1}{r}\frac{\partial}{\partial\theta}\left(\frac{\Gamma_\phi}{r}\frac{\partial V}{\partial\theta}\right)+\frac{\partial}{\partial z}\left(\frac{\Gamma_\phi}{r}\frac{\partial W}{\partial\theta}\right)$ $+\Gamma_\phi\frac{\partial(V/r)}{\partial r}-\frac{1}{r}\frac{\partial}{\partial r}(\Gamma_\phi V)-\frac{\rho UV}{r}+\frac{\Gamma_\phi}{r^2}\frac{\partial U}{\partial\theta}+\frac{1}{r}\frac{\partial}{\partial\theta}\left(\frac{2\Gamma_\phi U}{r}\right)$
W (z momentum)	μ	$-\frac{\partial p}{\partial z}+\frac{1}{r}\frac{\partial}{\partial r}\left(\Gamma_\phi r\frac{\partial U}{\partial z}\right)+\frac{1}{r}\frac{\partial}{\partial\theta}\left(\Gamma_\phi\frac{\partial V}{\partial z}\right)+\frac{\partial}{\partial z}\left(\Gamma_\phi\frac{\partial W}{\partial z}\right)$

U: Radial velocity component
V: Tangential velocity component
W: Axial velocity component

After finalizing the governing equations, it is necessary to provide auxiliary equations to estimate fluid properties and to specify appropriate initial and boundary conditions. These aspects are discussed in the next section.

2.2. AUXILIARY EQUATIONS

To close the set of model equations, it is necessary to specify equations to prescribe or describe fluid density and other fluid properties such as viscosity, diffusivity, thermal conductivity and heat capacity. It is possible to treat these properties either as constants or as functions of thermodynamic variables and/or compositions. For example, the dependence of fluid density on composition, temperature and pressure can be described by the following equation:

$$\rho=\frac{1}{\sum m_k/\rho_k}\quad\because\quad\rho_k=f_k(p,T)\tag{2.16}$$

For ideal gases, it is possible to write component density, ρ_k in terms of the molecular weight of component k, temperature, operating pressure and universal gas constant. For non-ideal fluids, one can use empirical correlations to represent variations of fluid density with temperature. The values of fluid viscosity, thermal conductivity and molecular diffusivity can be estimated using kinetic theory (Hirschfelder *et al.*, 1964). Kinetic theory allows one to estimate variations of these properties with temperature and pressure. Sometimes it is necessary to use empirical or semi-empirical formulae to estimate these properties while solving the basic conservation equations. For multicomponent flows, it is customary to use mixture properties as a mass fraction weighted average of the individual component properties, such as

$$\mu = \sum_k m_k \mu_k \qquad k = \sum_k m_k k_k \qquad C_{\rm p} = \sum_k m_k C_{{\rm p}k} \tag{2.17}$$

It is possible to use alternative formulations considering mole fractions rather than mass fractions. For most cases, mass fraction formulations will be adequate. An estimation of the diffusion coefficient (of component k) in a multicomponent mixture ($D_{k\rm m}$), however, is not straightforward. For mixtures of ideal gases, the diffusion coefficient in a mixture can be estimated as (Hines and Maddox, 1985)

$$D_{k\rm m} = \frac{1 - X_k}{\sum\limits_{j,j\neq k} X_j / D_{kj}} \tag{2.18}$$

where X_k is the mole fraction of component k and D_{k_j} is a binary diffusion coefficient for species k in species j. Pure component properties may be estimated by following standard practices (Reid *et al.*, 1987). Whenever possible, experimental values of transport properties and equations of state should be used. Typical values of the physical properties of different fluids are listed in Table 2.3. Data for pure compounds can be found in various handbooks (for example, Vargaftik, 1983; Yaws, 1995; Perry's Handbook, 1997). Data for mixtures (especially diffusion coefficients) are difficult to find. In the absence of experimental data, some help can be obtained from estimation methods. For dilute gases and gas mixtures, the kinetic theory of gases can be used to make reasonable estimates of transport properties (see, for example, Hirschfelder *et al.*, 1964). For liquids, theory is much less well developed. A recent review on theory and experiment may provide some assistance in estimating or measuring the required transport properties (Millat *et al.*, 1996).

2.3. BOUNDARY CONDITIONS

In order to solve the closed set of governing model equations, it is necessary to specify appropriate initial conditions and boundary conditions. For any reactor engineering problem, it will be necessary to select an appropriate solution domain, which is an important step in model formulation. The solution domain isolates the system being modeled from the surrounding environment. The influence of the environment on the flow processes of interest within the solution domain is represented by suitable formulations of boundary conditions. The solution domain, the co-ordinate system used to formulate the governing equations and the characteristics of the governing equations determine the boundary conditions requirements. Various commonly used boundary conditions are detailed here after a brief discussion on relating boundary conditions requirements with type of governing equations.

TABLE 2.3 Transport Properties (Most of the data are from Reid et *al.* (1987) and Perry's Handbook (1997))

	Viscosity[a] $\times 10^3$ Pa. s at 299 K	Thermal Conductivity[b] W $m^{-1}K^{-1}$ at 299 K	Heat Capacity[c] J kg^{-1} K^{-1} at 299 K	Binary Diffusivity[d], $\times 10^5$ m^2s^{-1} (atmospheric pressure)
Fluid				
Acetic acid	1.2		2184	
Acetone	0.34	0.175	2250	
Air	0.018	0.0262	1046	
Carbon dioxide	0.0145	0.0166	878	
Carbon monoxide	0.018		1046	
Chlorine	0.014	0.0089	489	
Hydrogen	0.0087	0.182	14644	
Nitrogen	0.0175	0.0260	1046	
Oxygen	0.02	0.0267	920	
Steam	0.0095	0.61	1841	
Toluene (L)	0.55	0.148	1840	
Water	0.9	0.608	4184	
System				
CO_2/N_2				1.69 at 298 K
H_2/NH_3				11.1 at 358 K
N_2/NH_3				3.32 at 358 K
O_2/H_2O				3.57 at 352 K
n-Heptane/Benzene				2.1×10^{-4} at 298 K
Benzene/n-Heptane				3.4×10^{-4} at 298 K
Water/Ethyl acetate				3.2×10^{-4} at 298 K
Ethyl acetate/Water				1.0×10^{-4} at 293 K

[a]Gases: $\sim 10^{-5}$ Pa. s; Water and many organic solvents: $\sim 10^{-3}$ Pa. s.
[b]Gases : $\sim 5 \times 10^{-3}$ to 0.1 $Wm^{-1}K^{-1}$; Non-metallic liquids : $\sim$0.1 to 1.0 $Wm^{-1}K^{-1}$; Metallic liquids : $\sim$10.0 to 100.0 $Wm^{-1}K^{-1}$.
[c]Gases : $\sim$1000 J kg^{-1} K^{-1}; Liquids : $\sim$1000 to 4200 J kg^{-1} K^{-1}.
[d]Gases : $\sim 10^{-5}$ to 10^{-4} m^2s^{-1}; Liquids : $\sim 10^{-11}$ to 10^{-8} m^2s^{-1}.

For any partial differential equation, initial and/or boundary conditions requirements depend on the direction of information propagation and the domain of dependence. Second-order partial differential equations are classified as elliptic, parabolic or hyperbolic. In elliptic equations, information propagates in all directions simultaneously. The solution domain is, therefore, a closed domain and the resulting solution is always smooth. In contrast, in hyperbolic equations, information propagates along characteristic directions with finite speed. These equations can, therefore, be solved using marching techniques. The solution may contain discontinuities (like shocks) because of the non-dissipative nature of these equations. For parabolic equations, the solution domain is open, but always yields a smooth solution due to its dissipative nature. A general, second-order partial differential equation in N independent variables $(x_1, x_2, \ldots, x_N)$ can be written:

$$\sum_{j=1}^{N}\sum_{k=1}^{N} A_{jk}\frac{\partial^2\phi}{\partial x_j \partial x_k} + H = 0 \tag{2.19}$$

This equation can be classified on the basis of eigenvalues, λ, of a matrix with entries A_{jk} (Fletcher, 1991). The eigenvalues (λ) are roots of the following equation:

$$\det\left[A_{jk} - \lambda\,\mathbf{I}\right] = 0 \tag{2.20}$$

where $\mathbf{I}$ is a unit vector. If any eigenvalue is zero, the equation is parabolic. If all eigenvalues are non-zero and are of the same sign, the equation is elliptic. If all eigenvalues are non-zero and all but one are of the same sign, the equation is hyperbolic. It should be noted that the coefficients A_{jk} might be functions of the dependent variable ϕ or independent variables. In such a case, the same equation may be locally parabolic, elliptic and hyperbolic depending upon the local conditions. In many cases, equations governing complex flow processes exhibit mixed properties and are difficult to formally classify under any particular type. The ideas discussed above should be kept in mind when formulating appropriate boundary conditions and when selecting appropriate numerical methods to solve the model equations. Commonly used boundary conditions are discussed below.

2.3.1. Inlet

For any model representing a flow process, the inlet boundary is a boundary through which the surrounding environment communicates with the solution domain. Generally, at such inlet boundaries, information about the velocity (or pressure), temperature and composition of the incoming fluid stream is assumed to be known. When the velocity components at the inlet are known, the inlet boundary conditions simply become:

$$U_{\text{in}} = U_{\text{set}} \qquad \phi_{\text{in}} = \phi_{\text{set}} \tag{2.21}$$

where subscript ‘set’ indicates known values. ϕ represents all the scalar variables of interest (temperature, species concentrations, physical properties and so on) except pressure. When the normal component of the velocity is known at the boundary, the boundary condition for pressure is not required since the velocity field depends on the pressure gradient and not on the absolute value of pressure.

It must be noted here that in most reactor simulations, the solution domain is restricted to the vessel, and generally flow within the feed pipes is not modeled. This means, that although volumetric flow rates are known accurately, the velocity distribution at the inlet is seldom known accurately. The most widely used practice is to use a knowledge of fully developed flow in pipes to specify the inlet velocity distribution. Thus, for laminar flow through a cylindrical inlet pipe, one can specify a parabolic velocity profile as a boundary condition at the inlet. However, if feed pipes have complex shapes, it will be necessary to develop an additional model to formulate appropriate inlet boundary conditions. Even with simple geometry like cylindrical pipes, in many reactor engineering applications the specification of inlet boundary conditions based on fully developed profiles may not be appropriate. To illustrate this, consider a simple example of a reactor vessel with a bottom inlet. In most cases, such an inlet pipe will have a bend very near to the entry in the reactor vessel (Fig. 2.2). Such a bend or any other pipe fitting will significantly change the velocity profile at the inlet defined at the vessel boundary. In such cases, either one has to include a significant portion of the feed pipe in the reactor simulation model or develop a separate model for the inlet pipe and use the results obtained from such a model to specify inlet boundary conditions near the vessel boundary.

When velocity components at the inlet boundary are not known, it is necessary to specify the pressure at the inlet boundary. Simplified equations can then be used (such as Bernoulli's equation) to calculate velocity at the inlet boundary (Fig. 2.3). For incompressible flow, if the specified total pressure at the inlet boundary is p_0, the

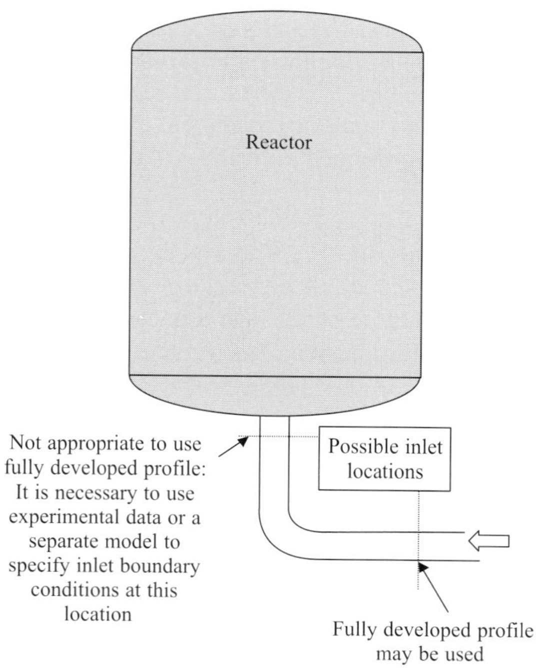

FIGURE 2.2 Typical arrangement of feed pipe to reactor vessel and location of inlet boundaries.

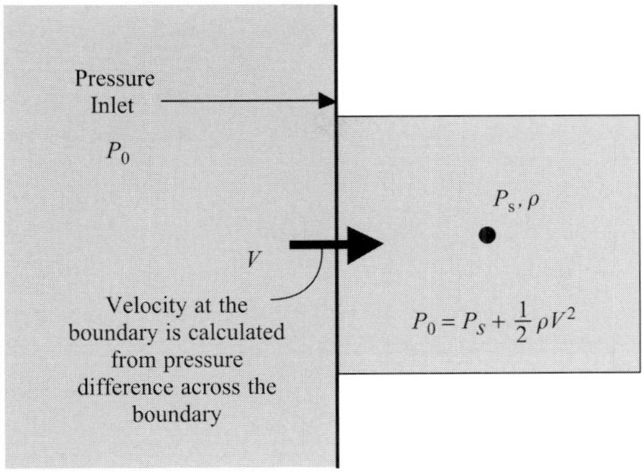

FIGURE 2.3 Inlet boundary conditions with unknown velocity.

inlet velocity is given by:

$$U_{\text{in}} = \left[\frac{2\,(p_0 - p_s)}{\rho}\right]^{1/2} \tag{2.22}$$

where p_s is the static pressure in the solution domain at the adjacent location of the inlet boundary. More complicated treatment will be necessary for compressible flows or for non-normal flows through the inlet pressure boundary. It must be kept in mind that the specified value of pressure at the boundary may lead to outflow from the boundary (when p_s is greater than p_0). It can, therefore, be used when it is not *a priori* known whether the flow enters or exits the solution domain at the open boundary under consideration. It can also be used as an outlet boundary condition (which may sometimes lead to inflow)!

2.3.2. Outlet

The surface of the solution domain through which the flow exits may be defined as the outlet. Normally the outlet boundary condition implies that gradients normal to the outlet boundary are zero for all the variables except pressure. If the direction normal to the outlet boundary is denoted by y, the outlet boundary conditions can be expressed as

$$\frac{\partial \phi}{\partial y} = 0 \tag{2.23}$$

It is not necessary to specify pressure at the outlet boundary.

Use of the outlet boundary condition is not appropriate when the gradients at the outlet boundary are not zero or when conditions downstream of the outlet boundary may influence flow within the solution domain (see Fig. 2.4, which shows inappropriate use of outlet boundary conditions). For such cases, it may be necessary to enlarge the solution domain to ensure that all the gradients vanish at the outlet boundary of the enlarged domain. Alternatively, a pressure boundary condition may be used (as discussed in the previous section). For the exit boundaries, static pressure is defined

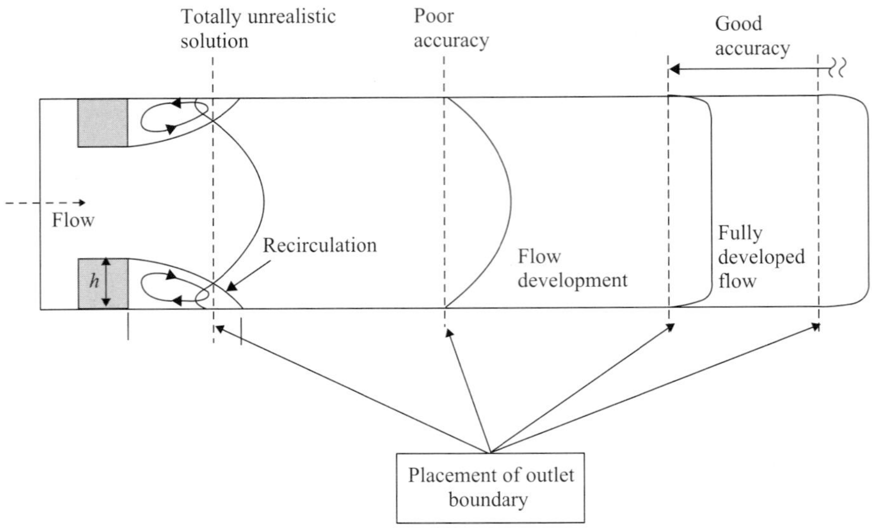

FIGURE 2.4 Location of outlet boundary condition.

instead of total pressure. For outflow through the boundary, this pressure is used to calculate the outflow velocities. If an inflow occurs through such a boundary, the kinetic energy of the incoming fluid is then assumed to be negligible.

For multiphase flows, it is possible to encounter a boundary of the solution domain through which one of the phases exits the domain but not the other (for example, the top surface of the bubble column reactor). Special boundary conditions need to be developed to represent such cases. These are discussed in Chapter 5.

2.3.3. Walls

At the impermeable wall boundaries of the solution domain, normally a 'no slip' boundary condition is employed. This is achieved by setting the transverse fluid velocity equal to that of the surface and setting the normal velocity to zero. Since the normal velocity at the wall is known, the value of pressure at the wall boundary is not required to be known. For species concentrations or temperatures, any of the following conditions can be specified at the wall boundaries:

- Surface temperature (or concentration) is specified.
- Heat (or mass) flux at the surface is specified.
- External heat transfer (or mass transfer) coefficient and external temperature (or concentration) at the surface is specified.

The specified heat or mass flux at the wall is then used to calculate the gradients of temperature or species concentrations at the wall by using the following equations:

$$q_{\mathrm{w}} = k \left.\frac{\partial T}{\partial n}\right|_{\mathrm{w}} \qquad j_{k\mathrm{w}} = \rho D_{k\mathrm{m}} \left.\frac{\partial m_k}{\partial n}\right|_{\mathrm{w}} \tag{2.24}$$

where q_w and j_{kw} are the specified heat and mass (of species k) flux at the wall. At the impermeable, inert and insulated wall, the gradients of temperature and species concentration are set to zero (zero flux condition). When external heat or mass transfer coefficients are specified, along with the external temperature or species concentration, the flux at the walls are equated to the flux in terms of these external transfer coefficients:

$$q_w = h_{ext}(T_{ext} - T_w) \qquad j_{kw} = k_{mext}(m_{kext} - m_w) \tag{2.25}$$

Schematic representation of these three possible boundary conditions at the wall is shown in Fig. 2.5 for the enthalpy/temperature equation. For systems with conjugate heat transfer, continuity of the temperature and the normal component of fluxes are specified at the walls. For systems with reactions occurring on solid surfaces, generally, accumulation of species at the solid surface is neglected and the diffusive flux at the wall is equated to the surface reaction rate.

2.3.4. Symmetry/Periodic/Cyclic

Recognizing the intrinsic symmetry of the flow process or the repetitious nature of the process equipment can minimize the size and extent of the solution domain. If such a possibility exists, fictitious boundaries may be used to define the solution domain with special boundary conditions imposed on these such fictitious surfaces. Some of the commonly encountered cases are discussed below.

If the flow process is symmetric or in other words contains a surface across which the flux of all quantities is zero, the extent of the solution domain can be reduced. Two examples of such symmetric flow processes are shown in Fig. 2.6. At a symmetry surface, the normal velocity is set to zero and the normal gradients of all variables, except normal velocity, are set to zero. This ensures that there is no convective or diffusive flux across the symmetry surface. It must be noted that symmetric construction of the process equipment under consideration does not guarantee that the underlying flow processes are also symmetric. Even if the solution domain is geometrically symmetric, the flow process of interest may not be so. One example of such a case is shown in Fig. 2.6. When the flow processes are not symmetric, it is necessary to

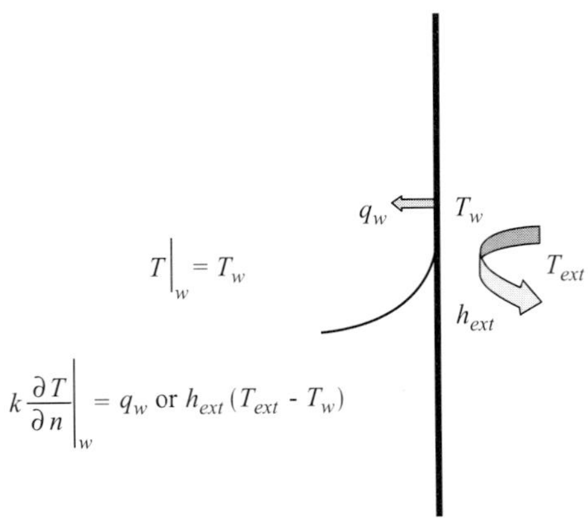

FIGURE 2.5 Wall boundary conditions for enthalpy/temperature equation.

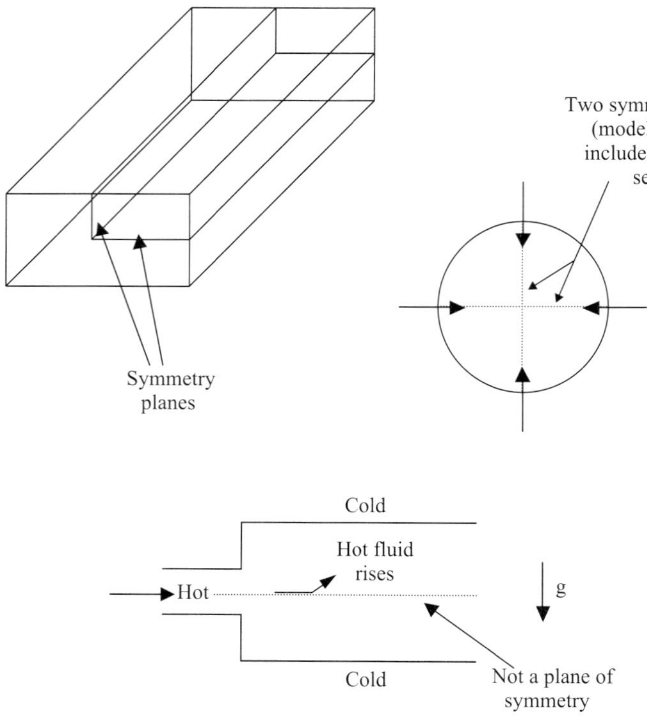

FIGURE 2.6 Examples of symmetric flows.

include the whole vessel as the solution domain. However, wherever possible, the existence of symmetry planes must be recognized to reduce the size of the solution domain.

When the physical geometry of the problem under consideration or the expected flow pattern has a cyclically repeating nature, cyclic or periodic boundary conditions can be used to reduce the size of the solution domain. Two types of cyclic boundary condition can be distinguished. The first is for rotationally periodic flow processes, where all the variables at corresponding periodic locations on the cyclic planes are the same. The second is for translationally periodic flow processes, where all the variables, except pressure, at corresponding periodic locations on the cyclic planes are the same. Examples of these two types are shown in Fig. 2.7. Such cyclic planes are in fact part of the solution domain (by the nature of their definitions) and no additional boundary conditions are required at these planes, except the one-to-one correspondence between the two cyclic planes.

2.4. DISCUSSION

The basic governing equations (2.1 to 2.10) along with appropriate constitutive equations and boundary conditions govern the flow of fluids, provided the continuum assumption is valid. To obtain analytical solutions, the governing equations are often simplified by assuming constant physical properties and by discarding unimportant

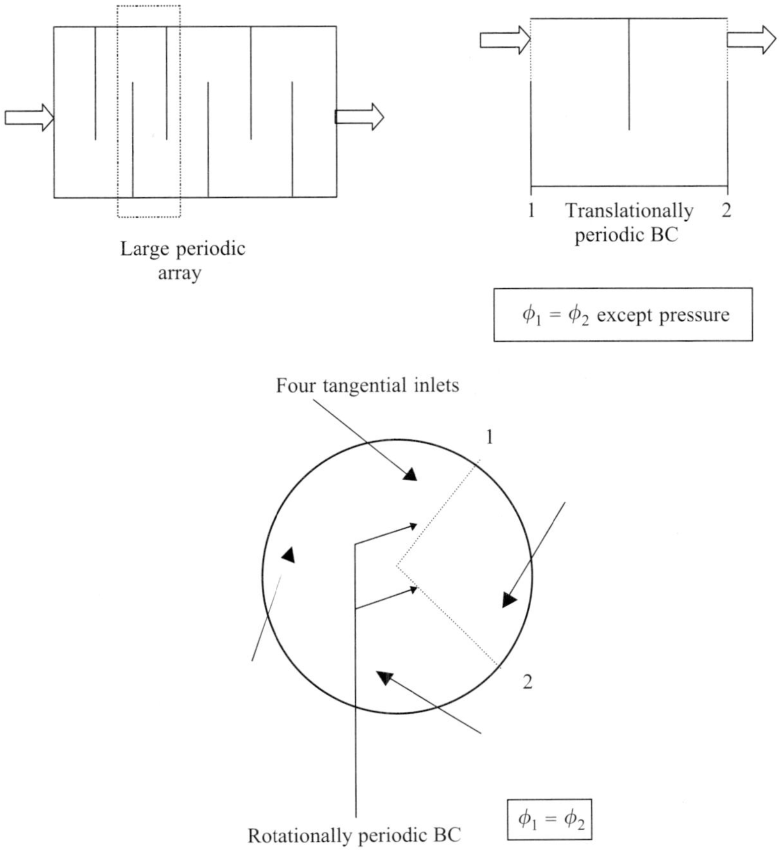

FIGURE 2.7 Flow processes with rotationally or translationally periodic boundaries.

terms (refer to Section 2.1.4). For example, many analytical solutions of the Euler equations are available (Lamb, 1932; Milne-Thompson, 1955; Frisch, 1995). Solutions of low Reynolds number hydrodynamics (creeping flows) are discussed by Happel and Brenner (1983) and Kim and Karrila (1991). For some laminar flow problems, analytical solutions can be obtained by asymptotic methods or by using scaling arguments (Leal, 1992). Despite these extensive efforts, for most practical flow problems, it is not possible to obtain analytical solutions.

Recent advances in numerical methods and algorithms allow solution of these governing equations using digital computers. The modeling of flow processes occurring in industrial equipment may, however, require additional modeling steps beyond the formulation of basic governing equations. Any engineer familiar with fabrication drawings of an industrial reactor will know the complexity and co-existence of a wide range of geometric and velocity scales within the reactor. An industrial reactor may contain several internals such as cooling coils, feed pipes, distributors and so on. Developing a single model to simulate all the flow processes occurring in such reactors is almost always impractical (if not impossible). More often than not the reactor engineer has to divide the overall problem into different components. Each component can then be modeled separately to learn about its fluid dynamics. At each stage, the reactor engineer has to recombine the understanding and knowledge gained during the modeling of these components to build the overall model. Of course, at each stage, the implications of considering the separate components and extrapolation of these results to formulate the overall model need to be constantly evaluated. The approach to modeling flow processes in complex industrial reactors is discussed further with the help of case studies in Parts III and IV.

Recent progress in computing technologies has resulted in an order of magnitude increase in our capacity to use and solve these basic equations to simulate complex flow processes. This may lead to thinking that given sufficient computing power, these equations can be solved numerically to make *a priori* predictions of any complex flow process. Unfortunately, this is NOT true, especially for those flow processes in which a reactor engineer will be interested.

A close examination of the basic equations will reveal that non-linearity is at the core of these equations and there are no general ways of solving non-linear problems. The non-linearity in the governing equations manifests in the form of turbulence under certain conditions (high Reynolds number or Grashoff number). Turbulence is the most complex fluid motion, making even its precise definition difficult. Despite tremendous progress in the last few decades, it is not yet possible to compute, from first principles, how much power one would need to pump a given volumetric flow of liquid through a pipe if the flow rate (Reynolds number) is high enough! In order to describe real-life, complex flow processes, it is, therefore, necessary to develop and use additional models to complement the basic governing equations discussed above. For reactor engineering applications, the problem of turbulence is further complicated by the presence of chemical reactions and by multiple phases. The modeling of turbulent flows, multiphase flows, and reactive flows, is discussed in detail in the following chapters.

2.5. SUMMARY

Governing equations describing the flow processes of continuous fluid are well established. These equations form the basis for further understanding and further attempts at modeling complex flow processes. In order to close the set of equations, it is necessary to provide appropriate constitutive equations, equations to estimate and represent the variation in properties of the fluids under consideration and the correct boundary conditions. The importance of boundary conditions cannot be overemphasized. Dimensional and order-of-magnitude analysis is often helpful in identifying important features of the flow process and may highlight possible simplifications. Even the simplest flow models may require numerical solutions. Typical flow processes relevant to reactor engineering are usually governed by strongly coupled, non-linear equations. Details of complexities arising due to these non-linearities, and numerical methods for solving these model equations are discussed in subsequent chapters of this part.

REFERENCES

Anderson, D.A., Tannehill, J.C. and Pletcher, R.H. (1984), "Computational Fluid Mechanics and Heat Transfer", Hemisphere, New York.

Bird, R.B. (1998), Viewpoints on transport phenomenon, *Korean J. Chem. Eng.*, **15**(2), 105–123.
Bird, R.B., Arnstrong, R.C. and Hassager, O. (1987), "Dynamics of Polymeric Liquids, Fluid Mechanics", Vol. **1**, 2nd edition, Wiley-Interscience, New York.
Bird, R.B. and Graham, M.D. (1998), General equation of Newtonian fluid dynamics, in "The Handbook of Fluid Dynamics", CRC Press, Boca Raton, FL.
Bird, R.B., Stewart, W.E. and Lightfoot, E.N. (1960), "Transport Phenomena", John Wiley & Sons, New York.
Brodkey, R.S. and Hershey, H.C. (1988), "Transport Phenomena: A Unified Approach", McGraw-Hill, New York.
Crochet, M.J., Davis, A.R. and Walters, K. (1984), "Numerical Simulation of Non-Newtonian Flow", Elsevier, Amsterdam.
Deen, W.M. (1998), "Analysis of Transport Phenomena", Oxford University Press, New York.
Fletcher, C.A.J. (1991), "Computational Techniques for Fluid Dynamics", Vols **1** and **2**, Springer Verlag, Berlin.
Frisch, U. (1995), "Turbulence: The Legacy of A.N. Kolmogorov", Cambridge University Press, Cambridge.
Happel, J. and Brenner, H. (1983), "Low Reynolds Number Hydrodynamics", Martinus Nijhoff, The Hague.
Hines, A.L. and Maddox, R.N. (1985), "Mass Transfer: Fundamentals and Applications", Prentice Hall, Engelwood Cliffs, NJ.
Hirschfelder, J.O., Curtiss, C.F. and Bird, R.B. (1964), "Molecular Theory of Gases and Liquids", John Wiley & Sons, New York.
Kim, S. and Karrila, S.J. (1991), "Microhydrodynamics: Principles and Selected Applications", Butterworth-Heinemann, Boston.
Lamb, H. (1932), "Hydrodynamics", 6th edition, Dover, New York.
Leal, L.G. (1992), "Laminar Flow and Convective Transport Processes", Butterworth-Heinemann, Boston.
Milne-Thompson, L.M. (1955), "Theoretical Hydrodynamics", 3rd edition, McMillan, New York.
Millat, J., Dymond, J.H. and Nieto de Castro, C. A. (1996), "Transport Properties of Fluids: Their Correlation, Predictions and Estimation", Cambridge University Press.
Perry, J.H., Gree, D.W. and Maloney, J.O. (1997), "Perry's Chemical Engineer's Handbook", 7th edition, McGraw Hill, New York.
Reid, R.C., Sherwood, T.K. and Prausnitz, J.M. (1987), "Properties of Gases and Liquids", 4th edition, McGraw Hill, New York.
Tanner, R.I. (1985), "Engineering Rheology", Clarendon Press, Oxford.
Taylor, R. and Krishna, R. (1993), "Multicomponent Mass Transfer", John & Wiley, New York.
Vargaftik, N.B. (1983), "Handbook of Physical Properties of Liquids and Gases: Pure Substances and Mixtures", Hemisphere, Washington.
Yaws, C.L. (1995), "Handbook of Transport Property Data: Viscosity, Thermal Conductivity and Diffusion Coefficients of Liquids and Gases", Gulf, Houston.

3 TURBULENT FLOW PROCESSES

3.1. INTRODUCTION

Turbulence is difficult to define precisely, although any reactor engineer may intuitively understand the differences in laminar and turbulent flow processes. Fluid motion is described as turbulent if it is irregular, rotational, intermittent, highly disordered, diffusive and dissipative. Turbulent motion is inherently unsteady and three-dimensional. Visualizations of turbulent flows reveal rotational flow structures (so called turbulence eddies), with a wide range of length scales. Such eddy motions and interactions between eddies of different length scales lead to effective contact between fluid particles which are initially separated by a long distance. As a consequence, heat, mass and momentum are very effectively exchanged. The rate of scalar mixing in turbulent flows is greater by orders of magnitude than that in laminar flows. Heat and mass transfer rates are also significantly higher in turbulent flows. Because of such effective mixing and enhanced rates of mass, momentum and heat transport, turbulence is often employed in chemical reactors to enhance performance. Turbulent flows are also associated with higher values of friction drag and pressure drop. However, more often than not, advantages gained with the enhanced transport rates are more valuable than the costs of higher frictional losses. It can be concluded that for many (if not most) engineering applications, turbulent flow processes are necessary to make the desired operation realizable and more efficient. It is, therefore, essential to develop suitable methods to predict and control turbulent flow processes.

Turbulence is the most complicated kind of fluid motion. There have been several different attempts to understand turbulence and different approaches taken to develop predictive models for turbulent flows. In this chapter, a brief description of some of the concepts relevant to understand turbulence, and a brief overview of different modeling approaches to simulating turbulent flow processes is given. Turbulence models based on time-averaged Navier–Stokes equations, which are the most relevant for chemical reactor engineers, at least for the foreseeable future, are then discussed in detail. The scope of discussion is restricted to single-phase turbulent flows (of Newtonian fluids) without chemical reactions. Modeling of turbulent multiphase flows and turbulent reactive flows are discussed in Chapters 4 and 5 respectively.

3.2. TURBULENCE: PHYSICAL PICTURE

Since a precise definition of turbulence is difficult, pictures and other visualizations of turbulent flows may give some idea of the complex characteristics of turbulence. Several such visualizations are available, including the famous painting 'The Deluge' by Leonardo da Vinci. Banerjee (1992) included several such pictures in his excellent paper on turbulence structures. Van Dyke (1982) published an album of fluid motion which is a 'must see' for any turbulence researcher. Several websites hold treasures of visual information on turbulence (see, for example, links listed at sites such as www.cfd-online.com and www.efluids.com). Pictures included in these resources show various aspects of turbulent flows and may give some intuitive understanding of turbulence.

Turbulence is intrinsically unsteady, even when constant boundary conditions are imposed. Velocity and all other flow properties fluctuate in a random and chaotic way. Turbulent fluctuations always have a three-dimensional spatial character. There have been many attempts to analyze and to construct a physical picture of turbulence, following several different approaches. These different approaches, broadly classified into three categories, are discussed in this section.

3.2.1. Statistical Approach

In this approach, the unsteady processes occurring in turbulent flows are visualized as a combination of some mean process and small-scale fluctuations around it. The typical time variation of fluid velocity at a point in a turbulent flow is shown in Fig. 3.1. In the statistical approach, an instantaneous velocity, U, is visualized as a mean velocity, $\bar{U}$ (shown by a horizontal line in Fig. 3.1) and fluctuations around it, u. Based on such an approach, the statistical theory of turbulence flows has been developed (see Hinze, 1975 and references cited therein). It has been the basis for most of the engineering modeling of turbulent flow processes. Some of the key concepts of the statistical approach are discussed below.

The large-scale motions (eddies) of turbulence are dominated by inertia effects. For these large-scale motions, viscous effects are negligible. Mean flow stretches these large eddies (in the form of vortices). Angular momentum is conserved during vortex stretching leading to a reduction in cross-section of these vortices. Thus, the process creates motions at smaller length scales (and also at smaller time scales). The stretching work done by the mean flow on large eddies provides the energy which maintains turbulence. The smaller eddies are themselves stretched by somewhat larger

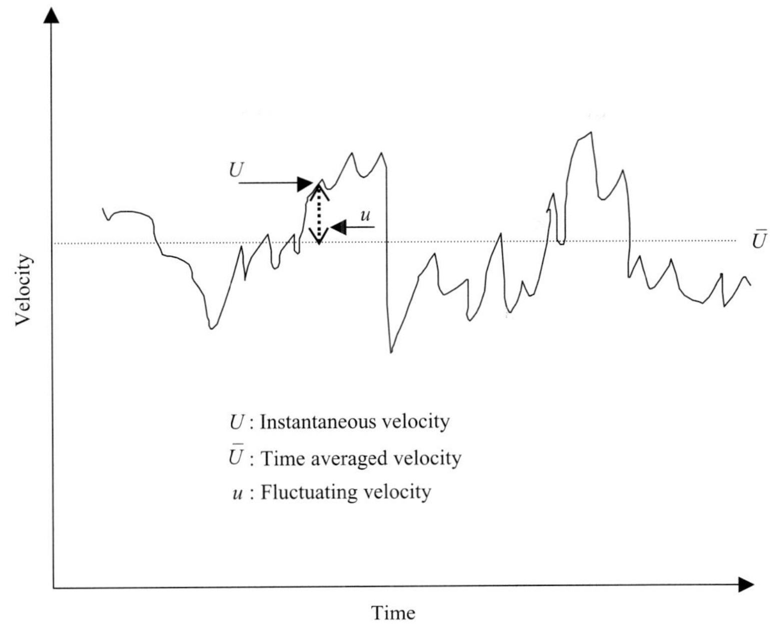

FIGURE 3.1 Typical point velocity behavior in turbulent flows.

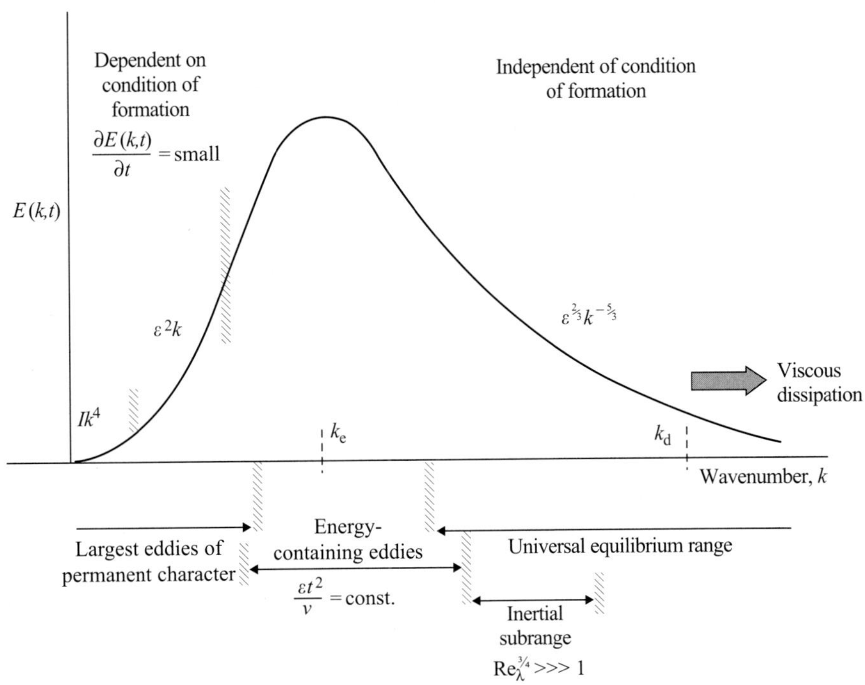

FIGURE 3.2 Energy spectrum for isotropic turbulence (from Hinze, 1975).

eddies and in this way, transfer energy to progressively smaller length scales (larger wave numbers). This process of energy transfer from large scales to small scales is termed as 'energy cascade'. As the length (and time) scales become sufficiently small, viscous effects start becoming important. For these small-scale motions, work is performed against the action of viscous stresses, so that the energy associated with the eddy motions is dissipated. This dissipation results in increased energy losses associated with turbulent flows. For many engineering flows, the smallest scales are of the order of 0.01 to 0.1 mm.

The structure of large eddies is highly flow dependent (and directional) due to their strong interaction with the mean flow. The diffusive action of viscosity tends to smear out directionality at small scales. At high mean flow Reynolds number, the smallest eddies are, therefore, non-directional or isotropic. For large enough Reynolds numbers, there exists an intermediate range of scales ('inertial sub-range') between these anisotropic large eddies and isotropic dissipative eddies. In this inertial sub-range, energy is transferred to smaller scales (higher velocity gradients) with negligible dissipation. As scale decreases below certain length scales (or velocity gradients increase beyond a certain limit), dissipation of kinetic energy by viscous stresses become dominant. Viscous stresses dissipate the kinetic energy and convert it to internal energy. The characteristic length scale at which viscous dissipation becomes important, is called the Kolmogorov scale. Kolmogorov and others (see Hinze, 1975) have described the process of 'energy cascade' in turbulent flows using spectral analysis. A typical energy spectrum of turbulent flows is shown in Fig. 3.2. k_e and k_d denote wave numbers of energy containing eddies and dissipative eddies, respectively. The $-5/3$ slope portion of the energy spectrum characterizes the presence of the inertial sub-range. Such spectral analysis has helped to quantify various scales occurring in turbulent flow processes and eventually to the development of computational models, which will be discussed in the following sections. The statistical approach has been used successfully for several applications. However, one of the most important objections to using the statistical approach to describe turbulent flows is that it totally ignores structures occurring within turbulent flows (see for example, Banerjee, 1992). An alternative approach based on turbulence structures is described below.

3.2.2. Structural Approach

Practitioners of this approach object to the ubiquitous averaging employed in the statistical approach, which obscures the structures present in the turbulent flows (high vorticity regions, bursts, streaks and so on). The presence of coherent structures in turbulent flows has long been recognized. Banerjee (1992) has given a lucid and very interesting account of the structural approach to studying turbulent flows. In any turbulent flow, such coherent structures exist. For some flows, these structures are more persistent and are not swamped by small-scale fluctuations. For such cases, obviously, the statistical approach may not be appropriate and a structure-based approach may be more fruitful. Banerjee (1992) cited examples where the structural approach can be used to develop quantitative, predictive models. However, in many flow situations, small-scale fluctuations and other factors shadow the coherent structures. In such cases, it is difficult to detect and quantify the characteristics of such structures. Moreover, a consistent theoretical framework to assimilate the random and deterministic elements of structures is lacking (structures are assumed to be randomly distributed in time and space but each occurrence is assumed to be governed by a locally deterministic cause). This approach is, therefore, not frequently used in the engineering modeling of turbulent flows.

3.2.3. Deterministic Approach

This is the latest approach to be used to understand turbulence, and is based on recent advances in the theory of non-linear problems and deterministic chaos. Here, attempts are being made to develop quantitative models for transition to turbulence. The tools developed and the results obtained by this approach so far look promising and may throw new light on the mechanism of transition (see Berge *et al.*, 1984 for a more detailed account of the deterministic approach). Efforts to date have been focused on simple systems and the transition to turbulence. The application of these ideas to fully developed turbulent flows has, however, not yet been seriously undertaken. It is not yet evident whether the understanding gained through this approach can be converted into successful predictive models for turbulent flows of practical interest. Reactor engineers, therefore, have to rely on a statistical approach to develop predictive models for most problems of interest.

Before examining approaches to developing predictive models, it will be useful to employ a statistical approach to quantify various relevant length and time scales of turbulent flows, keeping in mind the existence of coherent structures. Estimation of such length and time scales may allow an evaluation of different competing processes such as mixing, heat and mass transfer and chemical reactions. Broadly speaking, turbulent flows are characterized by two length scales: the integral scale, L, where the inertial sub-range begins, and the Kolmogorov length scale, λ_k, where the inertial sub-range ends, which are given by (Hinze, 1975):

$$L = \frac{3\pi}{4}\frac{\int_0^\infty E(k)/k\,dk}{\int_0^\infty E(k)\,dk} \tag{3.1}$$

$$\lambda_k = \left(\frac{\nu^3}{\varepsilon}\right)^{1/4} \tag{3.2}$$

where $E(k)\,dk$ is the turbulent kinetic energy contained in the wave number range k to $k + dk$, ν is the kinematic viscosity of the fluid and ε is the turbulent energy dissipation rate (which is defined later in this chapter). Each of these length scales is associated with corresponding velocity and time scales (see Hinze, 1975).

Generally, the integral length scale is proportional to the macroscopic length scale of the equipment (for example, about one tenth of the diameter for pipe flows; about half the blade width of an impeller in stirred reactors). The small scales are decided by the fluid viscosity and turbulence energy dissipation rate, ε. The small-scale motions exhibit universal characteristics and more or less behave in the same way in all flow processes. The integral scale motions interact with the mean flow field and strongly depend on the boundary conditions of the specific problem under consideration. These motions are sometimes called large eddies; eddy being a hypothetical construct to represent motions covering a small range of length scales. These large eddies are mainly responsible for the transport of momentum, mass and energy, and hence need to be adequately simulated by any turbulence model. Various approaches to modeling turbulent flows are discussed in the following sections.

3.3. MODELING APPROACHES

Although the structural and deterministic approaches to characterizing turbulence have demonstrated promising results, a deductive approach based on solution of the basic governing equations of the flow processes is the most widely used approach for engineering applications. The basic premise in modeling turbulence is that it can be understood within the continuum assumption of fluid dynamics. There are some experimental facts which might shed doubt on the validity of the assumption. For example, small amounts of long chain polymers have significant influence on turbulence properties (drag), even though the polymer molecules are well dispersed and have dimensions significantly smaller than the dissipation scales of turbulence (more about these scales later). Despite this, the continuum assumption has formed the basis for modeling turbulence over the last several decades and therefore will be accepted here for modeling turbulent flows relevant to reactor engineering.

Accepting the continuum assumption implies accepting the use of the same basic momentum conservation equations (discussed in Chapter 2) to describe turbulent flows. If this is the case, one may wonder why there is a need for any further modeling? One has only to solve the momentum conservation equations described earlier with appropriate boundary conditions to predict the desired flow characteristics at any value of Reynolds number. However, at large Reynolds numbers, the inherent non-linearity in these equations manifest in terms of turbulence, which is a three-dimensional, unsteady phenomenon as is previously described. No doubt, there exist a number of numerical methods and computer programs capable of solving three-dimensional, time dependent momentum equations. The main difficulty in solving the basic governing equations under turbulent conditions is the inability to resolve the wide range of spatial and temporal scales simultaneously. From the foregoing discussion about the scales, it can be shown that the distance between the large and small scales grows with increase in Reynolds number (as $Re^{3/4}$). Therefore, as the Reynolds number increases and the flow becomes more turbulent, the requirements on resolution become more and more stringent. The number of grid points and the smallness of the time steps required to resolve all the relevant time and space scales of turbulent motion push the computation of turbulent flows in industrial equipment beyond the realms of present computing capabilities. Estimates from various sources differ on the required mesh spacing and on when computer technology will have advanced to the point where turbulent flow calculations can be made from first principles. It appears that most engineering computations involving turbulent flow processes will have to rely on models of turbulent flows, at least for the foreseeable future. This is especially true for chemical reactor engineering applications, where, in addition to turbulence, there are many other complexities such as chemical reactions, multiple phases, complex geometry and so on.

It is sometimes argued that if Navier–Stokes equations can completely describe turbulent flows, it is futile to search for models which are simpler to solve and also retain a complete description of turbulent flows. Many reviews on turbulence modeling conclude by saying that we cannot calculate all the flows of engineering interest to the desired engineering accuracy with available turbulence models, which is of course true. However, the best modern computational models (and numerical methods) allow almost all the flows to be calculated to higher accuracy than the

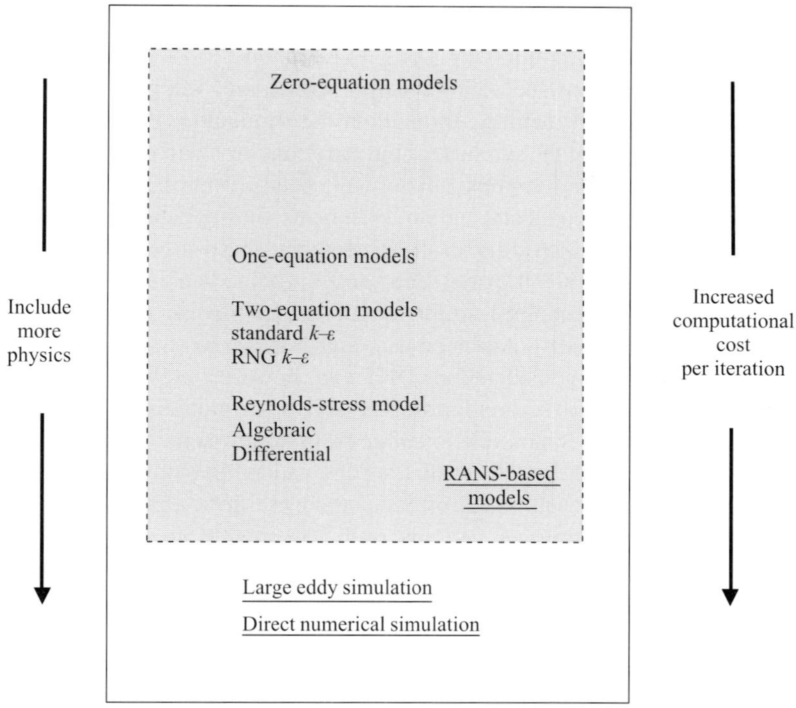

FIGURE 3.3 Modeling approaches for turbulent flows.

best-informed guess. This means that the methods are genuinely useful for engineering applications even though they cannot replace experiments. The major efforts in the area of turbulence modeling have been and are still directed towards developing tractable computational models of turbulent flows with reasonable demands on computational resources. Large numbers of models have been developed in the last three decades or so. These modeling approaches (which are summarized in Fig. 3.3) can be classified into three categories; direct numerical simulations (DNS), large eddy simulations (LES) and Reynolds-averaged Navier–Stokes equations (RANS). These three approaches are briefly reviewed. As one progresses from DNS to RANS, more and more of the turbulent motions are approximated and, therefore, require less computational resources.

3.3.1. Direct Numerical Simulation (DNS)

Direct numerical simulation, as the name implies, attempts to simulate all the dynamically important scales of turbulent flows, directly. It is based on the hypothesis that direct simulations may be carried out by artificially decreasing the Reynolds number to the point where important scales can be simulated accurately on existing computers. This is probably the most exact approach to turbulence simulation without requiring any additional modeling beyond accepting the Navier–Stokes equations to describe the turbulent flow processes. The result is equivalent to a single realization of a flow or a short duration laboratory experiment. It is also the simplest approach conceptually. In DNS, all the motions contained in the flow are resolved.

Specification of initial and boundary conditions is one of the most important and difficult steps in applying DNS. For example, it is necessary to provide inlet boundary conditions specifying the time variation of velocities at all the grid points lying on the inlet boundary, throughout the simulation. For DNS simulations, the usual application of the symmetry boundary condition will no longer be valid because small-scale motions in turbulent flows will not be symmetric. Since the approach aims to resolve all the spatial and temporal gradients, the application of DNS requires huge computational resources. It must be remembered that a large number of grid points are required to resolve small spatial scales and for each grid point, time history needs to be stored to make meaningful simulations. Thus, DNS generates a huge amount of data containing time history at each point, which may not be necessary for the engineering application under consideration. DNS can, however, provide valuable information about the interaction of small-scale and large-scale motions. Often, such information is very difficult or impossible to obtain from experiments. The information obtained from DNS can be helpful in evaluating and validating more approximate models and may lead to the development of better models. More details of the DNS approach and some applications can be found in Rogallo and Moin (1984), Kim *et al.* (1987), Reynolds (1990), Choi *et al.* (1994) and Leonard (1995) among others.

The DNS approach may also give useful information about the interaction of chemical reactions and turbulence. Such interactions are discussed in Chapter 5. In general, DNS generates a lot more information than that needed for typical reactor engineering applications. In order to use the information, a reactor engineer has to resort to some sort of averaging, and such averaging may introduce errors. When the accuracy of some of the input data to the model, such as reaction kinetics, is not very high, it may be worthwhile to explore alternative approaches, which are less exact than DNS but require much less computational resources. Lower demands on computational resources mean less turnover time (time required to complete the simulations) and more opportunities for engineering applications, provided the possible errors and their implications are fully recognized. Two such approaches are discussed below.

3.3.2. Large Eddy Simulations (LES)

Large eddy simulations are based on the hypothesis that the relevant scales in turbulent flows can be separated into large-scale and small-scale (sub-grid) components. It is assumed that such separation does not have a significant effect on the evolution of large-scale turbulent motions. The range of scales occurring in turbulent flows and their relationship with modeling approaches is shown schematically in Fig. 3.4. The large-scale motions are generally much more energetic than the small scale motions and are the main contributors to the transport of conserved quantities. LES attempts to simulate these large-scale motions more precisely than the small-scale motions. The small scales of turbulence are believed to be more universal in character than large scales, which facilitate their modeling. Therefore, in LES, large-scale motions are resolved rigorously and small-scale motions (large wave numbers) are modeled in lieu of being resolved. LES models are also three-dimensional and time-dependent but are much less costly (and more flexible) than DNS.

The maximum wave number resolved with the LES approach is chosen to lie in the inertial sub-range of the turbulence energy spectrum. The governing transport equations are derived either by filtering the Navier–Stokes equation or using volume

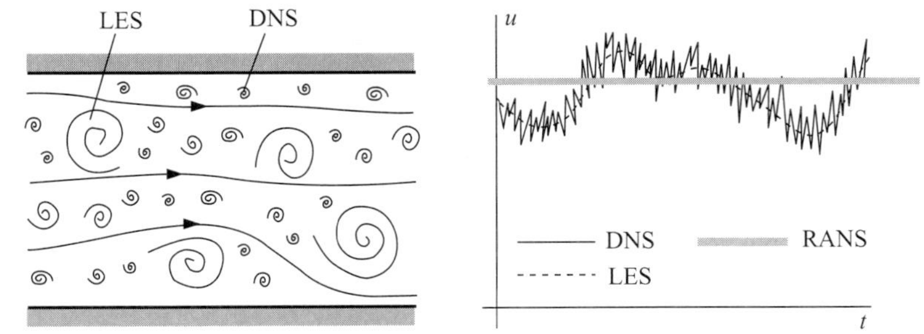

FIGURE 3.4 Schematic representation of scales in turbulent flows and their relationship with modeling approaches (adapted from Ferziger and Peric, 1995).

averaging concepts. Both methods lead to similar sets of governing equations. Any flow variable, ϕ, in the fluid domain, D, is decomposed into a large scale part, $<\phi>$ and a small scale part, ϕ'' as:

$$\phi = \langle\phi\rangle + \phi'' \quad \because \quad \langle\phi\rangle = \int_D G(x - x^*, \Delta)\phi(x^*)\, d^3x^* \tag{3.3}$$

where Δ is the characteristic filter scale and G is a filter function obeying the following property:

$$\int_D G(x - x^*, \Delta) d^3x^* = 1 \tag{3.4}$$

Several filters, such as Gaussian or piecewise continuous, are used. The filter function, G becomes a Dirac delta function in the limit of Δ tending to zero. Thus, direct simulations are recovered in the fine mesh limit. Such a filtering operation substantially reduces the amplitude of high wave number components of flow variable ϕ. Similar decomposition can also be made using the volume and surface averaging concepts. With this approach, the velocity associated with the face of a control volume is decomposed into a surface-averaged value and the fluctuation around the surface averaged value, similar to Eq. (3.3). It must be noted that unlike the traditional Reynolds averages (discussed in the next sub-section), in general, the time averages of these fluctuating components around filtered or surface-averaged quantities are not zero:

$$\overline{\langle\phi\rangle} \neq \langle\phi\rangle \qquad \overline{\phi''} \neq 0 \tag{3.5}$$

Fluctuations around the surface- or volume-averaged quantities generate additional terms in the governing transport equations which require further modeling to close the set of equations. These models (representing the effect of scales smaller than the characteristic filter scale) are called 'sub-grid scale' models (SGS). In principle, the characteristic length scale of a filter is not directly related to the grid size (grid size, obviously, cannot be larger than the filter scale). However, the name SGS has stuck and is used to denote these additional models. The additional terms appearing in the governing equations are generally classified into three groups, namely Leonard stresses, sub-grid scale cross-stresses and sub-grid scale Reynolds stresses (Leonard, 1974). Smagorinsky (1963) proposed the first sub-grid scale stress model. Several models have been proposed since then (Ferziger, 1976; Rogallo and Moin, 1984;

Hussaini *et al.*, 1990). Extensive research efforts have been made to evaluate these SGS models. Two of the main problems identified with different SGS models are (Speziale, 1998):

(1) the inability of SGS models to respond to changes in the local state of the flow, resulting in the need to make ad hoc adjustments in the model parameters. Turbulent channel flow, isotropic turbulence and more general homogeneously strained turbulent flows require values of the Smagorinsky constant that can differ by more than a factor of two;
(2) the generally poor correlation of SGS models with DNS at lower turbulence Reynolds numbers. Even for the simple case of isotropic turbulence, the Smagorinsky model correlates only at about the 50% level. (Note, for example, that the correlation between functions $y = x$ and $y = e^{-x}$ over the interval zero to one is more than 50% despite the fact that they are qualitatively different functions.)

Several attempts have been made to reduce or eliminate these problems. Development of SGS models is an active field of research and further details may be obtained by referring to Germano *et al.* (1991), Orszag *et al.* (1993) and Speziale (1998) among others.

The LES approach is capable of capturing time-dependent motions of large scale, which are averaged out in conventional turbulence models based on Reynolds-averaged equations. Small-scale motions exhibit more universal characteristics and, therefore, there is more hope of developing a generalized SGS model. Rigorous DNS simulations may assist such development. The LES approach has been used extensively to simulate turbulent flows with moderately high Reynolds numbers. More details of the LES approach and applications may be found in Reynolds (1990) and Ferziger (1995). More recently, attempts have also been made to apply LES to simulate more complex flows (for example, flow in stirred reactors, by Derksen and van den Akker, 1999). Despite these successes, LES is still computation intensive and suffers some of the disadvantages of DNS, such as difficulties in specifying boundary conditions and generating a huge amount of information, which may not be necessary for a reactor engineer. For steady state flows in particular, LES methods are still much more computation intensive than models based on Reynolds-averaged equations, which are discussed in the following sub-sections.

3.3.3. Reynolds-averaged Navier–Stokes Equations (RANS)

In this approach, an instantaneous value of any variable is decomposed into a mean, obtained by averaging over an appropriate time interval, and a fluctuating component:

$$\phi = \bar{\phi} + \phi' \tag{3.6}$$

The overbar denotes time averaging. The time averaged quantity is defined as:

$$\bar{\phi} = \frac{1}{\Delta t} \int_t^{t+\Delta t} \phi \, dt \tag{3.7}$$

The Reynolds averaging obeys the following property:

$$\bar{\bar{\phi}} = \bar{\phi} \qquad \bar{\phi'} = 0 \tag{3.8}$$

Equation (3.6) is substituted in the basic governing equations for ϕ and these are then time averaged to yield the governing equations for mean quantities (using Eq. (3.8)). For compressible turbulent flows, terms appearing in the Reynolds-averaged momentum equations are difficult to categorize according to the acceleration of the mean motion and apparent stresses. In such cases, the use of mass weighted averaging leads to compact expressions. Mass weighted averaging, also called Favre averaging, is defined as:

$$\bar{\phi} = \frac{\int_t^{t+\Delta t} \rho\phi \, dt}{\int_t^{t+\Delta t} \rho \, dt} \tag{3.9}$$

For flows in which density fluctuations are negligible, the formulations become identical. Favre-averaged quantities are not easily comparable with experimentally measured quantities, which are normally non-weighted time averages. For most chemical reactor engineering applications (except maybe combustion processes), classical Reynolds averaging is suitable.

The Reynolds-averaged form of the conservation equations of mass (overall) and momentum for an incompressible (constant density) fluid can be written as:

$$\nabla \cdot (\rho \bar{U}) = \sum_k \bar{S}_i \tag{3.10}$$

$$\frac{\partial}{\partial t}(\rho \bar{U}) + \nabla \cdot (\rho \bar{U}\bar{U} + \rho \overline{uu}) = -\nabla \bar{p} - \nabla \cdot \bar{\tau} + \rho g + \bar{F} \tag{3.11}$$

where the overbar indicates a time-averaged value. u is the fluctuating velocity. The terms appearing in Eq. (3.11) resemble those in Eq. (2.5) except for an additional term appearing on the left-hand side. These extra terms act as apparent stresses due to turbulent motions and are called Reynolds stresses or turbulent stresses and defined as:

$$(\tau_{ij})_{\text{turb}} = \rho \overline{u_i u_j} \tag{3.12}$$

The Reynolds-averaged form of conservation equation for a general variable ϕ can be written as:

$$\frac{\partial}{\partial t}(\rho \bar{\phi}) + \nabla \cdot (\rho \bar{U}\bar{\phi} + \rho \overline{u\phi'}) = \nabla \cdot (\bar{j_\phi}) + \bar{S}_k \tag{3.13}$$

where the additional term appearing on the left-hand side represents turbulent transport of ϕ.

In the Reynolds averaging approach, it is not necessary to resolve all the small-scale (spatial and temporal) phenomena since the variation of time-averaged quantities occurs at much larger scales (Fig. 3.4). This approach, therefore, requires much less computing resources than the LES or DNS approaches. However, not resolving the small-scale phenomena comes with an inherent problem, the so-called 'closure' problem. Time averaging of the basic governing equations of flow processes leads to the appearance of new terms in the governing equations, which can be interpreted as 'apparent' stress gradients and heat and mass fluxes associated with the turbulent motion. In principle, governing equations for these new terms can be derived, however, these equations contain further new unknown terms. It becomes, therefore, necessary to introduce a 'turbulence model', which relates the new unknown terms to known terms in order to close the set of governing equations. The process of closing the set of equations through a 'turbulence model' introduces some approximations and assumptions, which are discussed in the following subsection. Generally, for most engineering applications, averaged equations are 'closed' by employing first-order or second-order closures. The cost-to-benefit ratio for employing higher than second-order closures is generally not favorable.

Before discussing RANS-based models, which are commonly used for engineering simulations, it will be worthwhile here to examine the relationship between the three main approaches (DNS, LES and RANS). DNS results can be used to test and develop better sub-grid scale models, which can be used with LES simulations. Implications of the assumptions and approximations employed in RANS modeling can be evaluated using large eddy simulations. With advances in the development of massively parallel computing platforms and efficient computational schemes (for example, lattice Boltzmann methods introduced by Frisch *et al.*, 1986), more and more attempts are being made to employ LES or DNS to flow processes relevant to engineers. In recent years, attempts have been made to develop a consistent modeling framework which can switch over from RANS to LES and then to DNS continuously with increases in scale resolution employed in the computational model (refer to Speziale (1998) for a more detailed discussion). These studies should be used to understand the potential and the limits of RANS-based models. Judicious analysis and engineering creativity is essential to construct computational models to simulate complex industrial engineering flow processes. Some of the key models used to simulate turbulence with RANS equations are discussed below.

3.4. TURBULENCE MODELS BASED ON RANS

A turbulence model is a set of equations which express relations between unknown terms appearing in Reynolds-averaged governing equations with known quantities. Examination of Reynolds-averaged equations (Eqs (3.10) and (3.11)) reveals that there are four equations (one continuity and three momentum conservation equations) and thirteen unknowns (three mean velocities, mean pressure and nine Reynolds stresses). Similarly, for a general scalar variable, ϕ, there is one conservation equation (Eq. (3.13)) and four unknowns (mean value of general variable, $\bar{\phi}$, and three turbulent fluxes $\overline{u\phi'}$). The desired turbulence model has to develop a relationship between these extra unknown fluxes and known mean variables. RANS-based turbulence models can be grouped into two classes: one which uses the concept of turbulent or eddy viscosity and another which does not. Models pertaining to these two classes are discussed below. It is not the purpose of this section to present all models in sufficient detail that they can be used without consulting the original references. Instead, the most widely used two-equation model, namely the k–ε model will be described in sufficient detail to enable the reader to formulate a 'baseline' model and to appreciate major issues involved therein. Other models are briefly reviewed and key references are cited to assist user in selecting a turbulence model appropriate to the problem (objective) under consideration.

3.4.1. Eddy Viscosity Models

A large proportion of the models of Reynolds stress use an eddy viscosity hypothesis based on an analogy between molecular and turbulent motions. Accordingly, turbulent eddies are visualized as molecules, colliding and exchanging momentum and obeying laws similar to the kinetic theory of gases. This allows the description of Reynolds stresses:

$$-\overline{\rho u_i u_j} = \mu_\mathrm{T}\left(\frac{\partial U_i}{\partial x_j} + \frac{\partial U_j}{\partial x_i}\right) - \frac{2}{3}\delta_{ij}\left(\mu_\mathrm{T}\frac{\partial U_k}{\partial x_k} + \rho k\right) \tag{3.14}$$

Here, μ_T is referred to as turbulent or eddy viscosity, which, in contrast to molecular viscosity, is not a fluid property but depends on the local state of flow or turbulence. It is assumed to be a scalar and may vary significantly within the flow domain. k is the turbulent kinetic energy (normal turbulent stresses) and can be expressed as

$$k = \tfrac{1}{2}\overline{u_i u_i} \tag{3.15}$$

Substitution of Eq. (3.14) in the Reynolds-averaged momentum conservation equations (Eqs (3.11)) leads to a closed set, provided the turbulent viscosity is known. The form of the Reynolds-averaged momentum equations remain identical to the form of the laminar momentum equations (Chapter 2 and Table 2.2) except that molecular viscosity is replaced by an effective viscosity, μ_eff:

$$\mu_\mathrm{eff} = \mu + \mu_\mathrm{T} \tag{3.16}$$

By analogy with the kinetic theory of gases, turbulent viscosity may be related to the characteristic velocity and length scales of turbulence (u_T and l_T respectively):

$$\mu_\mathrm{T} \propto \rho u_\mathrm{T} l_\mathrm{T} \tag{3.17}$$

The turbulence models then attempt to devise suitable methods/equations to estimate these characteristic length and velocity scales to close the set of equations.

Several different models have been developed. Excellent reviews describing the relative merits and demerits of models pertaining to this class are available (Launder and Spalding, 1972; Rodi, 1984; Markatos, 1986; Nallaswamy, 1987). Some salient features, which will provide basic information and guidelines, are discussed here. Most simple models, called zero equation models, estimate characteristic length and velocity scales by algebraic equations. Prandtl (1925) proposed a mixing length hypothesis for two-dimensional boundary layer flows which relates turbulent viscosity to velocity gradient:

$$\mu_\mathrm{T} = \rho l^2 \left|\frac{\partial U}{\partial y}\right| \tag{3.18}$$

This hypothesis works surprisingly well for many boundary layer flows. Prandtl suggested the estimation of characteristic length (mixing length) of turbulence (l) by postulating it to be proportional to the distance from the nearest wall. Several variations of this model and several empirical corrections have been proposed over the years to account for the effect of low Reynolds number, transitional regime, mass transfer, pressure gradient, transverse curvature and three-dimensional flows (for example, see Cebeci and Abbott, 1975). The spreading rates and profiles of velocity, temperature and concentrations of a variety of boundary layer flows can be predicted satisfactorily. However, it is necessary to change the values of model parameters for different flows. This lack of universality indicates that these types of model fail to describe some important features of real flows. The mixing length hypothesis implies that the generation and dissipation of turbulence energy are in equilibrium everywhere. The role of convection and diffusion is ignored in these models. For most internal flows which are of interest to reactor engineers, it may be difficult to obtain satisfactory results using this class of models.

For such flows it is necessary to devise a model which relies on using partial differential equations for estimating both length scale and velocity scales of turbulence (two-equation model). Several such models have been proposed (Launder and Spalding, 1972; Rodi, 1984; Wilcox, 1993). Two-equation turbulence models are the simplest ones that promise success for flows in which length scales cannot be prescribed empirically and are, in general, the recommended first choice for simulating internal turbulent flows. There are several different two-equation models proposed in the literature. All of these models employ a modeled form of turbulent kinetic energy (modeling of the gradient diffusion term may, however, be different). The choice of the second model transport equation, from which the length scale is determined, is the main differentiating factor among these models. Instead of the length scale itself, generally a combination of turbulent kinetic energy, k and length scale, l_T, having the form:

$$z = k^m l_{\mathrm{T}}^n \tag{3.19}$$

is chosen as dependent variable, z. Some of the popular forms of z are:

- turbulence frequency of energy containing eddies $= f$ $(m = 1/2; n = -1)$
- time averaged square of the vorticity fluctuations $= W$ $(m = 1; n = -2)$
- turbulent energy dissipation rate $= \varepsilon$ $(m = 3/2; n = -1)$
- product of energy and length scales $= kl$ $(m = 1; n = 1)$

The modeled transport equations for z differ mainly in the diffusion and secondary source term. Launder and Spalding (1972) and Chambers and Wilcox (1977) discuss the differences and similarities in more detail. The variable, $z = \varepsilon$ is generally preferred since it does not require a secondary source, and a simple gradient diffusion hypothesis is fairly good for the diffusion (Launder and Spalding, 1974; Rodi, 1984). The turbulent Prandtl number for ε has a reasonable value of 1.3, which fits the experimental data for the spread of various quantities at locations far from the walls, without modification of any constants. Because of these factors, the k–ε model of turbulence has been the most extensively studied and used and is recommended as a baseline model for typical internal flows encountered by reactor engineers.

In the k–ε model of turbulence, turbulent viscosity is related to k and ε by the following equation:

$$\mu_{\mathrm{T}} = \frac{C_\mu \rho k^2}{\varepsilon} \tag{3.20}$$

where C_μ is an empirical coefficient. Therefore, in order to close the set of equations, it is necessary to obtain values for k and ε. Local values of k and ε can be obtained by solving their transport equations. Exact transport equations for k and ε can be derived from the Navier–Stokes equations (see, for example, Ranade, 1988 for such a derivation). Without going into details of exact transport equations, various terms appearing in exact equations of k and ε are interpreted by classifying them into four groups: convective transport, diffusive transport, generation and dissipation. Diffusive transport comprises a molecular as well as turbulent component. Velocity and pressure fluctuations contribute to the diffusive transport of turbulent kinetic energy as well as energy dissipation rates and are usually modeled using a gradient diffusion approximation. The turbulent diffusivity of k and ε are related to turbulent viscosity with additional empirical constants, which are known as turbulent Prandtl numbers for k and ε. Turbulent kinetic energy is generated by extracting energy from the mean flow, and the terms representing this are also modeled using the assumption of turbulent viscosity. The generation term in the transport equation for ε represents vortex stretching by mean flow and fluctuating flow. The dissipation term in the transport equation for k is simply equal to ε. The viscous dissipation term appearing in the equation for ε cannot be modeled separately. However, the difference between the generation and dissipation term can be modeled with the help of two additional empirical constants. The modeled form of transport equations for k and ε can be written (Launder and Spalding, 1972):

$$\frac{\partial(\rho k)}{\partial t}+\frac{\partial(\rho U_i k)}{\partial x_i}=\frac{\partial}{\partial x_i}\left(\frac{\mu_\mathrm{T}}{\sigma_k}\frac{\partial k}{\partial x_i}\right)+G-\rho\varepsilon \tag{3.21}$$

$$\frac{\partial(\rho\varepsilon)}{\partial t}+\frac{\partial(\rho U_i \varepsilon)}{\partial x_i}=\frac{\partial}{\partial x_i}\left(\frac{\mu_\mathrm{T}}{\sigma_\varepsilon}\frac{\partial \varepsilon}{\partial x_i}\right)+\frac{\varepsilon}{k}(C_1 G-C_2\rho\varepsilon) \tag{3.22}$$

where G is the turbulence generation term given by:

$$G=\tfrac{1}{2}\mu_\mathrm{T}\left[\nabla\bar{U}+(\nabla\bar{U})^\mathrm{T}\right]^2 \tag{3.23}$$

These transport equations contain four empirical parameters, which are listed in Table 3.1 along with the parameter appearing in Eq. (3.20). The values of these parameters are obtained with the help of experimental information about simple flows such as decay of turbulence behind the grid (Launder and Spalding, 1972). Before discussing the modifications to the standard k–ε model and its recent renormalization group version, it will be useful to summarize implicit and explicit assumptions underlying the k–ε model:

- Turbulence is nearly homogeneous.
- The spectral distributions of turbulent quantities are similar.
- Diffusion is of the gradient type with constant effective Prandtl numbers.
- High Reynolds numbers.

It must be remembered that since all the assumptions may not be valid for flows of practical interest, the model parameters are not truly universal but are functions of characteristic flow parameters. Several attempts have been made to enhance the applicability of the k–ε model by modifying these empirical parameters to suit the specific requirements of different types of flow. One of the weaknesses of the standard

TABLE 3.1 Parameters of the k–ε Model

Sr. No	Parameter	Standard k–ε	RNG k–ε
1	C_D	0.09	0.0845
2	C_1	1.44	1.42
3	C_2	1.92	$1.68 + \dfrac{C_D\eta^3(1-\eta/4.38)}{1+0.012\eta^3} \quad \because \quad \eta = \dfrac{k\sqrt{G/\mu_t}}{\varepsilon}$
4	σ_k	1.0	~ 0.7179 (high Re limit)*
5	σ_ε	1.3	~ 0.7179 (high Re limit)*

*The general expression for estimating effective Prandtl numbers for k and ε is:

$$\left|\frac{1/\sigma - 1.3929}{0.3929}\right|^{0.6321}\left|\frac{1/\sigma - 2.3929}{3.3929}\right|^{0.3679} = \frac{\mu}{\mu_T}$$

k–ε model is that it overpredicts turbulence generation in regions where the mean flow is highly accelerated or decelerated. Kato and Launder (1993) proposed a modified k–ε model to overcome this problem. It will not be possible to discuss all the proposed modifications of the k–ε model here. Launder and Spalding (1972), Rodi (1984), Markatos (1986) and Nallaswamy (1987) discuss these modifications, among others. More discussion on the influence of compressibility and other issues can be found in Wilcox (1993).

In recent years, renormalization group (RNG) methods have been used to formulate two-equation turbulence models. These methods are a general framework for model building in which the complex dynamics is described in terms of so-called 'coarse-grained' equations governing the large-scale, long-time behavior. The basic idea applied to turbulence modeling is the elimination of small-scale eddies by employing RNG methods. As the small-scale eddies are removed, the effective viscosity of the system is increased. Through the scale elimination procedure, RNG theory develops an equation for effective viscosity and the corresponding transport equations of k and ε (Yakhot and Orszag, 1986; Yakhot *et al.*, 1992). The overall form of the model closely resembles the standard k–ε model except for the values of the model parameters. The values of model parameters derived by RNG methods are also listed in Table 3.1. The main difference between the standard and RNG version lies in the equation of turbulent energy dissipation rate. In large strain rate flows, the RNG model predicts a lower turbulent viscosity (larger ε and lower k) than the standard model. Although the RNG model has been shown to perform better than the standard model for flows with high streamline curvature, vortex shedding etc., it has not yet been validated as extensively as the standard k–ε model.

The RNG version of the k–ε model has been extended to employ a differential form of the equation for calculating effective viscosity from a knowledge of k and ε (Fluent User Guide, Vol. 4, 1997):

$$\nu_{\text{eff}} = \nu\left(1 + \sqrt{\frac{C_\mu}{\nu}}\frac{k}{\sqrt{\varepsilon}}\right)^2 \tag{3.24}$$

This form allows extension to low Reynolds number and near wall flows, unlike the standard k–ε model, which is valid only for fully turbulent flows. Despite such an extension, the standard and RNG versions of k–ε models are normally valid for turbulent flows away from the walls. The presence of a wall alters turbulence in a non-trivial way, by damping turbulence in the region very close to the wall. At the outer part of the near-wall region, turbulence is rapidly generated due to the large gradient in mean velocity. Correct representation of the influence of walls on turbulent flows is an important aspect of simulating wall-bounded flows.

Numerous experiments have shown that the near-wall region can be divided into three layers (Fig. 3.5(a)).

(1) The innermost layer, called the viscous sub-layer in which flow is laminar-like and the molecular viscosity plays a dominant role;
(2) an intermediate buffer layer, where molecular viscosity and turbulence are equally important;
(3) the outer layer, called the fully turbulent layer, where turbulence plays a major role.

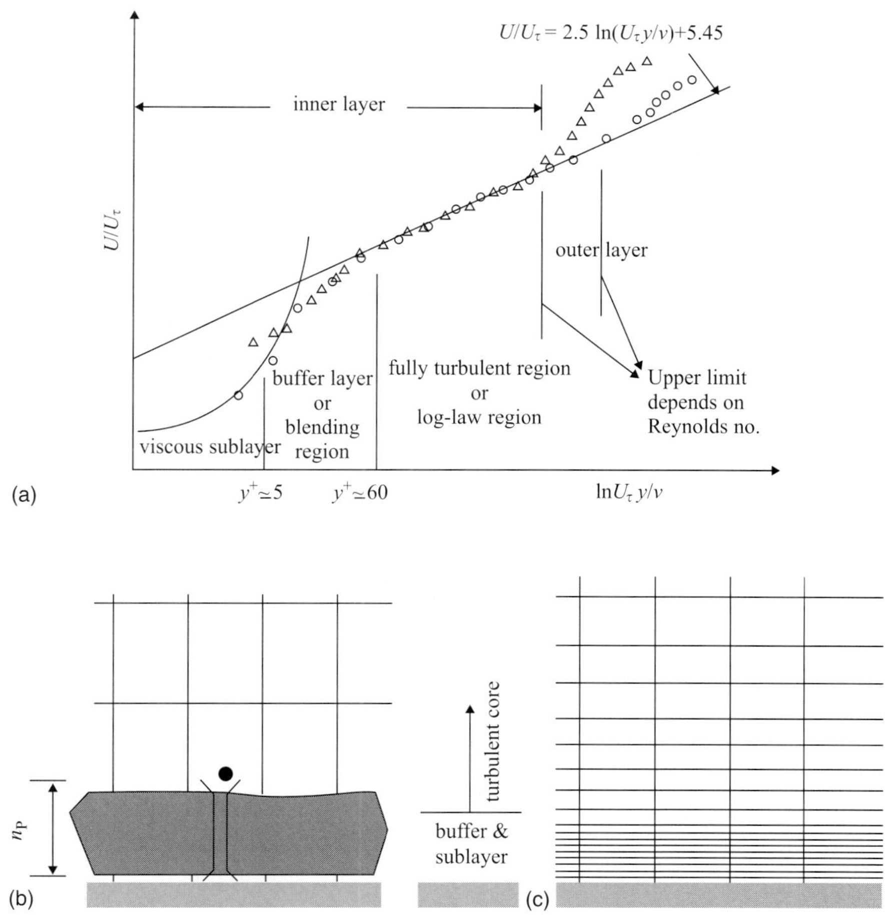

FIGURE 3.5 Near wall flows. (a) Flow structure near wall, (b) wall function approach, (c) low Re model approach (adapted from FLUENT user guide, Vol. 1).

There are two main approaches to modeling the near-wall region. In one approach, the so-called 'wall function' approach, the viscosity-affected inner regions (viscous and buffer layers) are not modeled. Instead, semi-empirical formulae (wall functions) are used to bridge the viscosity-affected region between the wall and the fully turbulent region. In another approach, special, low Reynolds number turbulence models are developed to simulate the near-wall region flow. These two approaches are shown schematically in Fig. 3.5(b) and 3.5(c).

In most high Reynolds number flows, the wall function approach gives reasonable results without excessive demands on computational resources. It is especially useful for modeling turbulent flows in complex industrial reactors. This approach is, however, inadequate in situations where low Reynolds number effects are pervasive and the hypotheses underlying the wall functions are not valid. Such situations require the application of a low Reynolds number model to resolve near-wall flows. For the low Reynolds number version of k–ε models, the following boundary conditions are used at the walls:

$$k = 0 \qquad \frac{\partial \varepsilon}{\partial n} = 0 \quad \text{or} \quad \varepsilon = \mu \left(\frac{\partial \bar{U}_t}{\partial n} \right)^2 \tag{3.25}$$

where U_t is the velocity component tangential to the wall and n is the co-ordinate normal to the wall. A number of low Reynolds number modifications to the k–ε model have been proposed (Chen and Patel, 1988; Wilcox, 1993; Hrenya and Sinclair, 1995). These models are too numerous to discuss here. Instead, the wall function approach, which is commonly used in reactor engineering applications, is briefly discussed below.

In the wall functions approach, a universal velocity profile of the form shown below is assumed to exist near the wall:

$$u^+ = \frac{1}{\kappa} \ln y^+ + B \tag{3.26}$$

where κ is the van Karmann constant (0.41), B is an empirical constant related to the thickness of the viscous sub-layer ($B \approx 5.2$ in a flat plate boundary layer) and u^+ and y^+ are defined as follows:

$$u^+ = \frac{U_t}{\sqrt{\tau_w/\rho}} \qquad y^+ = \frac{\rho\, n_P \sqrt{\tau_w/\rho}}{\mu} \tag{3.27}$$

where n_P is the normal distance of the considered node at point P from the wall (Fig. 3.5(b)). In addition, the flow is assumed to be in local equilibrium, which means that the production and dissipation terms are nearly equal. These assumptions then allow the use of coarse resolution at the wall. In fact, the wall function approach requires that the dimensionless distance of the adjacent grid node from the wall should be greater than 30 ($y^+ > 30$). For such a case, wall shear stress can be related to the tangential component of the velocity at the grid, as:

$$\tau_w = \frac{\kappa \rho C_\mu^{1/4} \sqrt{k}\, U_t}{\ln(y^+ E)} \tag{3.28}$$

For turbulent kinetic energy, k, the normal gradient at the wall is usually set to zero. By assuming the length scale near the wall, L to be given by:

$$L = \frac{\kappa n_{\mathrm{P}}}{C_\mu^{3/4}} \tag{3.29}$$

and by assuming equilibrium between production and dissipation, the turbulent energy dissipation rate at the node adjacent to the wall (denoted by subscript P, located at a normal distance n_P from the wall) can be computed without solving the transport equation for ε as:

$$\varepsilon_P = \frac{C_\mu^{3/4} k_P^{3/2}}{\kappa n_P} \tag{3.30}$$

It should be noted that the wall function approach is valid only when the first grid point adjacent to the wall (node P) is within the logarithmic region. For separated flows within the recirculation region and separation and reattachment regions, this condition may not be valid. To rectify this to some extent, several alternative wall functions have been proposed (see, for example, Amano, 1984). Generally, to simulate complex industrial reactors, wall functions are applied everywhere and the regions for which these may not be valid are assumed to be small. When the wall function approach is not applicable over a large portion of the wall boundaries, low Reynolds number models of turbulence should be used to resolve the finer details of near-wall flows.

In addition to representing the influence of walls on turbulence, adequate boundary conditions need to be specified to solve modeled equations of k and ε. At computational boundaries far from the wall, the following boundary conditions can be used (Ferziger and Peric, 1995):

- if the surrounding flow is turbulent:

$$\bar{U}\frac{\partial k}{\partial x} = -\varepsilon \qquad \bar{U}\frac{\partial \varepsilon}{\partial x} = -C_2\frac{\varepsilon^2}{k} \tag{3.31}$$

- in a free stream:

$$k = 0 \qquad \varepsilon = 0 \qquad \mu_{\mathrm{T}} = 0 \tag{3.32}$$

For the inlet boundary conditions, it will be necessary to specify values of k and ε. If available, experimental values should be used to set the inlet boundary conditions. If k is not known, it is generally estimated from a suitable guess of turbulence intensity (say 5%) at the inlet. The value of ε is usually estimated from a knowledge of k and assuming a characteristic length scale, L:

$$\varepsilon = \frac{k^{3/2}}{L} \tag{3.33}$$

The characteristic length used in the above equation may be taken as 0.07 times the equivalent pipe radius, in the absence of more information. If the Reynolds stress and mean velocities at the inlet are measured, ε can be estimated using the assumption of local equilibrium. The numerical implementation of these boundary conditions and numerical solution of two-equation turbulence models is discussed in Chapter 6.

3.4.2. Reynolds Stress Models

The two-equation models (especially, the k–ε model) discussed above have been used to simulate a wide range of complex turbulent flows with adequate accuracy, for many engineering applications. However, the k–ε model employs an isotropic description of turbulence and therefore may not be well suited to flows in which the anisotropy of turbulence significantly affects the mean flow. It is possible to encounter a boundary layer flow in which shear stress may vanish where the mean velocity gradient is non-zero and vice versa. This phenomenon cannot be predicted by the turbulent viscosity concept employed by the k–ε model. In order to rectify this and some other limitations of eddy viscosity models, several models have been proposed to predict the turbulent or Reynolds stresses directly from their governing equations, without using the eddy viscosity concept.

The exact transport equations for turbulent stresses can be derived from the Navier–Stokes equations, following similar procedures to those employed to derive the transport equations for turbulent kinetic energy. These transport equations contain several unknown correlations including the triple correlations of fluctuating velocities. It is, in turn, possible to derive transport equations for these triple correlations, which will, however, contain fourth-order correlations and so on. In general, however, triple and higher correlations are small in practical flows and a reactor engineer may not need to simulate them by transport equations. Therefore, for most reactor engineering flows, second-order closure, that is closing the transport equations for turbulent stresses, will be sufficient. Second-order closure models can be further classified into algebraic stress models (ASM) and differential Reynolds stress models (RSM). The starting point for both of these is the exact transport equation of turbulent stresses (these models can also be developed by a relaxation time approximation around an equilibrium model, Saffman, 1977). In order to understand the physical significance of the various terms appearing in these transport equations, the case of 2D boundary layers is considered here to avoid unnecessary complications. Multiplying each momentum transport equation by a fluctuating velocity component in the other direction and performing time averaging leads to the following equation:

$$\frac{D\overline{u'v'}}{Dt} = -\overline{v'^2}\frac{\partial U}{\partial y} - \frac{\partial}{\partial y}\left(\overline{u'v'^2} + \frac{\overline{p'u'}}{\rho}\right) + \overline{\frac{p'}{\rho}\left(\frac{\partial u'}{\partial y} + \frac{\partial v'}{\partial x}\right)} - 2\frac{\mu}{\rho}\sum_l \overline{\left(\frac{\partial u'}{\partial x_l}\frac{\partial v'}{\partial x_l}\right)} \tag{3.34}$$

Analogous to the transport equation of turbulence kinetic energy, k, the first term on the right-hand side represents 'production or generation', the second represents 'diffusion' and the final term represents 'dissipation'. The third term of the right-hand side, which has no counterpart in the k equation, represents 'redistribution'. It is the correlation between fluctuations in pressure and velocity gradients, which results in enhancement of velocity fluctuations in one direction at the expense of those in the other directions. It is necessary to model these terms in order to close the set of equations.

Production terms do not need any modeling since all the terms appearing there are calculated from the corresponding transport equations. The diffusional transport is assumed to be proportional to the spatial gradient of the stress component. Dissipation is usually assumed to take place isotropically in each of the three normal stress components, and is assumed to be zero in shear stress components. The redistributive action of pressure fluctuations can be represented by two groups of terms, one involving products of Reynolds stress and (ε/k), and the other containing products of stresses and mean velocity gradients (more discussion on precise details of these modeled terms can be found in Launder *et al.*, 1975; Launder, 1989). It must be noted that the approximations of dissipative or redistributive terms do not contain gradients of stress terms. Developers of algebraic stress models use this fact and attempt to eliminate convective and diffusive terms from the transport equations of turbulent stresses so as to derive a set of algebraic equations among the Reynolds stresses, the turbulence kinetic energy, the energy dissipation rate and mean velocity gradients. These algebraic equations can be expressed symbolically as

$$\overline{u_i u_j} = f\left(\overline{u_p u_q}, k, \varepsilon, \frac{\partial U_l}{\partial x_m}\right) \tag{3.35}$$

The precise form of the function varies depending on the approximated forms of the dissipative and redistributive terms and how the convective and diffusive transport terms are eliminated. Launder (1971) neglected the latter terms entirely while Rodi (1984) assumed that the convective transport is proportional to the transport of k with an equivalent assumption for the diffusion term. Rodi's algebraic stress model can be written:

$$\begin{aligned}
-\overline{u'u'} &= \frac{2}{3}k\mathrm{i}\left[1 - \frac{(1 - C_{2a})\,G/\varepsilon}{(G/\varepsilon) - (1 - C_{1a})}\right] \\
&\quad + \frac{1 - C_{2a}}{(G/\varepsilon) - (1 - C_{1a})}\frac{k}{\varepsilon}\left[-\left(\overline{u'u'}\cdot\nabla U + (\overline{u'u'}\cdot\nabla U)^T\right) - \frac{2}{3}G\mathrm{i}\right]
\end{aligned} \tag{3.36}$$

where i is the unit tensor and G is the generation of turbulent kinetic energy (given by Eq. (3.23)). The values of two additional model parameters, C_{1a} and C_{2a}, are reported as 2.2 and 0.45, respectively. The k and ε appearing in these equations can be obtained by solving the modeled transport equations of k and ε (Eqs (3.21) and (3.22)). Alternatively, one may use Reynolds stresses calculated by the above equations to calculate the generation term, G in the transport equations of k and ε. This practice will be more consistent and accurate. Note that Eq. (3.36) is an implicit equation for calculation of Reynolds stress since it appears on both sides of the equation. These implicit models can give rise to multiple solutions or singularities when solved iteratively. Therefore, several attempts have been made to develop explicit algebraic stress models (ASM) in recent years. For example, Gatski and Speziale (1993) developed a regularized, explicit algebraic stress model, which reduces to the k–ε model in the limit of homogeneous turbulence in equilibrium. These explicit ASM avoid multiple solutions and can, therefore, be recommended for simulations of complex turbulent flows. Gatski and Speziale (1993) and Speziale (1998) may be referred to for details of model equations and further analysis.

Wherever the convective and diffusive transport of Reynolds stresses are important (flows that are far from equilibrium), algebraic stress models may prove to be inadequate, and solution of the full transport equations of the Reynolds stresses may become necessary. Extensive efforts have been made to model the terms appearing in the exact transport equations of Reynolds stresses. The redistributive term has been the subject of most controversy and experimentation. Several different models have been proposed (Daly and Harlow, 1970; Hanjalic and Launder, 1972; Launder *et al.*, 1975; Reynolds and Cebeci, 1978; Launder, 1989). The current generation second-order closure models do not perform well when there are significant departures from equilibrium. It is a general feeling that it may require quite some time before these models are sufficiently well developed to perform better than simpler two-equation models (such as the k–ε model) for engineering problems. Recently attempts have been made to develop second-order closures that are suitable for non-equilibrium flows based on a relaxation time approximation around the non-equilibrium extension of the explicit ASM (Speziale, 1998). Speziale (1998) described this approach to formulate a consistent framework to integrate RANS (two equations to full second-order closure), LES and DNS based on such models. Such an approach looks promising and deserves further research. The details of Reynolds stress models are not included here, since most of the engineering flows may be adequately analyzed using modifications of two-equation turbulence models. Details of RSM can be found in above cited papers and references cited therein. A brief summary of the advantages and disadvantages of two-equation models (k–ε and RNG k–ε) and Reynolds stress models (algebraic and differential) is given in Table 3.2.

Apart from the models discussed and mentioned here, there are some more miscellaneous attempts to describe specific aspects of turbulence by phenomenological modeling. For example, Professor Spalding and his group have proposed the use of 'two-fluid' models of turbulence to describe the 'fragmentaryness' and 'intermittancy' of turbulent flows. The approach has shown some successes in simulating key features of jets and other flows (Spalding, 1983; Malin and Spalding, 1984), however, it is not adequately developed to use as a general approach. For some situations encountered in chemical reactors, such as combustion, this approach may be useful (see a review by Markatos, 1986).

It is important for a reactor engineer to select an appropriate turbulence model for the application at hand from the available turbulence models. It is also important that implications of assumptions underlying these models are adequately understood. It should be kept in mind that a more complex model does not necessarily mean a better model. The reactor engineer has to constantly evaluate implications of the underlying assumptions and performance of the model in light of whatever direct and indirect validation one can carry out and in light of the fulfillment of the simulation objectives. Generally, the two-equation, k–ε model can be recommended as a baseline model. When the interest is in simulating unsteady vortex shedding, the renormalization group version of the k–ε model may be used. In any case, be it the RNG model or the Reynolds stress models, it is always useful to first carry out simulations using the standard k–ε model. While doing this, a reactor engineer must, however, be careful in making appropriate corrections to the standard model to compensate for the known deficiencies of the standard model (such as for modelling axis-symmetric round jets). The predicted results of the two-equation model can then be used as an initial guess to start the simulations using more complex turbulence models. It must be noted that simulated results of many complex, industrial flow processes are more influenced by the employed grid resolution and discretization schemes than the underlying turbulence model. It is, therefore, necessary to clearly identify, monitor and control the influence of numerical issues on predicted results (these aspects are discussed in Chapters 6 and 7).

TABLE 3.2 Summary of Two-equation and Reynolds Stress Models

Model	Advantages	Disadvantages
Standard k–ε	• Simplest model to represent variation of turbulence length and velocity scales • Robust and economical • Excellent performance for many industrial flows • The most widely validated model	• More expensive than zero equation models • Assumes isotropic eddy viscosity • Performs poorly for: – some unconfined flows – rotating flows – non-circular ducts – curved boundary layers
RNG k–ε	• Performs better than standard model for some: – separated flows – swirling flows	• Assumes isotropic eddy viscosity • Not sufficiently validated so far
Algebraic Stress Models (ASM)	• Accounts for anisotropy • Combines generality of approach with the economy of the k–ε model • Good performance for isothermal and buoyant thin shear layers	• Restricted to flows where convection and diffusion terms are negligible • Performs as poorly as k–ε in some flows due to problems with ε equation • Not widely validated
Reynolds Stress Models (RSM)	• Most general model of all classical turbulence models • Performs well for many complex flows including non-circular ducts and curved flows	• Computationally expensive (seven extra PDEs) • Performs as poorly as k–ε in some flows due to problems with ε equation • Not widely validated

3.4.3. Scalar Transport Models

Turbulence is often employed to enhance the rates of mixing and transport processes. A reactor engineer is therefore interested in finding out the extent of turbulence generated in a reactor and its influence on other transport processes. The discussion of turbulence modeling so far has been restricted to the modeling of momentum conservation. It is necessary to account for turbulence, while modeling the species and enthalpy conservation equations. Species and enthalpy conservation, for most reactor engineering flows, are modeled using eddy viscosity type models. The Reynolds-averaged equation for a general scalar variable ϕ is Eq. (3.13). The third term on the left-hand side containing the correlation of fluctuating velocity and fluctuating scalar variable requires further modeling. In writing the time-averaged equations, density fluctuations were assumed to be insignificant. The correlation appearing in this equation is usually modeled using the gradient transport assumption:

$$\overline{u'\phi'} = -\frac{\nu_T}{\sigma_\phi}\nabla\phi \tag{3.37}$$

The parameter, σ_ϕ appearing in the above equation is the turbulent Prandtl number for ϕ. The value of turbulent Prandtl number is determined experimentally and is generally of the order of unity. The values of turbulent Prandtl number may also be estimated using RNG methods (Yakhot and Orszag, 1986). The Reynolds-averaged species as well as enthalpy conservation equations can be closed with the help of Eq. (3.37), provided that the closed form of the time-averaged source term is known. The modeling of time-averaged source terms for reactive flow processes will be discussed in the Chapter 5. Though it is possible to develop a transport equation for the correlation of scalar variable and fluctuating velocity by following the methods similar to those used for Reynolds stress models, gradient assumption is used in practice, for most of the engineering simulations.

The influence of a wall on the turbulent transport of scalar (species or enthalpy) at the wall can also be modeled using the wall function approach, similar to that described earlier for modeling momentum transport at the wall. It must be noted that the thermal or mass transfer boundary layer will, in general, be of different thickness than the momentum boundary layer and may change from fluid to fluid. For example, the thermal boundary layer of a high Prandtl number fluid (e.g. oil) is much less than its momentum boundary layer. The wall functions for the enthalpy equations in the form of temperature T can be written as:

$$\frac{(T_\mathrm{W} - T_\mathrm{P})\,\rho C_\mathrm{p} C_\mu^{1/4} k_\mathrm{P}^{1/2}}{q_\mathrm{w}} = \begin{cases} \mathrm{Pr}\,\dfrac{\rho y_\mathrm{P} C_\mu^{1/4} k_\mathrm{P}^{1/2}}{\mu} & \because \dfrac{\rho y_\mathrm{P} C_\mu^{1/4} k_\mathrm{P}^{1/2}}{\mu} < y_\mathrm{T}^* \\ \sigma_\mathrm{T}\left[\dfrac{1}{\kappa}\ln\left(E\dfrac{\rho y_\mathrm{P}^* C_\mu^{1/4} k_\mathrm{P}^{1/2}}{\mu}\right) + P\right] & \because \dfrac{\rho y_\mathrm{P} C_\mu^{1/4} k_\mathrm{P}^{1/2}}{\mu} > y_\mathrm{T}^* \end{cases} \tag{3.38}$$

where P is the 'pee function' given by (Launder and Spalding, 1974)

$$P = \frac{\pi/4}{\sin \pi/4}\left(\frac{A}{\kappa}\right)^{1/2}\left(\frac{\mathrm{Pr}}{\sigma_\mathrm{T}} - 1\right)\left(\frac{\sigma_\mathrm{T}}{\mathrm{Pr}}\right)^{1/4} \tag{3.39}$$

where Pr is the Prandtl number, A is van Driest's constant ($= 26$) and E is a wall function constant (~ 9 for smooth walls). y_T^* is dimensionless thermal sublayer thickness (the point of intersection of the linear law and the logarithmic law).

The modeled form of scalar transport equations can be used to simulate mixing and concentration fields within the reactor. Such computational models can, therefore, be used to link the reactor hardware and operating parameters with the mixing and residence time distribution, which will ultimately lead to estimation of reactor performance. A reactor engineer has to make appropriate selection of the turbulence model depending on the objectives under consideration. For example, for a heat transfer limited reactor, reactor hardware may be modified to install turbulence promoters. Unsteady vortices around these turbulence promoters may enhance the heat transfer rates and overcome heat transfer limitation. For such applications, capturing these vortices and simulating their influence on heat transfer rates is of primary importance. It is then necessary to select a turbulence model as well as its numerical implementation in such a way that it does not smear local structures such as vortices. If the interest is in estimating wall heat or mass transfer rates, it may be worthwhile to use more rigorous, non-equilibrium wall functions, which are sensitized to pressure gradient for better prediction of separated flows. For applications where the universal wall law is not valid, low Reynolds number turbulence models may be used at the expense of more computations. The reactor engineer may be interested in microscale flow characteristics near the feed nozzle in order to understand various selectivity issues in mixing sensitive reactions. An accurate simulation of energy dissipation rates is then of primary importance (these issues will be discussed in detail in the chapter on modeling reactive flow processes). When the objective is to quickly screen alternative reactor configurations to minimize overall mixing time (which is mostly dominated by the large-scale convective flows), it is sufficient to obtain the correct prediction of the mean velocity field. The choice of turbulence model is then not as critical as in some of the cases mentioned above.

For multiphase flow processes, turbulent effects will be much larger. Even operability will be controlled by the generated turbulence in some cases. For dispersed fluid–fluid flows (as in gas–liquid or liquid–liquid reactors), the local sizes of dispersed phase particles and local transport rates will be controlled by the turbulence energy dissipation rates and turbulence kinetic energy. The modeling of turbulent multiphase flows is discussed in the next chapter.

It must be realized that most of the available turbulence models obscure the actual physical processes such as eddies, high vorticity regions, large structures which stretch and engulf and so on. However, the cautious application and interpretation of turbulence models has proved to be a valuable tool in engineering research and design, despite their physical deficiencies. The other important issue one must remember concerns the appropriate selection of a turbulence model to achieve the required objectives. Launder (1989) argued the case of different turbulence models by drawing an analogy between these and a variety of transport machines: from bicycles, automobiles to airplanes. Just as each transport machine has its own role, different turbulence models can play mutually complementary roles in developing quantitative models for simulating turbulent flow processes. The discussion in this chapter, hopefully, provides a road map with which a reactor engineer can plan an exploration of the world of turbulence modeling. Specific case studies of the application of turbulence models to reactor engineering are discussed in Part IV of this book.

3.5. SUMMARY

Turbulence is a most complex fluid motion and has puzzled theoreticians and modelers for more than a century. Turbulence significantly enhances rates of mixing and other transport processes at the expense of more friction and energy losses. Many reactor technologies rely on these enhanced rates of transport processes via turbulence. It is, therefore, of crucial importance to develop turbulence models capable of making quantitative predictions. The wide range of length and time scales existing in turbulent flows poses a severe challenge to modelers. Several different approaches such as DNS (direct numerical simulations), LES (large eddy simulations) and RANS (Reynolds-averaged Navier–Stokes equations)-based models have been developed. Although DNS and LES offer valuable insight into turbulence and mechanisms of transport, for the foreseeable future, most reactor engineering flows have to rely on RANS-based models. It is noteworthy that the simple, two-equation k–ε model succeeds in expressing the main features of many turbulent flows by relying on just one characteristic length scale and time scale. This model is, therefore, recommended as a baseline model. More advanced RANS-based models such as Reynolds stress models (RSM) and non-linear extensions of k–ε models or RNG models deserve careful evaluation from the cost-to-benefit point of view for each case. It must be remembered that a more complex model does not necessarily mean a better model. Moreover, it should never be forgotten that all RANS-based models contain adjustable constants that need to be determined by fitting experimental data. All reactor engineers are aware of the dangers of extrapolating an empirical model beyond its data range. Although the turbulence models discussed here are not entirely empirical, none of the CFD simulations of 'new' turbulent flows should be accepted as they are, without rigorous error analysis and validation. Some aspects of error analysis and validation are discussed in Chapters 6 and 7. The new information obtained from DNS and LES approaches should be used to examine the limitations of RANS-based models and to guide their further development. Despite some of the deficiencies of turbulence models, the best modern computational models (and numerical methods) allow almost all flows to be calculated to higher accuracy than the best-informed guess. This means that these methods are genuinely useful for reactor engineering.

REFERENCES

Amano, R.S. (1984), Development of a turbulence near wall model, *Numer. Heat Transfer*, **7**, 59.

Banerjee, S. (1992), Turbulence structures, *Chem. Eng. Sci.*, **47**, 1793–1817.

Berge, P., Pomeau, Y. and Vidal, C. (1984), "Order within Chaos", John Wiley & Sons, Paris.

Cebeci, T. and Abbott, D.E. (1975), *AIAA J.*, **13**, 829.

Chambers, T.L. and Wilcox, D.C. (1977), Critical examination of two-equation turbulence closure models for boundary layers, *AIAA J.*, **15**(6), 821.

Chen, H.C. and Patel, V.C. (1988), Near-wall turbulence models for complex flows including separation, *AIAA J*, **26**, 641.

Choi, H., Moin, P. and Kim, J. (1994), Active turbulence control for drag reduction in wall bounded flows, *J. Fluid Mech.*, **262**, 75.

Daly, B.J. and Harlow, F.H. (1970), Transport equations in turbulence, *Phys. Fluids*, **13**, 2634.

Derksen, J. and van den Akker, H.E.A. (1999), Large eddy simulations on the flow driven by a Rushton turbine, *AIChE J*, **45**, 209–221.

Ferziger, J.H. (1976), Large eddy simulations of turbulent flows, *AIAA J.*, **14**, 76.

Ferziger, J.H. (1995), Large eddy simulation, in "Simulation and Modeling of Turbulent Flows", Cambridge University Press, New York.

Ferziger, J.H. and Peric, M. (1995), "Computational Methods for Fluid Dynamics", Springer Verlag, Berlin.

Frisch, U., Hasslacher, B. and Pomeau, Y. (1986), Lattice-gas automata for the Navier–Stokes equations, *Phys. Rev. Lett.*, **56**, 1505.

Gatski, T.B. and Speziale, C.G. (1993), On explicit algebraic stress models for complex turbulent flow, *J. Fluid Mech.*, **140**, 198.

Germano, M., Piomelli, U., Moin, P. and Cabot, W.H. (1991), A dynamic subgrid-scale eddy viscosity model, *Phys. Fluids*, **3**, 1760.

Hanjalic, K. and Launder, B.E. (1972), A Reynolds stress model of turbulence and its application to thin shear flows, *J. Fluid Mech.*, **52**, 609.

Hinze, J.O. (1975), "Turbulence", 2nd edition, McGraw–Hill, New York.

Hrenya, C.M. and Sinclair, J. (1995), Effects of particle phase turbulence in gas-solid flows, *AIChE J.*, **43**, 853–869.

Hussaini, M.Y., Speziale, C.G. and Zang, T.A. (1990), On the large eddy simulation of compressible isotropic turbulence, *Lecture Notes in Physics*, **357**, 354.

Kato, M. and Launder, B.E. (1993), The modeling of turbulent flow around stationary and vibrating square cylinders, *Proceedings of 9th Symposium on Turbulent Shear Flows*, Kyoto.

Kim, J., Moin, P. and Moser, R.D. (1987), Turbulence statistics in fully developed channel flows at low Reynolds number, *J. Fluid Mech.*, **177**, 133.

Launder, B.E. (1971), An improved algebraic stress model of turbulence, Imperial College, Mechanical Engineering Department Report, TM/TN/A/11.

Launder, B.E. and Spalding, D.B. (1972), "Lectures in Mathematical Models of Turbulence", Academic Press, London.

Launder, B.E. and Spalding, D.B. (1974), The numerical computation of turbulent flows, *Comput. Methods Appl. Mech. and Eng.*, **3**, 269.

Launder, B.E., Reece, G.J. and Rodi, W. (1975), Progress in the development of Reynolds stress turbulence closure, *J. Fluid Mech.*, **68**, 537.

Launder, B.E. (1989), Second-moment closure: present.... And future?, *Int. J. Heat Fluid Flow*, **10**, 282.

Leonard, A. (1974), On the energy cascade in large-eddy simulations of turbulent flows, *Adv. Geophys. A.*, **18**, 237.

Leonard, A. (1995), Direct numerical simulation, in "Turbulence and its Simulation", Springer Verlag, New York.

Malin, M.R. and Spalding, D.B. (1984), Calculations of intermittency in self-preserving free turbulent jets and wakes, CFDU Report, CFD/84/5, Imperial College, London.

Markatos, N.C. (1986), Computer simulation techniques for turbulent flows, in "Encyclopedia of Fluid Mechanics", Vol. 3, (Ed.) Chereminishoff, N.P., Gulf Publishing Co.

Nallaswamy, M. (1987), Turbulence models and their application to the predictions of internal flows: A review, *Computational Fluids*, **15**, 151.

Orszag, S.A., Staroselsky, I. and Yakhot, V. (1993), Some basic challenges for large-eddy simulation research, in "Large-Eddy Simulations of Complex Engineering and Geophysical Flows", Cambridge University Press, New York.

Prandtl, L. (1925) *Z. Angew. Math. Mech.*, **5**, 136.

Ranade, V.V. (1988), Design of multiphase reactors: measurements and modeling of flow structures in stirred vessels and design of loop reactors, PhD thesis, University of Bombay, India.

Reynolds, W.C. (1990), The potential and limitations of direct and large eddy simulations, in "Whither Turbulence? Turbulence at Cross Roads", Springer Verlag, Berlin.

Reynolds, W.C. and Cebeci, T. (1978), Calculation of turbulent flows, in "Turbulence topics in Applied Physics", Vol. **12**, 2nd edition, Springer Verlaag, Berlin.

Rodi, W. (1984), "Turbulence Models and their Application in Hydraulics", Delft, The Netherlands, IHRA.

Rogallo, R.S. and Moin, P. (1984), Numerical simulation of turbulent flows, *Ann. Rev. Fluid. Mech.*, **16**, 99–137.

Saffman, P.G. (1977), Results of a two-equation model for turbulent flows and development of relaxation stress model for application to staining and rotating flows, *Proceedings of Project SQUID Workshop on Turbulence in Internal Flows*, Hemisphere, New York, p. 191.

Smagorinsky, J. (1963), General circulation equipments with primitive equations, *Monthly Weather Rev.*, **93**, 99.

Spalding, D.B. (1983), Chemical reaction in turbulent fluids, *Physico Chem. Hydrodynamics*, **4**, 323–336.

Speziale, C.G. (1998), Turbulent modeling for time-dependent RANS and VLES: A review, *AIAA J.*, **36**(2), 173.

Van Dyke, M. (1982), *An Album of Fluid Motion*, The Parabolic Press, Stanford, CA.

Wilcox, D.C. (1993), "Turbulence Modeling for CFD", DCW Industries Inc., La Canada, California.

Yakhot, V. and Orszag, S.A. (1986), Renormalization group analysis of turbulence, I. Basic Theory, *J. Sci. Comput.*, **1**, 1.

Yakhot, V., Orszag, S.A., Thangam, S., Gtaski, T.B. and Speziale, C.G. (1992), Development of turbulence models for shear flows by double expansion technique, *Phys. Fluids A*, **4**(7), 1510.

4 MULTIPHASE FLOW PROCESSES

4.1. INTRODUCTION

Multiphase flow processes are key elements of several important reactor technologies. These technologies cover a wide range, from very large-scale operations such as fluid catalytic cracking reactors, to specialized reactors to produce high value, low volume specialty chemicals. The presence of more than one phase raises several additional questions for the reactor engineer. Multiphase flow processes exhibit different flow regimes depending on the operating conditions and the geometry of the process equipment. It is often necessary to develop tools to evaluate the operability of the multiphase flow process under specified conditions and to identify the operating regime. The fluid dynamics and transport processes occurring in multiphase reactors are especially sensitive to reactor configurations and operating conditions. Even small-scale hardware details such as the design of a feed nozzle or distributor may have a dramatic influence on the resulting flow structure. It is, therefore, of paramount importance to develop understanding and predictive tools to simulate multiphase flow processes to develop better reactor technologies.

The subject of the modeling of multiphase flow processes is quite vast and covers a wide range of sub-topics. It is virtually impossible to treat all the relevant issues in a single book, let alone in a single chapter. Here we attempt to provide a brief review of modeling approaches and cite the key references for further details. An attempt is made to provide sufficient information to develop a baseline model. The first section discusses various flow regimes and their key features. Various approaches to modeling these multiphase flow processes are then reviewed. Because of the importance of dispersed multiphase flows in reactor engineering, modeling of dispersed flows is discussed in more detail, in Section 4.2. Three basic approaches to modeling multiphase flows, namely, volume of fluid (VOF), Eulerian–Lagrangian (EL) and Eulerian–Eulerian (EE) are discussed with reference to dispersed flows. Some comments are made to guide the selection of an appropriate modeling approach. The topic of flow through porous media is discussed with specific emphasis on flow through fixed bed reactors. Some comments on developing tractable computational models of complex, multiphase flow processes are also included.

4.1.1. Types of Multiphase Flows

When two or more phases move relative to each other, these phases may exhibit a large number of possible flow regimes. There are several ways of classifying these multiphase flows. The simplest, first layer classification is according to the presence of thermodynamic phases: gas–liquid, gas–solid, gas–liquid–solid, liquid–liquid, liquid–solid and so on. Each component of these classes can then be grouped according to the flow regimes (topology of the flow). Broadly, flow regimes are classified as dispersed flows, mixed flows and separated flows (Ishii, 1975). In dispersed flows all the phases except one exist as dispersed (discontinuous) particles flowing through the continuous fluid. Examples of this flow regime include bubbles in liquid, solid particles in gas or liquid and liquid droplets in gas or other immiscible liquid. In separated flows, none of the phases exist in discontinuous particle form. All the phases flow in a semi-continuous mode with interfaces between the different phases. Examples of this flow regime include film flow, annular flow and jet flow. In mixed flow regimes, dispersed particles as well as semi-continuous interfaces exist together. Examples of this regime include droplet annular flow (where liquid flows in the form of an annular film over the pipe as well as suspended droplets in the gas core), bubbly annular flow (where some gas bubbles flow through the annular liquid film) and slug flow. Separated or mixed flow regimes may exist in trickle bed reactors. However, in most of the other reactors, dispersed flow regimes exist. Therefore, modeling of dispersed flows is discussed here in detail. The dispersed flow regime can be further divided into several sub-regimes. Some commonly encountered (in reactor engineering applications) gas–solid and gas–liquid flows are shown in Fig. 1.9. Key features of these different regimes are discussed here with reference to gas–solid and gas–liquid reactors.

In gas–solid reactors when solid particles are held stationary (so-called fixed bed reactor), gas flows through a porous medium comprising macropores existing between pellets or packed solid particles and micropores within the catalyst pellets (or other porous solids). Issues such as isotropy of the porous medium, initial distribution of gases, characteristics of solid particles, ratio of characteristic length scale of solid particles and that of the reactor and so on, influence the flow within fixed bed reactors. Support screens are often used to cover the bed of solid particles to avoid fluidization and carry-over of bed particles. These reactors are extensively used in process industries. Some examples and illustrative flow simulations are discussed in Chapter 13.

In other gas–solid reactors (fluidized reactors), gas is the continuous phase and solid particles are suspended within this continuous phase. Depending on the properties of the gas and solid particles, the geometry of the reactor and operating flow rates of gas and solid phases, several different sub-regimes of dispersed two-phase flows may exist as shown in Fig. 1.9. For relatively small gas flow rates, the reactor may contain a dense bed of fluidized solid particles. The bed may be homogeneously fluidized or gas may pass through the bed in the form of large bubbles. Further increase in gas flow rate decreases the bed density and the gas–solid contacting pattern may change from dense bed to turbulent bed, then to fast-fluidized mode and ultimately to pneumatic conveying mode. In all these flow regimes the relative importance of gas–particle, particle–particle and particle–wall interaction is different. It is, therefore, necessary to identify these regimes to select an appropriate mathematical model. Details of flow regime identification are discussed in Part IV while discussing the application of computational flow modeling to specific reactor types. In this chapter, governing equations for general flow types will be discussed.

For many gas–liquid or gas–liquid–solid reactors, the liquid phase is a continuous phase in which gas bubbles and solid particles are dispersed (bubble column or multiphase stirred tank reactors). Bubble column reactors may also exhibit different sub-regimes, namely homogeneous bubbly flow, churn-turbulent flow and slug flow depending on the geometry, operating conditions such as flow rates, pressure, temperature and physical properties of individual phases. The characteristics of these regimes are quite different from each other and each regime may require specialized models and boundary conditions. When there is further increase in gas flow rate, in some cases, frothing may occur. Beyond frothing, further increase in gas flow rate may make gas a continuous phase with liquid drops dispersed in it. When an additional flow-modifying element, such as the rotating impeller in stirred reactors, is present in the reactor, one may have to use a different classification for the flow regimes. See, for example, Fig. 1.8 for some flow regimes observed in a gas–liquid stirred tank reactor. As long as one phase exists as a continuous phase and the others as dispersed phases (this includes liquid–liquid and gas–liquid–liquid reactors), the general model equations discussed in the next section may be used.

Other special types of reactor may have different flow regimes specific to those particular configurations. For example, as mentioned earlier, in trickle bed reactors, liquid and gas flow through a packed bed of solid particles. Gas and liquid phases maintain a free interface and flow over solid particles. Several flow regimes may occur in such trickle bed reactors. It will not be possible to discuss modeling of flow in all these different types of multiphase reactors in a single chapter. Because of the importance of the dispersed flow regime, modeling of this flow regime is discussed here in detail. Modeling of other types of multiphase flow is briefly discussed and key references are cited for further reading. Some details are also discussed in Part IV of this book.

4.1.2. Modeling Approaches

It will be useful to discuss here different modeling approaches and some of the key issues in modeling multiphase flow processes. In general, there are three main issues one needs to address:

- Definition of 'phase'/Flow regime/Required resolution
- Formulation of governing equations
- Solution of governing equations

An obvious definition of 'phase' is 'thermodynamic state' (gas, liquid or solid). However, it is possible to define different 'phases' for computational purpose, although the thermodynamic state is not different. For example, while modeling dispersed gas–solid flows when there is a wide distribution of particle sizes, it is convenient to define multiple phases representing the solid phase. Each such phase may be associated with a specific narrow band of particle sizes, having more or less identical properties (such as drag coefficient). It is also sometimes useful to treat two thermodynamically distinct phases as one phase for computational purposes. For example, in a gas–liquid–solid slurry reactor, if the solid particles are fine enough to essentially follow liquid flow, it will be convenient to treat the liquid–solid mixture as a 'slurry' phase and model the three-phase system as a two-phase system (gas–slurry). Computational phases can even be defined based on local flow characteristics such as turbulent or irrotational fluid (Spalding, 1983). Judicious definition of computational phases and consideration of possible flow regimes are often the first crucial steps in selecting the modeling approach. Once the phases are defined, relevant flow regimes can be identified (see a brief discussion in the previous section, and Part IV). Depending on the required resolution, different modeling approaches may be used.

There are three main approaches for modeling multiphase flows:

(a) Volume of fluid approach (Eulerian framework for both the phases with reformulation of interface forces on volumetric basis).
(b) Eulerian framework for the continuous phase and Lagrangian framework for all the dispersed phases.
(c) Eulerian framework for all phases (without explicitly accounting for the interface between phases).

Basic concepts of these approaches are shown schematically in Fig. 4.1 and are briefly discussed below.

The first approach, the volume of fluid (VOF) approach, is conceptually the simplest. In this approach, the motion of all phases is modeled by formulating local, instantaneous conservation equations for mass, momentum and energy. Such local instantaneous conservation equations can be solved using appropriate jump boundary conditions at the interface. However, the interface between different phases may not remain stationary and imposing boundary conditions at such an interface becomes a very complicated moving boundary problem. To avoid this, instead of directly tracking the deforming and moving interface, the VOF approach tracks motion of all the phases, from which motion of the interface is inferred indirectly. All the interfacial forces, therefore, have to be replaced by smoothly varying volumetric forces. If the shape and flow processes occurring near the interface are of interest, the VOF approach should be used. Some interface-related forces, such as surface or adhesion forces, can be modeled accurately using this approach. This approach is, however, naturally limited to modeling the motion of only a few dispersed phase particles. For simulations of dispersed multiphase flows in large equipment, this approach is not suitable, as it requires huge computational resources to resolve flow

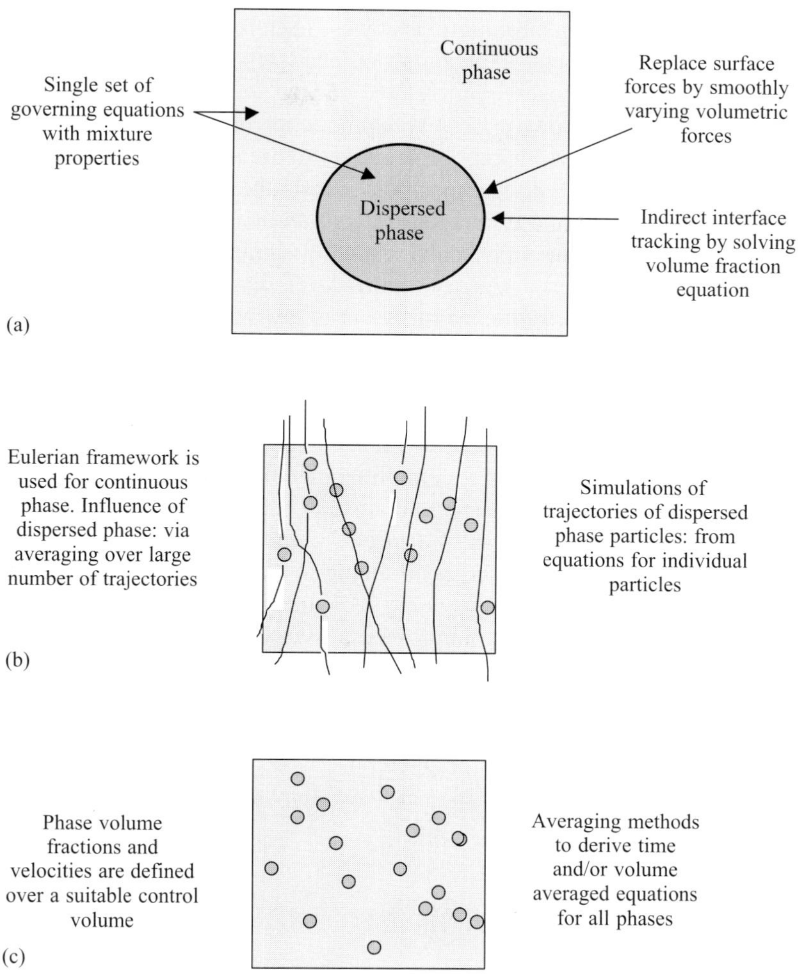

FIGURE 4.1 Modeling approaches for multiphase flows. (a) 'Volume of fluid' approach, (b) Eulerian–Lagrangian approach, (c) Eulerian–Eulerian approach.

processes around each dispersed phase particle. VOF-based models can be very useful as learning tools and can provide valuable information to develop appropriate closure models for Eulerian–Lagrangian and Eulerian–Eulerian approaches.

In the Eulerian–Lagrangian approach, explicit motion of the interface is not modeled. This means small-scale fluid motions around individual dispersed phase particles are not considered. Their influence is modeled indirectly while considering the motion of dispersed phase particles. In this approach, motion of the continuous phase is modeled using a Eulerian framework. The motions of dispersed phase particles (trajectories) are explicitly simulated in a Lagrangian framework. Averaging over a large number of trajectories is then carried out to derive the required information for the modeling of the continuous phase. In this approach, particle-level processes such as reactions, heat and mass transfer etc. can be simulated in adequate detail. In the case of turbulent flows, it is necessary to simulate a very large number of particle trajectories to obtain meaningful averages. Therefore, even with this approach, when the number of particles to be simulated increases, computational resources become stretched. The approach is, therefore, suitable for simulating dispersed multiphase flows containing a low ($<10\%$) volume fraction of the dispersed phases. For denser dispersed phase flows, it may be necessary to use a Eulerian–Eulerian approach.

The Eulerian–Eulerian approach models the flow of all phases in a Eulerian framework based on the interpenetrating continuum assumption. In this approach, trajectory simulations and averaging are not carried out at a computational level but are implicitly achieved at a conceptual level. The discrete character of the underlying process is, therefore, averaged out to provide a model involving a continuum associated with the dispersed phase particles. This approach is the most difficult one to understand conceptually, requiring extensive modeling efforts. Various averaging issues will have to be addressed while formulating the governing equations in this approach. If modeled successfully, this approach can be applied to multiphase flow processes containing large volume fractions of dispersed phase. It may, therefore, be extended to modeling and simulation of complex industrial multiphase reactors consisting of a large number of dispersed particles.

In a given situation, there is no simple answer to the question as to which of these approaches is preferable. Depending upon the complexity of the dispersed multiphase flows, more often than not, it may be necessary to use multiple modeling approaches to develop an adequate understanding of the flow processes under consideration. These three approaches are complementary in many respects (Berlemont *et al.*, 1995; Delnoij *et al.*, 1997). Application of these approaches to model dispersed multiphase flows is discussed below. Computational aspects of solving these model equations, including special treatment of interphase coupling terms, are discussed in Chapter 7.

4.2. MODELING DISPERSED MULTIPHASE FLOWS

Dispersed multiphase flows occur in a number of industrially important reactors including stirred tank reactors, fluidized bed reactors, bubble column reactors, combustors and so on. The modeler is often confronted with a complex flow process, in which some fundamental problems are still unsolved. In the simplest case, the reactor engineer has to deal with a one-way problem: prediction of particle trajectories or distribution in the known single-phase flow field. However, dispersed phase particles are not passive contaminants and the presence of these particles may influence the flow of the continuous phase. The level of interaction becomes especially complex for a turbulent flow field. When the size of the dispersed phase particle is very small or the mass loading of the particles is small, the influence of dispersed phase particles on the flow field of the continuous phase may be neglected. This is called one-way coupling. When the dispersed phase volume fraction is increased, the presence of dispersed phase will significantly affect the continuous phase flow field. This is called two-way coupling. If the particle number density is sufficiently large to allow direct particle–particle interactions, the modeler is faced with four-way coupling: continuous phase–dispersed phase particles–dispersed phase particles–continuous phase.

It is essential to examine the extent of coupling between dispersed and continuous phase to select an appropriate modeling approach. This is especially important for

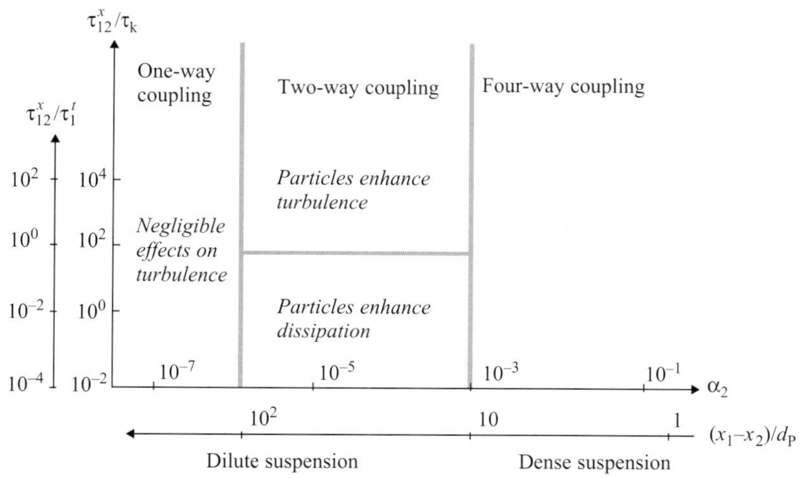

FIGURE 4.2 Coupling between phases in dispersed multiphase flows (from Elghobashi, 1991).

turbulent flows. The extent of coupling can be analyzed by examining relevant length and time scales. Elghobashi (1991) proposed a regime map for this purpose. His classification map is shown in Fig. 4.2. $(x_1 - x_2)/d_P$ denote the relative distance between the particles, which is approximately related to the volume fraction of the dispersed phase, α_2. τ^x_{12} is a particle relaxation time, which represents entrainment of the particles by the continuous phase (expressions for various relevant time scales for dispersed multiphase flows are listed in Appendix 4.1). When particle relaxation time is much smaller than the eddy lifetime experienced by the particle ($\tau^x_{12} \ll \tau^t_{12}$), particle motion is governed by continuous phase turbulence. In the other extreme, when ($\tau^x_{12} \gg \tau^t_{12}$), particle motion is only slightly affected by gas phase turbulence. When the collision time scale is much smaller than the particle relaxation time scale ($\tau^c_2 \ll \tau^x_{12}$), particle motion is governed by particle collisions. This is valid for dense dispersed multiphase flows. Similar analysis can also be carried out by comparing various characteristic length scales of motion with dispersed phase particle diameter (Gore and Crowe, 1989). Governing equations and boundary conditions for three modeling approaches are discussed below.

4.2.1. Volume of Fluid (VOF) Approach

Using the VOF approach, flow processes around individual dispersed phase particles are resolved unlike with EL or EE approaches. In this approach, the participating fluids share a single set of conservation equations. The governing equations can, therefore, be written:

$$\frac{\partial}{\partial t}(\rho) + \nabla \cdot (\rho U) = \sum_k S_k \tag{4.1}$$

$$\frac{\partial}{\partial t}(\rho U) + \nabla \cdot (\rho U U) = -\nabla \cdot \pi + \rho g + F \tag{4.2}$$

Discussions in Chapter 2 may be referred to for explanations of the various symbols. It is straightforward to apply such conservation equations to single-phase flows. In the case of multiphase flows also, in principle, it is possible to use these equations with appropriate boundary conditions at the interface between different phases. In such cases, however, density, viscosity and all the other relevant properties will have to change abruptly at the location of the interface. These methods, which describe and track the time-dependent behavior of the interface itself, are called front tracking methods. Numerical solution of such a set of equations is extremely difficult and enormously computation intensive. The main difficulty arises from the interaction between the moving interface and the Eulerian grid employed to solve the flow field (more discussion about numerical solutions is given in Chapters 6 and 7).

The volume of fluid (VOF) approach simulates the motion of all the phases rather than tracking the motion of the interface itself. The motion of the interface is inferred indirectly through the motion of different phases separated by an interface. Motion of the different phases is tracked by solving an advection equation of a marker function or of a phase volume fraction. Thus, when a control volume is not entirely occupied by one phase, mixture properties are used while solving governing Eqs (4.1) and (4.2). This avoids abrupt changes in properties across a very thin interface. The properties appearing in Eqs (4.1) and (4.2) are related to the volume fraction of the kth phase as follows:

$$\rho = \sum \alpha_k \rho_k \qquad C_\mathrm{p} = \frac{\sum \alpha_k \rho_k C_{\mathrm{p}k}}{\sum \alpha_k \rho_k} \tag{4.3}$$

The average of any other variable ϕ can also be written:

$$\phi = \frac{\sum \alpha_k \rho_k \phi_k}{\sum \alpha_k \rho_k} \tag{4.4}$$

The volume fraction of each fluid, α_k, is calculated by tracking the interface between different phases throughout the solution domain. Tracking of the interfaces between N different phases present in the system is accomplished by solving continuity equations for $N-1$ phases. For the kth phase, this equation has the following form (similar to scalar advection):

$$\frac{\partial \alpha_k}{\partial t} + (U_k \cdot \nabla)\alpha_k = S_{\alpha_k} \tag{4.5}$$

It must, however, be noted that the marker function or the volume fraction does not uniquely identify the interface. Several different interface configurations may correspond to the same value of volume fraction (Fig. 4.3). Several specialized techniques have been proposed to track the interface accurately (Rider and Kothe, 1995; Rudman, 1997). Some of these techniques are discussed in Chapter 7.

The VOF approach allows one to model various interfacial phenomena; for example, wall adhesion and surface (or interfacial) tension can be modeled rigorously using this approach. Brackbill *et al.* (1992) developed a continuous surface force (CSF) model to describe interfacial surface tension. CSF model replaces surface force by a smoothly varying volumetric force acting on all the fluid elements in the interface transition region. For two-phase flows (dispersed or secondary phase is denoted by subscript 2), surface force, F_{SF} can be written (Brackbill *et al.*, 1992):

$$F_{\mathrm{SF}} = 2\sigma\alpha_2\kappa n \tag{4.6}$$

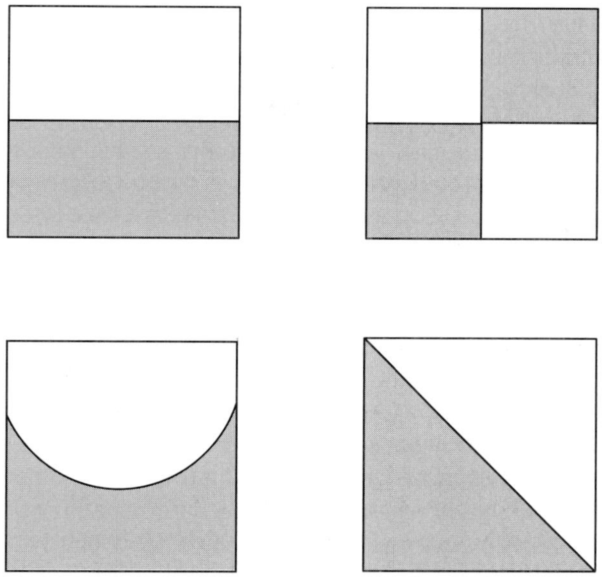

FIGURE 4.3 Possible interface configurations for the same value of volume fraction in the control volume (volume fraction = 0.5).

where σ is surface tension, κ is local curvature and n is the surface normal. The surface normal is defined as the gradient of the secondary phase volume fraction:

$$n = \nabla \alpha_2 \tag{4.7}$$

The local surface curvature is defined as

$$\kappa = \frac{1}{|n|}\left[\left(\frac{n}{|n|}\cdot\nabla\right)|n| - (\nabla \cdot n)\right] \tag{4.8}$$

The volume force described by Eq. (4.6) appears as a source in the momentum equation on the side of the interface corresponding to the secondary phase. In conjunction with this surface tension model, wall adhesion phenomena can also be modeled. The contact angle that the fluid is assumed to make with the wall is used to adjust the surface normal near the wall (Brackbill *et al.*, 1992). For accurate implementation of surface tension and wall adhesion phenomena, the solution method has to maintain a compact and sharp interface between phases. If care is taken in the numerical implementation, the VOF approach can simulate the deformation of shape of dispersed phase particles due to the surrounding flow (Delnoij, 1999). Thus, the VOF approach should be used when small-scale processes occurring near an interface separating the fluid particle from the continuous phase play a crucial role. Knowledge of these small-scale flow processes and the deformation of gas bubbles is crucial for accurate estimation of local mass and heat transfer rates near the dispersed phase particle. The main disadvantage of VOF is that it is computationally very demanding and, therefore, difficult to apply to dispersed multiphase flows containing a large number of dispersed phase particles. It may, however, serve as a useful learning tool for understanding details of dispersed multiphase flows. Recently, vigorous efforts have been made to use the VOF approach to simulate the motion of a few bubbles or a few particles to enhance the current understanding of the local flow characteristics around these dispersed phase particles (Stover *et al.*, 1997; Delnoij *et al.*, 1997; Krishna and van Baton, 1999). Due to computational constraints, most of these studies have been restricted to two-dimensional simulations, so that the quantitative agreement between predicted results and experimental data is not very satisfactory. Efforts are continuing to improve the underlying modeling of physics as well as its numerical implementation.

4.2.2. Eulerian–Lagrangian Approach

Using this approach, trajectories of dispersed phase particles are simulated by solving an equation of motion for each dispersed phase particle. Motion of the continuous phase is modeled using a conventional Eulerian framework. Depending on the degree of coupling (one-way, two-way or four-way), solutions of both phases interact with each other. For two-way or four-way coupling, an iterative solution procedure needs to be adopted. For four-way coupling, additional models to simulate particle–particle interactions also need to be incorporated while simulating the trajectories of dispersed phase particles. In simple, one-way coupling, a continuous phase flow field can be obtained independent of the motion of the dispersed phase. Using such a flow field, the trajectories of dispersed phase particles can be obtained by solving the equations of motion for dispersed phase particles.

Historically, the equation of motion of a single rigid sphere in a stagnant fluid was first studied by Stokes (1851). He derived the well-known drag formula based on this study. To examine issues other than the drag force, a good starting point may be the so-called BBO (Basset–Boussinesq–Oseen) equation (Gouesbet *et al.*, 1984). Tchen (1947) attempted to generalize the BBO equation to the case when the fluid is no longer at rest. Maxey and Riley (1983) developed equations of motion for a small rigid particle in a non-uniform flow. Development of the equation of motion for a rigid sphere which has non-stationary translational and rotational motion in a non-uniform flow is not a trivial problem. At present, a rigorous form of the equation of motion has been derived only in the case of creeping flow (Peirano, 1998). For general application, a modified form of the Maxey and Riley equation in the form of a general force balance over a single dispersed phase particle is used (Auton, 1983):

$$m_{\mathrm{P}}\frac{dU_{\mathrm{P}}}{dt} = F_{\mathrm{p}} + F_{\mathrm{D}} + F_{\mathrm{VM}} + F_{\mathrm{L}} + F_{\mathrm{H}} + F_{\mathrm{G}} \tag{4.9}$$

Here m_{P} and U_{P} represent the mass and velocity vector of the particle, respectively. The right-hand side represents the total force acting on the dispersed phase particle. The sum of forces due to continuous phase pressure gradient, F_{p}, and due to gravity, $\mathrm{F_G}$, can be written:

$$F_{\mathrm{p}} + F_{\mathrm{G}} = V_{\mathrm{P}}\nabla p - \rho_{\mathrm{P}} V_{\mathrm{P}} g \tag{4.10}$$

where p is pressure in the continuous phase and V_{P} is volume of the particle. The drag force, F_{D}, can be written:

$$F_{\mathrm{D}} = -\frac{\pi}{8} C_{\mathrm{D}}\rho_{\mathrm{C}} D_{\mathrm{P}}^{2} \mid U_{\mathrm{P}} - U_{\mathrm{C}} \mid (U_{\mathrm{P}} - U_{\mathrm{C}}) \tag{4.11}$$

where the subscript C denotes the continuous phase and P denotes the particulate phase. The drag force has been studied extensively. The drag coefficient, C_D, depends on the flow regime (particle Reynolds number) and the properties of the continuous phase. Several empirical correlations have been proposed for the estimation of the drag coefficient. For a single rigid sphere, the drag coefficient is usually approximated by the correlation proposed by Schiller and Naumann (1935):

$$C_D = \begin{cases} \mathrm{Re_P} < 1000 & \Rightarrow \quad 24/\mathrm{Re}(1 + 0.15\,\mathrm{Re}^{0.687}) \\ \mathrm{Re_P} \geq 1000 & \Rightarrow \quad 0.44 \end{cases} \tag{4.12}$$

$\mathrm{Re_P}$ is the particle Reynolds number:

$$\mathrm{Re_P} = \frac{\rho_C d_P |U_P - U_C|}{\mu_C} \tag{4.13}$$

$|U_P - U_C|$ represents the resultant slip velocity between the particulate and continuous phase. Some other commonly used drag coefficient correlations are listed in Appendix 4.2. For fluid particles such as gas bubbles or liquid drops, the drag coefficient may be different than that predicted by the standard drag curve, due to internal circulation and deformation. For example, Johansen and Boysen (1988) proposed the following equation to calculate C_D, which is valid for ellipsoidal bubbles in the range $500 < \mathrm{Re} < 5000$:

$$C_D = \frac{0.622}{1.0/Eo + 0.235} \quad \because \quad Eo = \frac{g|(\rho_P - \rho_C)|d_P^2}{\sigma} \tag{4.14}$$

Kuo and Wallis (1988) proposed a different equation for estimation of the drag coefficient, which is suitable for spherical and spherical cap bubbles. For the specific system under consideration, several specialized correlations may be used to estimate the drag coefficient. If the dispersed phase particles are not spherical, appropriate correction factors need to be introduced in these drag coefficient correlations (Clift *et al.*, 1978). It may also be necessary to correct the drag coefficient to account for the influence of a wall (Brenner, 1961). Most of these correlations have been developed for the motion of a single particle. When the dispersed phase volume fraction is high, the presence of other dispersed phase particles will affect the effective value of the drag coefficient. Several corrections have been proposed to account for the influence of the surrounding particles. Some of these are discussed in the section describing the Eulerian–Eulerian approach. Some drag coefficient correlations suitable for gas–liquid and gas–solid flows are discussed in Part IV while discussing the modeling of different reactor types.

Apart from the drag force, there are three other important forces acting on a dispersed phase particle, namely lift force, virtual mass force and Basset history force. When the dispersed phase particle is rising through the non-uniform flow field of the continuous phase, it will experience a lift force due to vorticity or shear in the continuous phase flow field. Auton (1983) showed that the lift force is proportional to the vector product of the slip velocity and the curl of the liquid velocity. This suggests that lift force acts in a direction perpendicular to both, the direction of slip velocity

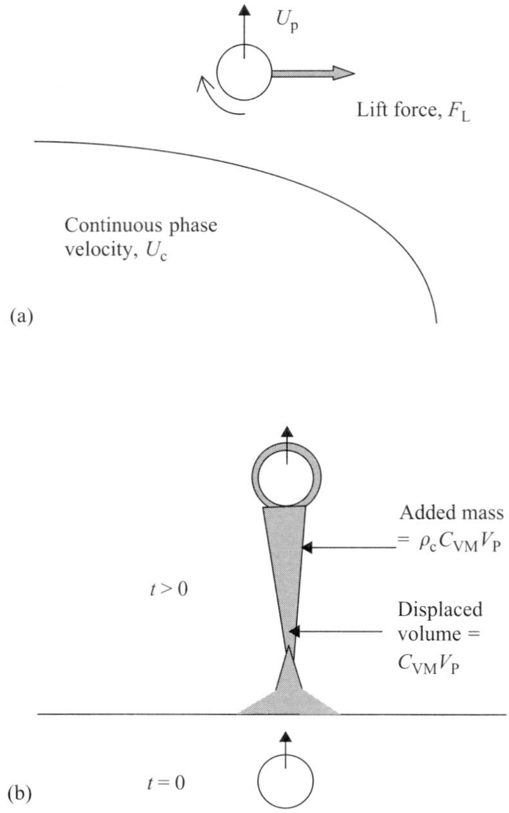

FIGURE 4.4 Lift (a) and virtual mass forces, (b) on dispersed phase particles.

and the direction of the curl of the continuous phase velocity field (Fig. 4.4). For locally homogeneous flows, the lift force is given by

$$F_L = -C_L \rho_C V_P (U_P - U_C) \times (\nabla \times U_C) \tag{4.15}$$

where C_L is an empirical lift coefficient. For potential flow and spherical particles, Drew and Lahey (1979) report the value of lift coefficient as 0.5. Recently Oesterle (1994) investigated lift forces in the Reynolds number range 1 to 1000, which is typical for reactor engineering applications. This study shows that lift forces are not negligible and tend to increase with increasing particle diameter. Two other situations may lead to transverse force: (1) when the dispersed phase particle is rotating and (2) when the particle is moving in the vicinity of a wall. Most studies related to these situations are restricted to small Reynolds number and have recently been summarized by Peirano (1998).

When a dispersed phase particle accelerates relative to the continuous phase, some part of the surrounding continuous phase also is accelerated. This extra acceleration of the continuous phase has the effect of added inertia or 'added mass' (Fig. 4.4).

This 'added mass' effect is modeled by introducing the virtual mass term, F_{VM}:

$$F_{\mathrm{VM}} = -\left(\frac{DI}{Dt} + I \cdot \nabla U_{\mathrm{C}}\right) \quad \because \quad I = C_{\mathrm{VM}} \rho_{\mathrm{C}} V_{\mathrm{P}} (U_{\mathrm{P}} - U_{\mathrm{C}}) \tag{4.16}$$

The material derivative, D/Dt, in this equation should be the derivative pertaining to the dispersed phase particle. The virtual mass coefficient, C_{VM}, may be a function of the volume fraction of neighboring bubbles. For a single dispersed particle, it is in the range 0.25 to 0.5. For gas–liquid flows, van Wijngaarden (1976) recommended following expression to estimate C_{VM}:

$$C_{\mathrm{VM}} = C_{\mathrm{VMP}}(1 + 2.78\alpha_{\mathrm{P}}) \tag{4.17}$$

where C_{VMP} indicates the value of C_{VM} for a single particle of dispersed phase.

There may be some additional forces, such as Basset force (due to development of a boundary layer around the dispersed phase particles), thermophoretic force (due to large temperature gradient) and Brownian force. The Basset force (denoted by F_{H} in Eq. 4.9) is relevant only for unsteady flows and in most cases, its magnitude is much smaller than the interphase drag force. Basset force involves a history integral, which is time-consuming to evaluate. Moreover, Basset force decays as t^{-n} with $n > 2$ (Mei, 1993) for intermediate time. Therefore, it is very often neglected while integrating the equation of motion of the particle. Picart *et al.* (1982) discussed specific conditions under which the Basset term may be neglected. For most reactor engineering flows, the other two forces, thermophoretic and Brownian forces, are also quite small compared to some of the terms discussed earlier.

Once the velocity field is calculated from the force balances discussed above, the trajectories of all the particles can be calculated using:

$$\frac{dx_i}{dt} = U_{\mathrm{P}i} \tag{4.18}$$

When simulating the trajectories of dispersed phase particles, appropriate boundary conditions need to be specified. Inlet or outlet boundary conditions require no special attention. At impermeable walls, however, it is necessary to represent collisions between particles and wall. Particles can reflect from the wall via elastic or inelastic collisions. Suitable coefficients of restitution representing the fraction of momentum retained by a particle after a collision need to be specified at all the wall boundaries. In some cases, particles may stick to the wall or may remain very close to the wall after they collide with the wall. Special boundary conditions need to be developed to model these situations (see, for example, the schematic shown in Fig. 4.5).

As particles move within the solution domain, solution of the force balance of each particle requires information about the flow field of the continuous phase. The continuous phase flow is described using the volume-averaged (overall) mass and momentum conservation equations:

$$\frac{\partial(\alpha_{\mathrm{C}}\rho_{\mathrm{C}})}{\partial t} + \nabla \cdot (\alpha_{\mathrm{C}}\rho_{\mathrm{C}} U_{\mathrm{C}}) = S_{\mathrm{C}} \tag{4.19}$$

$$\frac{\partial(\alpha_{\mathrm{C}}\rho_{\mathrm{C}} U_{\mathrm{C}})}{\partial t} + \nabla \cdot (\alpha_{\mathrm{C}}\rho_{\mathrm{C}} U_{\mathrm{C}} U_{\mathrm{C}}) = -\alpha_{\mathrm{C}} \nabla p - \nabla \cdot (\alpha_{\mathrm{C}} \tau_{\mathrm{C}}) + \alpha_{\mathrm{C}} \rho_{\mathrm{C}} g + S_{\mathrm{Cm}} \tag{4.20}$$

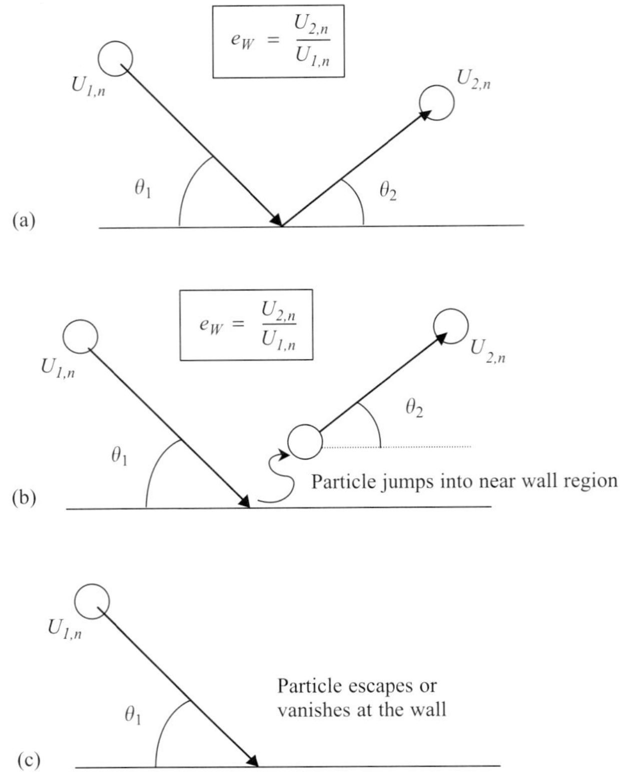

FIGURE 4.5 Wall boundary conditions for dispersed phase particles. (a) Reflection, (b) saltation, (c) particle escapes or vanishes.

where S_C and S_{Cm} are mass and momentum sources representing the exchange between dispersed phase particles and the continuous phase. Individual species and enthalpy conservation equations can be written analogously. For very low concentrations of small, dispersed phase particles, the influence of dispersed phase particles on the flow field of the continuous phase can be ignored. In such cases, equations for the continuous phase reduce to those of the single-phase conservation equations.

At moderate flow (mass) rates of dispersed phase particles, it is necessary to model the two-way coupling between continuous and dispersed phases. Such coupling occurs through volume fraction, α_C, and exchange source terms, S_C and S_{Cm}. The momentum exchange from dispersed phase particles to continuous phase is just the opposite of the momentum transfer rate due to drag, lift and virtual mass forces exerted by the continuous phase on the dispersed phase particles. These sources can be computed by summing the changes in momentum (or enthalpy or mass) of a particle as it passes through the control volume for continuous phase, over all the particles passing through that control volume. Suitable area and volume averaging methods need to be developed to formulate these coupling source terms. For such a coupled system, it is necessary to solve the governing equations of the dispersed and continuous phase iteratively until one obtains the converged solution. Two-way coupling was discussed recently by Delnoij *et al.* (1997) for gas–liquid bubbly flows and by Hoomans *et al.* (1998) for gas–solid flows. Interested readers are referred to these papers for more details of averaging and other coupling related issues. Some of these details are discussed in Chapter 7 when describing numerical methods to solve multiphase model equations.

If the volume fraction of the dispersed phase particles is high, particles may directly interact with each other by collisions and/or coalescence. The characteristic time of collisions between dispersed phase particles can be related to volume fraction, particle diameter and particle kinetic energy using the framework of kinetic theory. If the characteristic time of collisions is smaller than the particle response or relaxation time, the particles will not have adequate time to recover their own behavior between collisions. For such cases, four-way coupling will have to be accounted for. The four-way coupling problem, in its full generality, is still unsolved and is the object of much current research effort. Various approaches are used to tackle this problem. One can use a Eulerian framework in which collisions between particles are described using a kinetic theory approach. This approach is briefly discussed in the next section. Alternatively, particle–particle interactions can be included in a Lagrangian approach by considering particle collisions while simulating a large number of particles.

Several attempts have been made to simulate a large number of dispersed phase particles simultaneously (recently reviewed by Hoomans, 2000). These studies can be broadly divided into three approaches:

(1) Hard sphere approach
(2) Soft sphere approach
(3) Monte Carlo techniques

In a hard sphere approach, particles are assumed to interact through instantaneous binary collisions. This means particle interaction times are much smaller than the free flight time and therefore, hard particle simulations are event (collision) driven. For a comprehensive introduction to this type of simulation, the reader is referred to Allen and Tildesley (1990). Hoomans (2000) used this approach to simulate gas–solid flows in dense as well as fast-fluidized beds. There are three key parameters in such hard sphere models, namely coefficient of restitution, coefficient of dynamic friction and coefficient of tangential restitution. Coefficient of restitution is discussed later in this chapter. Detailed discussion of these three model parameters can be found in Hoomans (2000).

In a soft sphere approach, particles are allowed to overlap slightly. The contact forces are then calculated from the deformation history of the contact, using say a linear spring/ dashpot model. Xu and Yu (1997) and Mikami (1998) among others have used this approach to model gas–solid flows. In Monte Carlo simulations (Frenkel and Smith, 1996), a new overlap-free particle configuration is generated at each time step. The new configuration is accepted based on the change in system energy. Seibert and Burns (1998) used this method to simulate segregation phenomena in liquid–solid flows. In all these approaches, simultaneous simulation of a large number of particles stretches the limits of currently available computational resources. Despite the recent advances in devising efficient numerical techniques (to process collision events in an assembly of a large number of particles), application of these approaches is still more or less restricted to two-dimensional solution domains. These models may give useful information about particle–particle interactions. However, it is still difficult to apply these models to simulate large industrial multiphase reactors. As an alternative to simultaneously tracking many particles, it may also be possible to adapt a Lagrangian simulation, based on single-particle tracking using the 'double-solution' approach. In this approach, the trajectory of a single particle surrounded by a 'cloud of probability of collision' is simulated (Oesterle and Petitjean, 1993; Sommerfeld, 1995). A random process is used to decide when collisions may occur and particle characteristics are suitably modified to account for collisions. Even these models have not yet been applied to large multiphase reactors.

It may be noted that the discussion so far has not considered turbulent flow. When the continuous phase flow field is turbulent, its influence on particle trajectories needs to be represented in the model. The situation becomes quite complex in the case of two-way coupling between continuous phase and dispersed phase, since the presence of dispersed phase can affect turbulence in the continuous phase. The Eulerian framework may be more suitable to model such cases. Even when dispersed phase particles are assumed to have no influence on the continuous phase flow field, the trajectories of the particles will be affected by the presence of turbulence in the continuous phase. For such cases, it is necessary to calculate the trajectories of a sufficiently large number of particles using the instantaneous local velocity to represent the random effects of turbulence on particle dispersion.

The instantaneous velocity is equal to the mean velocity (which is known) plus a fluctuation velocity (which is unknown). Predictions using a turbulence model may give values of variance of the fluctuating velocity. The assumption of a Gaussian distribution for the fluctuations and a random value for fluctuation to be added to the mean velocity is not sufficient to obtain the instantaneous value. Instantaneous values should satisfy the Lagrangian correlation coefficient along the trajectory. Several models have been proposed to estimate the instantaneous velocity. See, for example, recent reviews by Sommerfeld (1993) and Gouesbet and Berlemont (1999). Two commonly used models to estimate instantaneous fluid velocity from the time-averaged flow field of the continuous phase are briefly discussed below:

(a) *Discrete random walk model.* In this model, the fluctuating component of the velocity is assumed to have a Gaussian distribution and is calculated by multiplication of a normally distributed random number and the local root mean square (rms) value of the velocity fluctuations. The same value of random number is used for the eddy lifetime (integral time scale). For each eddy lifetime, new value of random number is used. This stochastic process generates a correlation coefficient which linearly decreases from 1 at a delay equal to zero, to 0 at a delay equal to twice the eddy lifetime. Despite such a crude approximation for the correlation coefficient, this approach leads to reasonable results and has been widely used for a number of applications (Chen and Crowe, 1984; Sommerfeld, 1990).

(b) *Continuous random walk model.* In this model, the instantaneous fluid velocity is obtained by solution of a Langevin equation (Thomson, 1987), which may provide a more realistic description of turbulent eddies, although at the expense of greater computational effort. These models correlate the velocity fluctuation experienced by a particle at the new location with the fluctuation at the previous location using an exponentially decaying correlation function (Langevin velocity correlation function). In inhomogeneous turbulence, however, it has been found that the Langevin model fails and may lead to the accumulation of fluid particles in regions of low turbulence (Sommerfeld, 1993).

Berlemont *et al.* (1990) proposed a more sophisticated approach, the so-called 'correlation slaved approach', to estimate instantaneous velocity. They consider a correlation matrix, which evolves along the trajectory (also see, Gouesbet and Berlemont, 1999). Their model, however, needs much larger computational resources than the above two approaches.

Once the instantaneous velocity is obtained, particle trajectories can be simulated. To introduce two-way coupling, it is necessary to calculate the source terms in the balance equations of mass, momentum and energy for the continuous phase. With such source terms, the continuous phase flow field needs to be solved again, which is later used to calculate new trajectories. The number of iterations between turbulence and particulate modules to obtain convergence is typically three. However, in strongly coupled flows, convergence may be difficult to reach (Kohnen *et al.*, 1994).

The main advantage of using a Lagrangian framework for dispersed phase particles is that particle-level phenomena can be modeled rigorously. Species and enthalpy conservation equations for individual particles can be written:

$$\frac{d(m_\mathrm{P}\, m_k)}{dt} = S_k \tag{4.21}$$

$$\frac{d(m_\mathrm{P} C_\mathrm{P} h_\mathrm{P})}{dt} = S_h \tag{4.22}$$

The sources of interphase transport, S_k and S_h, can be formulated by considering particle-level phenomena, which will be of interest to the reactor engineers such as:

- heating or cooling of particles (simple heat balance over a particle);
- devolatilization (evaporation of volatile component from the solid particle);
- droplet vaporization;
- surface reaction (diffusion or kinetic controlled);
- coalescence and break-up.

It can be seen that in many of these particle-level phenomena, sources will be a function of continuous phase variables. Such a situation results in strong coupling between particle trajectory simulations and simulation of the continuous phase flow field. Detailed modeling of each of these can be accomplished following conventional practices and will not be discussed here. More information can be found in textbooks on chemical reaction engineering and heat and mass transport processes (Levenspiel, 1972; Westerterp *et al.*, 1984; Kuo, 1986; Kunii and Levenspiel, 1991).

Particle size distribution can conveniently be accommodated in a Lagrangian framework for dispersed phase particles. Detailed analysis of particle trajectories and particle-level phenomena can be very useful for the reactor engineer. Even for reactors where particle–particle interactions are significant and a Eulerian approach may be more suitable, modeling with a Lagrangian framework can provide limiting solutions as well as a basis for interpreting the Eulerian results from the particle perspective. Analysis of residence time and circulation time distribution within the reactor or massless particles can provide useful insight into the mixing process occurring within the reactor. Some of the possible applications of this approach are discussed in Parts III and IV.

4.2.3. Eulerian–Eulerian Approach

With this approach, even the dispersed phase is treated as a continuum. All phases 'share' the domain and may interpenetrate as they move within it. This approach is more suitable for modeling dispersed multiphase systems with a significant volume fraction of dispersed phase ($>10\%$). Such situations may occur in many types of reactor, for example, in fluidized bed reactors, bubble column reactors and multiphase stirred reactors. It is possible to represent coupling between different phases by developing suitable interphase transport models. It is, however, difficult to handle complex phenomena at particle level (such as change in size due to reactions/evaporation etc.) with the Eulerian–Eulerian approach.

For single-phase flows, rigorous basic transport equations are given in the form of mass, momentum and energy conservation (see Chapter 2). These equations are local, instantaneous equations and can be applied to all the volume and time domains under consideration. For multiphase flow processes, such local instantaneous field equations cannot be formulated without appropriate averaging. Several different averaging methods have been used. For example, Ishii (1975) and Drew (1983) used time averaging while Harlow and Amsden (1975), Rietema and van den Akker (1983) and Ahmedi (1987) used a volume averaging method. Besnard and Harlow (1988), Kataoka and Serizawa (1989) and Lahey and Drew (1989), among others, discussed various issues involved in the formulation of governing equations for multiphase flow processes. Recently, Enwald *et al.* (1996) discussed in detail the rigorous formulation of two-fluid model equations based on averaging techniques and corresponding closure laws. In this section, we present a general form of governing equations for dispersed multiphase flows, which will be suitable for further numerical solution, without going into details of their derivation.

The concept of volume fraction is introduced here heuristically without resorting to a rigorous treatment. With this approach, it is assumed that it is meaningful to conceive a volume fraction of phase k, α_k in any small volume of space at any particular time. If there are n phases in total, this gives:

$$\sum_{k=1}^{n} \alpha_k = 1.0 \qquad (4.23)$$

This means that there are sufficiently large numbers of dispersed phase particles in a volume characterized by the macroscopic length of the system.

The continuity equation for each phase can therefore be written:

$$\frac{\partial(\alpha_k \rho_k)}{\partial t} + \nabla \cdot (\alpha_k \rho_k U_k) = \sum_{p=1,p\neq k}^{n} S_{pk} \qquad (4.24)$$

where the subscript k denotes phase k. S_{pk} is the rate of mass transfer from the pth phase to the kth phase. This rate is based on a per unit volume of dispersion and not that of phase k. If it is based on the volume of phase k, it will be necessary to multiply it by the volume fraction of phase k, α_k. Summation of net mass transfer over all phases will be zero as there can be no net creation or destruction of mass.

The momentum balance for phase k can be written:

$$\frac{\partial(\alpha_k \rho_k U_k)}{\partial t} + \nabla \cdot (\alpha_k \rho_k U_k U_k) = -\alpha_k \nabla p - \nabla \cdot (\alpha_k \tau_k) + \alpha_k \rho_k g + F_k + F_g \qquad (4.25)$$

Here, F_k denotes the interphase momentum exchange terms between phase k and all other phases present in the system. Additional momentum sources, if any, and terms relevant to granular multiphase flows, are grouped together in F_g. It should be noted that pressure, p, is regarded as being shared by all the phases and, therefore, appears in the governing equations of all phases. The significance of the remaining terms in the equations is similar to those discussed for single-phase flow processes in Chapter 2.

Interphase coupling terms make multiphase flows fundamentally different from single-phase flows. The formulation of these terms and, therefore, of interphase exchange coefficients must proceed carefully, with attention being paid to the force balance for a single particle and to any possible inconsistencies. The interphase coupling terms must satisfy the following relation:

$$F_{kq} = -F_{qk} \tag{4.26}$$

The interphase coupling terms for phase k can be written:

$$F_k = \sum_{q=1}^{n} K_{kq}(U_q - U_k) + \sum_{q=1, q\neq k}^{n} S_{qk} U_{qk} \tag{4.27}$$

where K is the interphase momentum exchange coefficient. The second term represents the momentum transferred between phases due to mass transfer. This formulation automatically satisfies the constraint described by Eq. (4.26). In principle, the interphase momentum exchange terms should include all the relevant interphase forces described earlier in Section 4.2.2. To incorporate these forces, the particle volume included in expressions given earlier (Eqs (4.15) and (4.16)) must be replaced by the volume fraction of the dispersed phase. In most cases, the interphase drag force term dominates the other interphase forces such as lift force terms or virtual mass terms. When the dispersed phase density is much smaller than the continuous phase density (as with a bubble column reactor), the virtual mass effect may become significant. In such cases, special formulations will be necessary rather than those described by Eq. (4.27).

In order to clarify interphase momentum exchange terms, the case of two-phase flow is considered below. Let phase 1 be a continuous phase and phase 2 a dispersed phase. The interphase exchange force exerted in the i direction on the dispersed phase (phase 2) by the continuous phase can be modeled as

$$F_{2i} = -\frac{3\alpha_1\alpha_2\rho_1 C_\mathrm{D}\left(\sum_j (U_{2j} - U_{1j})^2\right)^{1/2}(U_{2i} - U_{1i})}{4d_p} \tag{4.28}$$

The sign of this force is decided by the sign of the difference in i directional velocities of the two phases (i directional slip velocity). This expression can be generalized to more than one dispersed phases in a straightforward way. C_D denotes the drag coefficient. The expressions given earlier (Eqs (4.12) and (4.14)) may be used to estimate the value of drag coefficient. Refer to Appendix 4.2 for some other commonly used correlations for estimating the drag coefficient. It is necessary to correct the estimation of drag coefficient to account for the non-spherical shape of the particle and for the presence of other particles. The presence of other particles will also modify the drag coefficient. For example, bubbles tend to follow one another's wake leading to reduction in the effective drag coefficient. Measurements by Tsuji *et al.* (1984) on two spheres in the Reynolds number range 100 to 200 can be expressed as

$$C_{\mathrm{D}} = C_{\mathrm{D0}}\left[1 - \left(\frac{d_{\mathrm{P}}}{L_{\mathrm{P}}}\right)^2\right] \tag{4.29}$$

where C_{D0} is the drag coefficient for a single particle of diameter d_{P} and L_{P} is the distance between the centers of the two spheres. Several correlations have been proposed to represent the influence of other particles on the drag coefficient (see a recent review by Enwald *et al.*, 1996 and Appendix 4.2). More information about drag coefficient correlations is included in Part IV when discussing the modeling of different reactor types.

For granular flows (fluid–solid flows), in which particle–particle interactions play a substantial role, it is necessary to introduce additional terms in the basic governing equations. Granular flows may exhibit several sub-regimes such as: (i) an elastic regime, in which the multiphase system behaves like an elastic solid and stress is strain dependent; (ii) a plastic regime, in which stress is independent of strain rate, typical for slow flow conditions; and (iii) a viscous regime, in which stress is dependent on strain rate (see Fig. 4.6 for a schematic representation of these regimes). Several models based on concepts ranging from elasticity to soil mechanics have been proposed. For reactor engineering, the kinetic theory of granular flows will be most useful to model fluid–solid flows in dilute to dense bed regimes. The kinetic theory of granular flows is based on similarities between the flow of a granular material, a population of particles with or without interstitial gas, and the molecules of gas. This treatment uses classical results from the kinetic theory of gases (Chapman and Cowling, 1970) to predict the form of transport equations for a granular material. One of the most complete works in the field of kinetic theory of granular flow is Jenkins and Richman (1985). Detailed discussion of the development of models of granular flow is beyond the scope of this book. Readers are referred to Gidaspow (1994) and some recent papers (Nieuwland *et al.*, 1996; Kuipers and van Swaaij, 1997; Peirano and Leckner, 1998). Kinetic theory based models introduce several additional terms in the solids stresses and, therefore, modify momentum conservation equations for

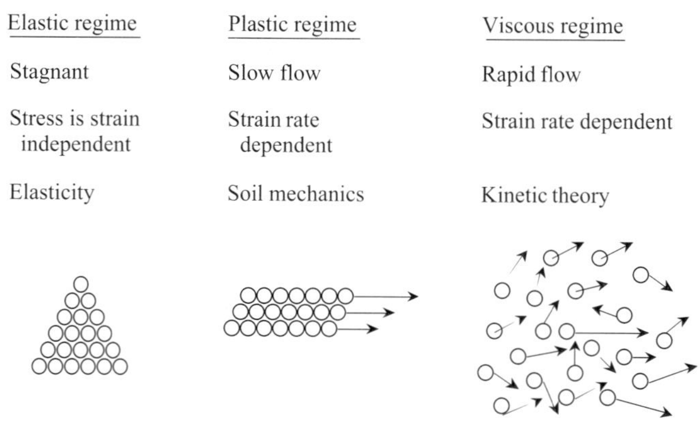

FIGURE 4.6 Schematic representation of different regimes of granular flow regimes.

solid phases. The solids stress can be written as:

$$\alpha_s \bar{\tau}_s = -P_s \bar{I} + 2\alpha_s \mu_s \bar{S} + \alpha_s \left(\lambda_s - \frac{2}{3}\mu_s \right) \nabla \cdot U_s \bar{I} \tag{4.30}$$

where P_s is solids pressure, μ_s is solids (shear) viscosity and λ_s is solids bulk viscosity. $\bar{S}$ is given by:

$$\bar{S} = \frac{1}{2}\left(\nabla U_s + (\nabla U_s)^{\mathrm{T}}\right) \tag{4.31}$$

In addition to these solids stresses, the solids momentum equation may have the following terms:

$$F_g = \sum_{l=1}^{n} K_{ls}(U_l - U_s) + S_s \tag{4.32}$$

The first term on the right-hand side represents momentum exchange between solid phases l and s and K_{ls} is the solid–solid exchange coefficient. The last term represent additional shear stresses, which appear in granular flows (due to particle translation and collisions). Expressions for solids pressure, solids viscosity (shear and bulk) and solid–solid exchange coefficients are derived from the kinetic theory of granular flows.

The solids pressure, P_s consists of a collisional and a kinetic part:

$$P_s = \sum P_{C,sn} + \alpha_s \rho_s \theta_s \tag{4.33}$$

where $P_{C,sn}$ is the pressure caused by collisions between the solid phases s and n and θ_s is the granular temperature. Granular temperature is a measure of the kinetic energy contained in the fluctuating velocity of particles, and is defined:

$$\theta_s = \frac{1}{3}\overline{u_s^2} \tag{4.34}$$

Several different expressions have been derived for solids pressure, solids shear viscosity and solids bulk viscosity, employing different approximations and assumptions while applying the kinetic theory of granular flows. Some of the commonly used equations are described below (see Gidaspow, 1994 and a review given by Peirano, 1998): Solids pressure:

$$P_s = \alpha_s \rho_s \theta_s (\omega + 2(1 + e_s)\alpha_s g_{0s}) \tag{4.35}$$

For dense suspensions (Gidaspow, 1994):

$$\omega = 1 \tag{4.36}$$

and for dilute suspensions, Bolio *et al.* (1995) used

$$\omega = \left(1 + \frac{d_s}{6\alpha_s D\sqrt{2}}\right) \tag{4.37}$$

e_s is the value of the restitution coefficient of solid particles (for elastic particles, the restitution coefficient is unity) and g_{0s} is a radial distribution function. The restitution coefficient is defined as the ratio of normal relative velocity after the collision and before the collision. The value of restitution coefficient may depend on particle size and relative velocity, however, generally it is assumed that it has a constant value for a given material. Measured restitution coefficients for different types of materials are given by Foerster *et al.* (1994). In the framework of the kinetic theory, the radial distribution function accounts for the increase in probability of collisions when the gas becomes denser. Analogously, when particles are closely packed (when motion is almost impossible), the radial distribution function tends to infinity. Chapman and Cowling (1970) derived an expression for the radial distribution function. However, this expression is not consistent with the asymptotic behavior of dense gases at extreme high concentrations. Several empirical correlations have been proposed. Lun and Savage (1986) proposed:

$$g_{0s} = \left(1 - \frac{\alpha_s}{\alpha_{s\,max}}\right)^{-2.5\alpha_s\,max} \tag{4.38}$$

Ogawa *et al.* (1980) proposed:

$$g_{0s} = \left(1 - \left(\frac{\alpha_s}{\alpha_{s,max}}\right)^{\frac{1}{3}}\right)^{-1}, \qquad \alpha_{s,max} = 0.65 \tag{4.39}$$

Ma and Ahmadi (1986) proposed a more complicated expression, which shows good agreement with simulations. However, in most engineering simulations, the above two empirical expressions are used and may be considered adequate.

Solids shear viscosity also comprises a kinetic contribution and collisional contributions. Commonly used expressions for viscosity are:

$$\mu_{s,coll} = \frac{4}{5}\alpha_s\rho_s d_s g_{0s}(1+e_s)\sqrt{\left(\frac{\theta_s}{\pi}\right)} \tag{4.40}$$

$$\mu_{s,kin} = \frac{10 d_s\rho_s(\theta_s\pi)^{1/2}}{96(1+e_s)g_{0s}}\left[1+\frac{4}{5}g_{0s}\alpha_s(1+e_s)\right]^2 \tag{4.41}$$

Bulk viscosity accounts for resistance of solid body to dilation and can be given as

$$\lambda_s = \frac{4}{3}\alpha_s\rho_s d_s g_{0s}(1+e_s)\left(\frac{\theta_s}{\pi}\right)^{1/2} \tag{4.42}$$

In the limit of maximum packing, granular flow becomes incompressible. Under such conditions, the kinetic contribution to viscosity is replaced by a friction contribution. Theories of soil mechanics may be used to estimate such friction contributions (Schaeffer, 1987).

The granular temperature, θ_s is obtained by solving its transport equation, which has the form:

$$\frac{3}{2}\left[\frac{\partial}{\partial t}(\rho_s\varepsilon_s\theta_s) + \nabla\cdot(\rho_s\varepsilon_s U_s\theta_s)\right] = \overline{\overline{\tau_s}} : \nabla U_s - \nabla\cdot(k_\theta\theta_s) - \gamma_\theta + \phi_{fs} + \phi_{ls} \tag{4.43}$$

where the first term on the right-hand side represents the generation of energy by the solid stress tensor, τ_s, the second term represents diffusion of energy (k_θ is the diffusion coefficient). The third term represents collisional dissipation of energy. The fourth and fifth terms represent energy exchange between fluid and solid, and solid and solid respectively. In order to close the equation set, it is necessary to develop expressions for new terms appearing in the governing equation of granular temperature. For these terms as well, several different alternative expressions have been derived (see Gidaspow, 1994 and a review by Peirano, 1998). Without discussing specific issues related to these different expressions, here we list some of the most commonly used expressions required to close the equation set. Granular temperature conductivity can be written:

$$\kappa_\theta = \frac{75\rho_s d_s\sqrt{\theta_s\pi}}{192(1+e_s)g_{0s}}\left[1+\frac{6}{5}\alpha_s g_{0s}(1+e_s)\right]^2 + 2\alpha_s^2\rho_s d_s(1+e_s)g_{0s}\sqrt{\frac{\theta_s}{\pi}} \tag{4.44}$$

Dissipation of energy due to inelastic collisions can be expressed in the form:

$$\gamma_\theta = 3(1-e_s^2)\alpha_s^2\rho_s g_{0s}\theta_s\left[\frac{4}{d_P}\sqrt{\frac{\theta_s}{\pi}} - \nabla U_s\right] \tag{4.45}$$

Energy exchange between the fluid and the solid phase is modeled as

$$\phi_{fs} = -3K_{fs}\theta_s \tag{4.46}$$

In order to fully understand the physical significance of various terms appearing in the governing equations of granular flows, the references cited above can be consulted. Detailed modeling of the various terms appearing in the granular flow equations is a fast developing field. It must be mentioned here that the modeler has to be careful to ensure consistency in all the different formulations when finalizing the complete set of governing equations. This is especially true when there are more than one solid phases (see Mathiesen (1997) and Mathiesen *et al.* (2000) for more discussion about the consistency in model formulations).

Other conservation equations (enthalpy and species) for multiphase flows can be written following a similar general format. For example, the enthalpy conservation equation is written:

$$\frac{\partial}{\partial t}(\alpha_k\rho_k h_k)+\nabla\cdot(\alpha_k\rho_k U_k h_k) = -\nabla\cdot q+(\tau_k:\nabla U_k)+\varepsilon_k\frac{Dp_k}{Dt}+\sum_{p=1}^{n}(Q_{pk}+S_{pk}h_{pk})+S_k \tag{4.47}$$

where h_k is the specific enthalpy of phase k and S_k is the source of enthalpy (for example, due to chemical reaction). Q_{pk} is the energy transfer between the pth and kth phase. $S_{pk}h_{pk}$ is the energy transfer associated with the mass transfer between p and k phases. Heat or mass transfer between phases must satisfy the local balance condition:

$$Q_{pk} = -Q_{kp} \qquad S_{pk} = -S_{kp} \tag{4.48}$$

The species conservation equation for multiphase flows can be written:

$$\frac{\partial}{\partial t}(\alpha_k\rho_k m_k^i) + \nabla\cdot(\alpha_k\rho_k U_k m_k^i) = \nabla\cdot(\alpha_k\rho_k D_k^i\nabla m_k^i) + \sum_{p=1}^{n}(S_{pk}) \tag{4.49}$$

where m_k^i is the mass fraction of species i in phase k. S_{pp} (mass transfer from phase p to phase p) is zero. The rate of energy or mass transfer between phases can be written:

$$Q_{pk} \text{ or } S_{pk} = (h_{pk} \text{ or } k_{pk})(\phi_p - \phi_k) \tag{4.50}$$

where the second term on the right-hand side represents the temperature or concentration driving force and the first term represents heat or mass transfer coefficient. An appropriate value of heat or mass transfer coefficient can be obtained by using suitable correlations of Nusselt number (in terms of Reynolds number and Prandtl number) or Sherwood number (in terms of Reynolds number and Schmidt number). Some typical correlations to estimate fluid–particle heat transfer coefficients and mass transfer coefficients are listed in Appendix 4.3. Evaporation of volatile fluid from dispersed phase particles needs special attention. Several different models with varying degrees of sophistication have been proposed. More often than not, semi-empirical models based on saturation and boiling temperatures along with time relaxation parameters are adequate to simulate evaporation processes in chemical reactors. In these models, source due to evaporation or condensation is generally expressed as

$$\dot{m}_v = \frac{r_v \alpha_l \rho_l (T_l - T_{\text{sat}})}{T_{\text{sat}}} \tag{4.51}$$

where T_{sat} is a saturation temperature and r_v is an empirical parameter controlling the rate of evaporation. See, for example, Theologos *et al.* (1997) on modeling the evaporation of liquid oil in the bottom section of a FCC riser reactor.

Boundary conditions for Eulerian multiphase flow models can be formulated using the usual practices discussed in Chapter 2. Some comments regarding special considerations for multiphase flows are included here. At impermeable walls, the usual ‘no slip’ boundary condition can be specified for the continuous phase. However, this condition will not be realistic for dispersed phase particles, which may slip along the wall if the particle size is bigger than the characteristic roughness scale of walls (Fig. 4.7). Sinclair and Jackson (1989) and Sommerfeld (1993) discussed the formulation of these boundary conditions in detail. For granular flows, Sinclair and Jackson (1989) formulated wall boundary conditions based on a microscopic model of particle collisions with the wall. They assumed that momentum flux transmitted to the boundary by collisions (product of the change of momentum per collision, collision frequency and the number of particles per unit area next to the wall) is equal to the tangential stress exerted by the particle adjacent to the wall. This leads to the following boundary condition:

$$\tau_{\text{sw}} = \frac{\pi \rho_s \overline{U_s} \psi \sqrt{\theta_s} \alpha_s}{2\sqrt{3}\alpha_{s\max}\left(1 - (\alpha_{s\max}/\alpha_s)^{-1/3}\right)} \tag{4.52}$$

where ψ is a specularity coefficient (equivalent to 1 minus the tangential restitution coefficient). For the granular temperature, a zero flux boundary condition is usually specified at the walls. Alternatively, it is possible to derive a boundary condition for granular temperature at the wall by equating the sum of the flux of granular temperature to the wall and the generation of granular temperature at the wall to the energy dissipation at the wall due to inelastic particle–wall collisions. Details may be found in Johnson and Jackson (1987).

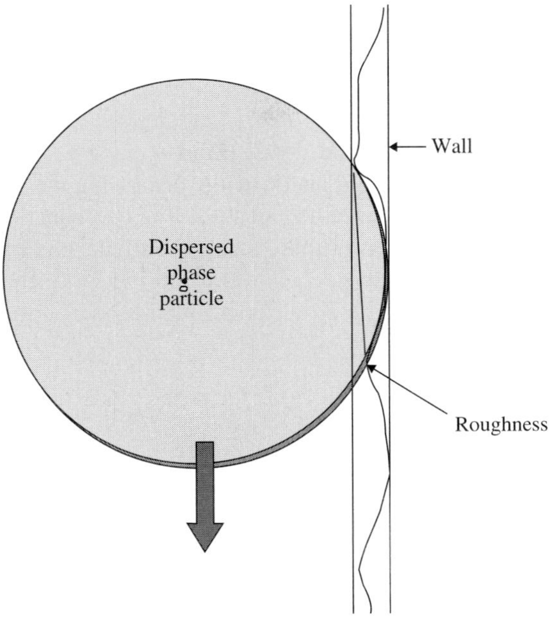

FIGURE 4.7 Dispersed phase particles may slip at wall.

The other situation which may require special treatment is a boundary of multiphase dispersion through which dispersed phase particles are allowed to escape, but not the continuous phase (for example, the top surface of gas–liquid dispersion in a bubble column reactor). The standard 'outlet' boundary conditions need to be suitably modified to represent the observed flow processes. It is possible to simulate the actual behavior by specifying appropriate sink near the top surface (see Ranade, 1998 and Chapter 11).

So far, discussion has been restricted to laminar multiphase flow processes. However, in most industrial multiphase reactors, flow processes are turbulent. Modeling multiphase turbulent flow processes is a fast developing field. Some recent developments and general modeling issues are briefly discussed here. The presence and motion of dispersed phase particle may affect the macroscopic turbulence field of the continuous phase as well as the microscale characteristics of this turbulence field. Depending on particle size, density (particle response time) and volume fraction of the dispersed phase, dispersed phase particles may enhance or suppress the turbulence. Particles may interact with microscale fluctuations of continuous phase and may damp the turbulence (suspension and oscillations of particles may dissipate the energy). Larger particles may enhance turbulence by extracting energy from macroscale fluctuations and by vortex shedding. Elghobashi (1991) proposed a regime map based on particle response time and the Kolmogorov time scale to identify the influence (damping/enhancement) and degree of coupling between turbulence regimes in multiphase flows (Fig. 4.2). This map may be used to estimate the extent of coupling between dispersed phase particles and turbulence.

Most attempts at modeling complex, turbulent multiphase flows rely on the practices followed for single-phase flows, with some ad hoc modifications to account for the presence of dispersed phase particles. For multiphase flows, several new correlations appear in time-averaged (RANS type) governing equations. Different models have been proposed to specifically represent turbulence in dispersed gas–liquid (reviewed by Ranade, 1995; Lahey, 1987; Lane *et al.*, 1999) and dispersed gas–solid flows (reviewed by Sommerfeld, 1993; Bolio *et al.*, 1995; Peirano, 1998). Some of these models are discussed in Part IV, while discussing the specific issues in modeling bubble column and fluidized bed reactors. The two-equation turbulence models (k–ε) form the basis for most of these studies. Turbulence in a continuous phase is usually modeled using transport equations for turbulent kinetic energy and turbulent energy dissipation rates. These transport equations are written in a form similar to single-phase flows:

$$\frac{\partial}{\partial t}(\alpha_k \rho_k \phi_k) + \nabla \cdot (\alpha_k \rho_k U_k \phi_k) = -\nabla \cdot \left(\alpha_k \frac{\mu_{\mathrm{T}k}}{\sigma_{\mathrm{T}k}} \nabla \phi_k \right) + S_{\phi k} \tag{4.53}$$

where ϕ_k can be turbulent kinetic energy or turbulent energy dissipation rate in phase k. The symbols $\mu_{\mathrm{T}k}$ and $\sigma_{\mathrm{T}k}$ have usual meanings of turbulent viscosity and turbulent Prandtl number for phase k. $S_{\phi k}$ is the corresponding source term for ϕ in phase k. Source terms for turbulent kinetic energy and dissipation can be written:

$$S_{kk} = \alpha_k[(G_k + G_{ke}) - \varepsilon_k] \tag{4.54}$$

$$S_{\varepsilon k} = \alpha_k \frac{\varepsilon_k}{k_k}[C_1(G_k + G_{ke}) - C_2 \varepsilon_k] \tag{4.55}$$

where G_k is generation in phase k and G_{ke} is extra generation (or dissipation) of turbulence in phase k. Generation due to mean velocity gradients, G_k can be calculated using the single-phase flow equation (Eq. (3.23)). Extra generation or damping of turbulence due to the presence of dispersed phase particles is represented by appropriate formulation for G_{ke}. Some formulations for G_{ke}, suitable for gas–liquid and gas–solid flows, are discussed in Part IV when discussing different reactor types. In the absence of adequate information, in many cases, extra generation terms are usually set to zero. Various attempts to develop models to represent extra generation or damping of turbulence are reviewed by Lahey (1987) and more recently, by Peirano and Leckner (1998). The turbulent viscosity, $\mu_{\mathrm{T}k}$, is calculated using the formula specified for single-phase flows (Eq. (3.20)). The values of parameters for the k–ε model are usually kept the same as those for the single-phase model (listed in Table 3.1). In principle, values of these parameters will be functions of particle loading and ratio of particle relaxation time to eddy lifetime (Lahey, 1987; Squire and Eaton, 1994). Cao and Ahmadi (1995) discussed the variation of parameter (C_μ) appearing in the expression for turbulent viscosity with volume fraction of dispersed phase. More research is needed to predict the continuous phase turbulence in multiphase flows accurately. The situation becomes even more difficult when modeling turbulence in the dispersed phase. Turbulence in the dispersed phase may be physically understood as the particle velocity fluctuations caused by collisions between particles and interactions with the continuous phase. These modeling attempts are discussed by Balzer *et al.* (1995), Simonin (1995) and Enwald *et al.* (1996).

In most practical applications of dispersed multiphase flows, the suspension consists of non-spherical particles having different diameters. The range of particle diameters or particle size distribution may (non-reactive fluidization of particles) or may not remain constant (bubble columns where gas bubbles may coalesce or break up and change the particle size distribution). It is necessary to adequately model the influence of particle size distribution on the fluid dynamics of multiphase flows. With the Lagrangian approach, the influence of particle size distribution can be readily included in the simulations. However, in a Eulerian–Eulerian approach, appropriate models and closures need to be developed. The three major approaches to accounting for the influence of particle size distribution (PSD) on fluid dynamics of multiphase flows are discussed below.

The first approach is an approximation, which relies on identifying an effective value of size of dispersed phase particle, which will behave in the same way as the population of dispersed phase particles with a specific PSD. Such an approach may give acceptable results if the PSD is narrow and smooth (uni-modal). There are many ways of defining a mean or an effective particle diameter for the suspension of particles. The mean volume-length diameter, the mean volume-surface diameter (Sauter mean diameter) and the mass mean diameter are the most commonly used mean diameters (Soo, 1990). According to Soo (1990), the mean volume diameter is suitable for the determination of volume fraction, whereas the mean surface diameter is relevant to physical mechanisms at the interface. Recently, Peirano and Leckner (2000) analyzed the fluid dynamics of gas–solid flows and concluded that for dilute suspensions (where collisional mechanisms can be neglected), if particle Reynolds numbers are smaller than 1, the mean volume-length diameter is the most representative. At higher Reynolds number (>1000), the mean volume-surface diameter is the most representative. For intermediate Reynolds number, the effective diameter smoothly varies from the mean volume-length to the mean volume-surface diameter. Such an effective diameter may be specified to simulate suspensions with narrow PSD.

When PSD is not smooth and wide (or is bi-modal), it is necessary to represent the dispersed phase by more than one fluid phase. The size distribution of dispersed phase particles is usually discretized into a few size groups. Each of these size groups is considered as an individual dispersed phase when simulating such multiphase flows. Several attempts have been made to develop a multiple solid phase granular flow model to simulate gas–solid flows with a wide size distribution of solid particles. Jenkins and Mancini (1987) extended the kinetic theory of granular flow to binary mixtures (assuming equal granular temperature). Gidaspow *et al.* (1996) and Magner (1996) extended this to binary mixtures with unequal granular temperature. Recently, Mathiesen *et al.* (2000) developed a generalized gas–solid model with multiple solid phases. They also discuss several consistency issues in formulating such a generalized model. Such a generalized model requires appropriate formulations of particle–particle drag coefficients, apart from consistent formulations of various previously discussed terms such as radial distribution function, solids pressure, solids viscosity and so on. It must be noted that computational requirements increase significantly with an increase in the number of solid phases. Mathiesen *et al.* (2000) reported results of simulations with three solid phases, which show encouraging agreement with experimental data. This approach shows promise, and deserves further investigation to explore applications to industrially relevant multiphase flows.

A similar approach can be used to simulate fluid–fluid flows such as gas–liquid or liquid–liquid. However, in such flows the dispersed phase particles can coalesce or break up during the flow, and the particle size distribution evolves as the flow develops. Therefore, to define multiple phases with specific ranges of particle diameters to represent the dispersed phase, it is necessary to develop models of coalescence and break-up to simulate the changes in particle size distribution. Recently Carrica *et al.* (1999) reported the development of such a model to simulate bubbly two-phase flows. They derived conservation equations for different bubble phases by representing an equation of bubble size distribution function as a multi-group scheme. An equation for bubble number density corresponding to each group can then be derived after incorporating appropriate coalescence and break-up models (see for example, Prince and Blanch, 1990 or Luo and Svendsen, 1996 for coalescence and break-up models). Carrica *et al.* (1999) used 15 groups for simulating bubbly flow around a surface ship. Thus, instead of solving transport equations for two phases, they need to solve transport equations for 16 phases, which requires much larger computational resources. The required resources will be increased by a factor more than the ratio of the number of transport equations in the model (8), because of the increase in the required number of iterations to converge. When the bubble size distribution makes significant contributions, it is necessary to adopt such an approach. As an alternative to such intensive simulations, an approximate model for coalescence and break-up may be developed by considering a bubble number density equation. Coalescence and break-up processes locally affect bubble number density. A local effective bubble diameter can then be found from bubble number density and gas volume fraction. This approach avoids having to solve an excessive number of transport equations and may give adequate representation of the variation of effective bubble size within the domain. Lane *et al.* (1999) recently used such an approach to simulate gas–liquid flows in stirred vessels.

The recent progress in experimental techniques and applications of DNS and LES for turbulent multiphase flows may lead to new insights necessary to develop better computational models to simulate dispersed multiphase flows with wide particle size distribution in turbulent regimes. Until then, the simulations of such complex turbulent multiphase flow processes have to be accompanied by careful validation (to assess errors due to modeling) and error estimation (due to numerical issues) exercise. Applications of these models to simulate multiphase stirred reactors, bubble column reactors and fluidized bed reactors, are discussed in Part IV of this book.

4.3. OTHER TYPES OF MULTIPHASE FLOWS

4.3.1. Flow Processes in Porous Media

Fixed bed reactors or packed bubble column reactors are examples of flow processes occurring in porous media, which are commonly encountered by reactor engineers. The problem of predicting fluid flow and the rates of mixing and other transport processes in such reactors is an important task for a reactor engineer. In general, two approaches are used to model the fluid dynamics of such reactors. The first one uses a lumped parameter approach and treats the irregular geometry of the packed region as an isotropic or non-isotropic porous media, characterized by a few lumped parameters. The second approach treats the geometrical intricacies of the packed region rigorously. Obviously, the second approach is computationally demanding and can be applied only to a small region of the reactor. It nevertheless can serve as a useful learning tool. These approaches are briefly discussed below.

In the lumped parameter approach, the packed region or the porous region is represented by introducing a suitable source or sink in the appropriate conservation equations. Most of the engineering simulations of flow through porous media (such as flow through fixed bed reactors or bundles of heat exchanger tubes) use this approach. The extra resistance offered by the porous medium to the flow can, for example, be represented by introducing a sink in the usual single-phase momentum conservation equations as:

$$\nabla p_{\mathrm{p}} = -\frac{\mu}{\beta}U - C\left(\frac{1}{2}\rho U|U|\right) \tag{4.56}$$

where β is a permeability and C an inertial resistance factor characterizing the porous media. The values of these two empirical constants need to be specified either from experimental data or by using the more rigorous models mentioned earlier. To model a packed bed reactor, usually the Ergun (1952) equation is used to estimate the values of characteristic parameters. Use of the Ergun equation leads to the following expressions for β and C:

$$\beta = \frac{D_{\mathrm{p}}^2}{150}\frac{\varphi^3}{(1-\varphi)^2} \qquad C = \frac{3.5}{D_{\mathrm{p}}}\frac{(1-\varphi)}{\varphi^3} \tag{4.57}$$

where D_{p} is particle diameter and φ is porosity. It is possible to use different values of these characteristic constants for different directions to represent the anisotropy of porous media. Any other empirical pressure drop correlation may be used instead of the Ergun equation. To model the porous region of complex shaped particles, such as fibers of glass wool, more complex equations or a look-up table may also be used.

The additional sink is added to the usual conservation equations corrected for the volume fraction of the porous media. The governing equations look similar to those for Eulerian multiphase flow processes (Section 4.2.2) except that the volume fraction of the porous medium is not a variable. In the enthalpy equation, it is possible to include influence of porous media by considering an effective thermal conductivity, k_{eff}, of the form:

$$k_{\mathrm{eff}} = \varphi k_{\mathrm{f}} + (1-\varphi)k_{\mathrm{s}} \tag{4.58}$$

where φ is a porosity. Subscripts f and s denote fluid and solid, respectively. It may also be necessary to include suitable modifications in the turbulence model to account for the different turbulence generation mechanism within the porous media. More often than not, the characteristic length scale of the porous region determines the characteristic length scale of the turbulence downstream of the porous region. The presence of porous media, therefore, decouples turbulence field upstream of porous region from the downstream. In such a situation, a length scale appropriate to the porous region under consideration may be used to estimate the desired turbulence quantities at the interface between the porous region and the downstream region.

Rigorous modeling of flow through porous media is very challenging, and recently, it has been explored as a learning tool. In this approach, microscopic flow processes are modeled in detail by considering a small periodic structure of the porous media. Geometrical details of solid regions and open regions are modeled rigorously. Therefore, although the governing equations become relatively simple (single-phase flow equations), the geometric modeling and grid generation become quite complicated. Computational demands also increase significantly. For example, Logtenberg *et al.* (1999) simulated flow and heat transfer in a fixed bed reactor by considering ten spherical particles in close contact. They had to use about 250 000 computational elements. Their model does not need any empirical parameters and could reproduce the flow and heat transfer behavior of a cluster of particles quite well. Such models will be very useful in developing a detailed understanding of microscopic flow structures in packed bed reactors and will complement lumped parameter models.

4.3.2. Separated Multiphase Flows

While discussing the flow through porous media in the above section, it was assumed that the open space is filled by a homogeneous continuous phase. It is possible to encounter situations in which more than one phase flows through packed beds. For example, in a typical absorption column/reactor, gas and liquid phase flow through the packed bed. For such a flow, there exists an interface between gas and liquid phases. Such a flow regime is called a separated flow regime. When gas and liquid phases are transported through conduits at high gas throughputs, an annular flow regime may exist in which liquid flows in the form of an annular film attached to the conduit walls and gas flows through the central core. This flow regime is also a separated flow regime. In a separated flow regime, several sub-regimes such as wavy flow may exist. To model such separated multiphase flows, it is necessary to use a volume of fluid (VOF) approach, since the interface between separated phases plays an important role. The basics of the VOF approach have already been discussed in Section 4.2.3. Application of VOF to simulate complex, separated multiphase flow have only recently started. Wehrli *et al.* (1997) and Casey *et al.* (1998) show some results of the application of VOF to simulate wavy flow over inclined solid surfaces. Considering the computational requirements of such simulations, the rigorous modeling of separated multiphase flows may be used as a learning tool and to developing semi-empirical lumped sub-models. Such lumped sub-models can then be used to simulate complex, multiphase flows through packed beds. The approach discussed for modeling flow through porous media may be extended to simulate multiphase flows through porous media. Details of modeling such packed bed or trickle bed reactors are briefly discussed in Chapter 13.

4.4. SUMMARY

Modeling multiphase flow processes is a complex and still developing subject. It is often an iterative process requiring multiple modeling frameworks to understand different aspects of the flow problem. The underlying physics is still inadequately known and a reactor engineer modeling complex multiphase flow processes often has to complement detailed modeling efforts with validation experiments and data analysis. It is indeed essential to use a hierarchy of models with an appreciation of 'learning' versus 'simulation' models to represent multiphase flow processes accurately. An appropriate methodology needs to be developed to systematically interpret the results obtained using different modeling frameworks. Ultimately, there is no substitute for the engineering judgement and creativity of a reactor engineer to develop a tractable computational model to simulate complex industrial multiphase flow processes.

REFERENCES

Acrivos, A. and Goddard, J.D. (1965), Asymptotic expansions for laminar-forced convection heat and mass transfer, *J. Fluid Mech.*, **23**, 273–291.

Ahmedi, G. (1987), On the mechanics of incompressible multiphase suspensions, *Adv. Water Res.*, **10**, 32.

Allen, M.P. and Tildesley, D.J. (1990), "Computer Simulations of Liquids", Oxford Science Publications, Oxford.

Auton, T.R. (1983), The dynamic of bubbles, drops and particles in motion in liquids, PhD Thesis, University of Cambridge, UK.

Balzer, G., Boelle, A. and Simonin, O. (1995), Eulerian gas–solid flow modeling of dense fluidized bed, Fluidization VIII, *Int. Symp. Of the Engineering Foundation*, Tours, p. 1125.

Berlemont, A., Desjonqueres, P. and Gouesbet, G. (1990), Particle Lagrangian simulation in turbulent flows, *Int. J. Multiphase Flow*, **16**, 19–34.

Berlemont, A., Simonin, O. and Sommerfeld, M. (1995), Validation of interparticle collision models based on large eddy simulations, AME/JSME Int. Conference of gas–solid flows, Hilton Head, SC 13–18 August, Proceedings FED, **228**, 359–369.

Besnard, D.C. and Harlow, F.H. (1987), Turbulence in multiphase flow, *Int. J. Multiphase Flow*, **10**, 32.

Besnard, D.C. and Harlow, F.H. (1988), Turbulence in multiphase flow, *Int. J. Multiphase Flow*, **14**(6), 679.

Bolio, E.J., Yasuna, J.A. and Sinclair, J.L. (1995), Dilute turbulent gas–solid flow in riser with particle–particle interactions, *AIChE J.*, **41**, 1375.

Brackbill, J.U., Kothe, D.B. and Zemach, C. (1992), A continuum method for modelling surface tension, *J. Computat. Phys.*, **100**, 335–354.

Brenner, H. (1961), The slow motion of sphere through a viscous fluid towards a plane surface, *Chem. Eng. Sci.*, **16**, 242.

Brian, P.L.T. and Hales, H.B. (1969), *AIChE J.*, **15**, 419.

Cao, J. and Ahmadi, G. (1995), Gas–particle two phase turbulent flow in a vertical duct, *Int. J. Multiphase Flow*, **21**, 1203.

Carrica, P.M., Drew, D.A., Bonetto, F. and Lahey, R.T. (1999), A polydisperse model for bubbly two phase flow round a surface ship, *Int. J. Multiphase Flow*, **25**, 257.

Casey, M., Lang, E., Mack, R., Schlegel, R. and Wehrli, M. (1998), Applications of CFD for process engineering at Sulzer, *Speedup J.*, **12**, 43–51.

Chapman, S. and Cowling, T.G. (1970), "The Mathematical Theory of Non–uniform Gases", Cambridge Mathematical Library, Cambridge.

Chen, P.P. and Crowe, C.T. (1984), On the Monte Carlo method for modeling particle dispersion in turbulence, *ASME Symp. Gas–Solid Flows*, p. 37.

Clift, R., Grace, J.R. and Weber, M.E. (1978), "Bubbles, Drops and Particles", Academic Press, New York.

Csnady, G.T. (1963), Turbulent diffusion of heavy particles in the atmosphere, *J. Atmos. Sci.*, **105**, 329–334.

Dalla Ville, J.M. (1948), "Micromeritics", Pitman, London.

Delnoij, E. (1999), "Fluid dynamics of gas–liquid bubble columns", PhD thesis, University of Twente, The Netherlands.

Delnoij, E., Lammers, F.A., Kuipers, J.A.M. and van Swaaij, W.P.M. (1997), Dynamic simulation of dispersed gas-liquid two-phase flow using a discrete bubble model, *Chem. Eng. Sci.*, **52**, 1429.

Drew, D.A. (1983), Mathematical modeling of two phase flow, *Ann. Rev. Fluid. Mech.*, **15**, 261.

Drew, D.A. and Lahey, R.T. (1979), Application of general consecutive principles to the derivation of multidimensional two phase flow equations, *Int. J. Multiphase Flow*, **5**, 243–264.

Elghobashi, S.E. (1991), Particle-laden turbulent flows: Direct simulation and closure models, *Appl. Sci. Res.*, **48**, 301–314.

Elghobashi, S.E. (1994), On predicting particle-laden turbulent flows, *Appl. Sci. Res.*, **52**, 309.

Enwald, H., Peirano, E. and Almstedt, A.E. (1996), Eulerian two phase flow theory applied to fluidization, *Int. J. Multiphase Flow*, **22**, 21.

Ergun, S. (1952), Fluid flow through packed columns, *Chem. Eng. Prog.*, **48**(2), 89.

Foerster, S.F., Louge, M.Y., Chang, H. and Allia, K. (1994), Measurements of the collision properties of small spheres, *Phys. Fluids*, **6**(3), 1108.

Frenkel, D. and Smith, B. (1996), "Understanding Molecular Simulations, from Algorithm to Applications", Academic Press, San Diego, CA.

Garside, J. and Al-Dibouni, M.R. (1977), Velocity voidage relationship for fluidization and sedimentation, *I&EC Proc. Des. Dev.*, **16**, 206.

Gidaspow, D. (1994), "Multiphase Flow and Fluidization", Academic Press, Boston.

Gidaspow, D., Huilin, L. and Magner, E. (1996), Kinetic theory of multiphase flow and fluidization validation and extension to binary mixture, *19th Int. Congress on Theoretical and Applied Mech.*, Kyoto, Japan, pp. 25–31.

Gore, R.A. and Crowe, C.T. (1989), Effect of particle size on modulating turbulent intensity, *Int. J. Multiphase Flow*, **15**(2), 279.

Gouesbet, G., Berlemont, A. and Picart, A. (1984), Dispersion of discrete particles by continuous turbulent motions. Extensive discussion of the Tchen's theory, using a two-parameter family of lagrangian correlation functions, *Phys. Fluids*, **27**(4), 827.

Gouesbet, G. and Berlemont, A. (1999), Eulerian and Lagrangian approaches for predicting the behavior of discrete particles in turbulent flows, *Prog. Energy Combustion Sci.*, **25**, 133–159.

Gunn, D.J. (1978), Transfer of heat or mass to particle in fixed and fluidized beds, *Int. J. Heat Mass Transf.*, **21**, 467–476.

Harlow, F.H. and Amsden, A.A. (1975), Numerical calculation of multiphase flow, *J. Computat. Physics*, **17**, 19.

Hoomans, B.P.B. (2000), Granular dynamics of gas solid two phase flows, PhD thesis, University of Twente, Enschede, The Netherlands.

Hoomans, B.P.B., Kuipers, J.A.M., Briels, W.J. and van Swaaij, W.P.M. (1998), Comment on the paper 'Numerical simulation of the gas solid flows in fluidized bed combining discrete particles method with computational fluid dynamics' by Xu, B.H. and Yu, A.B., *Chem. Eng. Sci.*, **53**, 2645.

Ishii, M. (1975), "Thermo–Fluid Dynamic theory of Two Phase Flow", Eyrolles.

Jenkins, J.T. and Richman, M.W. (1985), Grad's 13 moment system for a dense gas of inelastic spheres, *Arch. Ratio. Mech. Anal.*, **87**, 355–377.

Jenkins, J.T. and Mancini, F. (1987), Balance laws and constitutive relations for plane flows of a dense binary mixture of smooth, nearly elastic circular disks, *J. Appl. Mech.*, **54**, 27.

Johansen, S.T. and Boysen, F. (1988), *Metal. Trans.*, **19B**, 755.

Johnson, P.C. and Jackson, R. (1987), Frictional collisional constitutive relations for granular materials with application to plain shearing, *J. Fluid Mech.*, **176**, 67.

Kataoka, I. and Serizawa, A. (1989), Basic equation of turbulence in gas–liquid two phase flow, *Int. J. Multiphase Flow*, **15**(5), 843.

Kohnen, G., Ruger, M. and Sommerfeld, M. (1994), Convergence behavior for numerical calculations by the Eular/ Lagrange method for strongly coupled phases. *ASME Symp. On Numerical Methods in Multiphase Flows FED*, **185**, 191.

Krishna, R. and van Baton, J.M. (1999), Simulating the motion of gas bubbles in a liquid, *Nature*, **398**, 208.

Kuipers, J.A.M. and van Swaaij, W.P.M. (1997), Application of computational fluid dynamics to chemical reaction engineering, *Rev. Chem. Eng.*, **13**, 1–118.

Kunni, D. and Levenspiel, O. (1991), "Fluidization Engineering", John Wiley and Sons, New York.

Kuo, K.K.Y. (1986), "Principles of Combustion", John Wiley and Sons, New York.

Kuo, J.T. and Wallis, G.B. (1988), Flow of bubbles through nozzles, *Int. J. Multiphase Flow*, **14**, 547.

Lahey, R.T. (1987), Turbulence and phase distribution phenomena in two-phase flow. ICHMT International Seminar on Transient Phenomena in Multiphase Flow, Dubrovnik, Yugoslavia, May 24–30.

Lahey, R.T. and Drew, D.A. (1989), The three dimensional time and volume averaged conservation equations for two-phase flows, *Adv. Nucl. Sci. Technol.*, **20**, 1.

Lane, G.L., Schwarz, M.P. and Evans, G.M. (1999), CFD simulation of gas liquid flow in a stirred tank, *3rd Int. Symp. on Mixing in Industrial Processes*, Japan.

Levenspiel, O. (1972), "Chemical Reaction Engineering", 2nd edition, John Wiley and Sons, New York.

Levich, V.G. (1962), "Physicochemical Hydrodynamics", Prentice-Hall, Englewood Cliffs, NJ.

Logtenberg, S.A., Nijemeisland, M. and Dixon, A.G. (1999), Computational fluid dynamics simulations of fluid flow and heat transfer at the wall particle contact points in a fixed bed reactor, *Chem. Eng. Sci.*, **54**, 2433–2440.

Lun, C.K.K. and Savage, S.B. (1986), The effect of an impact velocity dependent coefficient of restitution on stresses developed by sheared granular materials, *Acta Mechanica*, **63**, 15.

Luo, H. and Svendsen, H.F. (1996), Theoretical model for drop and bubble breakup in turbulent flow, *AIChE J.*, **42**(5), 1225.

Ma, D. and Ahmadi, G.J. (1986), An equation of state for dense rigid sphere gases, *J. Chem. Phys.*, **84**(6), 3449.

Ma, D. and Ahmadi, G.J. (1989), A thermodynamical formulation for dispersed turbulence flows, *Int. J. Multiphase Flow*, **16**, 323.

Magner, E. (1996), Modeling and Simulation of gas/solid flow in curvilinear coordinates. PhD thesis, Telemark Institute of Technology, Norway.

Mathiesen, V. (1997), An experimental and computational study of multiphase flow behavior in circulating fluidized beds, PhD thesis, Norwegian University of Science and Technology, Norway.

Mathiesen, V., Solberg, T. and Hjertager, B.H. (2000), An experimental and computational study of multiphase flow behavior in a circulating fluidized bed, *Int. J. Multiphase Flow*, **26**, 387.

Maxey, M.R. and Riley, J.J. (1983), Equation of motion for a small rigid sphere in a non uniform flow, *Phys. Fluids*, **26**(4), 883.

Mei, R. (1993), History force on a sphere due to a step change in the free stream velocity, *Int. J. Multiphase Flow*, **19**, 509–525.

Mikami, T. (1998), Agglomeration fluidization of liquid/solid bridging particles and its control, PhD thesis, Tokyo University of Agriculture and Technology, Department of Chemical Engineering, Japan.

Molerus, O. (1980), A coherent representation of pressure drop in fixed beds and of bed expansion for particulate fluidized beds, *Chem. Eng. Sci.*, **35**(6), 1331–1340.

Morsi, S.A. and Alexander, A.J. (1972), An investigation of particle trajectories in two phase flow system, *J. Fluid Mech.*, **55**(2), 193–208.

Nelson, P.A. and Galloway, T.R. (1975), Particle to fluid heat and mass transfer in dense systems of fine particles, *Chem. Eng. Sci.*, **30**, 1–6.

Nieuwland, J.J., van Sint Annaland, M., Kuipers, J.A.M. and van Swaaij, W.P.M. (1996), Hydrodynamic modeling of gas/particle flows in riser reactors, *AIChE J.*, **42**(6), 1569.

Oesterle, B. (1994), Une etude de l'influence des forces transversales agissant sur les particles dans les ecoulements gaz–solide, *Powder Technol.*, **79**, 81.

Oesterle, B. and Petitjean, A. (1993), Simulation of particle–particle interaction in gas–solid flows, *Int. J. Multiphase Flows*, **19**, 199–211.

Ogawa, S., Umemura, A. and Oshina, N. (1980), On the equations of fully fluidized granular materials, *J. Angew. Math. Phys.*, **31**, 483.

Patel, M.K., Pericleous, K. and Cross, M. (1993), *Computat. Fluid Dyn.*, **1**, 161–176.

Peirano, E. (1998), Modeling and simulation of turbulent gas–solid flows applied to fluidization. PhD thesis, Chalmers University of Technology, Goteborg, Sweden.

Peirano, E. and Leckner, B. (1998), Fundamentals of turbulent gas solid flow applied to circulating fluidized bed combustion, *Proc. Energy Combustion Sci.*, **24**, 259–296.

Peirano, E. and Leckner, B. (2000), A mean diameter for numerical computations of polydispersed gas–solid suspensions in fluidization, *Chem. Eng. Sci.*, **55**(6), 1189–1192.

Picart, A., Berlemont, A. and Gouesbet, G. (1982), De l'infulence du terme de Basset sur la diepersion de particules discretes dans le cadre de la theorie de Tchen, *C.R. Acad. Sci., Paris, Series II*, **T295**, 305.

Prince, N.J. and Blanch, H.W. (1990), Bubble coalescence and breakup in air sparged bubble columns, *AIChE J.*, **36**, 1485.

Ranade, V.V. (1995), Computational fluid dynamics for reactor engineering, *Rev. Chem. Eng.*, **11**(3), 225–289.

Ranade, V.V. (1998), Multiphase reaction engineering, *Speedup J.*, **12**, 26–33.

Ranz, W.E. and Marshall, W.R. (1952), Evaporation from drops, *Chem. Eng. Prog.*, **48**, 141–146.

Richardson, J.F., Davidson, F. and Harrison, D. (eds) (1971), "Fluidisation", Academic Press, London and New York.

Richardson, J.F. and Zaki, W.N. (1954), Sedimentation and fluidization: part I, *Trans. Inst. Chem. Eng.*, **32**, 35.

Rider, W.J. and Kothe, D.B. (1995), Stretching and rearing interface tracking methods, Los Alamos National Laboratory (http://www.c3.lanl.gov/~wjr/pubs.html).

Rietema, K. and Van den Akker, H.E.A. (1983), On momentum equations in dispersed two phase system, *Int. J. Multiphase Flow*, **9**, 21.

Rimmer, P.L. (1968), Heat transfer from a sphere in a stream of small Reynolds number, *J. Fluid Mech.*, **32**, 1–7.

Rudman, M. (1997), Volume tracking methods for interfacial flow calculations, *Int. J. Num. Methods Fluids*, **24**, 671.

Schaeffer, D.G. (1987), Instability in the evolution equations describing incompressible granular flow, *J. Diff. Eq.*, **66**, 19–50.

Schiller, L. and Naumann, Z. (1935), *Z. Ver. Deutsch. Ing.*, **77**, 318.

Seibert, K.D. and Burns, M.A. (1998), Simulation of structural phenomenon in mixed-particle fluidized beds, *AIChE J.*, **44**, 528.

Simonin, O. (1995), Summerschool on 'Numerical modeling and prediction of dispersed phase flows', *IMVU*, Meserburg, Germany.
Sinclair, J.L. and Jackson, R. (1989), Gas–particle flow in a vertical pipe with particle–particle interactions, *AIChE J.*, **35**, 1473.
Soo, S.L. (1990), "Multiphase Fluid Dynamics", Science Press, Gower Technical, New York.
Sommerfeld, M. (1990), Numerical simulation of the particle dispersion in turbulent flow: the importance of particle lift forces and particle/wall collision models, in *Numerical Methods for Multiphase Flows*, Vol. **91**, ASME, New York.
Sommerfeld, M. (1993), Reviews in numerical modeling of dispersed two phase flows, *Proceedings of 5th Int. Symp. on Refined Flow Modeling and Turbulence Measurements*, Paris.
Sommerfeld, M. (1995), The importance of inter-particle collisions in horizontal gas–solid channel flows, in "Gas–solid Flows", ASME FED 228.
Spalding, D.B. (1983), Chemical reactions in turbulent fluids, *Physico Chem. Hydrodynamics*, **4**, 323–336.
Squire, K.D. and Eaton, J.K. (1994), Effect of selective modification of turbulence on two equation models for particle laden turbulent flows, *ASME J., Fluids Eng.*, **116**, 778.
Stokes, G.G. (1851), On the effect of the internal friction of fluids on the motion of pendulums, *Trans. Cambridge Phil. Soc.*, **9**, 8.
Stover, R.L., Tobías, C.W. and Denn, M.M. (1997), Bubble coalescence dynamics, *AIChE J.*, **43**, 2385–2392.
Tchen, C.M. (1947), Mean value and correlation problems connected with the motion of small particles suspended in a turbulent fluid, PhD thesis, Delft University of Technology, The Netherlands.
Theologos, K.N., Nikou, I.D., Lygeros, A.I. and Markatos, N.C. (1997), Simulation and design of FCC riser-type reactors, *AIChE J.*, **43**, 486–494.
Thomson, D.J. (1987), Criteria for the selection of stochastic models of particle trajectories in turbulent flows, *J. Fluid Mech.*, **180**, 529–556.
Tsuji, Y., Morikawa, Y. and Shiomi, H. (1984), LDV measurement of two phase air solid flow in vertical pipe: *J. Fluid Mech.*, **139**, 417–434.
Wehrli, M.B., Borth, J., Drtina, P. and Lang, E. (1997), Industrial applications of CFD for mass transfer processes, *Speedup J.*, **10**, 19–26.
Westerterp, K.R., van Swaaij, W.P.M. and Beenackers, A.A.C.M. (1984), "Chemical Reactor Design and Operation", 2nd edition, John Wiley and Sons, New York.
Wijngaarden, van L. (1976), Hydrodynamic interaction between gas bubbles in liquid, *J. Fluid Mech.*, **77**, 27–44.
Xu, B.H. and Yu, A.B. (1997), Numerical simulation of gas solid flow in a fluidized bed by combining discrete particle method with computational fluid dynamics, *Chem. Eng. Sci.*, **52**, 2785.

APPENDIX 4.1. TIME SCALES FOR DISPERSED MULTIPHASE FLOWS (FROM PEIRANO AND LECKNER, 1998)

Eddy lifetime or the integral time scale of turbulence can be expressed in the framework of the k–ε model as

$$\tau_1' = \frac{C_D k_1}{\varepsilon_1} \tag{A4.1.1}$$

Subscript 1 indicates continuous phase and 2 indicates dispersed phase. C_D is a parameter of the standard k–ε model (0.09), k_1 is turbulent kinetic energy and ε_1 is turbulent energy dissipation rate. The eddy lifetime seen by dispersed phase particles will in general be different from that for continuous phase fluid particles due to the so-called crossing-trajectory effect (Csnady, 1963). This can be expressed in the form:

$$\tau_{12}' = \frac{\tau_1'}{\sqrt{\left(1 + C_\beta 3|U_r|^2/2k_1\right)}} \tag{A4.1.2}$$

where U_r is relative velocity and C_β is a constant which depends on the type of flow. The particle relaxation time, which represents entrainment of particles by the continuous phase, is defined by

$$\tau_{12}^{x} = \frac{4d_P\rho_2}{3\rho_1 C_{DP}|U_r|} \qquad \text{(A4.1.3)}$$

where C_{DP} is the average drag coefficient for a single particle in a suspension. In the frame of a kinetic theory, the particle–particle collision time can be written:

$$\tau_2^{c} = \frac{d_P}{24\alpha_2 g_0}\left(\frac{\pi}{\theta_s}\right)^{1/2} \qquad \text{(A4.1.4)}$$

where θ_s is the granular temperature and g_0 is a distribution function defined in Section 4.2.2. Particle response time is defined as

$$\tau_p = \frac{\rho_2 d_p^2}{18\mu_1} \qquad \text{(A4.1.5)}$$

APPENDIX 4.2. CORRELATIONS FOR DRAG COEFFICIENT

A4.2.1. Drag Coefficient for Single Particle

Reference	Correlation			
Morsi and Alexander (1972)	$C_{DS} = \frac{A}{\text{Re}_s} + \frac{B}{\text{Re}_s^2} + C \quad \because \quad \text{Re}_s = \frac{\rho_C d_p\lvert U_p - U_C\rvert}{\mu_C}$			
	Re_s	A	B	C
	0–0.1	24	0	0
	0.1–1	22.73	0.0903	3.69
	<10	29.2	−3.9	1.222
	<100	46.5	−116.7	0.6167
	<1000	98.3	−2778	0.3644
Molerus (1980)	$C_{DS} = \frac{24}{\text{Re}_s} + \frac{4}{\sqrt{\text{Re}_s}} + 0.4$			
Patel *et al.* (1993)	$C_{DS} = \frac{24}{\text{Re}_s}\left(1 + 0.15\,\text{Re}_s^{0.687}\right) \qquad \text{Re}_s < 1000$			
Richardson *et al.* (1971)	$C_{DS} = \frac{24}{\text{Re}_s} \qquad \text{Re}_s < 0.2$			
	$C_{DS} = \frac{24.0}{\text{Re}_s} + \frac{3.6}{\text{Re}_s^{0.313}} \qquad 0.2 < \text{Re}_s < 500$			
	$C_{DS} = \frac{4.0}{9.0} \qquad \text{Re}_s > 500$			
Ma and Ahmadi (1989)	$C_{DS} = \frac{24}{\text{Re}_s}\left(1 + 0.1\,\text{Re}_s^{0.75}\right)$			
Dalla Ville (1948)	$C_{DS} = \left(0.63 + \frac{4.8}{\sqrt{\text{Re}_s}}\right)^2$			

Morsi and Alexander's (MA) correlation represents the single-particle drag curve accurately. Ma and Ahmadi's correlation predicts values comparable with the MA correlation. Molerus' correlation deviates from the MA correlation at higher Reynolds numbers. Patel's correlation is found to give a better fit with the MA correlation than Richardson's correlation. Dalla Ville's correlation overpredicts values of drag coefficient compared to the MA correlation.

A4.2.2. Drag Coefficient for Multi-particle Systems

Reference	Correlation
Molerus (1980)	$C_{DM} = \frac{24}{Re}\left(1 + 0.347\left(\frac{r_o}{\delta} + \frac{1}{2}\left(\frac{r_o}{\delta}\right)^2\right)_{\zeta=0.9}\right) + \frac{4}{\sqrt{Re}} + 0.4 + 0.565\left(\frac{r_o}{\delta}\right)_{\zeta=0.9}$ $\frac{r_o}{\delta} = \frac{1}{(\zeta/(1-\alpha)^{1/3}) - 1.0} \quad \because \quad \zeta = \text{packing parameter}$ $C_{DM} = \frac{4}{3\alpha}\left[\frac{150(1-\alpha)}{\alpha Re} + 1.75\right] \quad \alpha < 0.8$
Ergun (1952)	$C_{DS} = \frac{24}{Re_s}\left[1 + 0.15\, Re_s^{0.687}\right] \quad Re_s < 1000$
Richardson and Zaki (1954)	$C_{DS} = 0.44 \quad Re_s > 1000$ $C_{DM} = C_{DS}\alpha^{-2.65} \quad \alpha > 0.8$
Ma and Ahmadi (1989)	$C_{DM} = C_{DS}\left[\frac{1}{(1-((1-\alpha)/\alpha_{Smax}))^{2.5\alpha_{Smax}}}\right]$ $C_{DS} = \frac{24}{Re_s}\left[1 + 0.1\, Re_s^{0.75}\right]$
Garside and Al-Dibouni (1977)	$A = \alpha^{4.14}$ $B = 0.8\alpha^{1.28} \quad \alpha \leqslant 0.85$ $B = \alpha^{2.65} \quad \alpha > 0.85$ $f = 0.5\left[A - 0.06\, Re + \sqrt{0.0036\, Re^2 + 0.12\, Re(2B - A) + A^2}\right]$ $C_{DM} = \frac{1}{f^2}\left(0.63 + \frac{4.8}{\sqrt{(Re/f)}}\right)^2$
Modified Richardson and Zaki equation by Garside and Al-Dibouni (1977)	$n = \frac{5.1 + 0.27\, Re_s^{0.9}}{1 + 0.1\, Re_s^{0.9}}$ $C_{DM} = \frac{C_{DS}}{\alpha^{2(n-1)}}$

α: volume fraction of dispersed phase.

The Ergun equation with the Richardson and Zaki correlation (ERZ) gives continuous variation of the drag coefficient over the relevant range of dispersed phase volume fractions. The modified Richardson and Zaki correlation (MRZ) was also found to give a similar continuous variation of drag coefficient. The predictions of Molerus's correlation were found to be very sensitive to the values of packing parameters at a continuous phase volume fraction of about 0.4. Either ERZ or MRZ correlations may be used to represent the influence of other particles when simulating dense gas–solid flows.

APPENDIX 4.3. INTERPHASE HEAT AND MASS TRANSFER CORRELATIONS

System	Correlation	Reference
Solid or fluid particle, Re ~ 1	Nu or $\mathrm{Sh} = 2 + \mathrm{Pe}/2 \quad \because \quad \mathrm{Pe} = \mathrm{Re}\,\mathrm{Pr}$	Rimmer (1968)
Solid or fluid particle, high Pe and low Re	Nu or $\mathrm{Sh} = 0.997\,\mathrm{Pe}^{1/3} \quad \because \quad \mathrm{Pe} = \mathrm{Re}\,\mathrm{Pr}$	Levich (1962)
Solid or fluid particle, low Pe and low Re	Nu or $\mathrm{Sh} = 0.997\,\mathrm{Pe}^{1/3} + 0.992$	Acrivos and Goddard (1965)
Solid or fluid particle, high Re	Nu or $\mathrm{Sh} = 2 + 0.6\,\mathrm{Re}^{1/2}\,\mathrm{Pr}^{1/3}$	Ranz and Marshall (1952)
Solid particles, low Re	Nu or $\mathrm{Sh} = (4 + 1.21\,\mathrm{Pe}^{2/3})^{1/2}$	Brian and Hales (1969)
Particles at all Pe	Nu or $\mathrm{Sh} = 1 + (1 + \mathrm{Pe})^{1/3}$	Clift *et al.* (1978)
Granular flows/dense flows	$\mathrm{Nu} = (7 - 10\alpha_c + 5\alpha_c^2)(1 + 0.7\,\mathrm{Re}^{0.2}\,\mathrm{Pr}^{1/3}) + (1.33 - 2.4\alpha_c + 1.2\alpha_c^2)\,\mathrm{Re}^{0.7}\,\mathrm{Pr}^{1/3}$	Gunn (1978)
Dense flows	Nu or $\mathrm{Sh} = \dfrac{2\xi + \left\{\dfrac{2\xi^2(1-\alpha_c)^{1/3}}{\left[1-(1-\alpha_c)^{1/3}\right]^2} - 2\right\}\tanh\xi}{\left[\dfrac{\xi}{1-(1-\alpha_c)^{1/3}} - \tanh\xi\right]}$ $\xi = 0.3\left[(1-\alpha_c)^{-1/3} - 1\right]\mathrm{Re}^{1/2}\,\mathrm{Sc}^{1/3}$	Nelson and Galloway (1975)

Dimensionless numbers appearing in these correlations are as follows:

Re = Particle Reynolds number = $(\rho_c d_p U_r/\mu_c)$

Pr = Prandtl number = $(\mu_c C_p/k_c)$

Pe = Peclet number = Re Pr or Re Sc

Sc = Schmidt number = $(\mu_c/\rho_c D)$

The first five correlations predict limiting values of the Sherwood or Nusselt number as 2 and are mainly valid for single-particle or very dilute flows. The last two correlations predict Nusselt and Sherwood numbers lower than 2 for dense flows and should be used to simulate dense granular flows.

5 REACTIVE FLOW PROCESSES

5.1. INTRODUCTION

Modeling and analysis of reactive flow processes is the most important task carried out by chemical reactor engineers. A brief introduction to the classical reaction engineering approach to this task is given in Chapter 1. The concepts of residence time distribution and mixedness have been used extensively in the past to gain an insight into the interaction of flow, mixing and chemical reactions. Classical analysis based on these concepts, treats the chemical reactions in a rigorous way but makes some drastic assumptions about the underlying fluid dynamics. When the characteristic time scale of chemical reactions is comparable to or lower than the characteristic time scale for mixing, effective reaction rate is a complex function of mixing (and fluid dynamics) and chemical kinetics. Several idealized models, the so-called micromixing models, have been developed to treat such situations (some of which are discussed later in this chapter). These micromixing models require information about local turbulent kinetic energy and energy dissipation rates. It is, therefore, necessary to develop fluid dynamics based models of reactive mixing to enable better understanding and control over reactive flow processes. In many practical situations, even when reaction time scales are not smaller than mixing time scales globally, local hot spots may make reaction time scales smaller than local mixing time scales. Detailed CFD-based models need to be developed to understand the formation of such local hot spots and their effect on reactive flow processes. Even for slow reactive processes, CFD-based models are needed to establish relationships between several hardware-related issues (location, orientation and design of feed nozzles, distributors, internals and so on) and reactor performance. This chapter discusses various issues concerned with modeling approaches to reactive flow processes.

In any reactive flow process, molecular diffusion, which brings molecules of different species together, is essential for chemical reactions to occur. Mixing or some form of interspecies contact is essential for mutual molecular diffusion. Reactive flow processes are therefore controlled by fluid mechanics, mixing, diffusion and chemical reactions. Any useful mathematical model of reactive flow processes should give emphasis to all contributions in proportion to the importance of their effects. The interaction of these processes may lead to different reactor performances for the same chemical reaction. The same reaction rate (kinetics) may be classified as 'slow' or 'fast' depending on the relative rates of reactions and mixing. In principle, it is possible to represent all details of the reactive flow processes by the governing equations discussed in Chapter 2. These governing equations may be solved to get all the information, from the largest macroscopic space scale to the point where the fluid assumption itself breaks down, provided all the necessary data and boundary conditions are available.

The real question is how, in practice, this information can be obtained from the governing equations considering the severe constraints imposed by finite computer memory, storage and processing speeds. Even in the case of slow reactions, solutions to reactive flow processes require special techniques because of the presence of non-linear reaction sources. When reactions are fast, obtaining accurate solutions of even laminar reactive flow processes is extremely difficult (Oran and Boris, 1982). The presence of turbulence complicates the task of modeling reactive flow processes by an order of magnitude. The existence of widely different and interacting scales makes the task of formulating governing equations much more difficult than with laminar flow processes. It is necessary to understand the different steps occurring in turbulent reactive flow processes in order to examine the possibility of developing models suited to specific classes of flow processes. Though such models may lack universal applicability, they will still be valuable tools in modeling particular classes of reactive flow processes. The presence of more than one phase further complicates the modeling of reactive flow processes. It is necessary to judiciously combine conventional reaction engineering models developed for multiphase reactors with rigorous CFD-based models to achieve the relevant reactor engineering objectives.

In this chapter, modeling turbulent reactive flow processes and multiphase reactive processes is discussed. First, the following section discusses general aspects of mixing and defines various characteristic time scales for turbulent reactive flow processes. Different approaches to modeling single-phase reactive processes are briefly reviewed. More emphasis is given to modeling reactive flow processes in the liquid phase than in the gas phase. RANS-based phenomenological models and probability density function based models to simulate single-phase flows are then discussed in detail. In Section 5.3, modeling multiphase reactive processes is briefly discussed. Applications of these models to simulate different industrial reactors are discussed in Part III and Part IV.

5.2. TURBULENT REACTIVE MIXING

Traditionally reactor engineers analyze the mixing of fluids in terms of the degree of segregation (Levenspiel, 1972), a measure of mixing on the molecular scale.

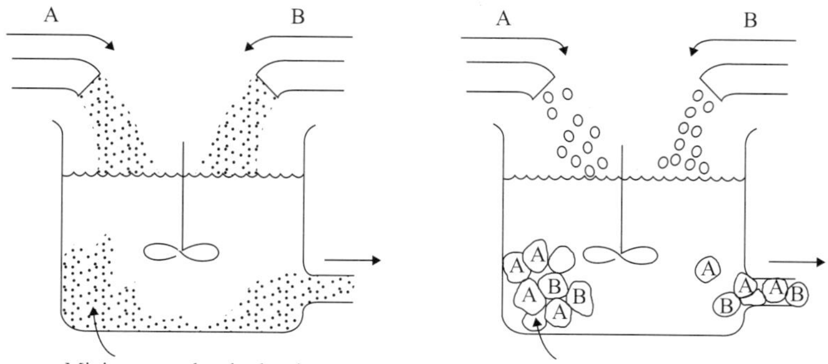

FIGURE 5.1 Macrofluid and microfluid Idealizations (from Levenspiel, 1972).

Two extremes of molecular mixing are traditionally known as microfluid and macrofluid. In microfluid, species are completely mixed on a molecular scale, while in macrofluid, there is no mixing on a molecular scale although the lumps of fluid are macroscopically well mixed. When miscible reactants are brought together to react in a reactor, the extent of mixing may control the reactor performance. Consider the case of a reactor carrying out reactions between two reactants A and B as shown in Fig. 5.1. Reactants A and B are introduced into the reactor in separate streams. Two extremes of microfluid and macrofluid may be considered. When reactants A and B are mixed on a molecular scale at a rate much faster than the reaction rate (microfluid), reaction will occur and the effective rate will be controlled by reaction kinetics. When reactants A and B are mixed macroscopically but are not mixed on a molecular scale (macrofluid), virtually no reaction can take place. Real systems will behave in an intermediate way, exhibiting A-rich and B-rich regions with partial segregation. In many fast reactions (compared to mixing) and high viscosity systems (such as polymerization reactions), the mixing process interacts with chemical reactions and may significantly influence the reactor performance (product distribution, product quality and so on). The traditional methods of finding the upper and lower limits on performance by employing the microfluid and macrofluid concepts are useful to guide the base-line design. Detailed fluid dynamics based modeling and simulations of interaction between mixing and chemical reactions may, however, lead to enhanced understanding and the capability to tailor the reactor performance. This chapter is restricted to the analysis of turbulent reactive mixing. Before discussing modeling approaches, it is useful to consider a physical picture of turbulent mixing and to estimate the relevant length and time scales to determine whether the reaction is 'fast' or 'slow'.

The basic concepts and physical picture of turbulence were discussed in Chapter 3. As discussed there, fluid motions of several scales co-exist in turbulent flows. Vortex stretching continuously forms small-scale fluid motions from large-scale motions. Kinetic energy is transferred to progressively smaller scales during this process. At the smallest scale, energy is irreversibly dissipated into heat at a rate ε, the turbulent energy dissipation rate. These smallest scales are called Kolmogorov scales and are defined as

$$\lambda_K = \left(\frac{\nu^3}{\varepsilon}\right)^{1/4} \qquad t_K = \left(\frac{\nu}{\varepsilon}\right)^{1/2} \tag{5.1}$$

where ν is kinematic viscosity (momentum diffusivity), λ_K is the length scale and t_K is the time scale. The strongly dissipative nature of fluid motions at these smallest scales indicates 'viscous mixing'. This formation of smaller scales constitutes the essence of mixing. Complete viscous mixing, however, does not ensure complete molecular mixing because in general, momentum diffusivity and molecular diffusivity are different. Molecular mixing is usually characterized by the Batchelor length scale, λ_B, which is the penetration depth of the scalar by diffusion in the Kolmogorov time scale, t_K and can be written:

$$\lambda_B = \frac{\lambda_K}{\sqrt{Sc}} \quad \because \quad Sc = \frac{\nu}{D} \tag{5.2}$$

where Sc is the Schmidt number and D is the molecular diffusion coefficient. For most gases, the Schmidt number is of the order of unity and therefore molecular mixing is as fast as viscous mixing. However, for most liquids, the Schmidt number is of the order 1000, which implies much slower molecular mixing. Typical energy and concentration spectra (and dissipation of turbulent kinetic energy and concentration fluctuations) for isotropic turbulence are shown in Fig. 5.2. The upper two curves are for turbulent kinetic energy and the lower two curves are for concentration fluctuations. It can be seen that the spectrum for concentration extends further to the right (towards scales smaller than Kolmogorov scales) than the energy spectrum (for systems with $\nu/D \gg 1$). For accurate simulation of mixing, it is necessary to resolve all the scales contributing to the dissipation of concentration fluctuations. This means that for simulations of reactive mixing in liquids, an even wider (than simulations of turbulent flows) range of length scales, encompassing inertial-convective, viscous-convective and viscous-diffusive sub-ranges, need to be modeled and resolved.

In order to gauge the relative importance and possible interaction between turbulence and chemical reactions, it is necessary to evaluate the various processes involved in reactive mixing. When a fluid element of different component (tracer) is added to the turbulent flow field, molecular mixing (and reaction, if possible) proceeds through several steps/mechanisms, some of which are listed below:

Step 1: convection by mean velocity
Step 2: turbulent dispersion by large eddies
Step 3: reduction of segregation length scale
Step 4: laminar stretching of small eddies
Step 5: molecular diffusion and chemical reaction

The fluid element of a tracer is transported within the solution domain by the mean flow field. During this process, turbulent fluctuating motions reduce the characteristic scales of 'lumps' of tracer (turbulent dispersion by large eddies). Generally, chemical engineers use the scale of segregation and intensity of segregation to characterize turbulent mixing (Danckwerts, 1953). The scale of segregation is a measure of the size of the unmixed lumps. Intensity of segregation is a measure of the difference in concentration between neighboring lumps of fluid. The lower the intensity of segregation the more the extent of molecular mixing. These two parameters are demonstrated qualitatively in Fig. 5.3 (for rigorous definitions, see Brodkey, 1975). Convection and turbulent dispersion by large eddies lead to macroscale mixing and do not cause any small-scale mixing. Fluid motions in the inertial sub-range reduce the characteristic

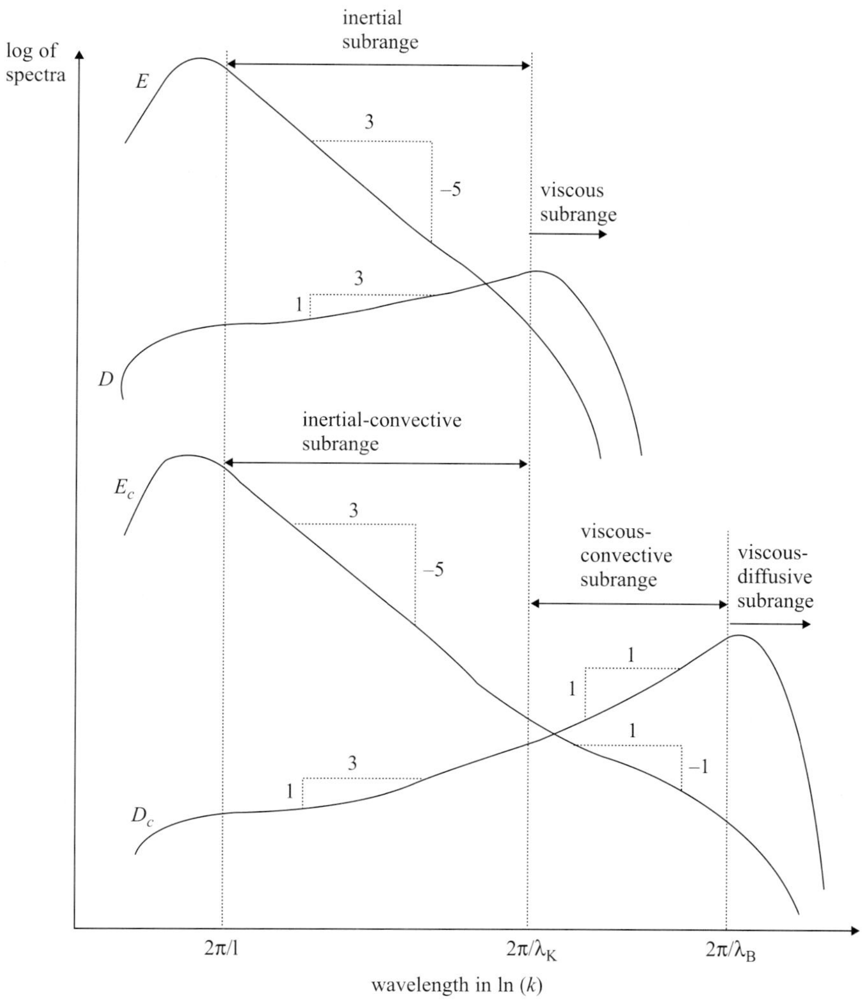

FIGURE 5.2 Energy and concentration spectra for isotropic turbulence (from Bakker, 1996).

scales of lumps of tracer via vortex stretching. This is step 3 mentioned above. Such a reduction in scale increases the interfacial area between segregated lumps of tracer fluid and the base fluid, which increases the rate of mixing by molecular diffusion. However, the increase in interfacial area resulting from inertial sub-range eddies may not be substantial. The mixing caused by this step is typically called 'meso-mixing'. Meso-mixing reduces the scale of mixing substantially but does not significantly affect the intensity of mixing. Engulfment and viscous stretching by Kolmogorov scale eddies lead to substantial increases in the interfacial area for molecular diffusion and therefore, contribute significantly to molecular mixing. A schematic representation of steps 3 and 4 is shown in Fig. 5.4. Inertial sub-range motions reduce the characteristic scale of mixing to the Kolmogorov length scale, λ_K. Viscous-convective motions (engulfment and stretching) create a large interfacial area for molecular diffusion and reduce the characteristic scales to Batchelor length scale, λ_B. The final step

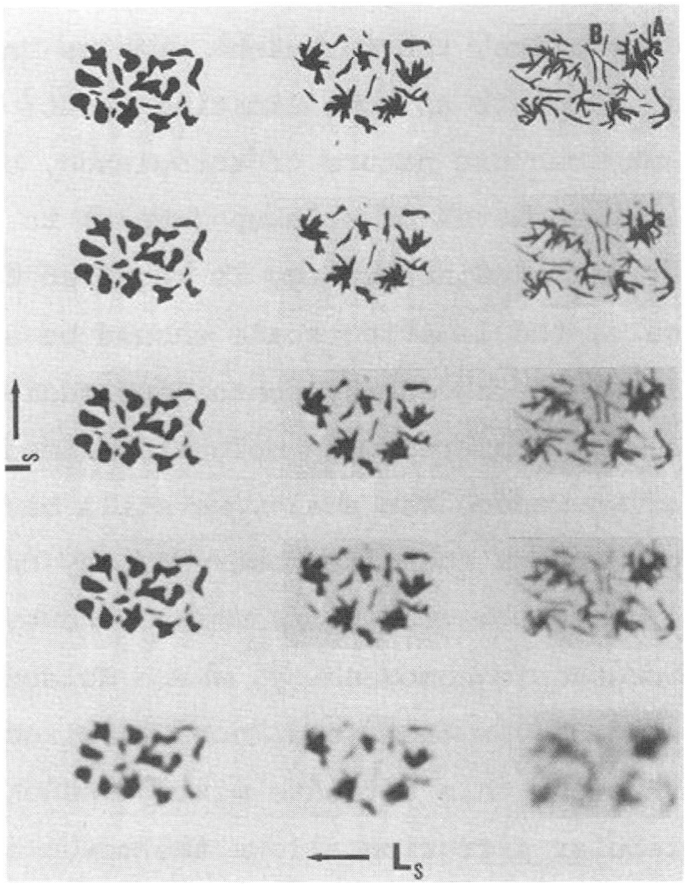

FIGURE 5.3 Scale and intensity of segregation (from Brodkey, 1975).

is a diffusion process through the interfacial area between layers of different fluids, accompanied by chemical reactions, if any. Molecular diffusion leads to complete mixing and dissipates concentration fluctuations.

In addition to an examination of length scales, it is useful to carry out quantitative examination of different relevant time scales of the mixing processes. Comparison of these time scales with the characteristic time scales of chemical reactions will be useful to determine the rate-controlling step in reactive flow processes.

The characteristic time scale for convection can be written:

$$\tau_c = \frac{L_R}{U_R} \quad \text{or} \quad \frac{V_R}{Q_R} \tag{5.3}$$

where L_R is the characteristic length scale and U_R the characteristic velocity scale of the reactor. The second term on the right-hand side is similar to the mean circulation time in the reactor, which is a ratio of reactor volume, V_R, and circulatory flow within the reactor, Q_R. The characteristic time for the turbulent dispersion may be estimated as the ratio of the square of the characteristic length scale of the reactor to the effective turbulent dispersion coefficient (Γ_D). Alternatively, it may be estimated as the ratio

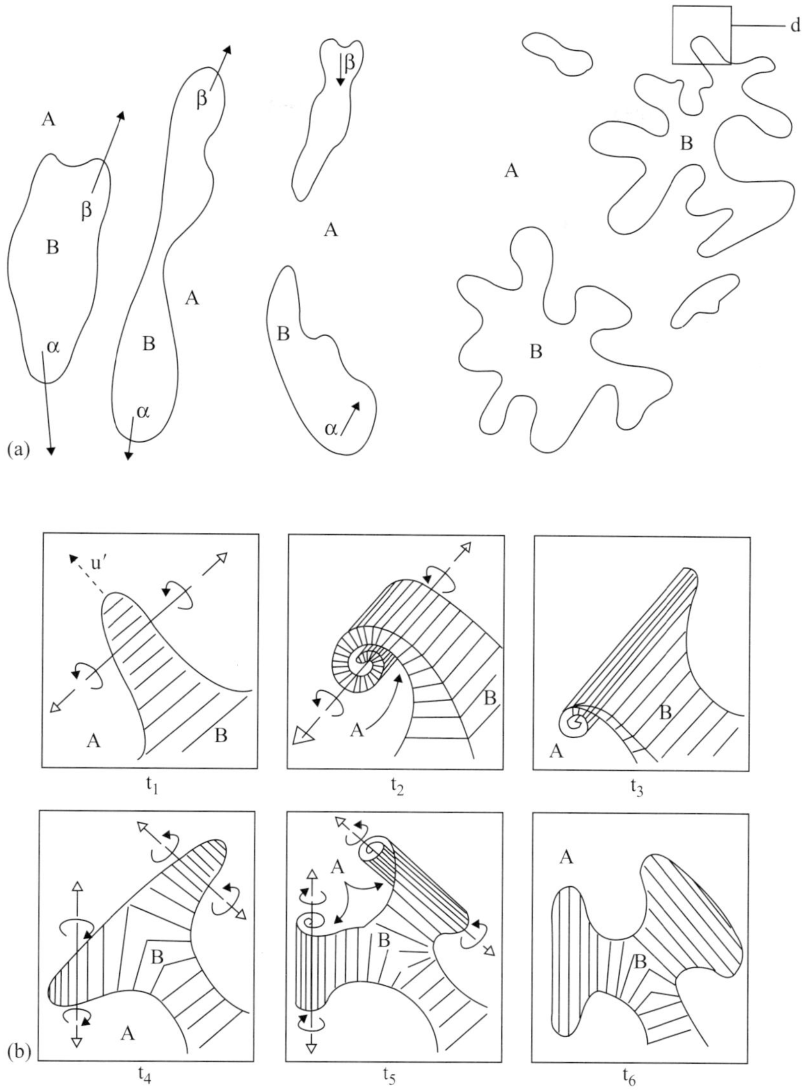

FIGURE 5.4 Schematic representation of small-scale mixing processes (from Baldyga and Bourne, 1984). (a) Reduction of length scale due to deformations within the inertial sub-range. (b) Creation of large interfacial area by vorticity acting on fluid elements of initial thickness of order λ_K.

of the characteristic length scale of the reactor to the square root of turbulent kinetic energy, k:

$$\tau_D = \frac{L_R^2}{\Gamma_D} \quad \text{or} \quad \frac{L_R}{\sqrt{k}} \tag{5.4}$$

An estimate of the effective turbulent dispersion coefficient for any reactor is generally difficult because of the spatial variation in the dispersion coefficient within the reactor. A first-level approximation may be based on average turbulence kinetic energy and turbulent energy dissipation rates. These two time scales representing convection and turbulent dispersion determine large-scale or macromixing in the reactor.

The last three steps control the small-scale or micromixing in the reactor. The characteristic time constant for the third step, that is for reduction in segregation scale (inertial-convective mixing), is (Corrsin, 1964; Baldyga, 1989)

$$t_{\mathrm{MS}} = \left(\frac{L_{\mathrm{s}}^2}{\varepsilon}\right)^{1/3} \tag{5.5}$$

where L_{s} is the segregation length scale and ε is the rate of dissipation of turbulent energy. The characteristic time for the engulfment step (t_{E}) can be estimated as (Baldyga and Bourne, 1989)

$$t_{\mathrm{E}} = 17.25\left(\frac{\nu}{\varepsilon}\right)^{1/2} \tag{5.6}$$

where ν is kinematic viscosity. This equation may be used for liquid systems with Schmidt number less than 4000. Alternatively, a modified form of Corrsin's equation can also be used (Pohoreki and Baldyga, 1993):

$$t_{\mathrm{E}} = 3.086\left(\frac{\nu}{\varepsilon}\right)^{1/2}(\ln \mathrm{Sc} - 1.27) \tag{5.7}$$

The diffusion time scale (t_{DS}) can be estimated as (Baldyga and Bourne, 1984)

$$t_{\mathrm{DS}} > \left(\frac{\nu}{\varepsilon}\right)^{1/2} \mathrm{arcsin}h\,(0.1\mathrm{Sc}) \tag{5.8}$$

where Sc is the Schmidt number, defined as the ratio of kinematic viscosity to molecular diffusivity.

These time scales of turbulent mixing processes need to be examined with reference to other important time scales of interest such as reaction time scale, average residence time and so on. While doing such an analysis, it may be easier to regroup these five steps into two categories: (1) macromixing processes, characterized by t_{macro} and (2) micromixing processes, characterized by t_{micro}. When one of the micromixing step is rate controlling, t_{micro} can be equated to the characteristic time scale of that particular micromixing step. It is also possible to define effective time scale when both step 3 and step 4 influence the micromixing process. This effective time scale can be expressed in the form (Ranade, 1993):

$$t_{\mathrm{eff}} = t_{\mathrm{MS}}\left\{1 + \frac{M-1}{M\left[e^{(M-1)t/t_{\mathrm{MS}}} - 1\right]}\right\} \tag{5.9}$$

where M is the ratio of t_{MS} and t_{E}. This effective time scale reduces to t_{E} for small values of time and to t_{MS} for small values of t_{E}. When there is an interaction between macromixing and micromixing processes, it is not possible to formulate a simple expression for characteristic time scale. The time scales discussed above are used to classify different reactive mixing models and to examine the available modeling approaches in the following section.

5.3. MODELING APPROACHES

Several factors determine the extent of influence of turbulence on effective rates of chemical reactions, including:

- whether reactants are premixed or non-premixed;
- rate of chemical reactions relative to the rate of scalar mixing;
- turbulence length scales relative to size of a reaction zone;
- multiple reactions/order of reactions.

Chemical reactions may also affect turbulence by releasing energy and modifying the fluid properties locally. The influence can be quite significant in variable density flows (e.g. combustion). Nevertheless, in many computational models of constant density reactive flow processes, it is implicitly assumed that chemical reactions do not affect scalar mixing rates.

Available reactor models can be classified according to their assumptions about the relative magnitudes of characteristic time scales of mixing (micromixing and macromixing) and reactive flow process (chemical reaction time scale, t_{kin} or residence time, τ). The relationship between suitability of different models and extent of macro- and micromixing is shown schematically in Fig. 5.5. When both, macro- and micromixing time scales are much smaller than the process time scale (high macro- and micromixing), ideal reactor models can safely be used (top right case in Fig. 5.5). When the rate of macromixing is slow but that of local micromixing is fast, the relevant mixing scale is intermediate between a micromixing scale and a reactor scale. Although reactants are locally mixed on a molecular scale, there is macroscopic segregation (top left case in Fig. 5.5). Cell balance models (Patterson, 1985; Middleton *et al.*, 1986) can be used to simulate such reactive flow processes. In these models, no special modeling efforts are generally necessary except for the special treatment demanded by extra non-linearity (due to the reaction source) present in the reactive systems. The governing equations discussed in Chapter 2 can be used to simulate the behavior of such systems.

When local micromixing is slow compared to the reaction time scale and the macromixing time scale is smaller than the process time scale, the performance of a reactive flow process is controlled only by the micromixing. In such cases, though there is no macroscopic segregation, reactants are not mixed on a molecular scale (see the right bottom case of Fig. 5.5). Several micromixing models have been developed to simulate such reactive flow processes. Some of the widely used models are:

- 'Engulfment Deformation Diffusion (EDD)' model of Baldyga and Bourne (1984).
- 'Interaction by Exchange with the Mean (IEM)' model of David and Villermaux (1987).
- 'Engulfment (E)' model of Baldyga and Bourne (1989).

These models are not discussed here and the cited papers may be referred to for details of model equations. When macroscale and microscale segregation exist together (bottom left case of Fig. 5.5), none of the cited models are adequate. For such systems, it is necessary to include detailed interaction of fluid mechanics, mixing and reactions in the mathematical model. Various modeling approaches to simulate reactive flow processes with macro- and microscale segregation are discussed briefly below.

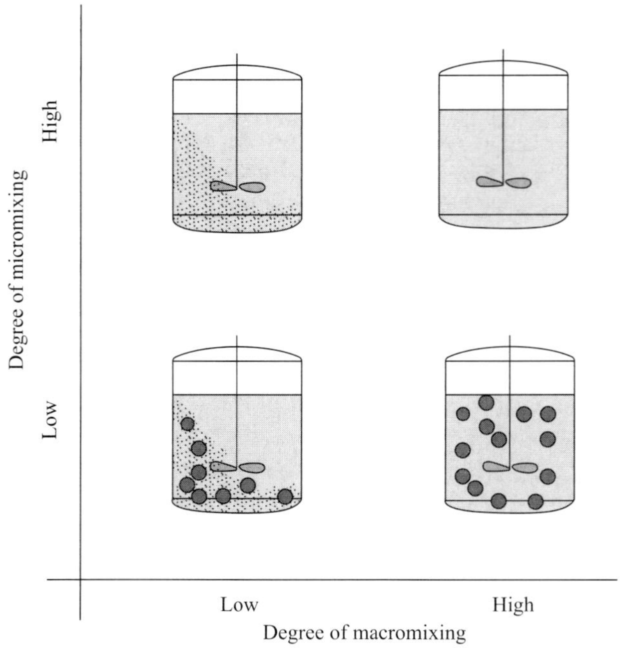

FIGURE 5.5 Extent of macromixing and micromixing and suitability of reactor models.

5.3.1. Direct Numerical Simulations (DNS)

As mentioned in Chapter 3, DNS involves full numerical simulation of the governing equations without approximations. Even in laminar reactive flow processes, space and time scales of relevant processes may range over many orders of magnitude. Such a wide range of time scales makes the governing equations quite 'stiff'. (In general, governing equations describing a flow process are termed 'stiff' if the process being modeled has a characteristic time of variation shorter than the time step one can afford.) Chemical reactions may cause very steep gradients locally. Resolving such gradients and handling the strongly coupled, non-linear governing equations may pose challenges even in laminar flow processes. Turbulence, which occurs on intermediate spatial scales, poses further problems in solving the governing equations. Despite the 'stiffness' of governing equations, DNS attempts to simulate reactive flow processes by resolving all the relevant space and time scales. Such rigorous DNS studies (see for example, Chakrabarti and Hill, 1997) have pointed out several characteristic features of reactive flow processes, such as:

(1) persistent tendency to initially segregate, with relatively thin reaction zones;
(2) scalar dissipation zone tracks well with the reaction zone, however, product concentration does not;
(3) reaction rate is highest in regions of greatest compressive strain rates;
(4) scalar variance decay is dominated by molecular dissipation and not by reaction.

Such an insight is useful for understanding the interaction of turbulence and chemical reactions and the influence of such interactions on effective rate and selectivity of chemical reactions. However, DNS may be carried out only for relatively simple geometry with moderate Reynolds number. Even then, huge computational resources are required. Some idea of the computational requirements imposed by the resolution demanded by DNS may be obtained by examining relevant dimensionless numbers. For direct simulations of reactive flow processes, in addition to resolving all the flow length scales from the integral to the Kolmogorov scale, scalar fields must be resolved up to Batchelor's scale. This means that the maximum wave number for the scalar field varies as:

$$k_{\max} \propto \mathrm{Sc}^{3/2}\mathrm{Re}^{3/4} \tag{5.10}$$

To make the matters worse, chemical reactions steepen scalar gradients and often, larger values of $k_{\max}$ need to be used. Since ($k_{\max} \times k_{\max} \times k_{\max}$) values must be stored in the computer memory for each field for each time step, application of DNS to reactive flow processes is limited to moderate Reynolds numbers and Schmidt numbers near unity. The Damkohler number (ratio of characteristic time scales of small-scale mixing and chemical reaction, see Chapter 2) is generally limited to values less than 30 to 50. Even if huge computational resources are available, the DNS approach is difficult to apply to the realistic geometry of industrial chemical reactors.

Moreover, practical reactive flow processes usually involve many interacting chemical species. These interactions are represented by many sets of coupled equations, which must be solved simultaneously. Before developing a model representing the entire reactive system, each individual process/chemical reaction must be understood and modeled separately. These sub-models can then be incorporated into the overall model, either directly or using a phenomenology. For reactive flow processes relevant to reactor engineers, it is often the case that various sub-models are not known adequately (for example, rates of chemical reactions or thermo-chemical data). It must be noted that, although DNS can provide valuable information about the interactions of flow processes and chemical reactions, it requires huge computational resources. When the accuracy of the required sub-models to carry out reactive flow simulations is inadequate, spending of huge computational resources on DNS is seldom justified. DNS, therefore, is not used to simulate complex industrial reactive flow processes. DNS, however, is an excellent tool for studying the fundamentals of turbulent reactive flow processes and for verifying other closure and phenomenological models of reactive flow processes.

5.3.2. Large Eddy Simulation (LES)

As discussed in Chapter 3, with LES, the smallest scale to be resolved is chosen to lie in the inertial sub-range of the energy spectrum, which means the so-called sub-grid scale (SGS) wave numbers are not resolved. As LES can capture transient large-scale flow structures, it has the potential to accurately predict time-dependent macromixing phenomena in the reactors. However, unlike DNS, a SGS model representing interaction of turbulence and chemical reactions will be required in order to predict the effect of operating parameters on say product yields in chemical reactor simulations. These SGS models attempt to represent an inherent loss of SGS information, such as the rate of molecular diffusion, in an LES framework. Use of such SGS models makes the LES approach much less computationally intensive than the DNS approach. DNS studies may be used to develop a suitable SGS model, which may, in turn, be used with an LES model to simulate complex reactive flow processes. The SGS models may also be developed based on phenomenological, micromixing models. The LES approach, therefore, may serve as a link between the more simplified moment closure/phenomenological models and DNS models. The overall computational demands of combining SGS models with LES simulations of complex industrial reactors may prove to be beyond the typical resources available to reactor engineers. It may be more effective to use Reynolds-averaged or phenomenological models in such cases.

5.3.3. RANS-based Models

By far, the most widely employed models for reactive flow processes are based on Reynolds-averaged Navier Stokes (RANS) equations. As discussed earlier in Chapter 3, Reynolds averaging decomposes the instantaneous value of any variable into a mean and fluctuating component. In addition to the closure equations described in Chapter 3, for reactive processes, closure of the time-averaged scalar field equations requires models for: (1) scalar flux, (2) scalar variance, (3) dissipation of scalar variance, and (4) reaction rate. Details of these equations are described in the following section. Broadly, any closure approach can be classified either as a phenomenological, non-PDF (probability density function) or as a PDF-based approach. These are also discussed in detail in the following section.

Apart from these three main approaches (DNS, LES and RANS), several attempts have been made to simulate reactive flow processes by using specialized micromixing models. These micromixing models are phenomenological and require empirical information to determine values of essential parameters (David and Villermaux, 1987; Ranade and Bourne, 1991). A typical model follows a lump of fluid in a Lagrangian frame that mixes with its environment following predetermined rules. Since the motion of a fluid element is tracked in a Lagrangian frame, chemical reactions occurring within the fluid element are treated without modeling. However, these micromixing models cannot be used as stand-alone models to simulate general reactive flow processes for the following reasons:

(1) these models require knowledge of mean velocity and turbulence fields;
(2) coupling between the micromixing time scale (see Section 5.1.1) and turbulence time scales is ambiguous; and
(3) extension to complex, inhomogeneous flows, where the environment contains partially reacted fluids, is difficult.

It is possible to eliminate some of these disadvantages of micromixing models by judiciously developing a composite modeling approach based on RANS and these micromixing models. Some such attempts are also discussed in the following section.

5.4. RANS-BASED MODELS OF REACTIVE FLOW PROCESSES

Reynolds-averaged equations for momentum transport, are already discussed in Chapter 3. For modeling reactive flow processes, in addition to the solution of overall mass conservation equation described in Chapter 3, it is necessary to solve conservation equations for individual species. Following the practices of Reynolds averaging, an instantaneous concentration of species k, C_k, can be written as the sum of time-averaged species concentration $\overline{C}_k$ and a fluctuation around the time average, C'_k. The time averaged conservation equation for species k can therefore be written:

$$\frac{\partial}{\partial t}\left(\rho \overline{C}_k\right) + \nabla \cdot \left(\rho \overline{U C_k} + \rho \overline{u' C'_k}\right) = \nabla \cdot \left(\overline{j_k}\right) + \overline{S}_k \qquad (5.11)$$

Note that unlike conventional molar units, concentration of species in the above equation is written in terms of mass fractions ($C_k = m_k$). Similar to the momentum equations discussed in Chapter 3, time averaging introduces unknown terms in the averaged equations. It is necessary to close the equation by modeling these unknown terms representing the turbulent flux of component k and the mean reaction rate. The scalar flux is dominated by the transport due to velocity fluctuations in the inertial sub-range of the energy spectrum. It is, therefore, primarily a term related to an integral scale of turbulence and is independent of molecular diffusivity. The gradient diffusion model is often employed to relate the scalar flux to the mean field:

$$\overline{u' C'_k} = \frac{\nu_T}{\sigma_{Tk}} \nabla \overline{C}_k \qquad (5.12)$$

where ν_T is turbulent momentum diffusivity and σ_{Tk} is turbulent Schmidt number for component k. Although the gradient diffusion assumption may fail in some situations, it is typically employed to carry out engineering simulations of complex reactive flow processes.

The most difficult term to close in Eq. (5.11) is the reaction rate term. Reaction rates are seldom formulated by considering all the elementary reactions. More often than not, the reactive system is represented by a lumped mechanism, considering only a few species. The case of m components participating in n independent chemical reactions is usually represented by two two-dimensional matrices ($m \times n$) of stoichiometric coefficients and order of reactions and two one-dimensional vectors (n) of frequency factors and activation energy. n chemical reactions are written:

$$\sum_{r=1}^{n} \sum_{k=1}^{m} z_{rk} C_k = 0 \qquad (5.13)$$

Stoichiometric coefficients (z_{rk}) are generally considered positive for products and negative for reactants. Each chemical reaction is associated with its kinetics representing dependence of net rate of reaction on concentrations of participating species and temperature. Dependence on concentrations of participating species is represented by order of reaction, 'o'. The rate is represented by two parameters, frequency factor, k_0, and activation energy, ΔE (see textbooks such as Levenspiel, 1972 for more discussion on these two parameters). The net rate of formation or consumption of component k due to reaction n is usually written:

$$R_{kn} = -z_{kn} k_{0n} e^{(-\Delta E_n / R'T)} \prod_{l=1}^{l=m} C_l^{o_{ln}} \qquad (5.14)$$

where z_{kn} is molar stoichiometric coefficient for species k in reaction n. k_{0n} and ΔE_n are frequency factor (pre-exponential factor) and activation energy for reaction n, respectively. R' is the universal gas constant. The product is taken over all participating reactants with o_{ln} is an order of reaction n with respect to reactant l. The net reaction source term for species k is calculated as a sum of the reaction sources over the n chemical reactions:

$$S_k = R_k = \sum_n R_{kn} \tag{5.15}$$

For any industrial reacting system, the relevant parameters appearing in the rate expression (Eq. (5.14)) need to be obtained by carrying out experiments under controlled conditions. It is necessary to ensure that physical processes do not influence the observed rates of chemical reactions. This is especially difficult when chemical reactions are fast. It may sometimes be necessary to employ sophisticated mathematical models to extract the relevant kinetic information from the experimental data. Some references covering the aspects of experimental determination of chemical kinetics are cited in Chapter 1. It must be noted here that in the above development, the intrinsic rate of all chemical reactions is assumed to follow a power law type model. However, in many cases, different types of kinetic model need to be used (for examples of different types of kinetic model, see Levenspiel, 1972; Froment and Bischoff, 1984). It is not possible to represent all the known kinetic forms in a single format. The methods discussed here can be extended to any type of kinetic model.

When chemical reactions are slow (with respect to mixing) it is not necessary to employ additional models to close the reaction source terms. For slow reactions (Da $\ll$ 1), turbulent mixing will be complete before the reaction can take place. The contributions of fluctuating concentrations may be neglected. Therefore, the time-averaged reaction source term can be related to the time-averaged temperature and species concentrations:

$$\overline{R_{kn}} = -z_{kn}k_{0n}e^{(-\Delta E_n/R'\overline{T})}\prod_l \overline{C_l^{o_{ln}}} \tag{5.16}$$

For fast and intermediate reactions, the time-averaged reaction source term will contain some additional terms. These additional terms need to be modeled to close the set of equations. For example, consider the case of a single second-order reaction with instantaneous rate given by

$$R = k_0 e^{-\Delta E/R'T} C_1 C_2 \tag{5.17}$$

The non-linearity in terms of concentrations and exponential factor containing temperature, make the task of closing the reaction source term quite difficult. Even for an isothermal system, the time-averaged reaction source term will contain a new term, the time average of the product of fluctuating concentrations ('c') of component 1 and component 2:

$$\overline{R} = k_0 e^{-\Delta E/R'\overline{T}}\left(\overline{C_1}\,\overline{C_2} + \overline{c_1 c_2}\right) \tag{5.18}$$

Closure models for terms like the second term in the bracket of the right-hand side are vital to the modeling of turbulent reactive flow processes. It must be noted that as the chemistry becomes more complicated, several such terms will appear, which will make the task of modeling more difficult. Various methods have been used to develop such closure models. These methods are classified into two groups, namely conventional closure models with or without using probability distribution functions

(PDF) and phenomenological models, which are not closure methods in the accepted sense.

5.4.1. Closure Models/PDF-based Models

If the chemical reactions are very fast compared to the mixing rate, it may be assumed that any mixed reactants are immediately reacted. No rate expression is therefore necessary. The simplest model to represent such cases is called the 'eddy break up (EBU) model' (Spalding, 1970; Magnussen and Hjertager, 1976). In the EBU model, the effective rate of chemical reactions is equated to the smaller of rate calculated based on kinetic model and that based on the eddy break-up rate. The eddy break-up rate is defined as the inverse of a characteristic time scale k/ε. Therefore, for fast reactions, the rate of consumption or formation is proportional to the product of density, mass fraction and the eddy break-up rate (ε/k). The model is useful for the prediction of premixed and partially premixed fast reactive flows. EBU, however, was originally developed for single-step chemical reactions. Its extension to multiple step reactive systems should be made with caution.

For complex chemistry, in many cases, a 'conserved scalar' or a 'mixture fraction' approach can be used, in which a single conserved scalar (mixture fraction) is solved instead of transport equations for individual species. The reacting system is treated using either chemical equilibrium calculations or by assuming infinitely fast reactions (mixed-is-reacted approach). The mixture fraction approach is applicable to non-premixed situations and is specifically developed to simulate turbulent diffusion flames containing one fuel and one oxidant. Such situations are illustrated in Fig. 5.6. The basis for the mixture fraction approach is that individual conservation equations for fuel and oxidant can be combined to eliminate reaction rate terms (see Toor, 1975 for more details). Such a combined equation can be simplified by defining a mixture

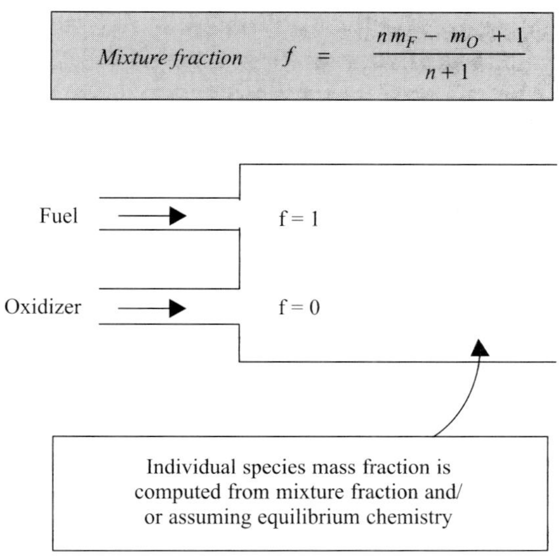

FIGURE 5.6 Mixture fraction approach.

fraction, f:

$$f = \frac{nm_F - m_O + 1}{n+1} \tag{5.19}$$

where m_F and m_O are mass fractions of fuel and oxidant, respectively and n is the number of moles of oxidizer required to burn one mole of fuel. Since the conservation equation of mixture fraction, f does not contain reaction terms the time-averaged equation can be readily obtained as

$$\frac{\partial}{\partial t}\left(\rho\bar{f}\right) + \frac{\partial}{\partial x_i}\left(\rho U_i\bar{f}\right) = \frac{\partial}{\partial x_i}\left(\frac{\mu_T}{\sigma_T}\frac{\partial \bar{f}}{\partial x_i}\right) \tag{5.20}$$

The time-averaged mixture fraction can be related to time-averaged values of local mass fractions of fuel and oxidant by using the time-averaged form of Eq. (5.19). It can be seen that a knowledge of time-averaged mixture fraction is not sufficient to obtain values of time-averaged fuel and oxidant mass fractions (one equation and two unknowns). In addition to average mixture fraction, if the variance of the mixture fraction is known, it is possible to obtain values of individual mass fractions of fuel and oxidant (see Toor, 1975; Jones and Whitelaw, 1982). The variance of mixture fraction can be obtained by solving its transport equation:

$$\frac{\partial}{\partial t}\left(\rho\overline{f'^2}\right) + \frac{\partial}{\partial x_i}\left(\rho U_i\overline{f'^2}\right) = \frac{\partial}{\partial x_i}\left(\frac{\mu_T}{\sigma_T}\frac{\partial \overline{f'^2}}{\partial x_i}\right) - 2\,\overline{u'f'}\frac{\partial \bar{f}}{\partial x_i} - 2D\overline{\left(\frac{\partial f'}{\partial x_i}\right)^2} \tag{5.21}$$

This equation contains three new terms, namely flux of scalar variance, production of variance and dissipation of scalar variance, which require further modeling to close the equation. The flux terms are usually closed by invoking the gradient diffusion model (with turbulent Schmidt number, σ_T, of about 0.7). This modeled form is already incorporated in Eq. (5.21). The variance production term is modeled by invoking an analogy with turbulence energy production (Spalding, 1971):

$$2\overline{u'f'}\frac{\partial \bar{f}}{\partial x_i} = -C_{g1}\upsilon_T\left(\frac{\partial \bar{f}}{\partial x_i}\right)^2 \tag{5.22}$$

where C_{g1} has a value of approximately 3. Spalding (1971) modeled the dissipation of variance as

$$2D\overline{\left(\frac{\partial f'}{\partial x_i}\right)^2} = C_{g2}\frac{\varepsilon}{k}\overline{f'^2} \tag{5.23}$$

where C_{g2} is about 0.2. Corrsin (1964) modeled the dissipation as a function of a scalar length scale and the rate of turbulence energy dissipation in isotropic turbulence:

$$2D\overline{\left(\frac{\partial f'}{\partial x_i}\right)^2} = \frac{2\overline{f'^2}}{4\left(L_s^2/\varepsilon\right)^{1/3} + (\nu/\varepsilon)^{1/2}\ln \mathrm{Sc}} \tag{5.24}$$

The scalar length scale, L_s, is assumed to be equal to $k^{3/2}/\varepsilon$ in the above expression. For systems with low values of Schmidt number, Corrsin's model reduces to that of Spalding, albeit with higher coefficient (0.5). Corrsin's model is found to be useful even for shear flow turbulence (Patterson, 1985). Detailed models of the variance dissipation rate are difficult to formulate in a general manner due to the large range of time/length scales involved. Fox (1995) proposed an alternative multiscale model. Most of the published models, however, use Eq. (5.23) to model the dissipation rate of scalar variance. Knowledge of mean mixture fraction and its variance is sufficient to calculate local values of fuel and oxidant mass fractions (Toor, 1975).

An alternative way of relating concentrations (mass fractions) of individual species to f is the assumption of chemical equilibrium. An algorithm based on minimization of Gibbs free energy to compute mole fractions of individual species from f has been discussed by Kuo (1986). The equilibrium model is useful for predicting the formation of intermediate species. If such knowledge of intermediate species is not needed, the much simpler approximation of 'mixed-is-burnt' can be used to relate individual species concentrations with f. In order to calculate the time-averaged values of species concentrations the probability density function (PDF) approach is used.

The probability density function, written as $p(f)$, describes the fraction of time that the fluctuating variable f takes on a value between f and $f + \Delta f$. The concept is illustrated in Fig. 5.7. The fluctuating values of f are shown on the right side while $p(f)$ is shown on the left side. The shape of the PDF depends on the nature of the turbulent fluctuations of f. Several different mathematical functions have been proposed to express the PDF. In presumed PDF methods, these different mathematical functions, such as clipped normal distribution, spiked distribution, double delta function and beta distribution, are assumed to represent the fluctuations in reactive mixing. The latter two are among the more popular distributions and are shown in Fig. 5.8. The double delta function is most readily computed, while the beta function is considered to be a better representation of experimentally observed PDF. The shape of these functions depends solely on the mean mixture fraction and its variance. The beta function is given as

$$p(f) = \frac{f^{\alpha-1}(1-\alpha)^{\beta-1}}{\int f^{\alpha-1}(1-\alpha)^{\beta-1}\,df} \tag{5.25}$$

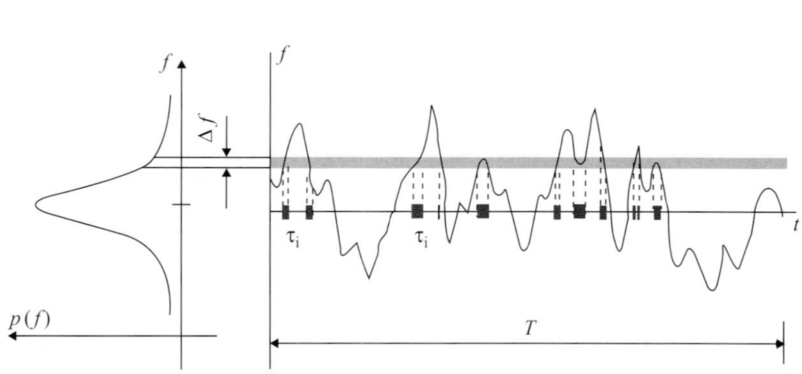

FIGURE 5.7 Graphical description of probability density function (PDF).

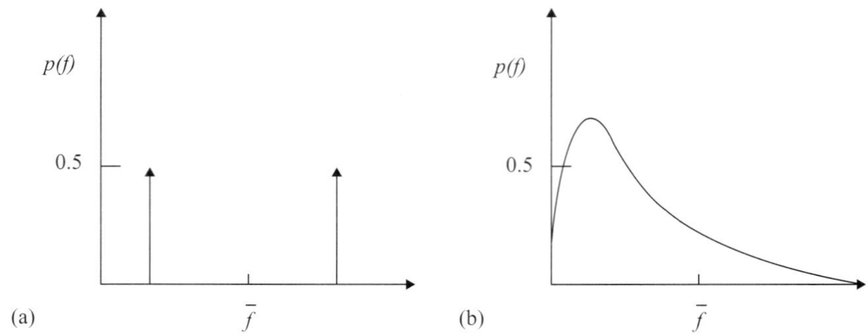

FIGURE 5.8 Shapes of commonly used probability density function. (a) Double delta function. (b) Beta function.

where α and β are given by:

$$\alpha = \bar{f}\left[\frac{\bar{f}\left(1-\bar{f}\right)}{\overline{f'^2}} - 1\right] \tag{5.26}$$

$$\beta = \left(1-\bar{f}\right)\left[\frac{\bar{f}\left(1-\bar{f}\right)}{\overline{f'^2}} - 1\right] \tag{5.27}$$

The time-averaged values of scalar variables, $\bar{\phi}_k$ (species mole fractions and temperature) is calculated as:

$$\overline{\phi_k} = \int_0^1 p(f)\phi_k(f)\,df \tag{5.28}$$

Thus, PDF and time-averaged values of individual species can be calculated if the mean values of mixture fraction (f) and mixture fraction variance ($\overline{f'^2}$) are known.

In several closure models, the covariance of two initially unmixed streams is related to the variance of a non-reactive scalar (Dutta and Tarbell, 1989). Many investigators have attempted to use the concept of probability density function (PDF) to evaluate higher order correlation appearing in time-averaged reaction source terms. The difficulties associated with the chemical reaction terms are thus shifted to computing the PDF of an inert scalar. The presumed PDF methods discussed above, assume a form for the PDF rather than computing it. From a computational standpoint, presumed PDF methods are straightforward extensions of moment closure methods. These methods also have been extended for non-adiabatic flow processes. In non-adiabatic processes, the local thermo-chemical state is not only related to mixture fraction but also to enthalpy. It is then necessary to employ a joint probability density function for mixture fraction and enthalpy. The presumed PDF methods have been widely employed in simulations of non-premixed combustion systems, and are mainstays of the engineering simulations of reactive flow processes (computational aspects of PDF-based models are discussed in Chapter 7). However, when there is more than one reaction involving finite-rate chemical reactions, the application of moment closure or presumed PDF methods becomes increasingly unreliable. These methods are also not suitable for modeling reactive processes with multiple feed points. Several other inherent limitations of these methods are discussed in detail by Fox (1996).

One of the ways to overcome the difficulties associated with these methods is to use full PDF methods. These methods obtain the PDF by solving a balance equation for the one-point, joint velocity composition PDF wherein the chemical reaction terms are in closed form (Pope, 1981). Unlike presumed PDF methods, full PDF methods do not require *a priori* knowledge of the joint composition PDF, and the effect of chemical reactions is treated exactly. The one-point, joint velocity composition PDF or the one-point joint composition PDF does not contain information about fluctuations in the velocity and composition gradients (two-point information). Therefore, appropriate models are necessary to represent these terms and viscous and scalar dissipation in the joint PDF. It is possible to formulate a PDF approach using either a Lagrangian or Eulerian framework. Details of full PDF modeling are discussed by Pope (1985), Tsai and Fox (1995) and Fox (1996) among others, and will not be discussed here. The Lagrangian full PDF methods provide a link with phenomenological micromixing models (Fox, 1998). These phenomenological models may offer a computationally less demanding alternative to the full PDF methods and may adequately represent liquid phase reacting flows. These non-PDF closure approaches are discussed in the following section.

5.4.2. Phenomenological (non-PDF) Models

A number of simple, non-distributed models of reactive mixing have been developed. The engulfment model (E) of Baldyga and Bourne (1989) and the interaction by exchange with the mean (IEM) model of David and Villermaux (1975) are two examples of many such attempts. Non-distributed models (which mostly use a Lagrangian framework to describe local phenomena occurring in discrete fluid lumps) have been used successfully to simulate the interaction of micromixing and chemical reactions. None of these models, however, can account for the effects of bulk circulation, large-scale dispersion and local mixing that lead to spatial distribution of segregation, conversion and yield in the reactor. These models cannot, therefore, be used to simulate any general, three-dimensional reactive flow processes. It is necessary to develop an appropriate framework, which combines the advantages offered by these phenomenological models with the potential of using them in a general Eulerian modeling framework. Some of these attempts are discussed here.

(a) ESCIMO model. The acronym stands for the main constituent concepts of the approach, namely engulfment, stretching, coherence, inter-diffusion and moving observer (Spalding, 1978). In this model, mixing and chemical reactions occurring in small-scale coherent 'folds' are considered. The folds are formed by the engulfment of one fluid by another, as a consequence of 'roll up' of vortex sheets. The first part of the ESCIMO approach involves the solution of equations describing mixing and chemical reactions within these coherent 'folds' (biographical part). The second part (demographic part) involves determination of the composition of the population of these 'folds', within the reactor. With this approach, the mixing, molecular diffusion and chemical reactions occurring within each fold can be modeled rigorously, which is similar to any non-distributed, Lagrangian (moving observer) micromixing model. The second part poses significant difficulties because it requires representing three-dimensional reactive flow processes. It requires repeated solutions of transport equations defining the probability of finding a fold of any specific group at the specific location (Spalding, 1983). This restricts the applicability of the ESCIMO approach to simple flow processes, such as a well-stirred reactor. Ma *et al.* (1982) proposed the concept of 'limited-migration' to address this problem partially. Although the approach shows a promising way of combining Lagrangian and Eulerian viewpoints to simulate reactive flow processes, applications of this approach are rather restricted and not sufficiently validated by comparison with experimental data.

(b) Flamelet models. In this approach, the complex chemistry calculations are decoupled from the turbulent flow description by introducing the concept of coherent 'flamelet'. Multi-component transport and chemical reactions can be modeled rigorously for the flamelet. The results of local flamelet analysis can then be incorporated in the overall calculation of the turbulent flow field (Libby and Williams, 1980; Liew *et al.*, 1984; Darabiha *et al.*, 1989). For practical applications, a flamelet library (a database) is constructed to provide the required specific information, such as the consumption rates per unit flamelet area. The mean reaction rate sources required for the calculation of mean flow and composition fields are computed by taking the product of rate per flamelet area and flamelet area per unit volume. The latter quantity is obtained by solving its transport equation, which requires further modeling effort (Darabiha *et al.*, 1989). In general, flamelet models are applicable to large Damkohler number systems (fast reactions) in which the typical turbulent scale is larger than the flame thickness. These models are therefore relevant to simulating IC engines and continuous flow combustors (at least for part of their operation). The flamelet approach has not been used to simulate liquid phase flow processes with fast reactions, for which multi-environment models may be more useful.

(c) Multi-environment models. In this approach, some of the micromixing models are extended to simulate interaction between macro- and micromixing by introducing the concept of multiple environments. Ritchie and Togby (1979) proposed a three-environment model; Mehta and Tarbell (1983) proposed a four-environment model. Ranade and Bourne (1991) have extended the engulfment model of Baldyga and Bourne (1989) to a general multi-environment model and have incorporated it in a Eulerian description of turbulent flow processes by developing transport equations for volume fractions of multi-environments. These models have the potential to simulate complex interactions between small-scale and large-scale reactive mixing. In the Ranade and Bourne (1991) model, the population of small-scale coherent fluid lumps (size of the order of the Kolmogorov length scale) is divided into N sub-groups (or environments). Each coherent fluid lump is assumed to have uniform concentration, implying that molecular diffusivity is not playing a significant role (a reasonable assumption for systems with Schmidt number <4000). The variations of concentration within these different sub-groups indicate incomplete micromixing and small-scale segregation. The large-scale mixing and transport of the small, coherent fluid lumps within the reactor (macromixing) is simulated using the general convective-dispersion transport equation in terms of general variable, ϕ:

$$\frac{\partial}{\partial t}(\rho\alpha_k\phi_k) + \frac{\partial}{\partial x_i}(\rho U_i\alpha_k\phi_k) = \frac{\partial}{\partial x_i}\left(\Gamma_\phi\alpha_k\frac{\partial}{\partial x_i}\phi_k\right) + S_{\phi_k} \tag{5.29}$$

where α_k is the volume fraction of sub-group (or environment) k. When general variable, ϕ, is unity, the equation reduces to the governing equation of the volume fractions of different environments. For species concentrations, general variable, ϕ, is equal to C_{mk}, which is the concentration of the mth species in environment k. The species concentration, C_{mk}, may change due to convection, turbulent dispersion, micromixing and chemical reactions. The latter two terms are represented by the source terms in these equations, which are modeled using an extension of the engulfment model (Ranade and Bourne, 1991):

$$S_{\alpha j} = E\alpha_j\alpha_{j+1} + 2E\alpha_{j+1}\sum_{i=1}^{j-1}\alpha_i - E\alpha_j\sum_{i=1}^{j-1}\alpha_i - E\alpha_j\sum_{i=j+2}^{N}\alpha_i \tag{5.30}$$

$$S_{cmj} = E\alpha_j\alpha_{j+1}C_{mj+1} + E\alpha_{j+1}\sum_{i=1}^{j-1}\alpha_i\left(C_{mi} + C_{mj+1}\right) - E\alpha_j C_{mj}\sum_{i=1}^{j-1}\alpha_i - E\alpha_j C_{mj}\sum_{i=j+2}^{N}\alpha_i + \alpha_j\gamma_{mj} \tag{5.31}$$

where γ_{mj} is the rate of production of component m due to chemical reactions occurring in the jth environment. The parameter, E is the reciprocal of a characteristic micromixing time scale (see Section 5.1).

This approach provides a flexible yet simple framework for modeling turbulent reactive flow processes. When micromixing is fast, that is, when E is large, small-scale mixing will make the concentrations in all sub-groups equal. This will reduce the model to a cell balance model. When macromixing is fast, the volume fractions of different sub-groups are the same all over the reactor and the model will reduce to the generalized engulfment model. In such cases, if the number of sub-groups is specified as two, the model reduces to that of Baldyga and Bourne (1989). At intermediate levels of micro or macromixing, the model is able to simulate the interaction of mixing and chemical reactions. The model is sensitive to the initial volume ratio of the segregated reactants, which has been experimentally observed. Many other closure models (for example, Patterson, 1985; Li and Toor, 1986; Dutta and Tarbell, 1989) do not possess this important property. The model also satisfies two important limits: the slow reaction (pure mixing) limit and the fast reaction limit (Ranade and Bourne, 1991). It has been compared with other published models by Ranade (1993). It has also been used successfully for simulating reactive mixing of series-parallel reactions in semi-batch stirred reactors by Ranade and Bourne (1991). More recently, a similar, four-environment model was used by Kolhapure and Fox (1999) to simulate mixing in a sensitive LDPE reactor. These authors have shown good agreement with the results obtained using this approach and those obtained with full PDF simulations. The methodology of combining multi-environment models with a computational fluid dynamics framework has recently been formalized by Fox (1998). This approach looks quite promising and suitable for simulating liquid phase fast chemical reactions in turbulent flow processes.

There are a few other non-PDF approaches to simulating reactive flow processes (for example, the linear eddy model of Kerstein, 1991 and the conditional moment closure model of Bilger, 1993). These approaches are not discussed here as most of the engineering simulations of reactive flow processes can be achieved by the approaches discussed earlier. The discussion so far has been restricted to single-phase turbulent reactive flow processes. We now briefly consider modeling multiphase reactive flow processes.

5.5. MULTIPHASE REACTIVE FLOW PROCESSES

In general, multiphase reactive flow processes are classified into three types according to the location of the reaction zone:

(a) Reactions occur in one of the participating phases (either in the bulk or near the interface). Several gas–liquid, liquid–liquid reactive processes fall into this category.
(b) Reactions occur on the surface of one of the participating phase. Catalytic reactions in gas–solid, liquid–solid and gas–liquid–solid reactive processes fall into this category.
(c) Reactions occur in one phase but products form another immiscible phase. Reactive crystallization, liquid phase reactions generating volatile products or soot formation fall into this category.

For multiphase reactive systems of types (a) and (b), at least one of the reactants has to reach the reaction zone from a different phase. In such systems, generally mass transfer between these two different phases (and its interaction with chemical reactions) is of primary importance and turbulent mixing is often of secondary importance. For such systems, modeling multiphase flows as discussed in Chapter 4 is directly applicable. The only additional complexity is the possibility of interaction between mass transfer and chemical reactions. The typical interphase mass transfer source for component k between phases p and q can be written (for the complete species conservation equation, refer to Chapter 4):

$$S_{kpq} = k_{Mpq}\underline{a}_{pq}\eta_{pq}\left(\Delta C_{kpq}\right) \tag{5.32}$$

where k_{Mpq} is the mass transfer coefficient, $\underline{a}_{pq}$ is an interfacial area per unit volume, η_{pq} is an enhancement factor representing interaction of mass transfer and chemical reactions, and ΔC_{kpq} is the net concentration driving force for mass transfer between phases p and q. For slow (compared to mass transfer rate) reactions, the enhancement factor will be unity. For fast reactions, the enhancement factor will be a function of reaction kinetics and concentrations.

The subject of mass transfer with chemical reactions has been well developed. Several excellent books discuss suitable models to estimate enhancement factors (Doraiswamy and Sharma, 1984; Westerterp *et al.*, 1984) to represent interactions between mass transfer and chemical reactions. Models have been developed to formulate expressions for the enhancement factor for a number of different reacting systems. In many situations, however, it is not possible to derive a closed form expression for the enhancement factor, which is applicable over all temperature ranges and compositions within the reactor. For such cases, it is recommended to use so-called 'look up' tables. A detailed local model for the interaction of mass transfer and chemical reactions can be developed and solved separately, to generate these enhancement factor 'look up' tables at various conditions. Efficient interpolation routines can then supply values of enhancement factor to the multiphase reactive flow model at the desired conditions (compositions and temperature). If an appropriate model is developed to simulate interaction between mass transfer and chemical reactions, such a model may be used within the general modeling framework (VOF, EL or EE) discussed in Chapter 4 to simulate multiphase reactive flow processes.

VOF-based models simulate the small-scale flow processes near the interface. It is possible to calculate the interfacial area from the simulated interface shape and orientation. Thus, VOF simulations may allow a detailed understanding of the interaction of mass transfer and flow processes around the interface. It must, however, be noted that quantitative agreement between VOF predictions and experimental data is not satisfactory for most cases relevant to reactor engineering. Therefore, although VOF simulations may be useful as learning tools, the application of VOF to simulate realistic reactive flow processes is not possible without first getting accurate predictions of flow field and interface shape. In a Eulerian–Lagrangian approach, particle-level phenomena can be modeled rigorously by developing species conservation equations for individual dispersed particles (Eqs (4.21) and (4.22)). The sources appearing in such particle conservation equations will have the form of Eq. (5.32). Interfacial area in such sources is computed from the effective diameter of the concerned dispersed phase particle. Different approaches to handling such systems have been discussed in the previous chapter. To simulate interphase mass transfer and reacting systems, it is necessary to consider two-way coupling between dispersed and continuous phase. The source terms (representing mass or heat transfer) computed from the particle trajectories need to be included in the governing equations of the continuous phase. If there is an interaction between mass transfer and chemical reactions, as discussed above, an appropriate local model needs to be considered when evaluating net sources due to mass transfer. For turbulent reactive multiphase flow processes, several stochastic trajectories must be used to compute an appropriate source term for the continuous phase equation. An instantaneous driving force for concentration (or temperature) will be a function of the instantaneous concentration (or temperature) of the continuous phase. Various ways of estimating the instantaneous velocity of the continuous phase have been discussed in Chapter 4. In principle, similar practices may be applied to estimate instantaneous concentration. However, considering the uncertainties in estimating interphase mass transfer coefficients and other related parameters, often time-averaged concentrations (or temperature) are used to formulate interphase mass transfer and reaction source terms.

In Eulerian–Eulerian (EE) simulations, an effective reaction source term of the form of Eq. (5.32) can be used in species conservation equations for all the participating species. The above comments related to models for local enhancement factors are applicable to the EE approach as well. It must be noted that interfacial area appearing in Eq. (5.32) will be a function of volume fraction of dispersed phase and effective particle diameter. It can be imagined that for turbulent flows, the time-averaged mass transfer source will have additional terms such as correlation of fluctuations in volume fraction of dispersed phase and fluctuations in concentration even in the absence of chemical reactions. If there is an interaction between chemical reaction and mass transfer, time averaging with an enhancement factor will introduce even more additional correlations. In most engineering simulations, however, the time-averaged source term is taken as the source term computed using time-averaged variables. The effort of developing additional closure models is generally not justified in the face of existing uncertainties in estimating mass transfer coefficient and interfacial area. There have been attempts to derive the transport equation for interfacial area rather than computing it from a knowledge of average volume fraction and the size of the dispersed phase particle (Kataoka *et al.*, 1992). Many engineering simulations, however, adopt the approach of calculating the mass transfer/reaction source term based on time-averaged variables and lumping all the effects of turbulence on mass transfer in the value of mass transfer coefficient, k_{Mpq}. Additional computational aspects of modeling multiphase reactive flow processes are discussed in Chapter 7. Some examples of CFD-based simulations of multiphase reactive flows are discussed in Parts III and IV.

When reactions occur on a surface, the effective rate of surface reaction may depend on the rates of various intermediate steps including:

- mass transfer of reactants to surface;
- adsorption of reactant species on the surface;
- surface chemical reactions;
- desorption of products from the surface; and
- mass transfer of these products from the surface to the bulk.

It is possible to formulate an expression for effective rate by analyzing relative rates of these different steps. Numerous reaction-engineering textbooks (for example, Levenspiel, 1972; Doraiswami and Sharma, 1984) discuss the formulation of effective rates and, therefore, it will not be discussed here. Such models of effective rate can be incorporated in the CFD framework by suitably modifying the source term (Eq. (5.32)). In many solid catalyzed processes, an effective rate of continuous phase reactions can be defined in terms of catalyst (solid) loading. In such cases, it is not necessary to model the surface reactions rigorously. The reaction sources appearing in the continuous phase can be directly formulated from a knowledge of volume fraction of solid phase. Some of these examples are discussed in Part III and IV.

The interaction of turbulent mixing and chemical reactions is relevant only to multiphase reactive processes of type (c) discussed at the beginning of this section. In this type, reactions take place in one phase. Therefore, if the reactions are fast compared to the mixing rate, turbulent mixing can affect the effective reaction rate, as discussed earlier in this chapter. The reaction part of such systems can be modeled using the methods discussed in Section 5.2. These systems, however, have additional complexity because of the formation of products which are thermodynamically more favorable to exist in a different immiscible phase. For example, in a reactive crystallization, homogeneous liquid phase reaction forms a product, which precipitates. In such a case, two approaches are possible. In the first, simpler approach, interphase mass transfer sources can be modeled as discussed above without any special treatment. Alternatively, in the second approach, the spontaneous nucleation process is represented by employing some empirical models. For example, Magnussen and Hjertager (1976) proposed a nucleation model to simulate soot formation in combustion processes. They developed a conservation equation for nuclei concentration by appropriate formulations of nuclei formation and consumption rates. Similar nucleation models can be developed to simulate reactive crystallization (Wei and Garside, 1997). Since most such models rely heavily on empirical information and are rather system-specific, these models are not discussed here. Depending upon the considered objectives of the flow model, the reactor engineer can formulate an appropriate model using the basic methodology discussed in this and the previous three chapters.

5.6. SUMMARY

Modeling turbulent reactive flow processes is a complex and still developing subject. Before undertaking detailed reactive mixing modeling, it is essential to carry out the analysis of various relevant time (and length) scales of the system under consideration. Such an analysis will be useful to evaluate different modeling approaches and to select the best-suited approach. For most liquid phase reactive processes, where reactions are fast compared to turbulent mixing, phenomenological models such as multi-environment models integrated within a CFD framework look promising. For many gas phase reactive processes like combustion, a mixture fraction approach with presumed PDF may be more suitable. Computationally intensive approaches like LES and DNS are more suitable as learning tools. These simulations can be fruitfully employed to validate some of the important issues of the other computationally less expensive models. For most multiphase reactive processes, interphase mass transfer plays the central role. Turbulent mixing is rarely important in such cases, except when reactions occur in one phase and form immiscible products. For such cases, models to simulate homogeneous turbulent reactive mixing are applicable. Additional models to simulate nucleation or to simulate transfer of immiscible product into another phase may be included. It must be remembered that the quality of results of reactive mixing simulations will depend on the quality of several input data such as rate constants, mass transfer coefficients, interfacial area and so on. These quantities are seldom known accurately for industrial processes under relevant operating conditions. Sensitivity with respect to values of input parameters must be examined before using the simulations for reactor engineering. Approaches to developing tractable computational models for simulating complex industrial reactive flow processes and ways of direct or indirect validation are discussed with examples in Parts III and IV.

REFERENCES

Baldyga, J. (1989), Turbulent mixer model with application to homogeneous, instantaneous chemical reactions, *Chem. Eng. Sci.*, **44**, 1175–1182.

Baldyga, J. and Bourne, J.R. (1984), A fluid mechanical approach to turbulent mixing and chemical reactions, *Chem. Eng. Commun.*, **28**, 243–258.

Baldyga, J. and Bourne, J.R. (1989), Simplification of micromixing calculations, *Chem. Eng. J.*, **42**, 83.

Bakker, R.A. (1996), Micromixing in chemical reactors, PhD thesis, Delft University of Technology, Delft, The Netherlands.

Bilger, R.W. (1993), Conditional moment closure for turbulent reacting flow, *Phys. Fluids A*, **5**(2), 436–444.

Brodkey, R.S. (1975), Mixing in turbulent field, in "Turbulence in Mixing Operation" (Ed. R.S. Brodkey), Academic Press, London.

Chakrabarti, M. and Hill, J.C. (1997), First order closure theories for series-parallel reaction in simulated homogeneous turbulence, *AICRE J.*, **43**, 902–912.

Corrsin, J. (1964), The isotropic turbulent mixer, *AIChE J*, **10**, 870.

Danckwerts, P.V. (1953), Continuous flow systems: distribution and residence times, *Chem. Eng. Sci.*, **2**, 1.

Darabiha, N., Giovangigili, V., Trouve, A., Candel, S.M. and Esposito, E. (1989), Coherent flame description of turbulent premixed ducted flames, in "Turbulent Reactive Flows", Springer-Verlag, New York.

David, R. and Villermaux, J. (1975), Micromixing effects on complex reactions in a CSTR, *Chem. Eng. Sci.*, **30**, 1309.

David, R. and Villermaux, J. (1987), Interpretation of micromixing effects on fast consecutive competing reactions in semi batch stirred tanks by a simple interaction model, *Chem. Eng. Commun.*, **54**, 333–352.

Doraiswamy, L.K. and Sharma, M.M. (1984), "Heterogeneous Reactions – Analysis Examples And Reactor Design", Vol. 2, John Wiley & Sons, New York .

Dutta, A. and Tarbell, J.M. (1989), Closure models for turbulent reacting flows, *AIChE J*, **35**, 2013.

Fox, R.O. (1995), The spectral relaxation model of the scalar dissipation rate in homogeneous turbulence, *Phys. Fluids*, **7**(5), 1082–1094.

Fox, R.O. (1996), Computational methods for turbulent reacting flows in chemical process industry, *Rev. Inst. Francais Petrole*, **52**, 215.

Fox, R.O. (1998), On the relationship between Lagrangian micromixing models and computational fluid dynamics, *Chem. Eng. Processing*, **37**, 521–535.

Froment, G.F. and Bischoff, K.B. (1984), "Chemical Reactor Analysis and Design," John Wiley & Sons, New York.

Jones, W.P. and Whitelaw, J.H. (1982), Calculation methods for turbulent reactive flows: A review, *Combust. Flame*, **48**, 1–26.

Kataoka, I., Besnard, D.C. and Serizawa, A. (1992), Basic equation of turbulence and modeling of interfacial transfer terms in gas-liquid two phase flow, *Chem. Eng. Commun.*, **118**, 221–236.

Kerstein, A.R. (1991), Linear eddy modeling of turbulent transport, *J. Fluid Mech.*, **231**, 361–394.

Kolhapure, N.H. and Fox, R.O. (1999), CFD analysis of micromixing effects on polymerization in tubular low density polyethylene reactors, *Chem. Eng. Sci.*, **54**, 3233–3242.

Kuo, K.K.Y. (1986), "Principles of Combustion", John Wiley & Sons, New York.

Levenspiel, O. (1972), "Chemical Reaction Engineering", 2nd edition, John Wiley & Sons, New York.

Li, K.T. and Toor, H.L. (1986), Turbulent reactive mixing with series parallel reaction, effect of mixing on yield, *AIChE J.*, **32**, 1312.

Libby, P.A. and Williams, F.A. (1980), "Fundamental Aspects in Turbulent Reacting Flows", Topics in Applied Physics, Vol. 44, Springer-Verlag, New York.

Liew, S.K., Bray, K.M.C. and Moss, J.B. (1984), A stretched laminar flamelet model of turbulent non-premixed combustion, *Combust. Flame*, **56**, 199.

Ma, A.S.C., Sun, R.L.T. and Spalding, D.B. (1982), Application of ESCIMO to the turbulent hydrogen-air diffusion flame, *19th Combustion Symposium*, Haifa.

Magnussen, B.F. and Hjertager, B.H. (1976), On mathematical models of turbulent combustion with special emphasis on soot formation and combustion, *16th International Symposium on Combustion*, Cambridge, MA.

Mehta, R.V. and Tarbell, J.M. (1983), Four environment models of mixing and chemical reaction, *AIChE J.*, **29**, 320.

Middleton, J.C., Pierce, F. and Lynch, P.M. (1986), Computation of flow field and complex reactions yield in turbulent stirred reactors comparison with experimental data, *Chem. Eng. Res. Des.*, **64**, 18.

Oran, E.S. and Boris, J.P. (1982), Detailed modeling of combustion systems, *Prog. Energy Combust. Sci.*, **7**, 1–72.

Patterson, G.K. (1985), "Mixing of Liquids by Mechanical Agitation", Gorden and Breach Science Publications, New York.

Pohoreki, R. and Baldyga, J. (1993), New model of micromixing in chemical reactor, *Int. Eng. Chem. Fund.*, **22**, 329.

Pope, S.B. (1981), Monte Carlo method for the PDF equations of turbulent reactive flow, *Combust. Sci. Technol.*, **25**, 159–174.

Pope, S.B. (1985), PDF methods for turbulent reactive flows, *Prog. Energy Combust. Sci.*, **11**, 119–192.

Ranade, V.V. (1993), Interaction of macro and micromixing in agitated reactors, in "Advances in Transport Processes", (Eds. R.A. Mashelkar and A.S. Mujumdar), Vol. 9, Elsevier, New York.

Ranade, V.V. and Bourne, J.R. (1991), Fluid mechanics and blending in agitated tanks, *Chem. Eng. Sci.*, **46**, 1883.

Ritchie, B.W. and Togby, A.H. (1979), A three environment micromixing model for chemical reactors with arbitrary separate feed streams, *Chem. Eng. J.*, **17**, 173.

Spalding, D.B. (1970), Mixing and chemical reaction in steady confined turbulent flames, in *13th Symposium on Combustion*, Salt Lake city, UT, 649.

Spalding, D.B. (1971), Concentration fluctuations in a round turbulent free jet, *Chem. Eng. Sci.*, **26**, 95–107.

Spalding, D.B. (1978), General theory of turbulent combustion, *J. Energy*, **2**, 16.

Spalding, D.B. (1983), Chemical reaction in turbulent fluids, *Physico Chem. Hydrodynamics*, **4**, 323–336.

Toor, H.L. (1975), The non-premixed reaction, in "Turbulence in Mixing Operations", Ed. R.S. Bradkey, Academic Press, New York.

Tsai, K. and Fox, R.O. (1995), Modeling multiple reactive scalar micromixing with the generalized IEM model, *Phys. Fluids*, **7**, 2820.

Wei, H. and Garside, J. (1997), CFD Modeling of precipitation, *Chem. Eng. Res. Des.*, **75**, 219–227.

Westerterp, K.R., Van Swaaij, W.P.M. and Beenackers, A.A.C.M. (1984), "Chemical Reactor Design & Operation", 2nd edition, John Wiley & Sons, New York.

6 NUMERICAL SOLUTION OF MODEL EQUATIONS

6.1. INTRODUCTION

Mathematical models of flow processes are non-linear, coupled partial differential equations. Analytical solutions are possible only for some simple cases. For most flow processes which are of interest to a reactor engineer, the governing equations need to be solved numerically. A brief overview of basic steps involved in the numerical solution of model equations is given in Section 1.2. In this chapter, details of the numerical solution of model equations are discussed.

In general, numerical solution of the governing transport equation replaces continuous information contained in the exact solution of partial differential equations by discrete information available at a finite number of locations (grid points). The values of all the dependent variables at these finite numbers of grid points are considered as basic unknowns. The task of a numerical method then becomes one of providing a set of algebraic equations for these unknowns and prescribing an algorithm to solve these algebraic equations. The algebraic equations (called discretized equations) involving the unknown values of dependent variables are derived from the governing partial differential equations. Some assumptions about how the unknown dependent variables change between grid points are necessary for such derivation. Generally, piecewise profiles are assumed, which describe variation over a small region around the grid point in terms of values at that grid point and the surrounding grid points. To facilitate this, the solution domain is divided into a number of sub-domains or computational cells (the process is called grid generation), so that a separate profile assumption can be associated with each computational cell.

For a given differential equation, there can be several different ways to derive the discretized equations (finite difference, finite volume, finite element). A brief introduction to these three methods is given in Chapter 1 (Section 1.2). As mentioned therein, finite volume methods ensure integral conservation of mass, momentum and energy over any group of control volumes and, of course, over the whole solution domain. This characteristic exists for any number of grid points (and not only for the limiting case of a large number of grid points) and is the most attractive feature from the reactor engineer's point of view. Thus, as a limiting case of one computational cell, the finite volume equations become equivalent to those written for the ideal, completely mixed reactor (with which most reactor engineers are quite familiar). This book, therefore, discusses details of the finite volume method. This chapter is restricted to discussing application of the finite volume method to solve the general conservation equations discussed in Chapter 2. Applications to solve more complex model equations (like those governing multiphase flows or reactive mixing) are discussed in the next chapter.

Before discussing the finite volume method, it is worthwhile to examine the desired properties of the numerical solution method, which are summarized below:

(a) Consistency: In a consistent method, the error between the discretized equation and the exact equation (called the truncation error) tends to zero, as the grid spacing tends to zero. Truncation error is usually proportional to a power of the grid spacing, Δx and/or the time step Δt. It is usually estimated by employing Taylor series expansions to recover the original equation plus the remainder, which represents the truncation error. If the most important term in such a remainder is proportional to $(\Delta x)^n$ or $(\Delta t)^n$, the method is termed an nth order approximation. For any consistent method, n should be greater than zero.
(b) Stability: Having consistent approximations does not guarantee that the solution of the discretized equations system will become the solution of an exact equation in the limit of small step size. In any numerical method, errors appear in the course of solution process. It is essential to ensure that the numerical method does not magnify these errors (such a method is said to be stable). Stability of the numerical method is difficult to determine especially for non-linear problems. To ensure stability, many numerical methods need to impose limits on the time step or need to employ under-relaxation practices. Some of these issues are discussed later.
(c) Convergence: If the solution of the discretized equations tends to the exact solution of the differential equations as the grid spacing tends to zero, the numerical method is said to be convergent. For linear problems, consistency and stability are the necessary and sufficient conditions for convergence. For non-linear problems, however, convergence is usually checked by carrying out numerical solutions for a number of successively refined grids. Usually a consistent and stable numerical method leads to a grid-independent solution.

Besides examining these properties of numerical methods, specific efforts need to be made to assess the accuracy of numerical solutions of flow processes. Various types of errors and possible ways of estimating and controlling these errors are discussed in Section 6.5. Application of a finite volume method to solve partial differential equations and specific algorithms to treat pressure–velocity coupling are discussed in Sections 6.2 and 6.3, respectively.

6.2. FINITE VOLUME METHOD

In the finite volume method, discretized equations are obtained by integrating the governing transport equations over a finite control volume (CV). In this section, general aspects of the method are briefly discussed using a generic conservation equation for quantity, ϕ. Patankar (1980), Versteeg and Malalasekara (1995) and Ferziger and Peric (1995) may be referred to for a more detailed description.

Let us consider the task of solution of a generic transport equation of the following form in a two-dimensional solution domain:

$$\frac{\partial(\rho\phi)}{\partial t} + \nabla \cdot (\rho U \phi) = \nabla \cdot \left(\Gamma_\phi \nabla \phi\right) + S_\phi \tag{6.1}$$

The first step is to divide the solution domain into a finite number of control volumes or computational cells (grid generation). Two types of grid, namely, structured and unstructured grids, were briefly introduced in Section 1.2 (and are illustrated in Fig. 1.12). Methods of grid generation will not be discussed in this book. Some of the references useful for grid generation and some of the available grid generation tools are cited in Chapters 7 and 8, respectively. For the purpose of discussing the finite volume method, here we consider a simple, structured grid arrangement. Different methods can be employed to generate a structured computational grid (that is to select positions of computational nodes and boundaries of computational cells). However, usually boundaries of computational cells are decided as a first step and then a computational node is assigned at the center of each computational cell or control volume (CV) (as shown in Fig. 6.1a), rather than selecting node positions in a first step and assigning cell faces at the midpoints of each pair of nodes (Fig. 6.1b). It is important to note that CVs should not overlap and each CV face should be unique to the two CVs, which lie on either side of it. Here we illustrate the procedure using a Cartesian grid. A typical finite volume grid and notation is shown in Fig. 6.2.

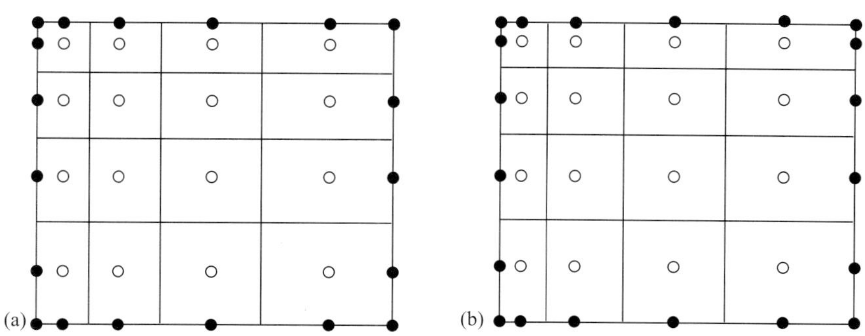

FIGURE 6.1 Finite volume grid, nodes centered in control volumes (left) and faces centered between nodes (right).

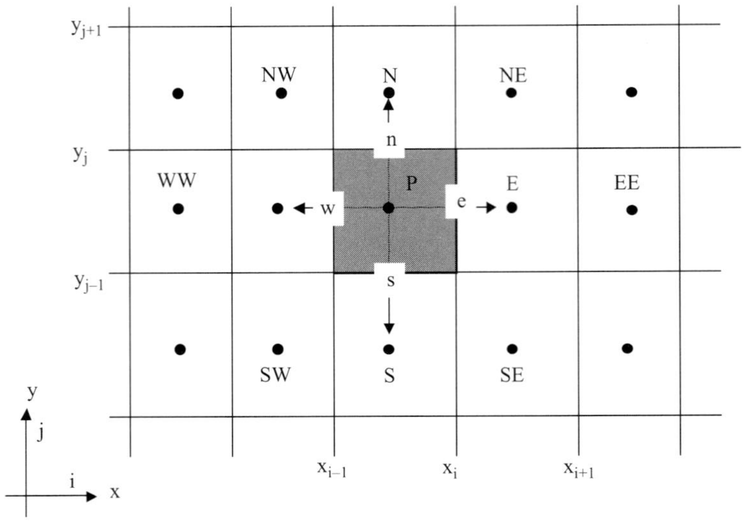

FIGURE 6.2 Typical finite volume CV and the notation used for a Cartesian grid.

6.2.1. Discretization of Governing Model Equations

The governing transport equations are integrated over each computational cell (employing a divergence theorem) and over the considered time interval Δt:

$$\int_{t}^{t+\Delta t}\left\{\int_{V}\frac{\partial(\rho\phi)}{\partial t}dV+\int_{S}\rho U\phi\cdot n\,dS=\int_{S}\Gamma_{\phi}\nabla\phi\cdot n\,dS+\int_{V}S_{\phi}dV\right\}dt \qquad (6.2)$$

where integration over V denotes volume of a computational cell and S denotes surface of a computational cell. In order to discuss the main issues of the finite volume method, let us first consider a steady state problem. For such a case, the outer integral over time and the first term of Eq. (6.2) will vanish. The second term is the net convective flux of quantity ϕ through the boundaries of a control volume. The third term is the net diffusive flux. To calculate convective and diffusive fluxes, one needs to know $(\rho U\phi)$ or $(\Gamma_{\phi}$ grad $\phi)$ everywhere on all the surfaces bounding the considered control volume. This information is not available since the values of all the variables are known only at the computational nodes. It is, therefore, necessary to make approximations while estimating the flux through the surface of computational cells. The fourth term in Eq. (6.2) represents the volumetric source (or sink). Usually all terms in the governing equations which cannot be classified as in the first three terms, are accommodated in such a source term. Approximations also need to be invoked to estimate such volume integrals.

To carry out the integration step shown in Eq. (6.2) on a computational cell, two levels of approximation need to be invoked. At the first level, the surface (or volume) integral is approximated in terms of the variable values at one or more locations on the cell face (within the CV). At the second level, the variable values at these locations are approximated in terms of the values at the computational nodes (cell centers). A judicious compromise between simplicity, ease of implementation, accuracy and computational efficiency has to be made while selecting these two levels of approximation. For the first level of approximation, normally a simple second-order approximation is used to replace the surface or volume integrals. Therefore, a surface integral is approximated as a product of the integrand at the cell face center and the cell face area. Similarly, a volume integral is approximated as the product of the mean value of the integrand over the CV (approximated as the value at the cell center) and the CV volume. To illustrate these approximation practices, consider the CV centered on a node P. Flux through the CV boundary denoted 'e' (east face of CV) in Fig. 6.2, F_e, can be written:

$$F_e = \int_{S_e} f \, dS \tag{6.3}$$

where f is the component of the convective or diffusive vector in the direction normal to face e and S_e is the area of face e. Invoking the second-order approximation, F_e can be written:

$$F_e = f_e S_e \tag{6.4}$$

where f_e is the value of the integrand at the center of face e. Alternative second-order approximations for F_e are possible, which may write F_e in terms of f_{ne} and f_{se} (f_{ne} and f_{se} are values of the integrand at the north-most point and south-most point of the east face, respectively). Simpson's rule may then be used to represent F_e in terms of f_e, f_{ne} and f_{se} as a fourth-order approximation. It must be noted that values of the integrand are normally not available at cell faces and, therefore, need to be obtained by interpolation. To preserve the accuracy of the above approximation, interpolation should also use at least the same or higher order approximation. Considering this, in most cases, it is sufficient to use the second-order approximation given by Eq. (6.4).

The volume integrals can be approximated as follows:

$$S_\phi = S_{\phi P} V_P \tag{6.5}$$

where $S_{\phi P}$ is the value of source term S_ϕ at the cell center P, and V_P is the volume of the computational cell centered around node P. A higher order approximation of this volume integral will require the values of ϕ at more locations than just the center. Since only the values at cell centers will be available, correspondingly higher order interpolation schemes need to be used to retain the accuracy of these volume integrals. Here again, normally it is sufficient to use the second-order approximation represented by Eq. (6.5). These approximations allow one to write Eq. (6.2) in the following form (steady state equation for the two-dimensional Cartesian grid shown in Fig. 6.2):

$$\begin{aligned} &S_e (\rho U \phi)_e - S_w (\rho U \phi)_w + S_n (\rho V \phi)_n - S_s (\rho V \phi)_s \\ &= S_e \left(\Gamma \frac{d\phi}{dx}\right)_e - S_w \left(\Gamma \frac{d\phi}{dx}\right)_w + S_n \left(\Gamma \frac{d\phi}{dx}\right)_n - S_s \left(\Gamma \frac{d\phi}{dx}\right)_s + S_{\phi P} V_P \end{aligned} \tag{6.6}$$

The second level of approximation concerns estimating the values of variables and gradients of variables (normal to cell faces) at locations other than computational nodes (cell centers). Such an approximation will then result in a set of linear algebraic equations. It must be noted that the source terms appearing in Eq. (6.6), that is $S_{\phi P}$, will generally be non-linear. It is necessary to linearize such source terms in order to formulate a set of linear algebraic equations. A generic source term linearization can be expressed as

$$S_{\phi P} V_P = S_C^{\phi} + S_P^{\phi} \phi_P \tag{6.7}$$

The assumption of a linear profile between the neighboring nodes offers the simplest approximation of the gradient at the face lying between those nodes. For example, the gradient of ϕ at face e can be written:

$$\left(\frac{\partial \phi}{\partial x}\right)_e = \frac{\phi_E - \phi_P}{x_E - x_P} \tag{6.8}$$

For a uniform Cartesian grid, this approximation is of second-order accuracy. Even for a non-uniform grid, the error reduction with respect to grid refinement is similar to that of a second-order approximation. Higher order polynomials can be used to estimate the required gradients. For example, a fourth-order approximation for the gradient at face e on the uniform Cartesian grid can be written:

$$\left(\frac{\partial \phi}{\partial x}\right)_e = \frac{27\phi_E - 27\phi_P + \phi_W - \phi_{EE}}{24\Delta x} \tag{6.9}$$

Such higher order approximation for the gradient makes sense, only if the integrals are also approximated using higher order approximations. For most complex flow simulations, second-order approximation of the gradient (given by Eq. (6.8)) is considered satisfactory.

Velocity and other variables at cell faces can be obtained by employing suitable interpolation practices. Numerous alternative interpolation methods have been developed. Generically, a value of general variable ϕ at the cell face can be expressed in terms of two neighboring nodes and one additional upstream node (the need to include an additional upstream node is discussed later in this chapter). For example, the value of ϕ at cell face e can be written:

$$\phi_e = \begin{cases} \beta_1\phi_P + \beta_2\phi_E + \beta_3\phi_W & \because \quad U_e > 0 \\ \beta_1\phi_E + \beta_2\phi_P + \beta_3\phi_{EE} & \because \quad U_e < 0 \end{cases} \tag{6.10}$$

where β are coefficients dependent on the interpolation method (refer to Fig. 6.2 to clarify the notation of node points), which obey the following restriction:

$$\beta_1 + \beta_2 + \beta_3 = 1 \tag{6.11}$$

Substitution of gradient terms (Eq. (6.8)), interpolated values and the linearized source term in Eq. (6.6) gives the discretized form of Eq. (6.6) for a uniform grid:

$$a_P\phi_P = a_E\phi_E + a_W\phi_W + a_{WW}\phi_{WW} + a_N\phi_N + a_S\phi_S + a_{SS}\phi_{SS} + S_C^{\phi} \tag{6.12}$$

where,

$$a_E = D_e - (\beta_2 F_e) \tag{6.13}$$

$$a_W = D_w + (\beta_1 F_w - \beta_3 F_e) \tag{6.14}$$

$$a_{WW} = \beta_3 F_w \tag{6.15}$$

$$a_N = D_n - (\beta_2 F_n) \tag{6.16}$$

$$a_S = D_s + (\beta_1 F_s - \beta_3 F_n) \tag{6.17}$$

$$a_{SS} = \beta_3 F_s \tag{6.18}$$

$$a_P = a_E + a_W + a_N + a_S + a_{WW} + a_{SS} - S_P^\phi + (F_e - F_w + F_n - F_s) \tag{6.19}$$

$$F = S(\rho U) \quad \text{or} \quad S(\rho V) \tag{6.20}$$

$$D = S\frac{\Gamma_\phi}{\Delta x} \quad \text{or} \quad S\frac{\Gamma_\phi}{\Delta y} \tag{6.21}$$

When deriving these expressions, it was assumed that velocity at all the cell faces is positive. In other cases, suitable modifications to include appropriate upstream nodes (in place of ϕ_{WW} and ϕ_{SS}) should be made. It can be seen that the continuity equation indicates that the last term inside the bracket of Eq. (6.19) will always be zero for constant density flows. The behavior of numerical methods depends on the source term linearization employed and interpolation practices. Before these practices are discussed, a brief discussion of the desired characteristics of discretization methods will be useful. The most important properties of the discretization method are:

- Conservativeness: To ensure the overall conservation of ϕ, the flux of ϕ leaving a CV across a given face, must be equal to the flux of ϕ entering the adjacent CV through the same face. Therefore, the flux through the common face must be represented by one and the same expression in adjacent CVs.
- Boundedness: Numerical solution methods must respect the physically consistent bounds on variable values (bounded by minimum and maximum boundary values when there is no source). An essential requirement of boundedness is that all the coefficients of the discretized equation should be of the same sign and (usually) positive. If this condition is not satisfied, it is possible to observe unphysical 'wiggles' in the solution. It can be seen from Eqs. (6.13) to (6.18) that some of the coefficients may become negative if values of β are not chosen carefully. For example, a_E can become negative if $F_e > (D_e/\beta_2)$. It must also be noted that source term linearization practices should ensure that S_P^ϕ is always negative in order to possess the boundedness property (otherwise the value of a_P may become negative). Diagonal dominance of the discretized equations is a desirable feature for satisfying the 'boundedness' criterion. Scarborough (1958) gave a sufficient condition for diagonally dominant set of equations as:

$$\frac{\sum |a_{nb}|}{a_P} \begin{cases} \leqslant 1 \text{ at all nodes} \\ < 1 \text{ at least at one node} \end{cases} \tag{6.22}$$

  Diagonal dominance and all positive coefficients ensure boundedness. Special procedures are invoked to ensure the boundedness of many higher order schemes, which otherwise, may produce wiggles and unbounded solutions. Some of these methods are discussed in the following.
- Transportiveness: Transportiveness can be illustrated by considering the distribution of ϕ in the vicinity of its source. The contours of constant ϕ are shown in Fig. 6.3 for different values of Peclet number (ratio of strengths of convection and diffusion, Pe = F/D). For a process with zero Peclet number (pure diffusion), contours of constant ϕ are circular and therefore conditions

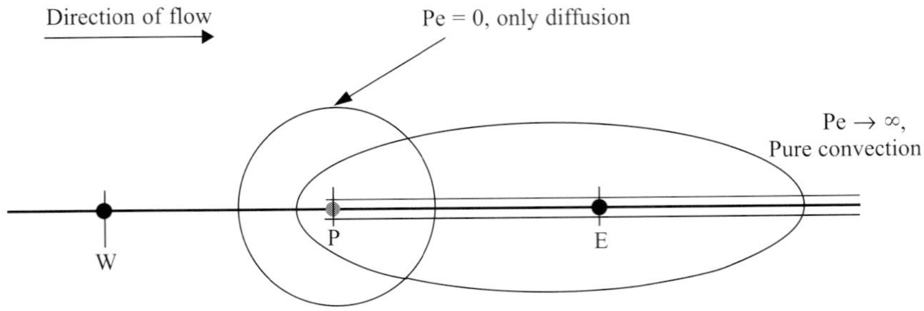

FIGURE 6.3 Distribution of ϕ around its source. (from Versteeg and Malalasekara, 1995. Printed with permission from the Publishers.)

at node P will be influenced not only by upstream conditions at W but also by all the conditions further downstream (node E). As the value of Peclet number increases (more convection), directionality of influence becomes increasingly biased towards the upstream direction. This means that conditions at node E are strongly influenced by those at P but conditions at P will experience only a weak influence from those at node E. At the extreme case of infinite Peclet number, the constant ϕ contours are completely stretched in the direction of flow and conditions at node E will not influence those at node P. Discretization schemes must respect the transportiveness property (directionality of influence) of flow processes.

Source term linearization and interpolation practices to estimate cell face values are discussed with reference to these desirable properties of the discretization method.

(a) Source term linearization

The linearization of source term, $S_{\phi P}$ should be a good representation of the S and ϕ relationship. Depending on the functional form of $S_{\phi P}$, there are several different ways of formulating coefficients S_C^{ϕ} and S_P^{ϕ} of Eq. (6.7). Patankar (1980) discussed various linearization practices and recommended the following method:

$$S_{\phi P} = S_{\phi P}^{*} + \left(\frac{dS_{\phi P}}{d\phi}\right)^{*} (\phi_P - \phi_P^{*}) \tag{6.23}$$

where * indicates the guess value or the previous iteration value. This linearization practice is recommended provided that the source term decreases with increasing ϕ. Thus, the coefficients of linearized source terms can be written:

$$S_C^{\phi} = \left[S_{\phi P}^{*} - \left(\frac{dS_{\phi P}}{d\phi}\right)^{*} \phi_P^{*}\right] V_P \qquad S_P^{\phi} = \left(\frac{dS_{\phi P}}{d\phi}\right)^{*} V_P \tag{6.24}$$

This formulation ensures that the slope of the linearized source term representation (Eq. (6.7)) is the same as the slope of the non-linear source term at node P, and is always negative. It must be noted that linearization with steeper slopes normally leads to slower convergence. For detailed discussion of the effect of source term linearization on convergence, and on the handling of source terms with non-negative slope with ϕ, see Patankar (1980).

(b) Interpolation practices

Some commonly used interpolation practices are discussed here. A simple and straightforward approximation to the value at the CV face center is linear interpolation between the two nearest nodes. At location e on a Cartesian grid (Fig. 6.2), general interpolation coefficients (β) for such a scheme can be written:

$$\beta_1 = (1 - \lambda_e) \qquad \beta_2 = \lambda_e \qquad \beta_3 = 0 \tag{6.25}$$

where the linear interpolation factor, λ_e is defined as

$$\lambda_e = \frac{x_e - x_P}{x_E - x_P} \tag{6.26}$$

Interpolation with Eq. (6.25) is second-order accurate. This approximation is called the 'central differencing scheme' (CDS).

It can be seen that the central differencing scheme discussed above is conservative. The coefficients of CDS satisfy the Scarborough criterion. However, for uniform grid ($\lambda_e = 0.5$), when the Peclet number is higher than 2, the coefficients a_E will become negative [$F_e > (D_e/\beta_2)$]. This violates the boundedness requirements and may lead to physically unrealistic solutions. At all values of Peclet number, CDS retains the same directionality of influence and, therefore, does not possess the transportiveness property. To gain the transportiveness property, several differencing schemes have been proposed. The simplest is the first-order upwind differencing scheme (UDS), which approximates the value of ϕ_e by retaining only the upstream influence (with reference to Eq. (6.10)):

$$\beta_1 = 1 \qquad \beta_2 = 0 \qquad \beta_3 = 0 \tag{6.27}$$

It can be seen that this UDS is conservative and transportiveness is built into the formulation. It is the only discretization scheme which unconditionally satisfies the boundedness criteria and therefore, never leads to 'wiggles'. Unfortunately, the scheme is only first-order accurate and is numerically diffusive. This numerical diffusion is magnified in multidimensional problems if the flow is oblique to the grid. The rapid variations in the variables will be smeared out and since the rate of error reduction is only first order, very fine grids are required to obtain an accurate solution. In order to exploit the higher accuracy of CDS, several combinations of CDS and first-order UDS have been proposed (for example, hybrid differencing schemes and power law differencing schemes). In all these combined schemes, CDS is used as long as Peclet numbers are less than 2. For larger Peclet numbers, either the standard UDS or the power law variant is used (Patankar, 1980). These combined schemes are also unconditionally bounded and therefore widely used in various computational codes. However, the accuracy in terms of Taylor series truncation error is still only of first order.

Several attempts have been made to employ higher order interpolation schemes. One of the most popular schemes is QUICK (quadratic upstream interpolation for convective kinetics), proposed by Leonard (1979). In this scheme, the face value of ϕ is obtained by a quadratic function passing through two bracketing nodes (on each side of the face) and a node on the upstream side (Fig. 6.4). The formulae for

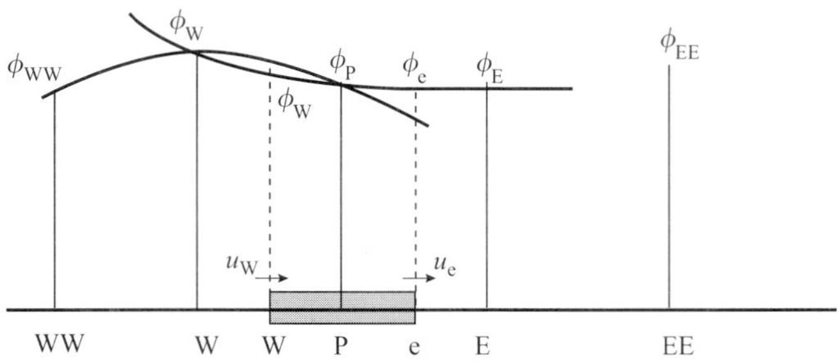

FIGURE 6.4 Quadratic profiles used in QUICK scheme.

estimating ϕ_e using Eq. (6.10) can be written:

$$\beta_2 = \frac{\lambda_e (\Delta x_w + \lambda_e \Delta x_e)}{\Delta x_e + \Delta x_w} \qquad \beta_3 = -\frac{\lambda_e (1 - \lambda_e) \Delta x_e^2}{\Delta x_w (\Delta x_e + \Delta x_w)} \qquad \beta_1 = 1 - \beta_2 - \beta_3 \tag{6.28}$$

For the uniform grid, the coefficients of the three nodal values involved in the interpolation become 3/8 for the downstream point, 6/8 for the first upstream node and $-1/8$ for the second upstream node. This scheme is more complex than CDS and it extends the computational molecule by one more node in each direction (the conventional tri-diagonal methods are, therefore, not directly applicable. See the discussion in the following subsection). The scheme has a third-order truncation error and was made popular by Leonard (1979). The transportiveness property is built into the scheme by considering two upstream and one downstream node. However, the main coefficients of the discretized equations are not guaranteed to be positive. This may lead to instability and may lead to unbounded (wiggles) solutions under certain conditions.

Several attempts have been made to reformulate the QUICK and other higher order schemes to ensure the boundedness property. One way to achieve this is to place the troublesome negative coefficients in the source term to alleviate the stability problems (see for example, Hayase *et al.*, 1992 and references cited therein). Other attempts include modifications of higher order schemes either based on flux limiting or based on slope limiting (see Leveque, 1996 for a recent review). It will be instructive to examine the various discretization schemes using the so-called 'normalized variable diagram' to understand and to compare these modifications. Depending on the direction of normal velocity at the face, the locally normalized variable is defined as

$$\tilde{\phi} = \frac{\phi - \phi_U}{\phi_D - \phi_U} \tag{6.29}$$

where subscript D, U and C denote downstream, upstream and central node, respectively. It can be seen that normalized values of ϕ at downstream and upstream nodes are 1 and 0, respectively (Fig. 6.5). Because of this, all the discretization schemes can now be written in terms of the normalized variable at the center node. Most of the widely used discretization schemes are shown in Fig. 6.6 in terms of the normalized variable diagram (NVD). Leonard (1988) has shown that any linear NVD characteristic which passes through the second quadrant may produce unphysical oscillations (CDS, QUICK). Characteristics, which pass through the fourth quadrant (below point O), are artificially diffusive. Characteristics, which pass above point

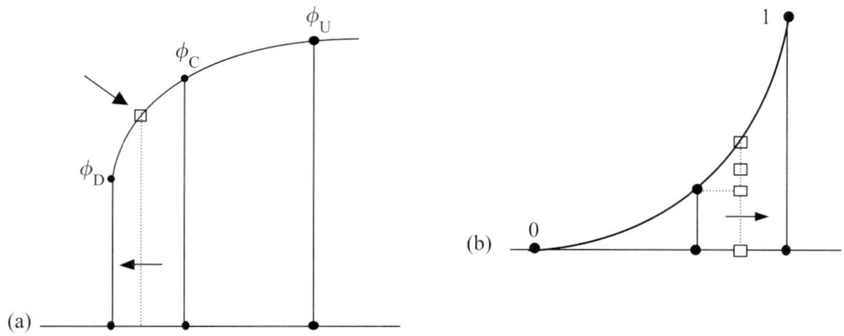

FIGURE 6.5 Node variables in the vicinity of a CV Face (at broken line . . . .)

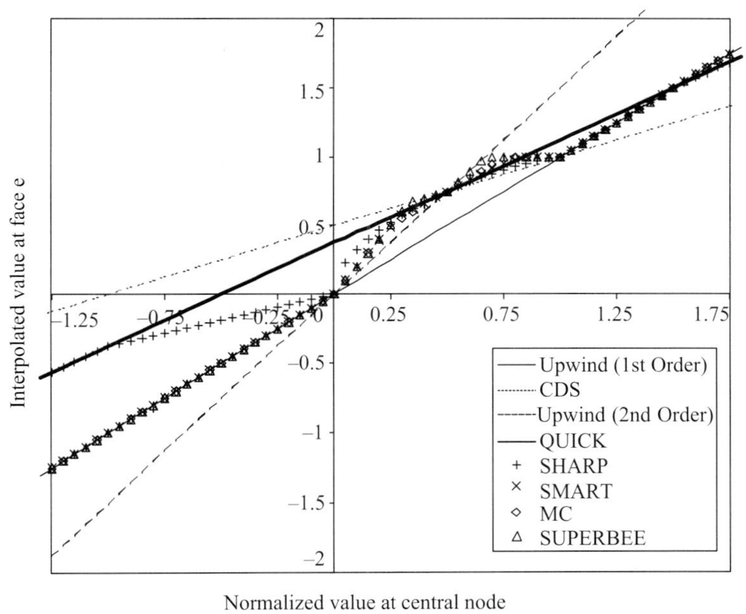

FIGURE 6.6 Discretization schemes on normal variable diagram.

P (1, 1), are oscillatory in two dimensions (second-order upwinding; for details of second-order upwinding schemes, see Shyy *et al.*, 1992). Characteristics passing through point Q (0.5, 0.75) have second-order accuracy (third order, if the slope at Q is 3/4). Thus, NVD can be used to evaluate different discretization schemes as well as devise new ones.

Van Leer (1977) introduced a monotized centered (MC) scheme. The SUPERBEE scheme is specifically developed to handle discontinuities (Roe, 1985). Gaskell and Lau (1988) proposed a SMART (sharp and monotonic algorithm for realistic transport) scheme, and Leonard (1988) proposed the SHARP (simple high accuracy resolution program) scheme based on modifications of QUICK to preserve boundedness. These schemes are also shown in Fig. 6.6. All of these schemes try to avoid non-physical oscillations by introducing modifications around the basic QUICK scheme. The SUPERBEE limiter tends to be overcompressive, meaning that it tends to steepen up smooth profiles into discontinuities. For this reason, it is useful for preserving discontinuities but inappropriate for problems with smooth solutions. The desire to use higher order discretization schemes must be balanced against the limitations imposed by the complexity of the problem being solved, the availability of computing resources, the stability and convergence of the solution algorithm and the capacity to tolerate non-physical over- and undershoots. Among the various schemes, QUICK (and its modifications SHARP or SMART) and second-order upwind differencing schemes look more attractive from the point of view of accuracy and ease of implementation. For complex multiphase flows, the flow field may exhibit extreme sensitivity to the gradients of the dispersed phase volume fraction. In such cases, a hybrid or power law scheme advocated by Patankar (1980) may be a better choice, at least while initiating the simulations from an arbitrarily guessed flow field.

Using one of the suitable discretization schemes discussed above, it is possible to relate values of variables and their gradient at CV faces to the node values. It is also necessary to use suitable interpolation schemes to estimate other relevant quantities like effective diffusion coefficients, (Γ) at required locations. Either algebraic mean or harmonic mean can be used to estimate the value of effective diffusion coefficients at cell faces. For example, the effective diffusion coefficient at face e can be written (for a uniform grid):

$$\Gamma_{\phi e} = \frac{\Gamma_{\phi P} + \Gamma_{\phi E}}{2} \quad \text{or} \quad \frac{2\Gamma_{\phi P}\Gamma_{\phi E}}{\Gamma_{\phi P} + \Gamma_{\phi E}} \tag{6.30}$$

The harmonic mean to estimate effective diffusion coefficients (second expression on RHS of Eq. (6.30)) can handle abrupt changes in values of Γ_ϕ without requiring an excessively fine grid in the vicinity of the change (see Patankar, 1980 for more details).

The foregoing discussion allows one to formulate a set of algebraic equations comprising one algebraic equation for each CV (per variable). However, CVs having one or more faces coinciding with the boundaries of the solution domain may require special treatment. The discussion on implementation of boundary conditions within the framework of the finite volume method is postponed until Section 6.3.3. Methods for the solution of algebraic equations resulting from the discretization process are discussed below.

6.2.2. Solution of Algebraic Equations

After implementing all the boundary conditions, one obtains one algebraic equation per node (per variable), which relates the variable value at the node to the values of variables at several neighboring nodes. The numbers of equations and unknowns are equal and, therefore, the system is well defined and closed. The algebraic equation for any CV has the following form:

$$a_P\phi_P = \sum_l a_{nb}\phi_{nb} + S_{\phi C} \tag{6.31}$$

where P denotes the node at which the governing equation is approximated, nb denotes neighboring nodes and the index l covers all the neighboring nodes involved in discretized approximation. The coefficients (a_P and a_{nb}) and the source term, $S_{\phi C}$, are estimated using the initial guess or previous iteration values. The node P and its neighbors appearing in the above equation form the so-called computational molecule. Examples of computational molecules are shown in Fig. 6.7. Before discussing the solution of algebraic equations of the form (6.31), it will be useful to introduce the concept of under-relaxation.

It must be remembered that linear algebraic equations of the form (6.31) are approximate forms of the original non-linear discretized equations. The overall iterative procedure of repeatedly solving linearized equations to obtain solutions of non-linear equations is susceptible to divergence, especially when these are coupled with equations of other variables. In order to control the magnitude of change during each iteration, an under-relaxation parameter, α_ϕ is introduced:

$$\phi_{\mathrm{P}}^{\mathrm{new}} = \alpha_\phi \phi_{\mathrm{P}}^{\mathrm{new}} + \left(1 - \alpha_\phi\right) \phi_{\mathrm{P}}^{*} \tag{6.32}$$

where $\phi_{\mathrm{P}}^{\mathrm{new}}$ is the solution of Eq. (6.31) and * indicates the guess value or the previous iteration value. The under-relaxation parameter, α_ϕ, takes a value between zero and one. Lower values of under-relaxation parameter lead to more stable but slower convergence. The optimum value of under-relaxation parameter is problem dependent. Generally, small values are used during the early iterations, which are gradually increased as convergence is approached. Converged results are independent of the values of under-relaxation parameters. Instead of explicitly applying under-relaxation as shown in Eq. (6.32), it is more efficient to combine Eqs (6.31) and (6.32) to form the modified equation (Patankar, 1980):

$$\left(\frac{a_{\mathrm{P}}}{\alpha_\phi}\right) \phi_{\mathrm{P}} = \sum_{l} a_{\mathrm{nb}} \phi_{\mathrm{nb}} + S_{\phi \mathrm{C}} + (1 - \alpha_\phi) \left(\frac{a_{\mathrm{P}}}{\alpha_\phi}\right) \phi_{\mathrm{P}}^{*} \tag{6.33}$$

The diagonal dominance of such a modified discretized equation set is increased since the coefficient of ϕ_{P} in the modified equation is larger than that in Eq. (6.31) while other coefficients remain the same. This formulation has a positive effect on many iterative solution methods and is, therefore, recommended.

The system of linear algebraic equations (Eq. (6.31) or (6.33)) can be written in matrix notation:

$$A\phi = B \tag{6.34}$$

where A is a square matrix (since the number of equations and unknowns must be equal), ϕ is a vector of unknown variable values at the grid nodes and B is the vector containing the remaining terms. The matrix A is usually a sparse matrix (most

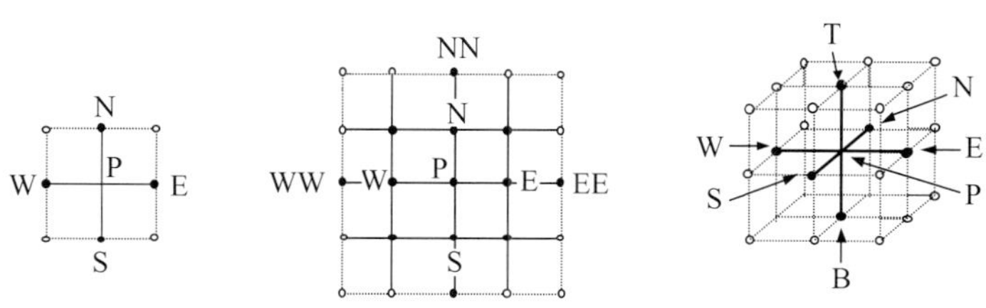

FIGURE 6.7 Example of computational molecules.

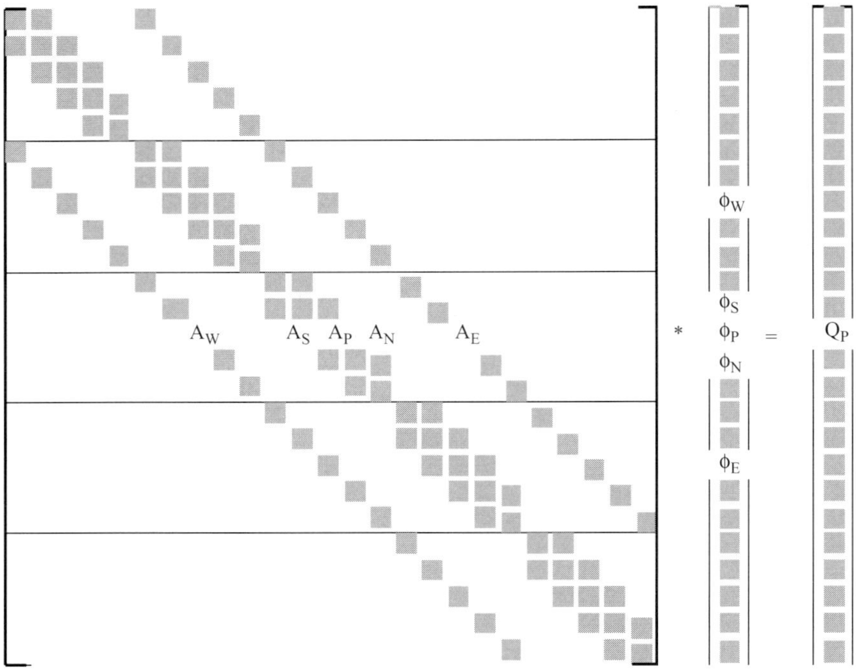

FIGURE 6.8 Structure of the matrix for a five-point computational molecule.

of the elements are zero). The structure of matrix A depends on the ordering of variables in vector ϕ and the size of the computational molecule. For the case of a five-point computational molecule, the structure of A is shown in Fig. 6.8. For the unstructured grid, the coefficient matrix A remains sparse, however, it no longer has a banded structure. Different types of solvers are, therefore, needed for structured and unstructured grids. In this section, some of the methods used to solve algebraic equations resulting from the structured grid are discussed. Details of solvers suitable for unstructured grid can be found in Saad and Schultz (1986). General information about the solution of algebraic discretized equations may be found in Ferziger and Peric (1995).

Direct methods of solution of linear algebraic equations are essentially matrix inversion algorithms (Gauss elimination, LU decomposition etc. Details of these methods can be found in Press *et al.*, 1992). These methods have large memory requirements and are computationally expensive for a large number of equations. These methods become especially inefficient when solving linearized non-linear equations. Iterative methods are based on repeated application of a relatively simple algorithm (a Jacobi point by point method or line by line methods) leading to eventual convergence. If each iteration is inexpensive and the required number of iterations is small, an iterative method will be more efficient than the direct method. For many CFD problems, this is usually the case. The other advantage of iterative methods is that only non-zero coefficients of the equations need to be stored in core memory. Some of the basic methods which can be used with iterative solvers are the Gauss-Siedel method, successive over-relaxation (SOR) and the tri-diagonal matrix algorithm (TDMA). The TDMA is actually a direct solver for the one-dimensional problem if the value at one node is a function of only its neighboring two nodes. It is, however, widely used in a line-by-line fashion to solve multidimensional CFD problems (where the value at a node is a function of more than two neighboring nodes). Proper choice of sweeping the lines on which TDMA is applied can accelerate the overall convergence rate (for example, marching the lines from upstream to the downstream direction). When higher order discretization schemes are used (QUICK or second-order upwind schemes), the TDMA method can be applied only by incorporating a large number of neighboring contributions in the source term. Understandably, the performance of TDMA deteriorates for such cases, resulting in slower convergence. A more generalized version of TDMA known as the penta-diagonal algorithm (for a set of linear equations containing five non-zero elements per equation) is available (see Fletcher, 1991).

For even larger computational molecules (arising in multidimensional problems with complex body fitted grids), Stone (1968) proposed a strongly implicit procedure (SIP). Schneider and Zedan (1981) developed an improved version of this method called modified SIP or MSIP. Details of these methods may be found in the cited references and in Anderson *et al.* (1984) and Peric (1987). These methods may also act as a basis for developing additional methods to accelerate convergence, such as conjugate gradient (Golub and van Loan, 1990) or multi-grid methods (Hackbusch, 1985; Peric *et al.*, 1988; Sathyamurthy and Patankar, 1994). Several acceleration methods based on additive correction philosophy have been proposed (for example, Hutchinson and Raithby, 1986; Kelkar and Patankar, 1989). In additive correction philosophy, a correction to the current solution field is sought, so that the corrected solution obeys global conservation within the considered sub-region. Combination of the correction methods and multi-grid methods may also be effectively used to accelerate the convergence. Multi-grid methods are more like useful strategies than specific methods. Within the multi-grid framework, several choices of such parameters as number of grid levels, number of iterations on each grid level, the order in which various levels are visited, interpolation between various levels, may be made to construct different methods. The rate of convergence, of course, will depend on the choice of these parameters. These details will not be discussed here and may be found in the cited references.

6.3. FINITE VOLUME METHOD FOR CALCULATION OF FLOW FIELD

The discussion in the previous section assumed that the velocity field required to calculate the necessary coefficients of the discretized equations was somehow known. However, generally, the velocity field needs to be calculated as part of the overall solution procedure by solving momentum conservation equations. The governing equations are discussed in Chapters 2 to 5. The basic momentum transport equations governing laminar flow are considered here to illustrate the application of the finite volume method to calculation of the flow field. The governing equations can be written:

$$\frac{\partial}{\partial t}(\rho V)+\nabla\cdot(\rho VV) = -\nabla p+\nabla\cdot\left(\mu\left(\nabla V+\nabla V^{\mathrm{T}}\right)+\left(\kappa-\frac{2}{3}\mu\right)\delta_{ij}\left(\nabla\cdot V\right)\right)+\rho g \tag{6.35}$$

It can be seen that since momentum equations are vector equations, the convective and diffusive terms in the equations appear more complicated than the generic transport equations discussed in the previous section. The convective terms are non-linear and the viscous terms contain more than one term. However, all of these terms can be discretized using the methods discussed in the previous section. All the extra non-zero terms not conforming to the generic equations are usually combined in the form of a source term. It must also be noted that all the three momentum equations are strongly coupled because each velocity component appears in all three momentum equations. This coupling can also be handled by the techniques of iterative solution discussed earlier. The unique feature of momentum equations, which distinguish them from the generic transport equation discussed earlier, is the role played by the pressure. The pressure gradients appear in the source terms of the momentum equations but there is no obvious equation to obtain the pressure. The pressure field is indirectly specified via the continuity equation. It is, therefore, necessary to calculate the pressure field in such a way that the resulting velocity field satisfies the continuity equation. Special treatments are needed to convert the indirect information in the continuity equation into a direct algorithm to calculate pressure (algorithms to treat pressure–velocity coupling). Some widely used algorithms are discussed in this subsection. Since the principal variable in momentum equations is a vector, it allows more freedom in the choice of variable arrangements on the grid.

6.3.1. Co-located and Staggered Grid Arrangement

Basic features of grids used for numerical solution are discussed in Section 6.2. When all the variables are stored at the same set of grid nodes, the arrangement is termed as 'colocated'. It is, however, not necessary that all the variables share the same grid. It is possible, and sometimes advantageous, to use different locations for storing values of different velocity components and pressure (staggered grid). The two types of grid arrangement are shown in Fig. 6.9. 'Colocated' seems to be an obvious choice, which has significant advantages in complicated solution domains. However, straightforward application of the finite volume method discussed earlier for momentum equations using the colocated grid fails to recognize the difference between a checkerboard pattern and uniform pressure fields. The staggered grid arrangement is proposed to suit the natural coupling of pressure and velocity. In this arrangement, the velocity field is stored at the faces of CV around a pressure node. In such an arrangement, the pressure and diffusion terms are very naturally approximated by a central difference approximation without interpolation. Also the evaluation of mass fluxes in the continuity equation (on the faces of a pressure CV) is straightforward. With a staggered grid arrangement, the natural coupling between pressure and velocity fields helps to avoid some types of convergence problems and oscillations in the pressure field. Because of these advantages, the staggered grid arrangement has been used extensively to solve momentum equations. In recent years, more and more problems with complex geometry have been tackled using non-orthogonal grids. The staggered grid arrangement for equations in generalized coordinates is complicated because it introduces additional curvature terms, which are difficult to treat numerically. Thus, improved pressure–velocity coupling algorithms were developed which enable the use of colocated grids to solve momentum equations. Most commercial CFD codes now use colocated arrangements.

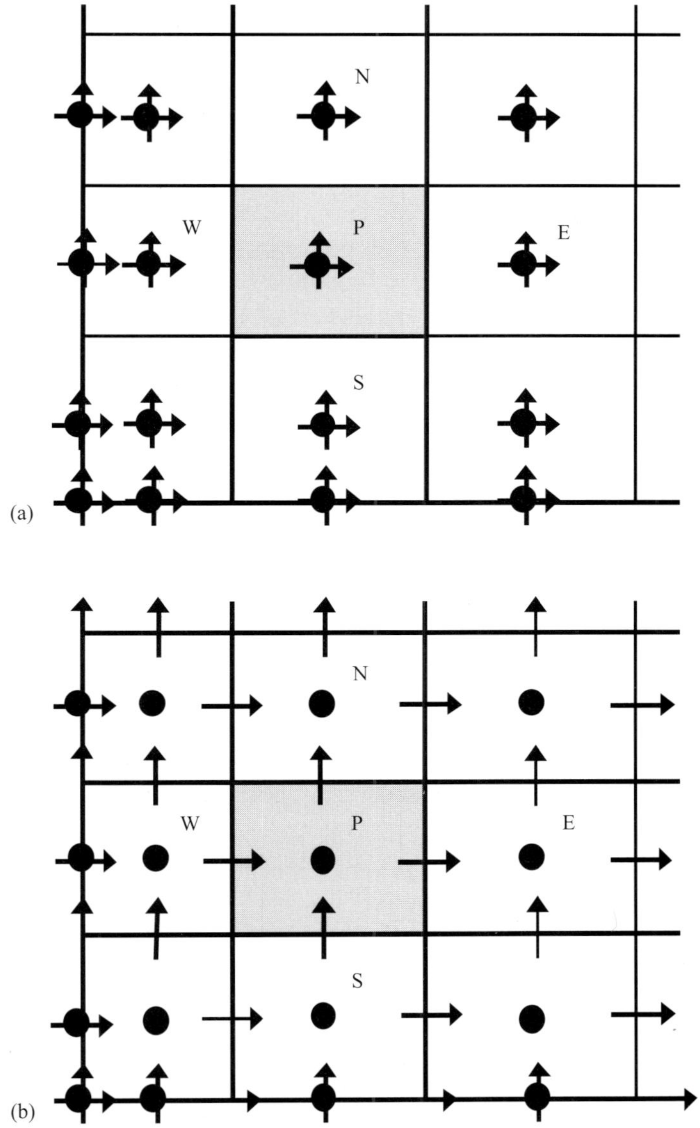

FIGURE 6.9 (a) Co-located and (b) Staggered grid arrangements.

6.3.2. Algorithms to Treat Pressure–Velocity Coupling

The momentum and continuity equations can be combined to derive an equation for pressure. For example, for constant density and viscosity fluid, the continuity equation can be used to simplify the divergence of the momentum equation (Eq. (6.35)) to yield an equation for pressure:

$$\frac{\partial}{\partial x_i}\left(\frac{\partial p}{\partial x_i}\right) = -\frac{\partial}{\partial x_i}\left[\frac{\partial\left(\rho U_i U_j\right)}{\partial x_j}\right] \tag{6.36}$$

This elliptic pressure equation can be solved by the methods discussed earlier. It is important to note that the numerical approximations of this equation must be consistent with the approximations used in discretizing the original momentum and continuity equations. For example, the outer derivative of pressure in Eq. (6.36) comes from the continuity equation, while the inner derivative arises from momentum equations. These outer and inner derivatives must be discretized using the corresponding schemes used for discretizing the continuity and momentum equations, respectively. Violation of this constraint may lead to incorrect solution of the continuity equation. To maintain consistency, generally the pressure equation is derived directly from the discretized momentum and continuity equations rather than approximating Eq. (6.36). Several methods have been proposed to estimate the pressure field. The most widely used methods for incompressible flows, which are relevant to reactor engineering applications, are implicit or semi-implicit pressure correction methods. In these methods, pressure or pressure correction (or both) equations are derived from the discretized momentum and continuity equations, and used to enforce mass conservation at each iteration (or time step). Some of these methods are briefly discussed below.

One of the popular methods proposed by Patankar and Spalding (1972) is called SIMPLE (semi-implicit method for pressure linked equations). In this method, discretized momentum equations are solved using the guessed pressure field. The discretized form of the momentum equations can be written:

$$a_{\mathrm{P}} U_{i\mathrm{P}}^{*} = \sum a_{\mathrm{nb}} U_{i\mathrm{nb}}^{*} + S_{\mathrm{U}_i}^{*} - V_{\mathrm{P}i}\left(\frac{\delta p^{*}}{\delta x_i}\right) \tag{6.37}$$

where $(\delta / \delta x_i)$ indicates a discretized version of spatial derivative and * indicates the guess value or the value obtained from the previous iteration. $V_{\mathrm{P}i}$ is the volume of CV around the node P. The velocity values obtained by solving these equations will not satisfy the continuity equation since the correct pressure field will not be known beforehand. In order to correct the fields obtained, SIMPLE proposes corrections of the form:

$$U_{i\mathrm{P}} = U_{i\mathrm{P}}^{*} + u_{i\mathrm{P}}' \qquad p = p^{*} + p' \tag{6.38}$$

The discretized versions of the momentum equations and Eq. (6.38) lead to discretized equations in terms of velocity and pressure correction:

$$a_{\mathrm{P}} u_{i\mathrm{P}}' = \sum a_{\mathrm{nb}} u_{i\mathrm{nb}}' - V_{\mathrm{P}i}\left(\frac{\delta p'}{\delta x_i}\right) \tag{6.39}$$

The corrected velocities are assumed to satisfy continuity equations. If the corrected velocity expressions (Eq. (6.38)) are substituted in the discretized continuity equation, pressure correction equations can be derived. However, velocity corrections as given by Eq. (6.39) involve velocity corrections at neighboring nodes and unless some approximations are made, it is not possible to obtain the desired pressure correction equations. In SIMPLE algorithm, the first term comprising velocity corrections at the neighboring nodes is neglected to yield a simplified expression for velocity corrections:

$$u_{i\mathrm{P}}' = -\frac{V_{\mathrm{P}i}}{a_{\mathrm{P}}}\left(\frac{\delta p'}{\delta x_i}\right) \tag{6.40}$$

For a staggered grid arrangement, velocity correction can be related to pressure corrections at the two nodes around it:

$$u'_{\mathrm{e}} = \left(\frac{V_{\mathrm{P}}}{a_{\mathrm{P}}\delta x_i}\right)\left(p'_{\mathrm{P}} - p'_{\mathrm{E}}\right) \tag{6.41}$$

Substitution of this velocity correction into the discretized form of the continuity equation then leads to a pressure correction equation of the following form:

$$a_{\mathrm{P}}p'_{\mathrm{P}} = \sum a_{\mathrm{nb}}p'_{\mathrm{nb}} + S^*_{\mathrm{M}} \tag{6.42}$$

where S_{M} is the mass imbalance and * indicates the value obtained from the currently available values of variables. The coefficients of this discretized equation, a_{P} and a_{nb}, can be obtained with the help of Eq. (6.40). Equation (6.42) can be solved to obtain the pressure correction field. Once the pressure correction field is known, Eq. (6.40) can be used to obtain velocity corrections. Equation (6.38) can then be used to obtain the corrected pressure and velocity field. The gross assumption of neglecting velocity corrections at the neighboring nodes (first term of Eq. (6.39)), however, has detrimental consequences on the overall performance of the algorithm. The corrected pressure and velocity fields need to be under-relaxed in order to maintain the stability of the algorithm. As mentioned earlier, under-relaxation is a way to control the change in the variable values during the iterative processes. Such under-relaxation for the pressure and velocity field may considerably reduce the rate of convergence. Several methods have been proposed to enhance the rate of convergence.

van Doormal and Raithby (1984) proposed a variation of SIMPLE, called SIMPLEC (SIMPLE consistent). In this method, instead of neglecting the first term of the right-hand side of Eq. (6.30), it is assumed that the order of magnitude of the velocity corrections at the neighboring nodes will be the same as that of the node under consideration. This assumption is more consistent and leads to the following equation for velocity correction:

$$u'_{i\mathrm{P}} = -\frac{V_{\mathrm{P}i}}{\left(a_{\mathrm{P}} - \sum a_{\mathrm{nb}}\right)}\left(\frac{\delta p'}{\delta x_i}\right) \tag{6.43}$$

The overall algorithm is exactly the same as that of SIMPLE, the only exception being that Eq. (6.43) is used instead of Eq. (6.40) to derive the discretized pressure correction equation. The more consistent approximation proposed in SIMPLEC reduces the need for under-relaxing the pressure.

Patankar (1980) proposed a revised SIMPLE algorithm called SIMPLER (SIMPLE revised). In SIMPLER, the velocity correction part of the SIMPLE algorithm is retained. However, instead of using the pressure corrections to calculate the pressure field, the SIMPLER algorithm uses a separate pressure equation to calculate the pressure field. The discretized momentum equation can be written:

$$a_{\mathrm{P}}U_{i\mathrm{P}} = \sum a_{\mathrm{nb}}U_{i\mathrm{nb}} + S_{\mathrm{U}_i} - V_{\mathrm{P}i}\left(\frac{\delta p}{\delta x_i}\right) \tag{6.44}$$

If Eq. (6.44) is substituted into the discretized continuity equation, a discretized equation of the pressure field can be obtained which will be similar to Eq. (6.42) in form. The coefficients of this pressure equation and pressure correction equation will also be the same. The source terms, however, will be different. In the pressure equation the source terms are calculated in terms of pseudo-velocities, which can be written (drawing an analogy with the earlier derivation):

$$\hat{U}_{i\mathrm{P}} = \frac{\sum a_{\mathrm{nb}} U_{i\mathrm{nb}} + S_{\mathrm{U}_i}}{a_{\mathrm{P}}} \tag{6.45}$$

Since no terms are omitted when deriving the pressure equation used by SIMPLER, the resulting pressure field corresponds with the velocity field. Therefore, unlike SIMPLE, the correct velocity field results in the correct pressure field. Consequently, SIMPLER does not require under-relaxation of pressure and performs significantly better than SIMPLE.

Issa (1986) proposed a two-step corrector algorithm called PISO (pressure implicit with splitting of operators). In this algorithm, the first corrector step is the same as that of the SIMPLE algorithm. The corrected velocity and pressure fields are used to derive the second correction equation. For this second step, the first term in the right-hand side of Eq. (6.39) containing the neighboring velocity corrections is calculated from the first correction step. Application of the discretized continuity equation to the corrected velocities leads to the second pressure correction equation. The coefficients of the second pressure correction equation are the same as those of the first correction equation. The source term, however, contains terms containing neighboring velocity corrections. Details of the derivation of this second correction equation may be found in Issa (1986) and Versteeg and Malalasekara (1995).

Several variants of the SIMPLE family of algorithms have been proposed. Various studies comparing relative performances of these algorithms are available (for example, Jang *et al.*, 1986; Braaten and Shyy, 1987; Wanik and Schnell, 1989; McGuirk and Palma, 1993). It must be noted that there is no single algorithm, which may be identified as the best algorithm for all types of problems. The performance of any algorithm depends on the flow conditions, the degree of coupling between various equations, the amount of under-relaxation used and sometimes, also on details of the numerical technique used to solve the algebraic equations (direction of sweeps and so on). In general, when momentum equations are not coupled with a scalar variable, the PISO algorithm performs better than SIMPLE or SIMPLEC. When such a coupling exists, PISO may show no significant advantage over the other methods. SIMPLER and SIMPLEC have proven to be robust and efficient in strongly coupled problems. Both of these are superior to SIMPLE in many flows. It is, however, difficult to single out a superior algorithm between SIMPLER and SIMPLEC. General experience suggests that SIMPLER is more robust and more suitable for complex applications like multiphase flows.

The solution algorithm for this class of methods can be summarized as follows:

1. Momentum equations are solved using the guessed (or available from the previous iteration) velocity and pressure field.
2. The pressure correction equation is solved and the velocity field is corrected using the derived pressure correction field. For PISO, a second pressure correction equation is solved to correct the pressure and velocities again.

For SIMPLER, the pressure equation is solved based on the updated velocity field.

3. Scalar equations (if any) are then solved using the corrected velocity field (for example, k and ε equations when solving the k–ε model of turbulence or the enthalpy equation when solving non-isothermal flows).
4. Fluid properties are updated (if not constants).
5. Return to step 1 until a converged solution is obtained.

The algorithms discussed so far can be applied directly when staggered grids are used. In staggered grids, the cell face values required for assembling the discretized continuity equation are available readily and contain the pressure gradient terms naturally. For the colocated grid, however, some modifications to these algorithms are required to avoid oscillations in the pressure field. Although these oscillations can be filtered out (van der Wijngaart, 1990), to devise a compact pressure correction equation similar to those discussed earlier, it is necessary to consider corrections to cell face velocities rather that node velocities (where the values are naturally available in colocated grids). The corrections to cell face velocities can be derived following the methods discussed earlier, the only difference is that the coefficient a_P in Eq. (6.40) are not the nodal values, as in the staggered arrangement, but are interpolated cell center values. This procedure may appear unnatural compared to direct application of the staggered arrangement, however, as mentioned in the previous sub-section, a colocated grid arrangement is preferable for flow simulations in complex geometry. Details of the derivation of pressure correction equations and application of SIMPLE-like algorithms to colocated grids may be found in Lilek and Peric (1995) and Ferziger and Peric (1995) among others. In general, the performance of SIMPLE-like algorithms (convergence rate, dependence on under-relaxation factors, computing costs etc.) is similar for staggered and colocated grid arrangements. The difference between solutions obtained with different variable arrangements is much smaller than the discretization error.

The overall solution procedure and other finer details of under-relaxation and convergence criteria are briefly discussed in Section 6.5. It is useful to briefly discuss the implementation of commonly encountered boundary conditions when solving flow field equations.

6.3.3. Implementation of Boundary Conditions

Mathematical formulations of various boundary conditions were discussed in Section 2.3. These boundary conditions may be implemented numerically within the finite volume framework by expressing the flux at the boundary as a combination of interior values and boundary data. Usually, boundary conditions enter the discretized equations by suppression of the link to the boundary side and modification of the source terms. The appropriate coefficient of the discretized equation is set to zero and the boundary side flux (exact or approximated) is introduced through the linearized source terms, S_C and S_P. Since there are no nodes outside the solution domain, the approximations of boundary side flux are based on one-sided differences or extrapolations. Implementation of commonly encountered boundary conditions is discussed below. The technique of modifying the source terms of discretized equation can also be used to set the specific value of a variable at the given node. To set a value at node P, the components of the linearized source terms, S_C and S_P, are set to very large values, like ($\phi_{set}\ 10^{30}$) and (-10^{30}) respectively. In such a case, the right and left sides of the discretized equation (Eq. (6.12)) are dominated by these large terms yielding approximately:

$$\left(\approx 10^{30}\right)\phi_P = \left(\approx 10^{30}\right)\phi_{set} \tag{6.46}$$

This fixes the value of variable ϕ at node P to ϕ_{set}. This method can also be used to simulate solid obstacles within a solution domain by fixing ϕ_{set} to zero. The system of discretized equations can then be solved as usual without considering the obstacles separately.

Convective fluxes are usually specified at the inlet boundaries (and set to zero at impermeable walls and the symmetry axis). Upwind approximations can usually be used. For the staggered grid arrangement, the velocity node is located at the boundary surface. The velocity at such a node on the boundary is then directly specified without the need for solving the discretized equation. For colocated grids, the specified inlet velocity is used to calculate the convective flux from the cell face coinciding with the inlet boundary. For diffusive fluxes, either the flux or the boundary value of the variable is specified. If the boundary value is specified, diffusive fluxes are evaluated using one-sided approximations for normal gradients. If the flux is specified, it is used to calculate the flux, and an approximation to the flux in terms of nodal values can be used to calculate the boundary value of the variable. For the zero gradient boundary condition, no term needs to be added to the source term.

For a staggered grid arrangement, a knowledge of pressure is not required at the boundaries on which the normal velocity is specified. At such boundaries, zero gradient boundary conditions should be used for pressure correction and pressure equations. When boundary pressure is specified, the pressure correction at the boundary needs to be set to zero. When a colocated grid arrangement is used, the boundary pressure needs to be known in order to calculate pressure forces appearing in the momentum equations. This is normally obtained by extrapolation. In most cases, linear extrapolation is sufficient. It must be noted that for incompressible flows, the absolute value of pressure (and, therefore, of pressure correction) is not relevant; only differences in the pressure are meaningful. Usually, the pressure is set to a fixed reference value at a suitable grid point and pressure values at all other nodes are calculated relative to this reference value.

At the outlet, extrapolation of the velocity to the boundary (zero gradient at the outlet boundary) can usually be used. At impermeable walls, the normal velocity is set to zero. The wall shear stress is then included in the source terms. In the case of turbulent flows, wall functions are used near walls instead of resolving gradients near the wall (refer to the discussion in Chapter 3). Careful linearization of source terms arising due to these wall functions is necessary for efficient numerical implementation. Other boundary conditions such as symmetry, periodic or cyclic can be implemented by combining the formulations discussed in Chapter 2 with the ideas of finite volume method discussed here. More details on numerical implementation of boundary conditions may be found in Patankar (1980) and Versteeg and Malalasekara (1995).

6.4. FINITE VOLUME METHOD FOR UNSTEADY FLOWS

To compute unsteady flows, the time derivative terms in the governing equations need to be discretized. The major difference in the space and time co-ordinates lies in the direction of influence. In unsteady flows, there is no backward influence. The governing equations for unsteady flows are, therefore, parabolic in time. Therefore, essentially all the numerical methods advance in time, in a step-by-step or 'marching' approach. These methods are very similar to those applied for initial value problems (IVPs) of ordinary differential equations. In this section, some of the methods widely used in the context of the finite volume method are discussed.

For unsteady flows, discretization schemes need to be devised to evaluate the integrals with respect to time (refer to Eq. (6.2)). The control volume integration is similar to that in steady flows discussed earlier. The most widely used methods for discretization of time derivatives are two-level methods. In order to facilitate further discussion, let us rewrite the basic governing equation as an ordinary differential equation with respect to time by employing the spatial discretization schemes discussed earlier:

$$\frac{d\phi}{dt} = f(t, \phi) \tag{6.47}$$

By integrating with respect to time between two grid points, one obtains:

$$\int_{n}^{n+1} \frac{d\phi}{dt}\, dt = \phi^{n+1} - \phi^{n} = \int_{n}^{n+1} f(t, \phi)\, dt \tag{6.48}$$

Since the variation of ϕ with time is not known, some approximations are necessary to evaluate the integration of the function. Four commonly used approximations are detailed below (shown schematically in Fig. 6.10).

(a) Explicit Euler: Integral is evaluated using the value of ϕ available at the previous node:

$$\int_{n}^{n+1} f(t, \phi)\, dt = \Delta t f(t_n, \phi_n) \tag{6.49}$$

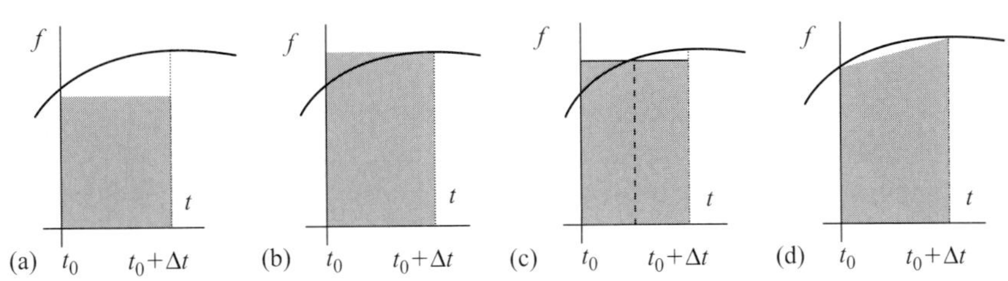

FIGURE 6.10 Approximation of time integral. (a) Explicit, (b) Implicit, (c) Mid-point, (d) Trapezoid.

(b) Implicit Euler: Integral is evaluated using the value of ϕ available at the next node:

$$\int_{n}^{n+1} f(t,\phi)\,dt = \Delta t f(t_{n+1},\phi_{n+1}) \tag{6.50}$$

(c) Mid-point rule: Integral is evaluated using the value of ϕ available at the mid-point:

$$\int_{n}^{n+1} f(t,\phi)\,dt = \Delta t f(t_{n+\frac{1}{2}},\phi_{n+\frac{1}{2}}) \tag{6.51}$$

(d) Trapezoid rule: Integral is evaluated using linear interpolation:

$$\int_{n}^{n+1} f(t,\phi)\,dt = \Delta t \frac{1}{2}\left[f(t_n,\phi_n) + f(t_{n+1},\phi_{n+1})\right] \tag{6.52}$$

The first method is an explicit method while the remaining three are implicit methods (to varying degree). The Euler explicit and implicit methods are first-order accurate (errors are proportional to Δt) while the remaining two methods are second-order accurate (errors are proportional to Δt^2). Explicit methods have minimum requirements for memory and computations but are unstable at larger time steps. Implicit methods may require an iterative solution (and more memory) to obtain the values at the new time step but are much more stable. Apart from the two-level methods discussed here, there are multi-level methods such as the Runge–Kutta methods and Adams methods. Detailed discussion of these methods can be found in Press *et al.* (1992). For computational flow modeling, if the spatial discretization is second-order accurate, two-level methods for integration with respect to time will generally be sufficient, and are widely used. For special purposes, when higher order spatial discretization is used (for example, in large eddy simulations), higher order schemes can be used. Here we discuss application of two-level methods to solve the generic unsteady transport equation (Eq. (6.1)).

Integration of first term of Eq. (6.1) over a computational cell and over a time interval can be written as:

$$\int\int_V \frac{\partial(\rho\phi)}{\partial t} dV\,dt = \left(\phi_{\mathrm{P}}^{n+1} - \phi_{\mathrm{P}}^{n}\right)\rho\,\Delta V \tag{6.53}$$

The procedure for evaluating integrals of the remaining terms of Eq. (6.1) over a control volume remain the same as discussed earlier. To evaluate integration with respect to time, it will be necessary to employ one of the two-level methods discussed above. As mentioned earlier, generally all the terms appearing in Eq. (6.1) are linearized when carrying out discretization. Linearization simplifies the task of time integration. Integration of ϕ with respect to time can then be written (considering the example of a term containing ϕ_{E}):

$$\int a_{\mathrm{E}}\phi_{\mathrm{E}}\,dt = a_{\mathrm{E}}\left[\theta\phi_{\mathrm{E}}^{n+1} + (1-\theta)\,\phi_{\mathrm{E}}^{n}\right]\Delta t \tag{6.54}$$

where θ is a parameter controlling the degree of implicitness. Zero implies an explicit scheme, and one implies a fully implicit scheme (0.5 corresponds to the Crank–Nicholson scheme). Carrying out such a procedure for all terms of the governing transport equation, a discretized equation similar to Eq. (6.11), is obtained for the unsteady simulations:

$$a_P\phi_P^{n+1} = \sum_{nb} a_{nb}\left[\theta\phi_{nb}^{n+1} + (1-\theta)\,\phi_{nb}^{n}\right] + \left(a_P^0 - \sum_{nb}(1-\theta)\,a_{nb} + (1-\theta)\,S_P\right)\phi_P^n + S_{C\phi} \tag{6.55}$$

where

$$a_P = \theta\sum_{nb} a_{nb} + a_P^0 - \theta S_{P\phi} \qquad a_P^0 = \rho\frac{\Delta V}{\Delta t} \tag{6.56}$$

For physically realistic and bounded results, it is necessary to ensure that all the coefficients of the discretization equation are positive. This requirement imposes restrictions on the time step that can be used with different values of θ. It can be seen that a fully implicit method with θ equal to unity is unconditionally stable. Detailed stability analysis is rather complex when both convection and diffusion are present. In general, simplified criteria may be used when an explicit method is used in practical simulations:

$$\Delta t < \frac{\Delta x_i}{U_i} \quad \text{or} \quad \frac{\Delta x^2}{2\Gamma_\phi} \tag{6.57}$$

These criteria can be interpreted as no fluid particle (information) can propagate more than one grid length in a single time step. If the details of development from the initial guess to the final steady state are not important and only the final steady state is of interest, such a restriction on the time step may limit the rate of convergence. In such a case, implicit methods are advantageous. Since implicit methods are unconditionally stable, large time steps can be used and it might suffice to do a single iteration per time step. Such a pseudo-time-marching approach can be conveniently used to obtain steady state solutions to complex flow problems. Pseudo-time-marching is analogous to employing an under-relaxation. Pseudo-time-marching uses the same time step for all CVs, which is equivalent to using a different under-relaxation factor for each CV; use of a constant under-relaxation factor for all CVs is equivalent to applying a different time step for each CV. Typical steps in applying SIMPLE-like algorithms to solve unsteady flow problems are summarized in Fig. 6.11. Within a single time step it may be necessary to carry out several iterations to obtain an adequately converged solution of the governing equations. Within each such iteration, there may be internal iterations to solve algebraic equations. Some issues related to the overall performance of such a solution procedure are discussed in the next chapter.

6.5. APPLICATION OF FINITE VOLUME METHOD

Implementation of the basic steps of the finite volume method discussed above to solve the governing equations of a flow model requires development of a computer

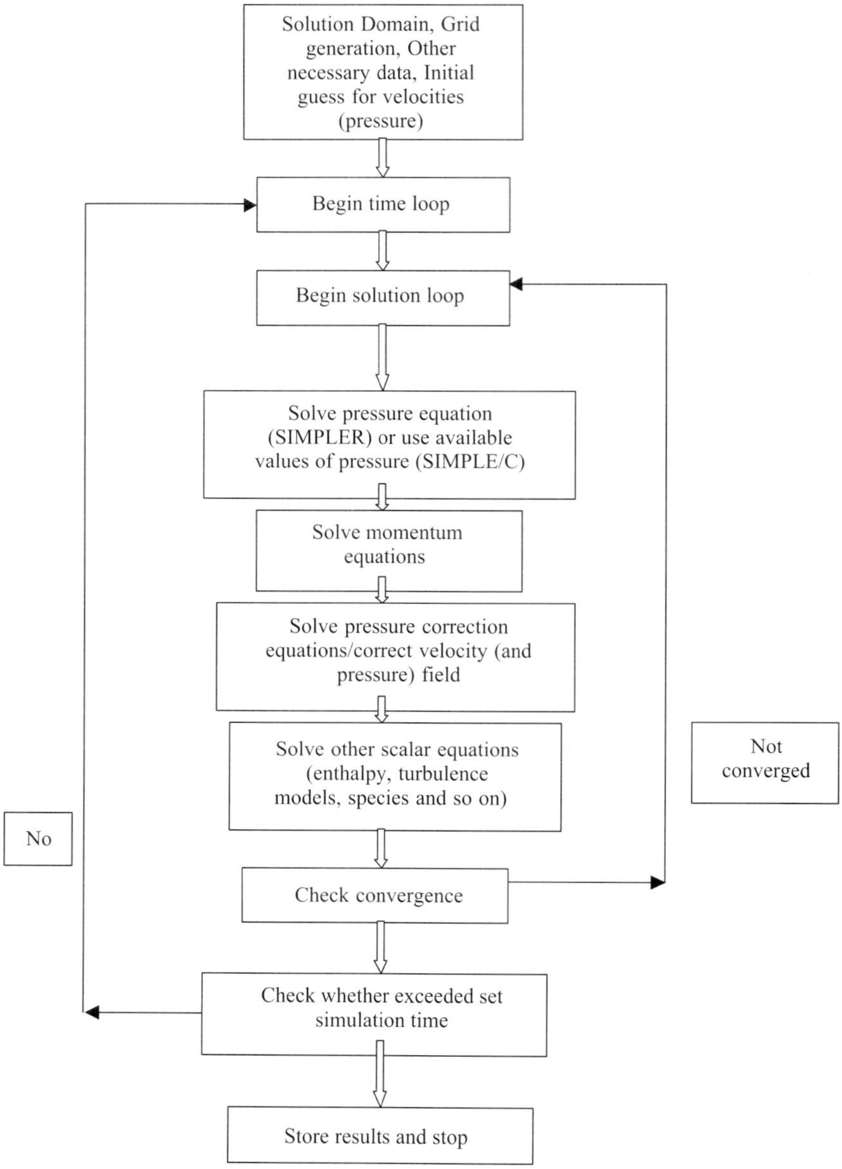

FIGURE 6.11 SIMPLE family of algorithms for unsteady flows.

program. Development of a computer program involves many issues and is outside the scope of this work. It is assumed that suitable computational tools are available to a reactor engineer. Key issues which need to be considered when selecting suitable computational tools, are discussed in Chapter 8. In this section, various issues relevant to computational flow simulations are discussed with the help of a simple example. Consider a cubical vessel with rectangular inlet and outlets as shown in Fig. 6.12a. Geometrical and other details are given in Table 6.1. Simulations were carried out for four different viscosity fluids (in the range 0.001 Pa.s to 100 Pa.s) to determine the possible influence of viscosity on the numerical solution of model equations.

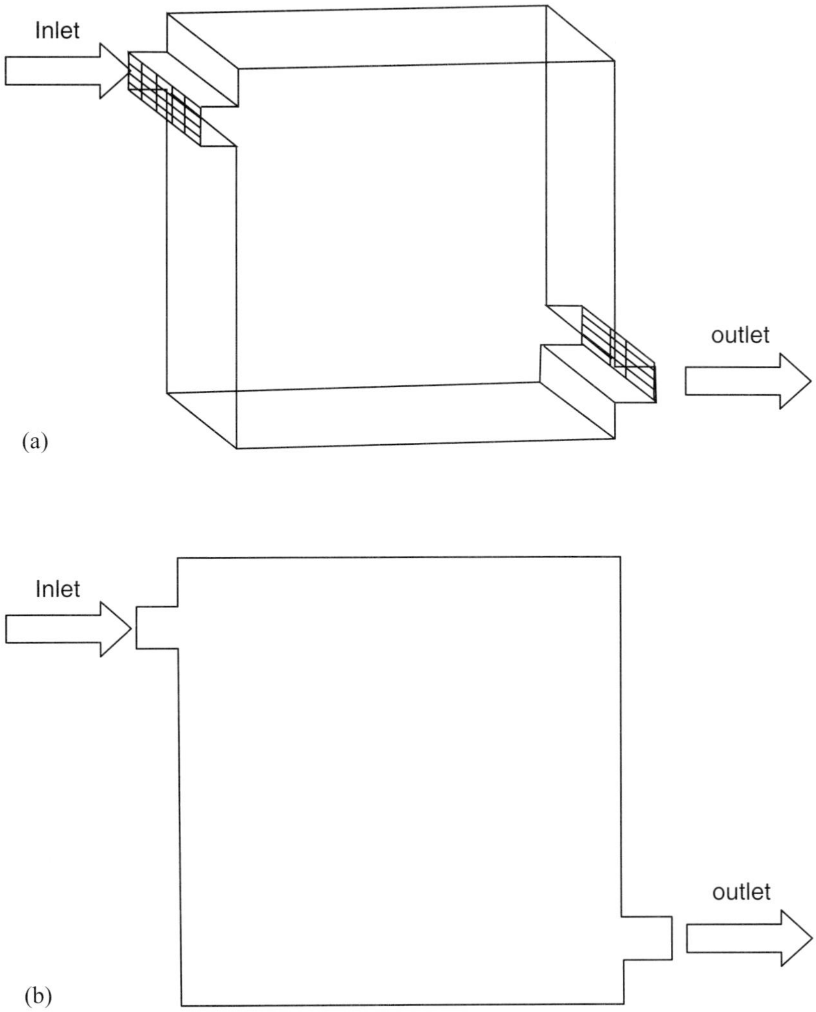

FIGURE 6.12 Outline of vessel (isometric and two-dimensional approximation).

TABLE 6.1 Data Used for Simulation Example

Three-dimensional vessel (Fig. 6.12a):
Volume = 1 m^3
Length = Depth = Breadth = 1 m
Inlet area = 0.1 × 1.0 = 0.1 m^2
(Distance between top edge of inlet to vessel edge = 0.1 m)
Outlet area = 0.1 × 1.0 = 0.1 m^2
(Distance between bottom edge of outlet to vessel bottom = 0.1 m)
Two-dimensional approximation (Fig. 6.12b):
Depth = 0.01 m
Inlet velocity = 1 m s^{-1}
Fluid viscosity = 0.001 Pa.s, 1 Pa.s, 10 Pa.s and 100 Pa.s

6.5.1. Solution Domain and Computational Grid

The first task in initiating a numerical simulation is to select an appropriate solution domain and formulate appropriate boundary conditions to specify the influence of the environment on flow processes in the considered solution domain. Flow in a cubical vessel with rectangular inlet and outlet can be conveniently modeled by considering a two-dimensional geometry, if the end effects are assumed not to be important. In any case, it can be seen that the most important flow processes occur in the x–y plane. It is, therefore, useful to examine various numerical issues such as the required number of grids, discretization schemes etc., by carrying out two-dimensional simulations. If necessary, after identifying an adequate number of grid points, a complete three-dimensional simulation may be carried out to verify the adequacy of the two-dimensional approximation. A two-dimensional solution domain was therefore considered for numerical simulation of the flow in a cubical vessel (Fig. 6.12b).

The next issue is the formulation of appropriate boundary conditions. The availability of suitable boundary conditions may also affect the decision concerning the extent of the solution domain. Obviously in practice, the inlet and outlet of any vessel will be connected to the associated pipe work. It is essential to decide the extent of the solution domain in such a way that it does not affect the simulated results. Generally for high velocity inlets, conditions in the process vessel do not affect the flow characteristics of the inlet pipe, and therefore it is acceptable to set the inlet boundary conditions right at the vessel boundary. More often than not, some piping at the outlet section may have to be considered if the outlet boundary condition is to be used. Alternatively, one may use constant pressure boundary conditions. Possible boundary conditions and solution domain are shown in Fig. 6.13. Before examining the influence of the solution domain on the simulated results, it is necessary to identify an adequate number of grids to resolve all the major features of the flow.

Flow simulations in the simplest solution domain (Fig. 6.13a) were carried out with different numbers of grids: 10×10, 20×20, 40×40, 80×80. Commercial CFD code, FLUENT (Fluent Inc., USA) was used for these simulations. Since the geometry of the proposed solution domain was simple, it was possible to generate a suitable computational grid using the tools provided within FLUENT, and a separate grid generation tool was unnecessary. For all of these four grid levels, uniform grids were used. Typical grids used for simulations (for the 40×40 case) are shown in Fig. 6.14. Typical flow results in the form of vector and contour plots are shown in Fig. 6.15. The influence of grids on predicted results is shown in Fig. 6.16. All of these results were obtained for fluid with viscosity 100 Pa.s. It can be seen that there is almost no change in the predicted results for grids beyond 40×40. Therefore, 40×40 grids (for square geometry) were used to examine the influence of length of the outlet pipe and corresponding boundary conditions. Comparison of predicted results for different configurations is shown in Fig. 6.17. Since the difference in predicted results with and without outlet pipes is not significant, for all further simulations, a solution domain without extensions of inlet or outlet pipes was considered.

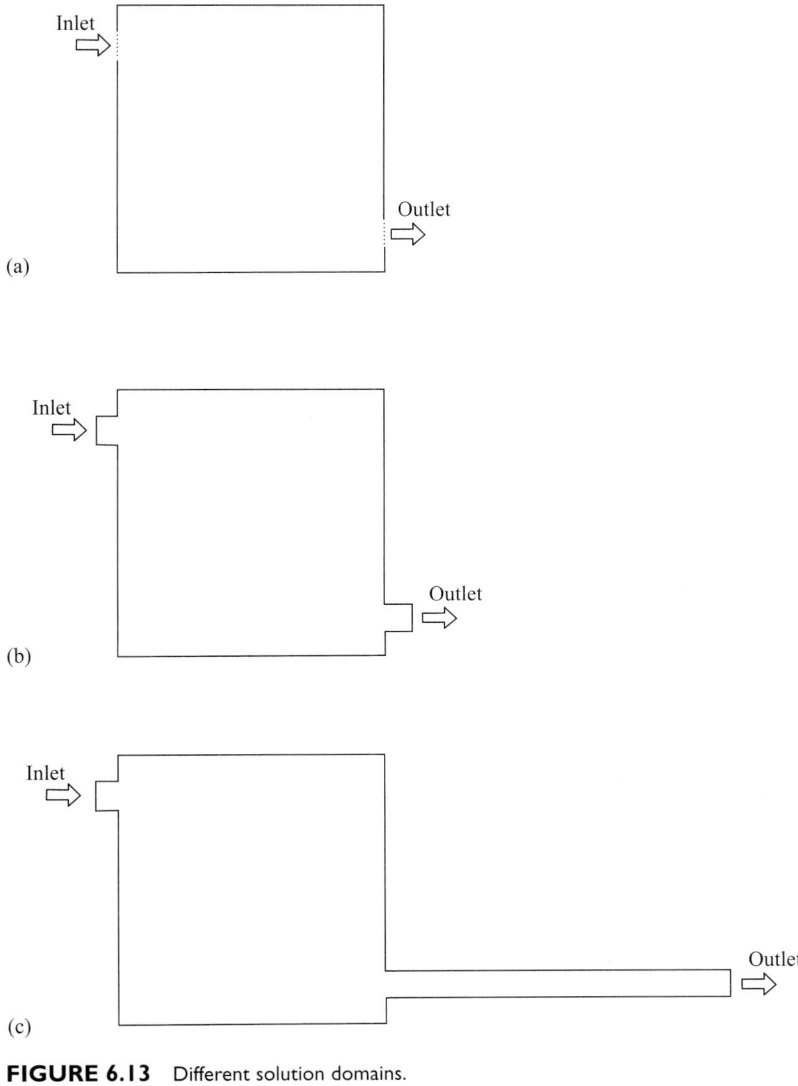

FIGURE 6.13 Different solution domains.

6.5.2. Convergence and Error Analysis

As mentioned in the earlier part of this chapter, the overall solution procedure is iterative and an adequate degree of convergence needs to be ensured before further processing of simulated results. Usually a measure of how closely each discretized equation is balanced is used to decide convergence. For this, generally the imbalance in the governing equations is summed over all computational cells in the solution domain. Such a sum is called the residual and for a general conservation equation can be written (from Eq. (6.12)):

$$R = \sum_{\text{all nodes}} \left| a_{\mathrm{E}}\phi_{\mathrm{E}} + a_{\mathrm{W}}\phi_{\mathrm{W}} + a_{\mathrm{WW}}\phi_{\mathrm{WW}} + a_{\mathrm{N}}\phi_{N} + a_{\mathrm{S}}\phi_{\mathrm{S}} + a_{\mathrm{SS}}\phi_{\mathrm{SS}} + S_{\mathrm{C}}^{\phi} - a_{\mathrm{P}}\phi_{\mathrm{P}} \right| \tag{6.58}$$

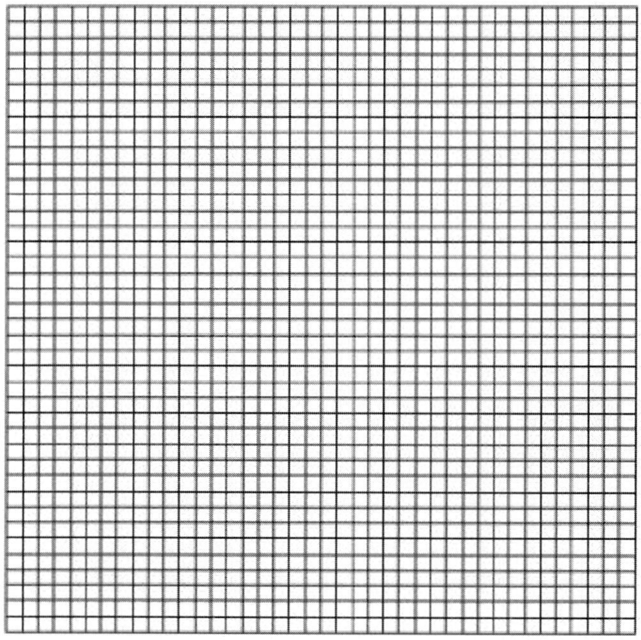

FIGURE 6.14 Typical grid used for simulations (40 × 40).

The residuals (R) for each of the governing equations need to be reduced to an adequately low level. Definition of an 'adequate' degree of convergence may be problem dependent. In general, an examination of the history of residuals and variables at key locations, along with the integral balances may provide a good indication of the degree of convergence. The convergence behavior of a numerical method depends on several factors discussed in this chapter. For a given algorithm and discretization scheme, values of the under-relaxation factor control the rate of convergence.

For the problem considered in the previous sections, the influence of under-relaxation factors on the reduction in residuals is shown in Fig. 6.18. It can be seen that up to a certain limit, as the under-relaxation factor increases, the rate of residual reduction increases. However beyond a certain limit, further increase in under-relaxation parameters may lead to divergence (see, for example, results for an under-relaxation parameter of 0.85, where residues increase with further iterations). For an under-relaxation parameter of 0.6 (for velocities), residual and variable history are shown in Fig. 6.19. These profiles and an examination of integral balances indicate that adequate convergence occurs in about 150 iterations. Further simulations lead to further reduction in residuals, however, the predicted results are almost independent of the actual value of residuals beyond 150 iterations. This fact further confirms that convergence level obtained at 150 iterations (with an under-relaxation parameter of 0.6) was satisfactory. Comparison of the converged results obtained using different under-relaxation parameters confirms that the value of under-relaxation parameter has no influence on the converged results. After ensuring adequate convergence, it is important to examine possible errors in the simulated results.

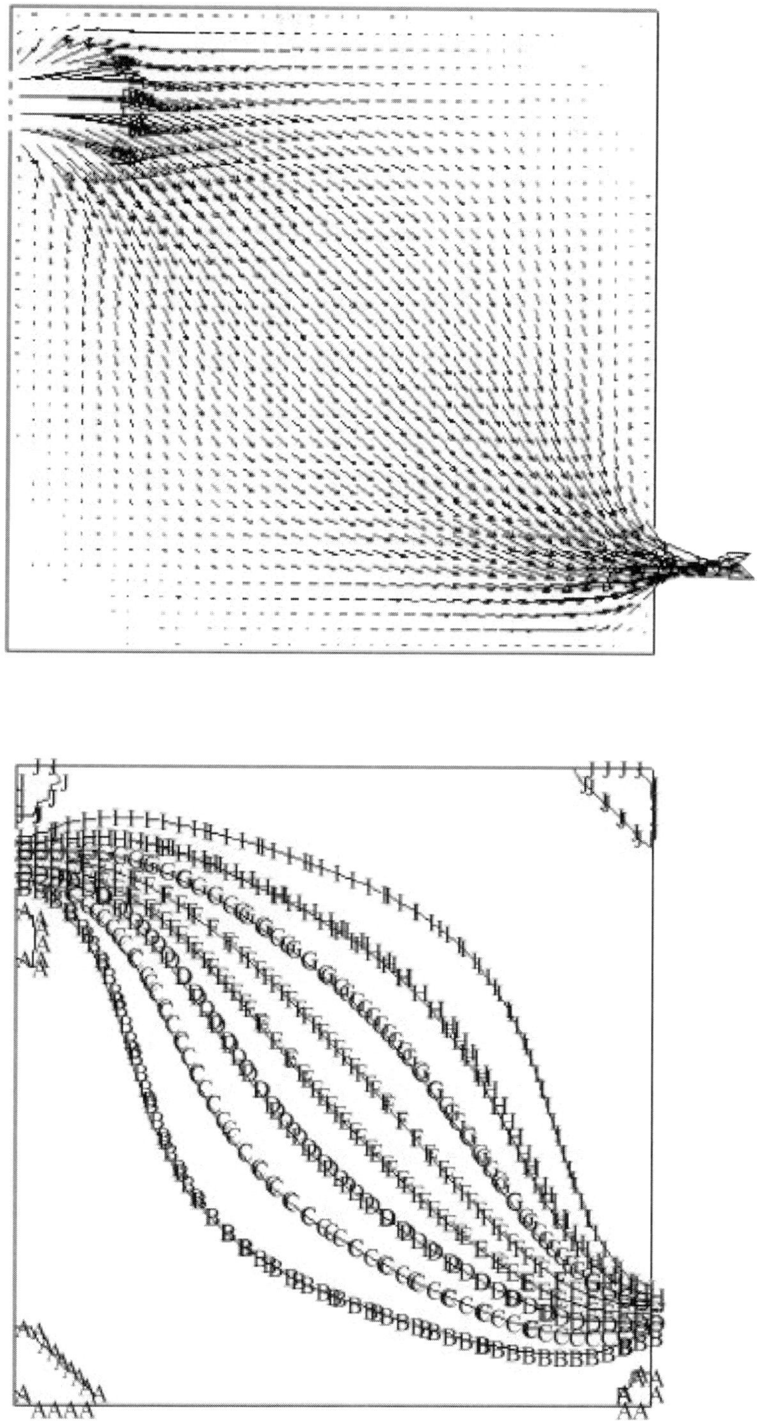

FIGURE 6.15 Typical simulation results; Grid: 40 × 40. Vector: maximum length 1 m s^{-1}. Contours of stream function: 10 uniform contours between 0 to 0.001 (Lowest level: A; Highest level: J).

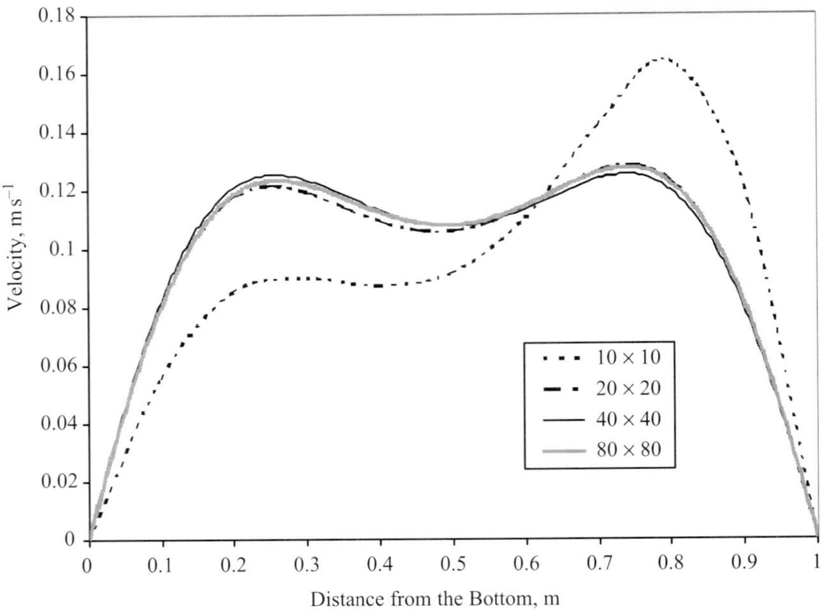

FIGURE 6.16 Influence of grid size of predicted results (Velocity profile at $x = 0.5$ m).

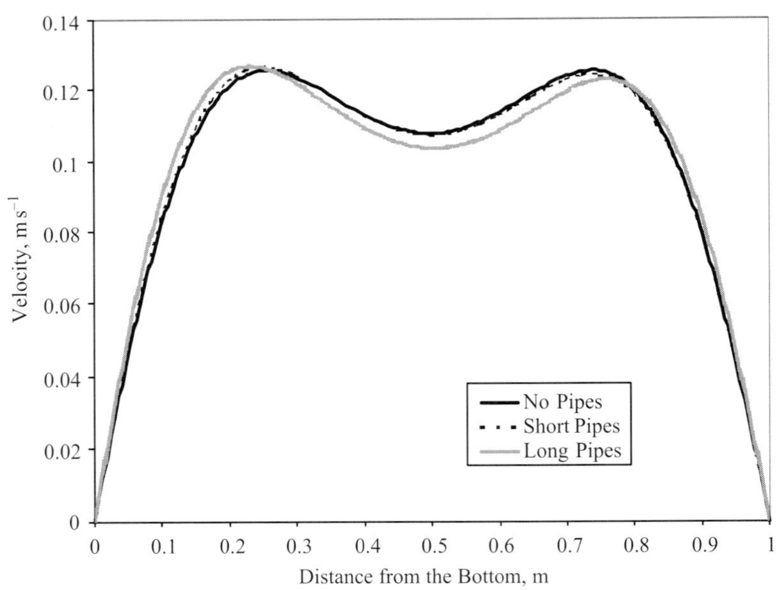

FIGURE 6.17 Influence of solution domain of predicted results (Velocity profile at $x = 0.5$ m; Grid: 40×40).

There are several ways of evaluating possible errors in the simulated results. Values of residuals in the discretized equations are one of the indicators of errors. In addition, it is often useful to examine integrated fluxes of the quantity of interest (for example, mass flow rate) and compare them with the expected values. For example,

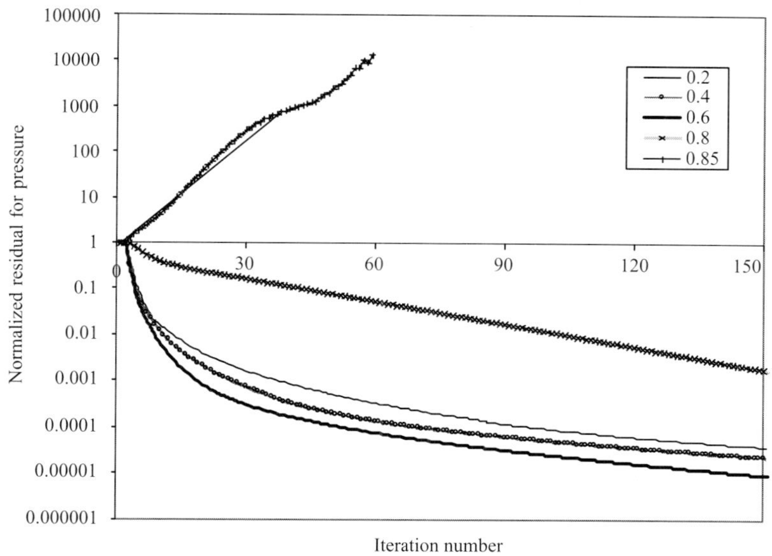

FIGURE 6.18 Influence of under-relaxation parameters on convergence (Pressure residual; Grid: 40 × 40).

in the case considered, net mass flow passing through any constant I plane should be equal to the inlet mass flow rate. Simulated results reveal that computed net mass flow rate is the same as the inlet flow rate, indicating adequate convergence. All the results discussed so far were obtained with a first-order upwind differencing scheme. In order to assess the quality of results, simulations were carried out for two higher order schemes: a second-order upwind method and QUICK (with SMART limiter to prevent non-physical oscillation). The predicted profiles at the mid-I plane of the base case are compared with the results of these two cases in Fig. 6.20. It can be seen that the difference in predicted results of the three discretization schemes is not significant. Thus, simulated results are not dependent on any of the numerical parameters: number of grids, discretization schemes, convergence criterion and so on. After ensuring this, further evaluation of simulated results can be done with the help of experimental data, if available. After such validation, the computational model may be used to understand the flow process under consideration. Here we illustrate the possible use of the computational model to understand the influence of the fluid viscosity on the fluid dynamics of the considered configuration.

6.5.3. Simulations with Low Viscosity Fluid

Starting with simulations of fluid with viscosity 100 Pa.s, further simulations were carried out for fluids with viscosity 10 Pa.s, 1 Pa.s and 0.001 Pa.s. Initially all simulations were carried out for 40 × 40 grids. Typical predicted results are shown in Figs 6.21 and 6.22. It can be seen that fluid viscosity has a pronounced influence on fluid dynamics. As the viscosity decreases, the penetration depth of the incoming jet increases, leading to circulatory flow within the domain. For lower viscosity fluids, much sharper profiles exist within the solution domain. It will be of interest

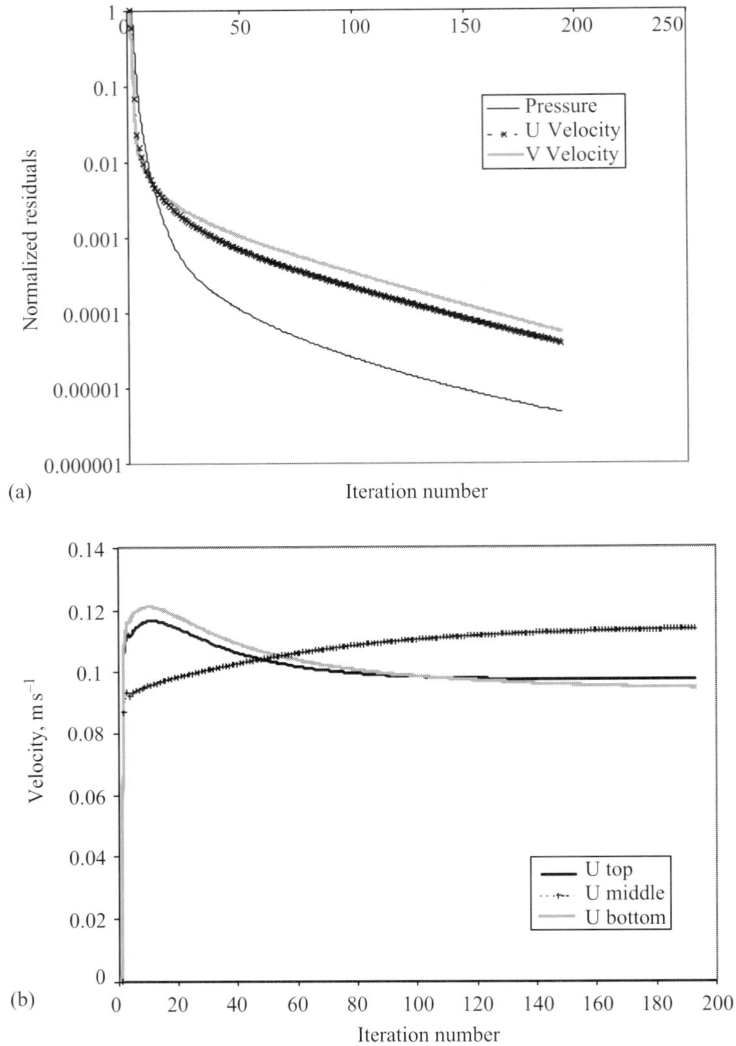

FIGURE 6.19 Residual and variable history (Under-relaxation factor for velocity = 0.6; Grid: 40 × 40). (a) Residuals; (b) Velocity (top: $J = 36$; middle: $J = 22$; bottom: $J = 7$).

to examine whether the conclusion of grid adequacy is valid for the low viscosity fluids. Predicted results for the lowest viscosity fluids, obtained with different grids, are shown in Fig. 6.23. It can be seen that the predicted results are functions of grid size and are no longer grid independent even for the finest grid size used (640 × 640). This can be understood with reference to the phenomenon of turbulence discussed in Chapter 3. For a fluid with viscosity of 0.001 Pa.s, the set boundary conditions generate flow with sharp gradients, through which flow instability and turbulence sets in. In turbulent flow widely different scales co-exist and flow becomes inherently unsteady. It can be seen that even 400 000 computational cells turn out to be inadequate to capture all the small-scale features of turbulence (without using unsteady state equations). It may be necessary to use an appropriate turbulence model in such a

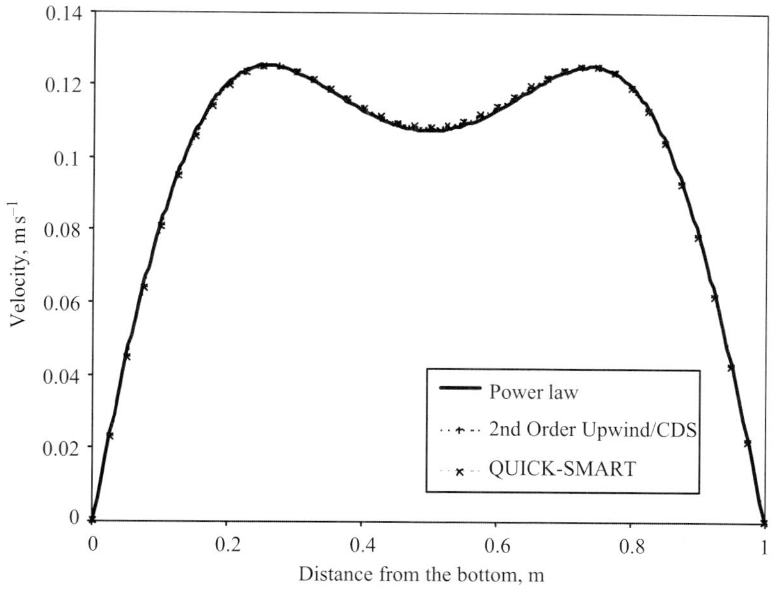

FIGURE 6.20 Influence of discretization scheme on predicted results (Velocity profile at $x = 0.5$; Grid: 40×40).

case. The solution of model equations describing turbulent and other complex flows is discussed in the next chapter.

6.6. SUMMARY

The finite volume method ensures integral conservation of mass, momentum and energy and is, therefore, attractive for reactor engineering applications. The steps in applying the finite volume method to solve transport equations are listed below.

- Select appropriate solution domain (and boundary conditions).
- Divide the selected domain into an adequate (which may be verified by examining the grid dependence of predicted results) number of computational cells.
- Obtain a set of discretized equations by integrating transport equations over computational cells. This step requires use of various discretization and interpolation schemes.
- Select an appropriate algorithm to treat the various couplings and non-linearities.
- Select a corresponding method to solve the linearized algebraic equations.
- Implement these methods in a computer program and obtain results.
- Evaluate the results obtained.

Each of these steps has been discussed in detail in this chapter. Generally, second-order approximations for interpolation are adequate. Various second-order schemes and their modified versions to minimize non-physical 'wiggles' were discussed.

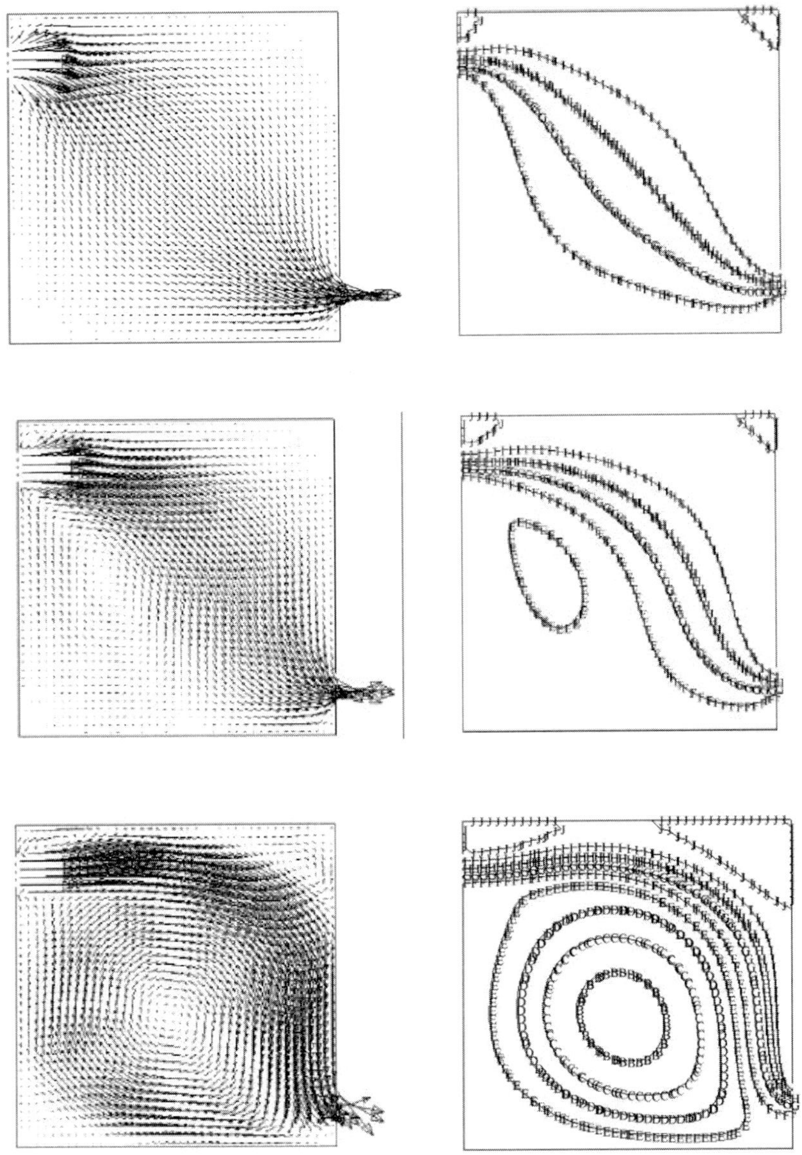

(a) (b) (c)

FIGURE 6.21 Influence of viscosity (Vector plots; contours of stream function: $A = -0.001$ and $J = 0.001$). Viscosity (a) 100 Pa.s; (b) 10 Pa.s; (c) 1 Pa.s.

The QUICK discretization scheme along with SMART or SHARP modifications, is recommended. Various algorithms for treating pressure–velocity coupling were discussed. The performance of these algorithms depends on flow conditions, degree of coupling between various equations, under-relaxation parameters and so on. Our experience of using the SIMPLER algorithm for a wide variety of reactors indicates that it is quite robust and efficient. A cubical reactor was considered to demonstrate

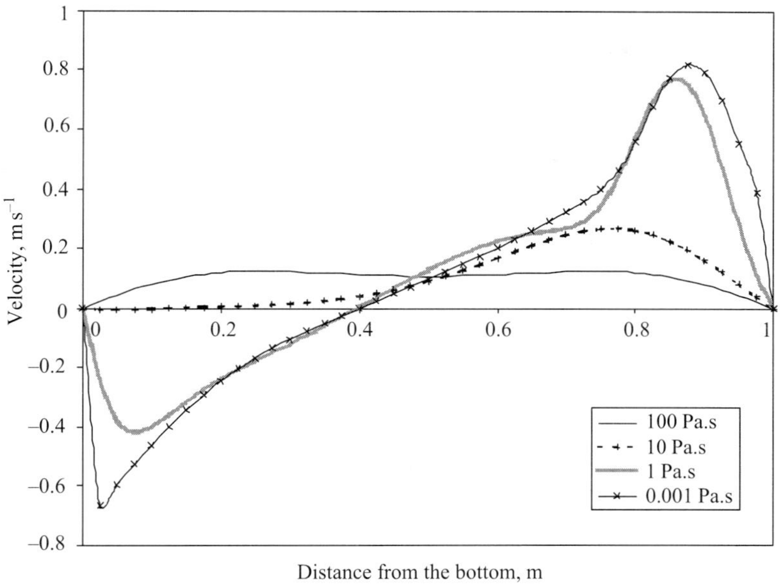

FIGURE 6.22 Influence of viscosity (U profile at $x = 0.5$; Grid: 40×40).

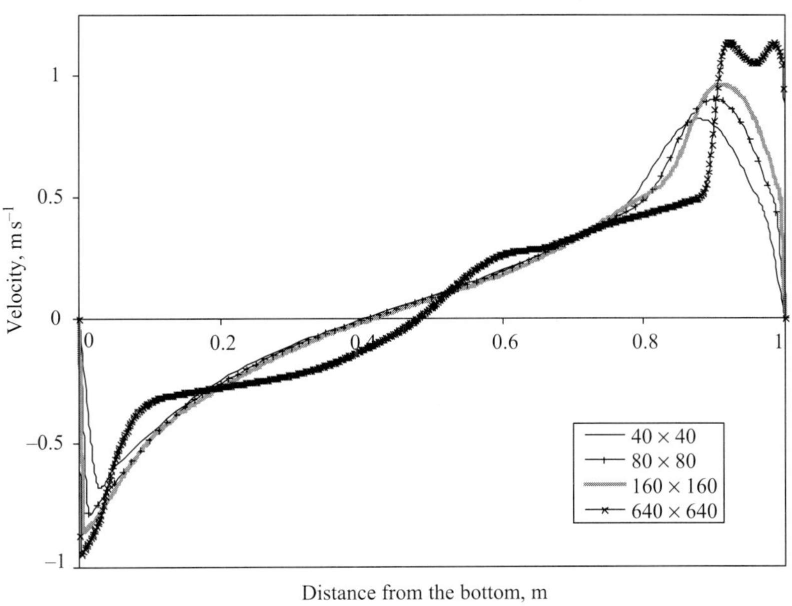

FIGURE 6.23 Influence of grid size for low viscosity fluid ($\mu = 0.001$ Pa.s).

application of the finite volume method to flow simulations. Various aspects of practical flow simulations (including post-processing) were illustrated with the help of this example. Difficulties in obtaining grid-independent results for the case of turbulent flows were illustrated. The solution of model equations describing turbulent and other complex flows is discussed in the next chapter.

REFERENCES

Anderson, D.A., Tannehill, J.C. and Pletcher, R.H. (1984), "Computational fluid Mechanics and Heat Transfer", Hemisphere, New York.

Braaten, M.E. and Shyy, W. (1987), Study of pressure correction methods with multigrid for viscous flow calculations in non-orthogonal curvilinear co-ordinates, *Numerical Heat Transfer*, **11**, 417–442.

Ferziger, J.H. and Peric, M. (1995), "Computational Methods For Fluid Dynamics", Springer-Verlag, Berlin.

Fletcher, C.J. (1991), "Computational Techniques for Fluid Dynamics", Vols I and II, Springer-Verlag, Berlin.

Gaskell, P.H. and Lau, A.K.C. (1988), Curvature – compensated convective transport: SMART, A new boundedness preserving transport algorithm, *Int. J. Numerical Methods Fluids*, **8**(6), 617–641.

Golub, G.H. and van Loan, C. (1990), "Matrix Computations", Johns Hopkins University Press, Baltimore.

Hackbusch, W. (1985), "Multi-grid Methods and Applications", Springer, Berlin.

Hayase, T., Humphrey, J.A.C. and Grief, R. (1992), A constantly formulated QUICK scheme for fast and stable convergence using finite volume iterative calculation procedures, *J. Computat. Phys.*, **98**, 108–118.

Hutchinson, B.R. and Raithby, G.D. (1986), A multigrid method based on additive correction strategy, *Numerical Heat Transfer*, **9**, 511–537.

Issa, R.I. (1986), Solution of the implicitly discretized fluid flow equations by operator splitting, *J. Computat. Phys.*, **62**, 40–65.

Jang, D.S., Jetli, R. and Acharya, S. (1986), Comparison of the PISO, SIMPLER and SIMPLEC algorithms for the treatment of the pressure velocity coupling in steady flow problems, *Numerical Heat Transfer*, **19**, 209–228.

Kelkar, K.M. and Patankar, S.V. (1989), Development of generalized block correction procedure for the solution of discretized Navier–Stokes Equation, *Comput. Phys. Commun.*, **53**, 329–336.

Leonard, B.P. (1979), A stable and accurate convective modeling procedure based on quadratic upstream interpolation, *Comput. Methods Appl. Mech. Eng.*, **19**, 59–98.

Leonard, B.P. (1988), Third-order multidimensional monotonic Euler/ Navier Stokes Solver, Draft for First National Fluid Dynamic Conference, Cincinnati, Ohio, July 1988.

Leveque, R.J. (1996), High-resolution conservative algorithms for advection in incompressible flow, *SIAM J. Numer. Anal.*, **33**, 627–665.

Lilek, Z. and Peric, M. (1995), A fourth order finite volume method with colocated variable arrangement, *Comput. Fluids*, **24**, 239–252.

McGuirk, J.J. and Palma, J.M.L.M. (1993), The efficiency of alternative pressure-correction formulations for incompressible turbulent flow problems, *Comput. Fluids*, **22**, 77.

Patankar, S.V. (1980), "Numerical Heat Transfer and Fluid Flow", Hemisphere, Taylor & Francis Group, New York.

Patankar, S.V. and Spalding, D.B. (1972), A calculation procedure for heat, mass and momentum transfer in three-dimensional parabolic flows, *Int. J. Heat Mass Transfer*, **15**, 1787.

Peric, M. (1987), Efficient semi-implicit solving algorithm for nine-diagonal co-efficient matrix, *Numerical Heat Transfer*, **11**, 251–279.

Peric, M., Kessler, R. and Scheuerer, G. (1988), Comparison of finite volume numerical methods with staggered and collocated grids, *Comput. Fluids*, **16**(4), 389–403.

Press, W.H., Flannery, B.P., Teukolsky, S.A. and Velyerling, W.T. (1992), "Numerical Recipes – The Art of Scientific Computing", Cambridge University Press, Cambridge.

Roe, P.L. (1985), Some contributions to the modeling of Discontinuous flows, in "Lecture Notes in Applied Mathematics", Vol. 22, Springer-Verlag, Berlin, pp. 163–193.

Saad, Y. and Schultz, M.H. (1986), GMRES: a generalized residual algorithm for solving non-symmetric linear systems, *SIAM J. Sci. Stat. Comput.*, **7**, 856–869.

Sathyamurthy, P.S. and Patankar, S.V. (1994), Block-correction based multigrid method for fluid-flow problems, *Numerical Heat Transfer*, **25B**, 375–394.

Scarborough, J.B. (1958), "Numerical Mathematical Analysis", 4th edition, Johns Hopkins University Press, Baltimore.

Schneider, G.E. and Zedan, M. (1981), A modified strongly implicit procedure for the numerical solutions of field problems, *Numerical Heat Transfer*, **4**, 1–9.

Shyy, W., Thakur, S. and Wright, J. (1992), Second-order upwind and central differencing schemes for recirculating flow computations, *AIAA J.*, **30**, 923–932.

Stone, H.L. (1968), Iterative solution of implicit approximations of multidimensional partial differential equations, *SIAM, J. Numer. Anal.*, **5**(3), 530–558.

van der Wijngaart, R.J.F. (1990), Composite grid techniques and adaptive grid refinement in CFD, Report ClaSSiC-90-07, Dept. of Computer Science, Stanford University.

van Doormal, J.P. and Raithby, G.D. (1984), Enhancements of the SIMPLE method for predicting incompressible flows, *Numerical Heat Transfer*, **7**, 147–163.

van Leer, B. (1977), Towards the ultimate conservative difference scheme, IV, a new approach to numerical convection, *J. Comput. Physics*, **23**, 276–299.

Versteeg, H.K. and Malalasekara, W. (1995), "An Introduction to CFD", Longman Scientific & Technical, Harlow.

Wanik, A. and Schnell, U. (1989), Some remarks on the PISO and SIMPLE algorithms for steady flow, *Comput. Fluids*, **17**, 555.

7 NUMERICAL SOLUTION OF COMPLEX FLOW MODELS

A reactor engineer frequently encounters turbulent, multiphase and reactive flows, which are more complex than those discussed in the previous chapter. In this chapter, modifications or special techniques/algorithms required to extend the finite volume method to handle such complexities are discussed. In addition, some of the practical issues involved in carrying out numerical simulations of complex flow models are also discussed.

7.1. SIMULATION OF TURBULENT FLOWS

Mathematical models for simulating turbulence are discussed in Chapter 3. Here the scope is restricted to simulations of RANS-based turbulence models. Information about numerical methods relevant to LES and DNS may be found in the references cited in Chapter 3. For RANS-based turbulence models, in addition to Reynolds-averaged momentum and continuity equations, governing equations for the additional turbulence variables such as turbulent kinetic energy or turbulent energy dissipation rate, need to be solved. Algorithms and methods discussed in the previous chapter can be directly applied to solve these model equations. Usually, turbulence model equations are solved after correcting the pressure and velocity fields (refer the overall solution procedure shown in Fig. 6.11) in each iteration. For example, when turbulent flows are simulated using the two-equation, k–ε model of turbulence, the governing equations for k and ε are solved using the methods discussed for general scalar equations. It must be noted that the magnitudes of source terms appearing in the governing equations for k and ε are significant and must be treated carefully for good convergence behavior. Since both k and ε will always be positive, the source term must be linearized to ensure the non-negativity of k and ε. One of the simplest ways to linearize these source terms is to express the ratio of ε and k in terms of turbulence viscosity:

$$\frac{\varepsilon}{k} = \frac{C_{\mathrm{D}}\rho k}{\mu_{\mathrm{T}}} \tag{7.1}$$

When initiating the calculations, turbulent viscosity is set to a small value (usually the same as the molecular viscosity). Linearized source terms for k and ε can then be written:

$$S_{\mathrm{C}k} = V_{\mathrm{cell}} G \qquad S_{\mathrm{P}k} = -V_{\mathrm{cell}} \rho \left(\frac{C_{\mathrm{D}}\rho k}{\mu_{\mathrm{T}}} \right) \tag{7.2}$$

$$S_{\mathrm{C}\varepsilon} = V_{\mathrm{cell}} C_1 G \left(\frac{C_{\mathrm{D}}\rho k}{\mu_{\mathrm{T}}} \right) \qquad S_{\mathrm{P}\varepsilon} = -V_{\mathrm{cell}} \rho \left(\frac{C_{\mathrm{D}}\rho k}{\mu_{\mathrm{T}}} \right) C_2 \tag{7.3}$$

When wall functions are used to specify wall boundary conditions, it is important to suitably linearize the source terms appearing in momentum equations by following the practices discussed in the previous chapter.

In many turbulent flow simulations, it is useful to carry out the first few iterations without considering the turbulence model. This allows some flow field to develop within the solution domain. The solution of turbulence model equations are then activated and the whole set of equations are solved until the desired convergence is obtained. It is often useful to set some small values to turbulent kinetic energy and dissipation rates when initiating their solution. For more complex turbulence models (non-linear k–ε models, algebraic or differential Reynolds stress models), it is always desirable to obtain preliminary results using the standard k–ε model, which is quite robust. It is often observed that the number of computational cells and discretization schemes have more significant impact on the simulated results than the choice of turbulence model. Measures should therefore be taken to assess the adequacy of the grid employed and the discretization scheme. It must be noted that usually the application of wall functions imposes some constraints on the location of the nearest grid node from the wall. The validity of these assumptions must be verified by examining simulated results.

Some prior knowledge of the expected flow field always helps to estimate the required under-relaxation techniques and to evolve suitable solution strategies. In some cases exhibiting complex interactions, it is helpful to temporarily switch off the solution to some of the equations. The progress of error reduction can be monitored and controlled by adjusting several parameters of the numerical method (such as direction of sweeps of algebraic solver, internal iterations of different variables and so on). The importance of ensuring adequate convergence was mentioned in the previous chapter. It is even more crucial in simulating turbulent flows. Often in complex turbulent flows, the user may have to employ lower values of under-relaxation factor. Such low values will force slow changes in the predicted flow field, sometimes indicating an apparently converged behavior. It is important to verify the degree of convergence by comparing the history of key variables at different points as well as the history of some relevant integrated flow measure (such as volume-averaged turbulent energy dissipation rate).

In order to illustrate some of the issues relevant to simulations of turbulent flows, here we consider the same example discussed in the previous chapter. As noted there, for low viscosity fluids, it is difficult to obtain grid-independent results. The reason is that with the given boundary conditions, the flow is turbulent for low viscosity fluids and requires an extremely large number of grids to resolve the small-scale features completely. To avoid the need for using an excessively large number of grid points, one may use a turbulence model (at the expense of information about the small-scale features) and obtain grid-independent results for the mean flow field. To illustrate this, the standard k–ε model was used to carry out simulations of the flow of low viscosity fluid (0.001 Pa.s) in the cubical reactor discussed in the previous chapter. Profiles of velocity and turbulent kinetic energy at $x = 0.5$ m predicted with different numbers of grids are shown in Fig. 7.1. It can be seen that with the turbulence model, the predicted results become almost grid-independent if the number of computational cells are more than 25 600 (160×160). It is useful to examine the variation of predicted volume-averaged turbulence characteristics (energy dissipation rate and kinetic energy) with the inverse of the number of computational cells (shown in Fig. 7.2). It can be seen that predicted characteristics obtained with a 160×160 grid are quite close to the values extrapolated to an infinite number of computational cells, which confirms the earlier conclusion of grid independence.

In order to bring the considered example closer to the reactor-engineering field, a case with a downward pumping impeller in the vessel was considered. The presence of a downward pumping impeller was approximated by specifying a uniform downward velocity at the impeller location (Fig. 7.3). Two different values of velocity, 1 ms^{-1} and 5 ms^{-1}, were specified. The influence of the number of computational cells on the predicted flow for the case with an impeller (with downward velocity 5 ms^{-1}) was examined. The results are shown in Fig. 7.4. It can be seen that even with the impeller, 160×160 grids are adequate to simulate the turbulent flow. Thus, all subsequent simulations were carried out using this grid. It can be seen that with a downflow impeller, the volume-averaged turbulent energy dissipation rate is substantially higher (compare Figs 7.2 and 7.4). The predicted flow field (velocity vectors, contours of stream function and contours of turbulent kinetic energy) for a downward velocity of 5 ms^{-1} is shown in Fig. 7.5. It can be seen that because of the asymmetric inlet, the flow field is not symmetric around $x = 0.5$ m. The influence of the impeller downward velocity on the volume-averaged turbulent characteristics is shown in Fig. 7.6.

The case of an impeller downward velocity of 5 $m\,s^{-1}$ was further investigated to examine the influence of turbulence models and discretization schemes. The influence of discretization schemes on predicted results (with the standard k–ε model) is shown in Fig. 7.7. It can be seen that with a sufficiently fine grid, the influence of the discretization scheme is not significant. Additional simulations reveal that for the coarser grid there is a significant difference in the predicted results of different discretization schemes. The difference diminishes as the number of computational cells increases. The influence of the turbulence model employed on predicted results is shown in Fig. 7.8. It can be seen that the predictions by standard and RNG versions of k–ε models are almost the same. The predictions of the Reynolds stress model are, however, significantly different from these two models. This illustrates the importance of appropriate selection of turbulence model and the

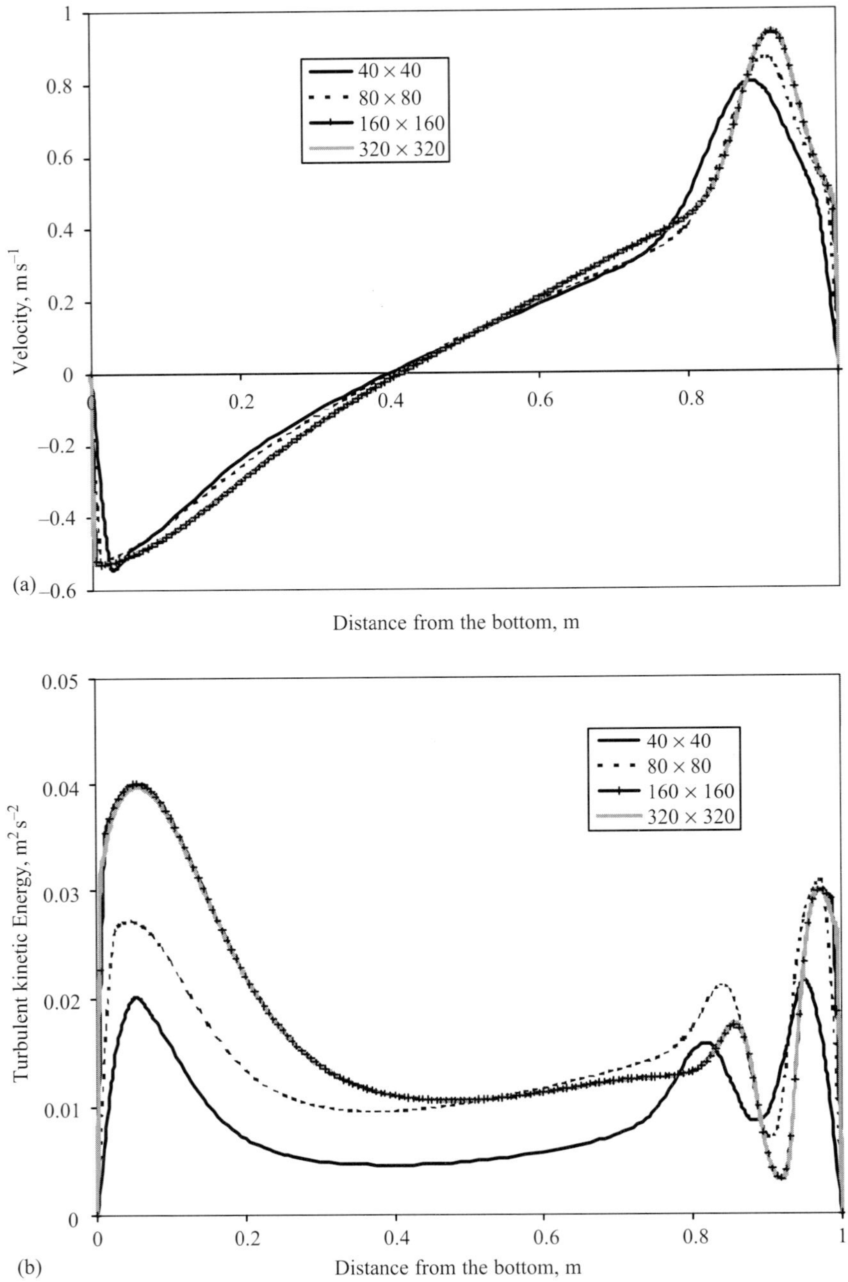

FIGURE 7.1 Influence of grid size on predicted results. (a) *U*-profile at $x = 0.5$ m, (b) *k*-profile at $x = 0.5$ m.

necessity for validation of the computed results. It should be emphasized that a mathematically more complex model does not necessarily guarantee better predictions. A suitable turbulence model should be selected by considering the specific flow characteristics (refer to the discussion in Chapter 3). The example discussed here

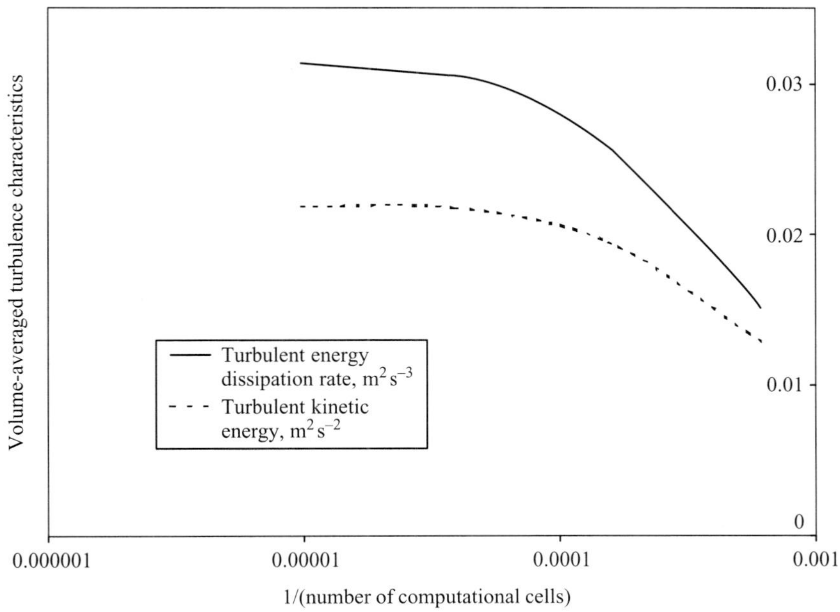

FIGURE 7.2 Influence of grid size on volume averaged turbulent characteristics.

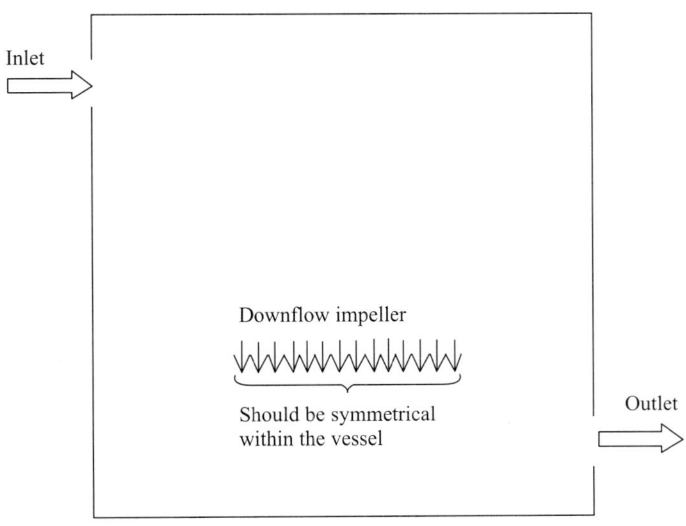

FIGURE 7.3 Configuration with downflow impeller.

also illustrates the importance of detailed analysis and post-processing of simulated results. Not only for turbulent flows but also for any complex flow-modeling problem, before one uses simulated results, systematic error analysis based on numerical experiments as well as some experimental validation is essential. Examples of the validation of single-phase flows generated by different impellers are discussed in Chapter 10.

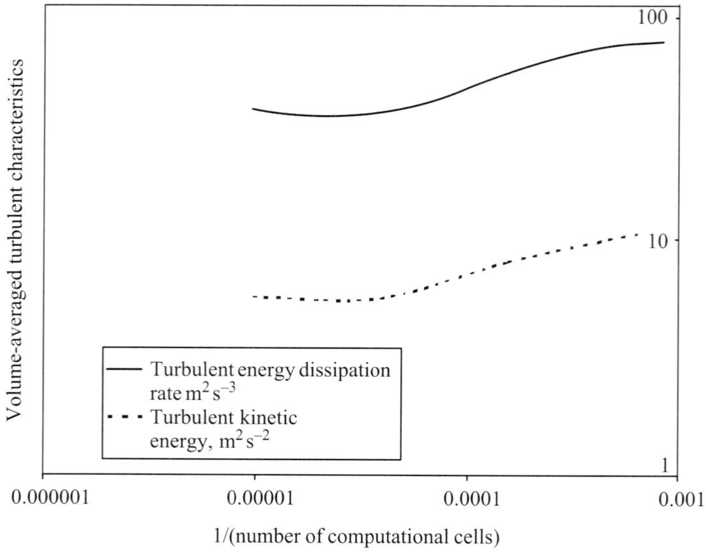

FIGURE 7.4 Influence of grid size on volume averaged turbulent characteristics with impeller.

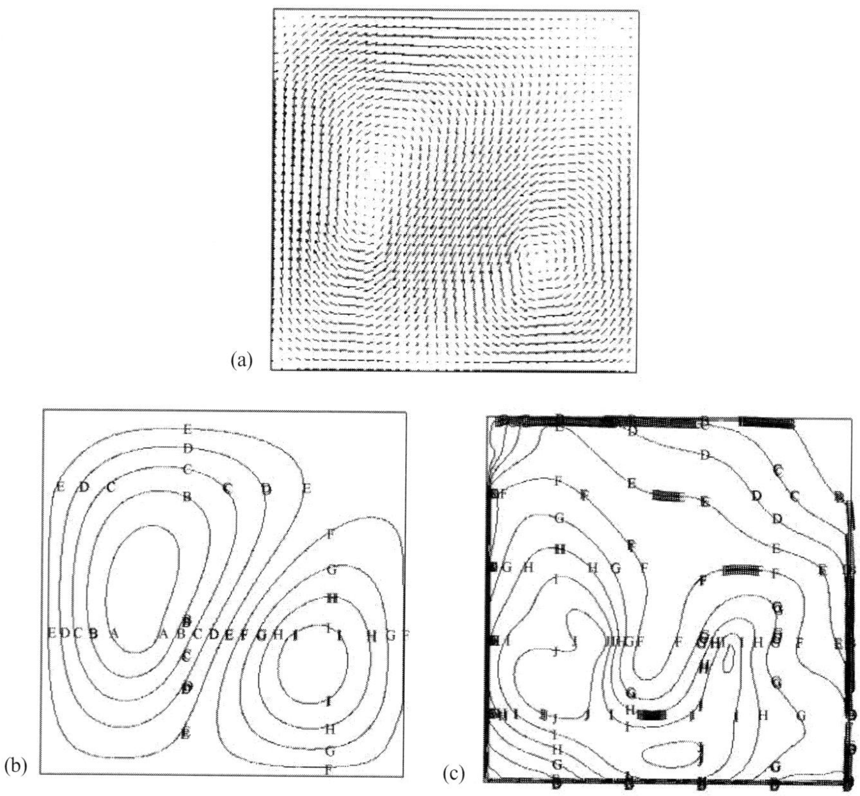

FIGURE 7.5 Predicted flow field with two equation turbulence model (standard k–ε model). (a) Vector plot, (b) Contours of stream function (−0.01 [A] to 0.01 [J]), (c) Contours of turbulent kinetic energy (0 [A] to 0.01 [K]).

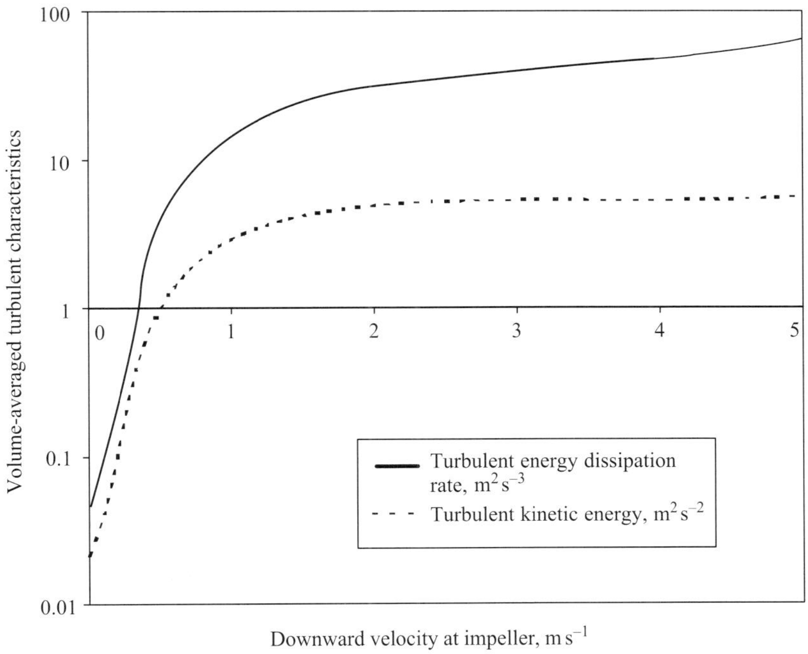

FIGURE 7.6 Influence of impeller velocity on volume-averaged turbulent characteristics.

7.2. SIMULATION OF MULTIPHASE FLOWS

Mathematical models governing multiphase flows are discussed in Chapter 4. As mentioned earlier, multiphase flows may exhibit several different flow regimes, and different modeling approaches are used to simulate these different flow regimes. Three basic modeling approaches, namely (1) volume of fluid approach (VOF), (2) Eulerian–Lagrangian (EL), and (3) Eulerian–Eulerian (EE) and the corresponding basic transport equations governing multiphase flows were discussed in Chapter 4. Although the basic finite volume method is applicable to simulation of multiphase flows, each of these approaches requires different features and special algorithms to solve the governing equations. Some of these issues are briefly discussed here.

7.2.1. Volume of Fluid (VOF) Approach

In the VOF approach, the present phases share a single set of conservation equations as discussed in Chapter 4. The essential feature of the VOF model is that it simulates the motion of a fluid–fluid interface embedded in the overall motion. It is important to maintain a compact interface thickness (one computational cell thick) to realize accurate simulations. VOF methods employ a marker function $F(x,t)$ (or a volume fraction) that uniquely identifies the fluid under consideration. A unit value for F indicates a cell completely filled with one phase, whereas a zero value indicates a cell containing only the other phase. Therefore, computational

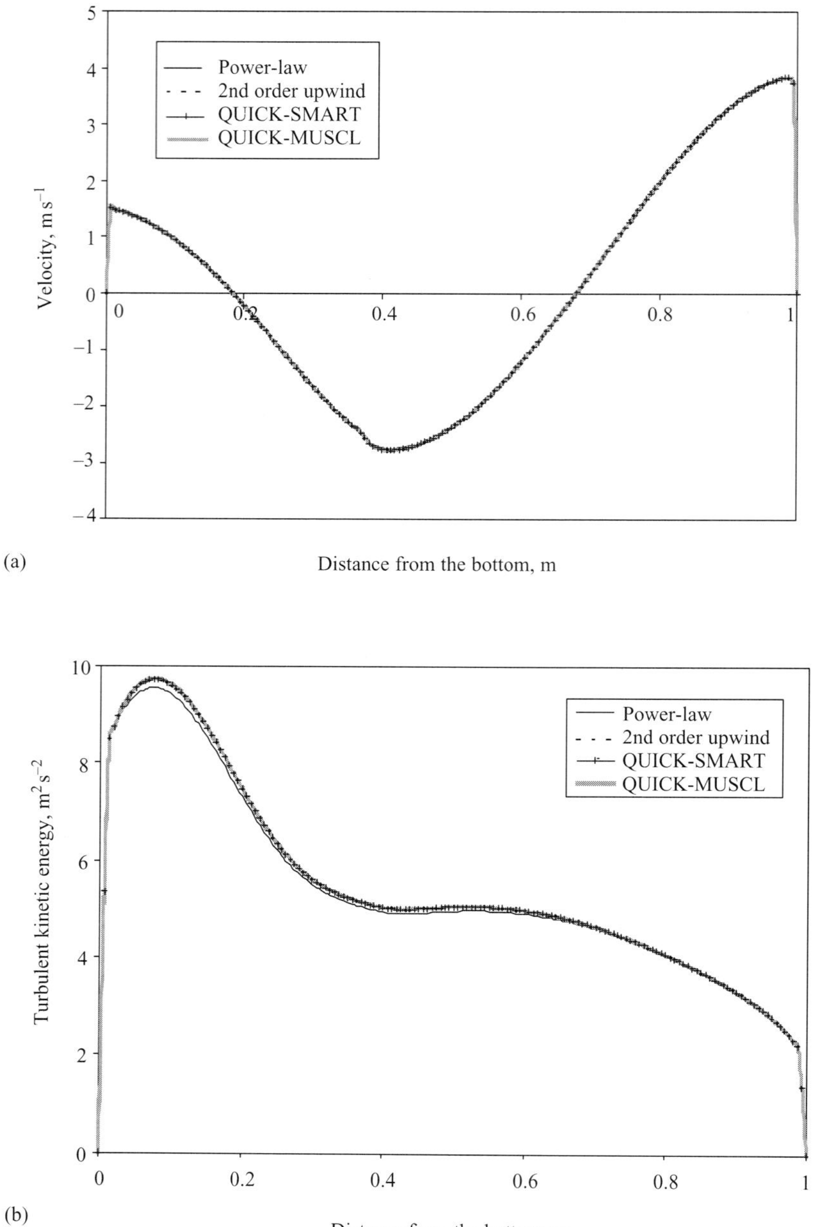

FIGURE 7.7 Influence of discretization schemes on predicted results. (a) U velocity at $x = 0.5$ m, (b) Turbulent kinetic energy at $x = 0.5$ m.

cells with intermediate values of F contain an interface between phases. The motion of the interface is tracked by solving the transport (advection) equation of F given by

$$\frac{\partial F}{\partial t} + (U \cdot \nabla) F = 0 \tag{7.4}$$

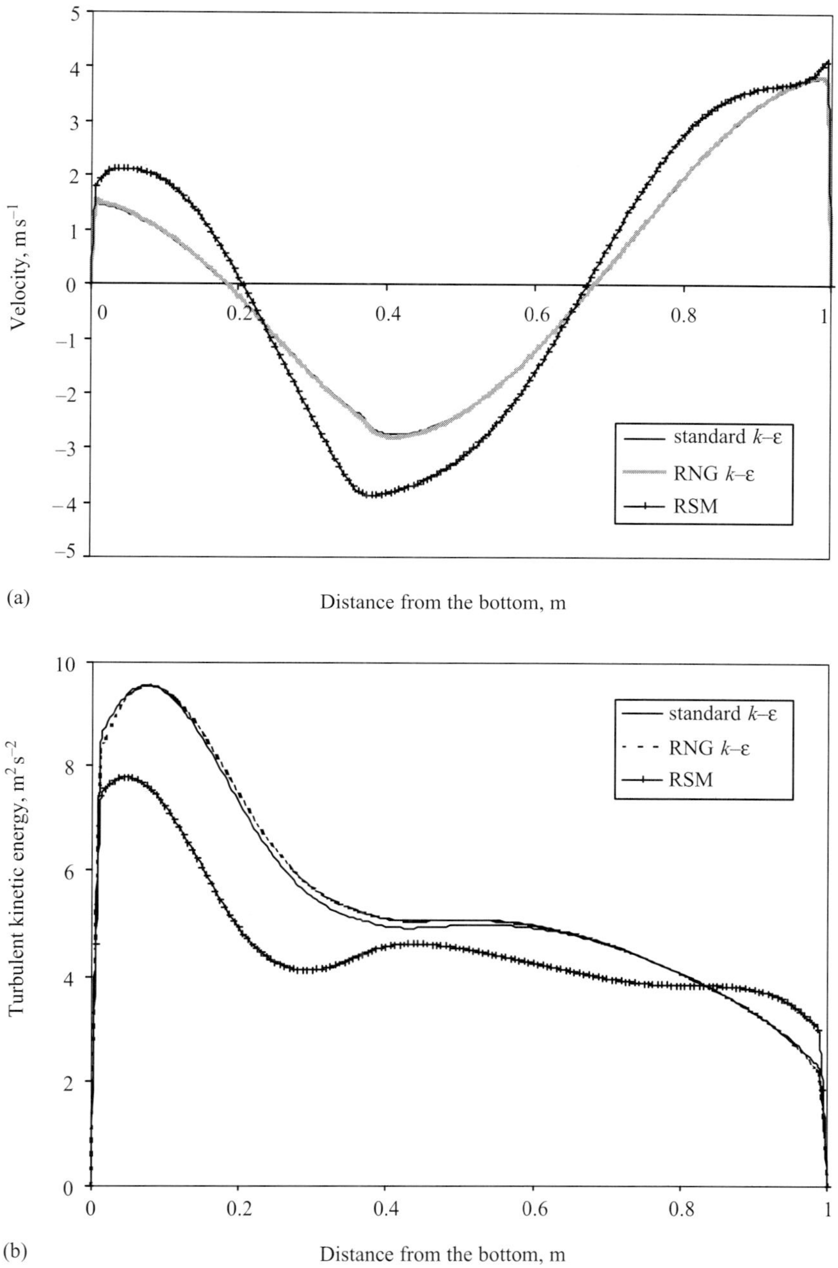

FIGURE 7.8 Influence of turbulence model on predicted results. (a) U velocity at $x = 0.5$ m/s, (b) Turbulent kinetic energy at $x = 0.5$ m.

The position of the interface between phases is inferred from the values of marker function. The discretized form of this equation relates the value of F at the new time level with its previous time-level value and to the fluxes of F through the cell faces. Approximations used in calculating these cell fluxes may lead to smearing of the fluid–fluid interface, which has to be minimized during numerical simulations. Several

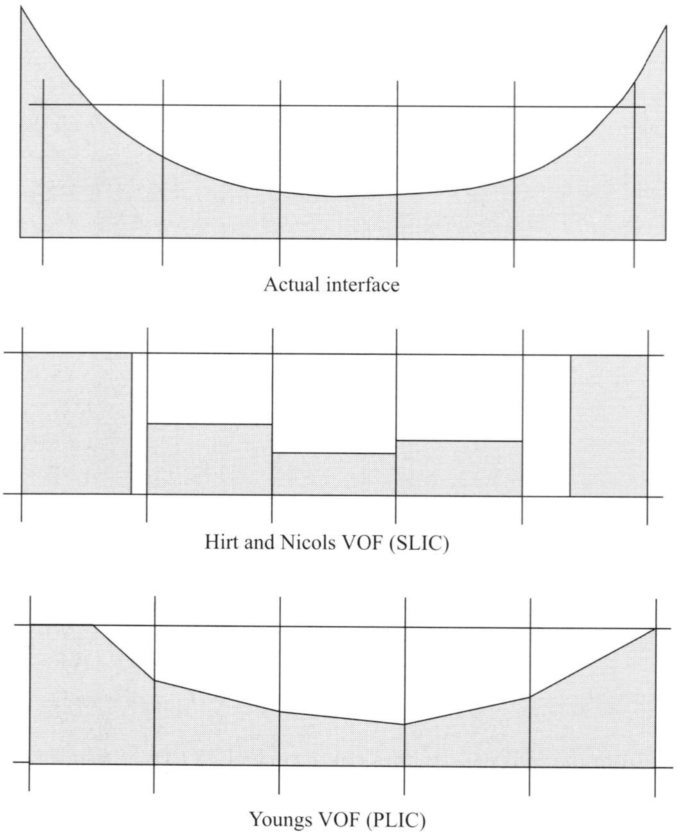

FIGURE 7.9 VOF interface reconstruction methods.

techniques such as SLIC (simple line interface calculation) and PLIC (piecewise linear interface calculation) have been developed to minimize computational smearing of the interface (see Rider and Kothe, 1995, for a review).

One of the most popular VOF methods is that due to Hirt and Nichols (1981). This method uses an approximate interface reconstruction that forces the interface to align with one of the co-ordinate axis, depending on the prevailing direction of the interface normal. A schematic diagram of reconstruction of a two-dimensional interface is shown in Fig. 7.9. To compute fluxes in a direction parallel to the reconstructed interface, upwind fluxes are used. Fluxes in a direction perpendicular to the reconstructed interface are estimated using a donor–acceptor method. In a donor–acceptor method, a computational cell is identified as a donor of some amount of fluid from one phase and another neighbor cell is identified as the acceptor of that donated amount of fluid. The amount of fluid from one phase that can be convected (donated) across a cell boundary is limited by the minimum of the filled volume in the donor cell or the free volume in the acceptor cell. This minimizes numerical diffusion at the interface.

The PLIC method is much more accurate than the SLIC method discussed above (Rider and Kothe, 1995; Rudman, 1997). In PLIC, an interface within a computational cell is approximated by a straight-line segment with a slope determined from the interface normal (Fig. 7.9). This interface normal is calculated from the gradient of volume fraction (using a nine-point computational molecule in two dimensions). The line segment cuts the computational cell in such a way that the fractional fluid volume is equal to the value of marker function at that cell. The resulting fluid polygon is then used to determine fluxes through any cell face. Implementation of the PLIC method (calculation of face fluxes) proposed by Youngs (1982) is shown graphically in Fig. 7.10 for one specific interface configuration. Sixteen possible different configurations, depending on the orientation of the interface with respect to the co-ordinate axis, have been identified. For any specific configuration, formulae similar to those shown in Fig. 7.10 can be derived to calculate cell fluxes.

Apart from the identification of interface and calculation of cell fluxes, an appropriate computer implementation of interfacial tension is also one of the key elements in carrying out realistic VOF simulations. Most studies have implemented the continuum surface force (CSF) model of Brackbill *et al.* (1992) to describe interfacial tension. As discussed in Chapter 4, the CSF model replaces the interfacial force by a smoothly varying volumetric force acting on all fluid elements in the interface transition region (see Eq. (4.6)). The local surface curvature appearing in this equation can be calculated from the unit normal at the interface between phases (see Eq. (4.8); Kothe *et al.*, 1991; Delnoij, 1999). For additional details of numerical implementation, the original references should be consulted. It is sufficient to emphasize here that the accuracy of the CSF model depends on sharpness of the interface maintained by the interface-tracking model. Preferably, the sharpness of the interface should be maintained at around the order of the cell width [$O(\delta x)$].

Apart from the interface tracking and forces due to interfacial tension, conventional numerical techniques developed for single-phase flow simulations are used to solve the relevant transport equations. As mentioned earlier, controlling numerical diffusion and smearing of the interface are key issues in realistic VOF-based simulations. The size of computational cells and discretization schemes, therefore, significantly affect the predicted results. To illustrate VOF simulations, the formation of gas bubbles through an orifice sparger was simulated. The considered geometry, computational grid and other necessary data are shown in Fig. 7.11. Simulations were carried out in an unsteady mode. To simulate transients accurately, it is necessary to ensure adequate convergence at each time step. Typical predicted results 0.12 s after the introduction of gas from the nozzle are shown in Fig. 7.12. It can be seen that the discretization scheme has a substantial influence on the predicted shape and rise velocity of bubbles. Similar observations were made by Delnoij (1999). The computational requirements of VOF-based simulations are much higher than those of Eulerian–Eulerian or Eulerian–Lagrangian approaches. In most cases, accurate simulations of interfacial phenomena require simulations in three-dimensional domains, which further increases computational demands. For example, detailed two-dimensional VOF simulations carried out by Krishna and van Baten (1999) showed significant discrepancies in the observed and predicted bubble rise velocities. Most VOF-based simulations are, therefore, restricted to a few large fluid particles. Despite this, VOF-based simulations can be used as useful learning simulations to gain insight into the interaction of continuous flow field and deformation and interfacial processes of large fluid particles. Some examples are discussed in Part IV.

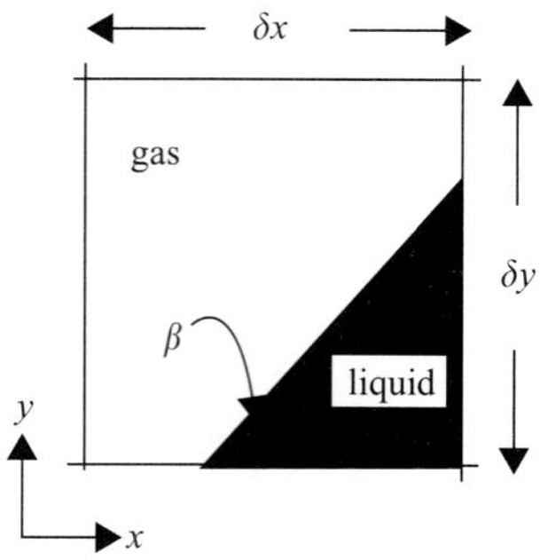

Side fractions:

$$S_{\text{top}} = 0$$

$$S_{\text{right}} = \sqrt{F(i,j) \cdot 2 \cdot \tan\beta}$$

$$S_{\text{left}} = 0$$

$$S_{\text{bottom}} = \sqrt{F(i,j) \cdot 2 \cdot \cot\beta}$$

$$\beta = \tan^{-1}\left(\frac{-n^x}{n^y}\right)$$

Fluxes through the four cell faces:

$$\text{If } u_{\text{top}} > 0$$

$$\text{If } u_{\text{top}} \cdot \delta t \leq \left(1 - S_{\text{right}}\right) \cdot \delta y$$

$$F_{\text{top}} = 0$$

else

$$F_{\text{top}} = \frac{1}{2}[u_{\text{top}} \cdot \delta t - (1 - S_{\text{right}}) \cdot \delta y]^2 \cot\beta$$

$$\text{If } u_{\text{right}} > 0$$

$$\text{If } u_{\text{right}} \cdot \delta t \geq S_{\text{bottom}} \cdot \delta x$$

$$F_{\text{right}} = F(i,j) \cdot \delta x \cdot \delta y$$

else

$$F_{\text{right}} = \frac{1}{2} u_{\text{right}} \cdot \delta t \left[2 - \frac{u_{\text{right}} \cdot \delta t}{S_{\text{bottom}} \cdot \delta x}\right] S_{\text{right}} \cdot \delta y$$

$$\text{If } u_{\text{bottom}} > 0$$

$$\text{If } u_{\text{bottom}} \cdot \delta t \geq S_{\text{right}} \cdot \delta y$$

$$F_{\text{bottom}} = F(i,j) \cdot \delta x \cdot \delta y$$

else

$$F_{\text{bottom}} = \frac{1}{2} u_{\text{bottom}} \cdot \delta t \left[2 - \frac{u_{\text{bottom}} \cdot \delta t}{S_{\text{right}} \cdot \delta x}\right] S_{\text{bottom}} \cdot \delta x$$

$$\text{If } u_{\text{left}} > 0$$

$$\text{If } u_{\text{left}} \cdot \delta t \leq (1 - S_{\text{bottom}}) \cdot \delta x$$

$$F_{\text{left}} = 0$$

else

$$F_{\text{left}} = \frac{1}{2}[u_{\text{left}} \cdot \delta t - (1 - S_{\text{bottom}}) \cdot \delta x]^2 \tan\beta$$

FIGURE 7.10 Young's VOF method to determine cell face fluxes (from Delnoij, 1999).

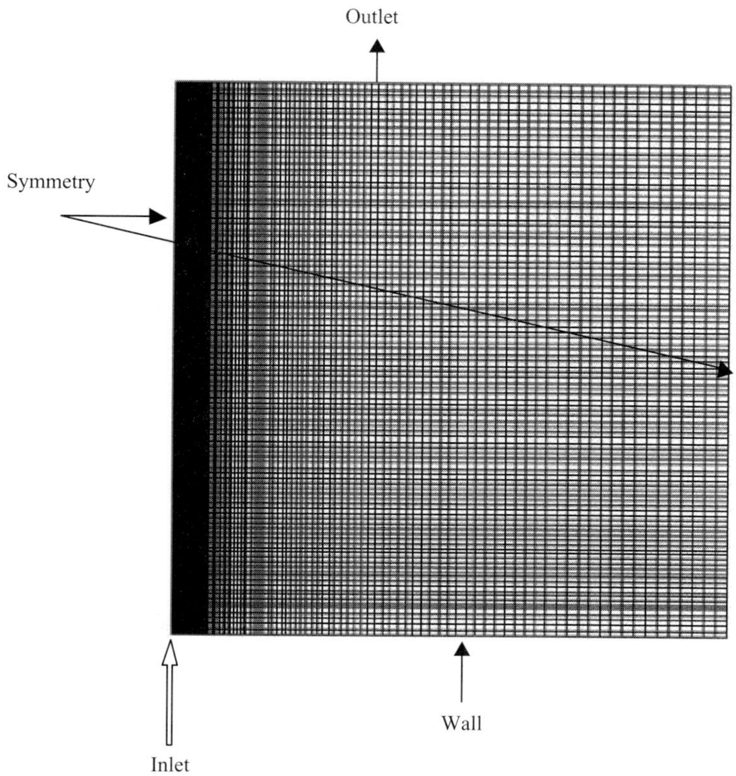

FIGURE 7.11 Geometry and grid used for VOF simulation (Domain size: 0.1 m × 0.1 m; inlet nozzle width = 0.001 m; inlet gas velocity = 0.2 ms^{-1}).

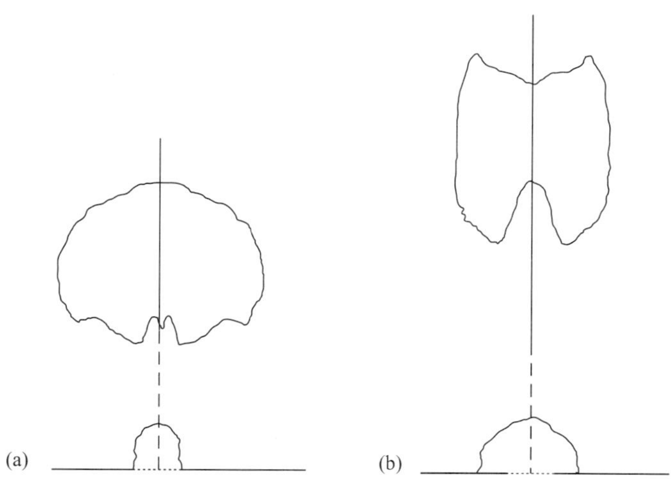

FIGURE 7.12 Results of VOF simulations at 0.12 s (influence of differencing scheme). (a) Power law. (b) QUICK (SUPERBEE).

7.2.2. Eulerian–Lagrangian Approach

In this approach, the finite volume methods discussed in the previous chapter can be applied to simulate the continuous fluid (in a Eulerian framework). Various algorithms for treating pressure–velocity coupling, and the discussion on other numerical issues like discretization schemes are applicable. The usual interpolation practices (discussed in the previous chapter) can be used. When solving equations of motion for a continuous fluid in the presence of the dispersed phase, the major differences will be: (1) consideration of phase volume fraction in calculation of convective and diffusive terms, and (2) calculation of additional source terms due to the presence of dispersed phase particles. For the calculation of phase volume fraction and additional source terms due to dispersed phase particles, it is necessary to calculate trajectories of the dispersed phase particles, in addition to solving the equations of motion of the continuous phase.

To calculate dispersed phase particle trajectories it will be necessary to solve a set of coupled ordinary differential equations (Eqs. 4.1 and 4.9). Any standard initial value ODE solvers can be used for this purpose. These methods are not discussed here. Necessary details may be found in texts such as *Numerical Recipes* (Press *et al.*, 1992). When calculating the trajectories of dispersed phase particles, any other auxiliary equations to account for heat transfer or chemical reactions can also be solved following similar procedures. Care must be taken to ensure that the time steps used for integration are sufficiently small and the trajectory integration is adequately time accurate. It is often necessary to use different time steps to simulate transients in the continuous flow field and trajectories of dispersed phase particles.

Although the methods discussed in the previous chapter and standard ODE solvers can be used to carry out simulations of dispersed multiphase flows using a Eulerian–Lagrangian approach, some important issues deserve additional comments. Use of different time steps for different processes is one important issue. If direct interaction among dispersed phase particles is considered (collisions and bouncing of particles), then it may be necessary to use three different time steps: (1) Δt_F to resolve transients in the macroscopic flow of the continuous phase; (2) Δt_P to estimate forces acting on dispersed phase particles (during this time interval, the macroscopic flow field of continuous phase may be assumed to be constant); and (3) Δt_T to update positions of dispersed phase particles (during this time interval, forces acting on particles may be assumed to be constant. Particle velocities and positions may, however, change due to particle collisions). These three time scales are shown schematically in Fig. 7.13 for a case of a gas–liquid flow. The sequence of collisions needs to be processed one collision at a time. Obviously for each collision, the collision time will be different and needs to be computed after identifying the two colliding (for binary collisions) particles. Efficient numerical techniques such as neighbor list techniques have been developed to minimize computations for the identification of two colliding particles causing the next collision (see Hoomans *et al.*, 1996; Delnoij, 1999 for more details). To account for collisions between dispersed phase particles, both soft particle (for example, Tsuji *et al.*, 1993) and hard particle (for example, Hoomans *et al.*, 1996) models have been used. Collisions act as an important mechanism to transport momentum and energy, in the case of gas–solid flows. For dispersed gas–liquid flows, however, the contribution of collisions to momentum transport may be neglected (Delnoij *et al.*, 1999). In such a case, it may be sufficient to use two time steps, one to update the flow field of the continuous phase and the other for trajectory calculations.

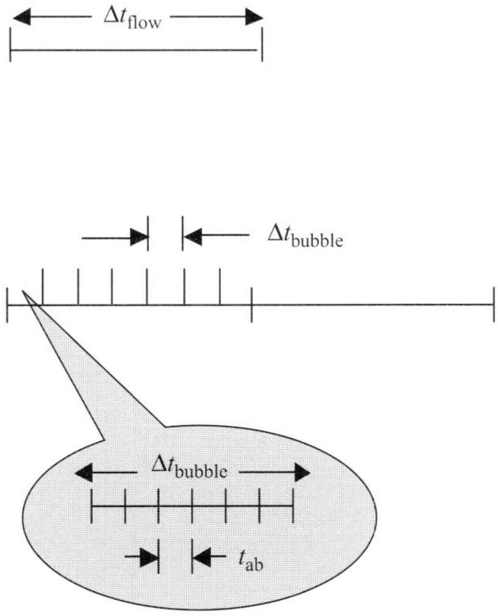

FIGURE 7.13 Time steps used for Eulerian–Lagrangian simulations. Δt_{flow}: Time step used to resolve macroscopic liquid flowfield, Δt_{bubble}: Time step used to estimate forces acting on bubbles (macroscopic liquid flowfield is assumed to be constant), t_{ab}: Time step used to displace bubbles and to account for collisions. Forces acting on bubbles are assumed to be constant.

Trajectory calculations require the calculation of net force acting on the dispersed phase particles. To calculate such a net force, local values of pressure, continuous phase velocities, partial and substantial derivative of pressure and partial and substantial derivatives of continuous phase velocities need to be available at the center of mass position of dispersed particles. However, these Eulerian variables and their derivatives are known only at discrete nodes in the computational domain. Therefore, suitable interpolation should be used to obtain the required values at the particle location, using the previously obtained solution of the continuous phase flow equations. As a first-level approximation, a continuous phase velocity may be taken as a computational cell based velocity for all locations within the cell. The accuracy of the results, however, will be significantly influenced by this assumption. A better assumption would be to use appropriate area or volume averaging. The concept may be illustrated by considering a two-dimensional example as shown in Fig. 7.14. The local value of a quantity f at the center of mass of the dispersed phase particle (f_{P}) can be calculated using

$$f_{\text{P}} = \frac{1}{\Delta x \Delta y} \sum_{n=1}^{4} A_n f_n \tag{7.5}$$

with f_n being some Eulerian quantity at node n, and A_n representing an area:

$$\begin{aligned} A_1 &= (\Delta x - \delta x)(\Delta y - \delta y) \qquad & A_2 &= \delta x(\Delta y - \delta y) \\ A_3 &= \delta y(\Delta x - \delta x) \qquad & A_4 &= \delta x \delta y \end{aligned} \tag{7.6}$$

Extension of these formulae for volume averaging in three-dimensional Eulerian–Lagrangian simulations is straightforward.

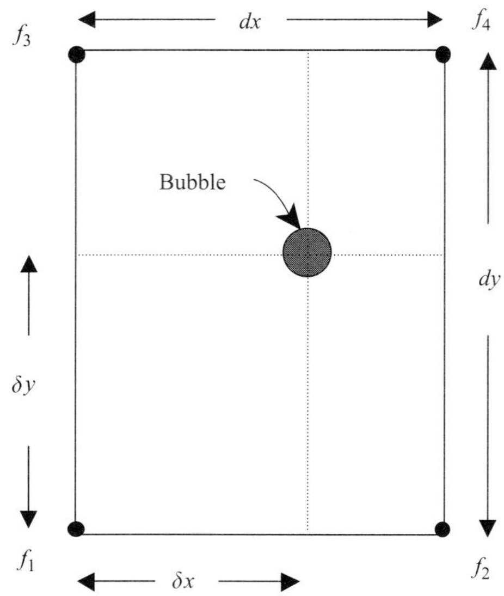

FIGURE 7.14 Area weighting of node values (f_n) (Refer Eqs. (7.5) and (7.6)).

So far, discussion has focused on simulating one-way coupling between continuous and dispersed phases. To simulate two-way coupling between multiple phases, iterative procedures need to be employed. The overall procedure is as follows:

- Solution of the continuous phase flow field (in the absence of dispersed phase).
- Calculation of trajectories of dispersed phase particles.
- Recalculation of continuous phase flow using the interphase exchange of momentum, heat and mass determined from trajectory calculations.
- Recalculation of dispersed phase trajectories in the modified continuous flow field.
- Repetition of the previous two steps until convergence is achieved.

For the calculation of continuous phase flow in the presence of dispersed phase particles, again several averaging procedures need to be employed. The volume fraction of the continuous phase in a computational cell is calculated by subtracting the ratio of volume occupied by dispersed phase particles and the volume of the computational cell from unity:

$$\varepsilon_{\mathrm{c}} = 1 - \frac{\sum\limits_{i \in \mathrm{cell}} V_{\mathrm{p}i}}{V_{\mathrm{cell}}} \qquad (7.7)$$

When calculating continuous phase volume fraction, it is very important to account for the possibility of dispersed phase particles overlapping with more than one computational cell. The volume occupied by such particles needs to be distributed over the respective cells. Calculation of the exact distribution of the volume of the dispersed phase particles to the respective cells may become computationally intensive when several particles are considered. Equations to distribute the volume of dispersed phase particles to different computational cells are illustrated in Fig. 7.15 for the two-dimensional case. Delnoij (1999) proposed some approximations based on the lengths

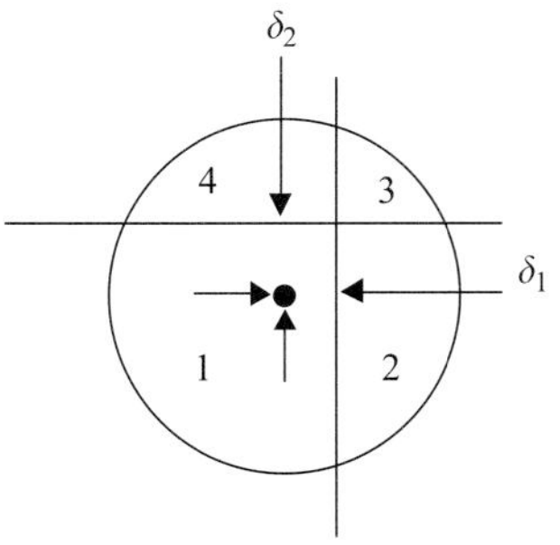

$$A_3 = \delta_1\delta_2 - \frac{1}{2}R_p\left[\delta_1\sqrt{1-\left(\frac{\delta_1}{R_p}\right)^2} + \delta_2\sqrt{1-\left(\frac{\delta_2}{R_p}\right)^2}\right.$$
$$\left. -R_p\left(\arccos\left(\frac{\delta_1}{R_p}\right) - \arcsin\left(\frac{\delta_2}{R_p}\right)\right)\right]$$

$$A_3 + A_4 = R_p\left[R_p\arccos\left(\frac{\delta_2}{R_p}\right) - \delta_2\sqrt{1-\left(\frac{\delta_2}{R_p}\right)^2}\right]$$

$$A_3 + A_2 = R_p\left[R_p\arccos\left(\frac{\delta_1}{R_p}\right) - \delta_1\sqrt{1-\left(\frac{\delta_1}{R_p}\right)^2}\right]$$

$$A_1 + A_2 + A_3 + A_4 = \pi R_p^2$$

FIGURE 7.15 Distribution of particle volume into surrounding Eulerian cells (two-dimensional case).

of common edge segments of adjacent computational cells on which dispersed phase particles overlap:

$$A_1 = \frac{\pi}{4}\left(R_\mathrm{p}+\delta_1\right)\left(R_\mathrm{p}+\delta_2\right) \qquad A_3 = \frac{\pi}{4}\left(R_\mathrm{p}-\delta_1\right)\left(R_\mathrm{p}-\delta_2\right)$$
$$A_2 = \frac{\pi}{4}\left(R_\mathrm{p}-\delta_1\right)\left(R_\mathrm{p}+\delta_2\right) \qquad A_4 = \frac{\pi}{4}\left(R_\mathrm{p}+\delta_1\right)\left(R_\mathrm{p}-\delta_2\right) \tag{7.8}$$

Numerical experiments indicate that such an approximation may be acceptable for most engineering simulations. These approximations may be extended to three-dimensional simulations by considering volumes instead of areas.

The momentum transfer rate from the dispersed phase particles to the continuous phase is the opposite of the sum of all the forces exerted by the continuous phase on the dispersed phase:

$$S_{cm}V_\mathrm{cell} = \sum_{i\in\mathrm{cell}}\left(F_{\mathrm{D}i} + F_{\mathrm{L}i} + F_{\mathrm{VM}i}\right) \tag{7.9}$$

$S_{cm}$is the net source due to dispersed phase particles (Eq. (4.11)). F_D, F_L and F_VM are drag, lift and virtual mass forces (Section 4.2.1). It must be noted that Eq. (7.9) assumes that the volume-averaged momentum transfer (from the dispersed phase) for a computational cell is equivalent to the sum of local momentum transport rates of all the dispersed phase particles within that computational cell. In principle, local momentum transport rate for each dispersed phase particle (at its center of mass) must be distributed to all the surrounding nodes of the continuous phase (Fig. 7.14). Since the local values of continuous phase properties are obtained by the reverse procedure, this method will ensure momentum conservation rigorously (as Newton's third law is strictly obeyed). Suitable area or volume averaging (similar to Eqs. (7.5) and (7.6)) can be employed to implement this method.

It should be noted here that although Eulerian–Lagrangian simulations do not require substantially new algorithms, the overall solution procedure is complex and interdependent. Computational load increases substantially as the number of dispersed phase particles increases. The usual considerations of number of computational cells, discretization schemes etc. will be important in multiphase flows as well. Advanced post-processing tools are generally required to interpret and to use the simulated results. Validation becomes a complex task since the simulated results are functions of several underlying sub-models and numerical approximations (constitutive equations of interphase transport equations, various interpolations from continuous to dispersed and vice versa). In most cases, available experimental data is of time-averaged quantities (such as velocity or volume fraction profiles). Calculation of time-averaged quantities from full transient simulations is memory intensive. Special procedures need to be employed during transient simulations to allow calculation of time-averaged quantities. For most dispersed phases, true time-averaged quantities (independent of further increase in averaging time) require long computational times (a few days to weeks of dedicated CPU time on reasonably powerful processors are common). Obviously, before one initiates such lengthy calculations, several numerical experiments should be carried out to finalize the appropriate selection of parameters.

Since Eulerian–Lagrangian simulations involve many different numerical parameters (choices of integration of trajectory calculations, method of accounting for the influence of turbulence on particle trajectories and so on) in addition to the usual numerical issues, it is difficult to discuss these issues here in detail. To illustrate the results of a Eulerian–Lagrangian simulation, the case of the reactor with a downward impeller is considered. Gas is introduced through a sparger located below the impeller. Net flow of liquid through the reactor was set to zero for these simulations. The location of the sparger and boundary conditions used for the simulations are shown in Fig. 7.16. Trajectories of gas bubbles introduced from the sparger were modeled using two methods: (1) a discrete random walk with no velocity interpolation within computational cells; and (2) a continuous random walk with velocity interpolation within computational cells. Simulations were carried out until the predicted results are almost independent of additional time steps. Predicted results (in the form of iso-lines of gas volume fraction) are shown in Fig. 7.17. Both the methods predict accumulation of gas near the 'eyes' of circulation loops. Although the predicted overall gas volume fraction from these two methods is not significantly different, trajectories and local details are quite different. It is indeed essential to validate (either directly or indirectly) predictions of such complex multiphase flow simulations before they are used for engineering applications. Examples of such validation are discussed when describing applications of the Eulerian–Lagrangian approach to simulating gas–liquid flows in bubble column reactors in Chapter 11.

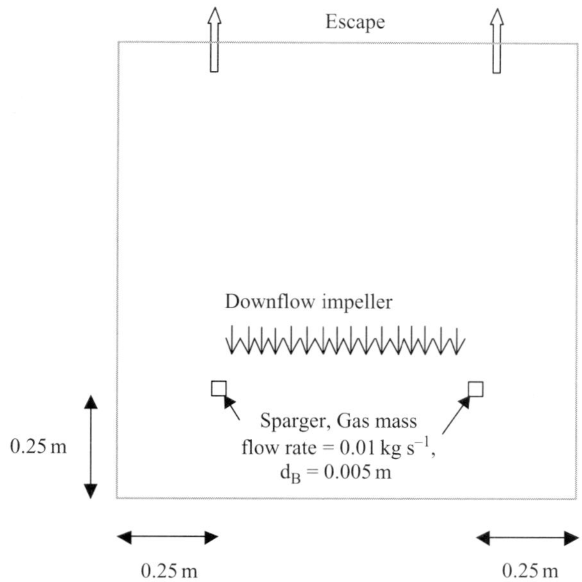

FIGURE 7.16 Geometry and boundary conditions used for Eulerian–Lagrangian simulations.

With a Eulerian–Lagrangian approach, processes occurring at the particle surface can be modeled when simulating particle trajectories (for example, the process of dissolution or evaporation can be simulated). However, as the volume fraction of dispersed phase increases, the Eulerian–Lagrangian approach becomes increasingly computation intensive. A Eulerian–Eulerian approach more efficiently simulate such dispersed multiphase flows.

7.2.3. Eulerian–Eulerian Approach

In this approach, the governing equations are formulated based on the concept of interpenetrating continua. The governing equations are discussed in Chapter 4. It can be seen that the form of governing equations is similar to that for single-phase flows. Simulation of multiphase flows, however, requires solution of a larger number of equations (governing as well as auxiliary). The increase in the number of equations may not increase the difficulty of obtaining solutions. The main difficulties in simulating multiphase flows lie in handling the pressure–velocity coupling and non-linearity and strong coupling between various equations, which cause extremely slow convergence.

For single-phase flows, pressure is shared by three momentum equations and requires special algorithms to compute the pressure field. Most of these algorithms (discussed in the previous chapter) use one continuity equation and three momentum equations to derive pressure and/or pressure correction equations. However, for multiphase flows, there is more than one continuity equation. Answers to questions such as which continuity equation should be used to derive pressure equations are not obvious. As discussed in the previous chapter, it is customary to employ iterative techniques to solve single-phase flow equations. Such iterative techniques can, in principle, be extended to simulate multiphase flows. In practice, however, the process

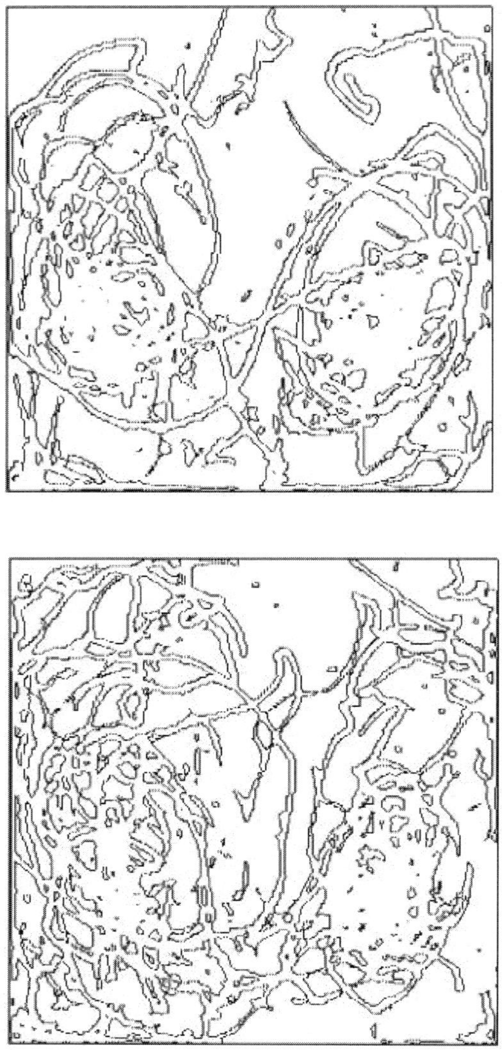

(a)

(b)

FIGURE 7.17 Eulerian–Lagrangian simulations; iso-lines of gas volume fraction of 0.0002. (a) Discrete random walk without velocity interpolation, (b) Continuous random walk with velocity interpolation.

is often found to converge with intolerable slowness. A suitable remedy to accelerate convergence needs to be devised, and some possible ways of overcoming these difficulties are discussed here.

Several alternatives may be used to derive suitable pressure or pressure correction equations. In this section, we will discuss a specific option based on the work of Spalding (1980) and Carver (1984). This option has been used to simulate gas–liquid flows in stirred vessels (Ranade and van den Akker, 1994) and bubble columns (Ranade, 1992; 1997) and was found to be quite robust. The method is illustrated here for two-fluid models. It can be extended to more than two phases following the same general principles. The overall method is an extended version of the SIMPLER

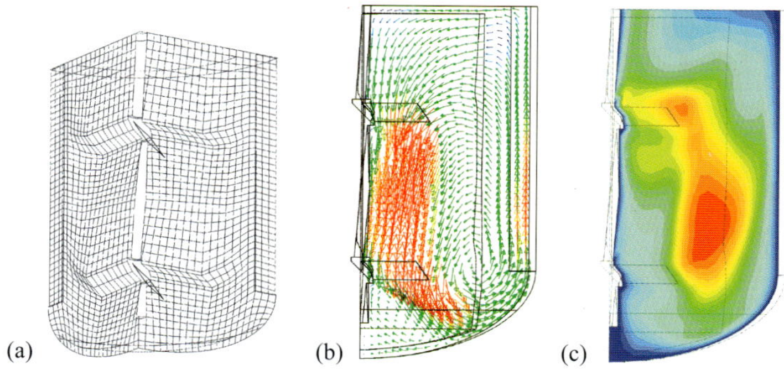

FIGURE 9.3 Sample of simulation results for a two pitched blade turbine (legend not shown due to confidentiality constraints). (a) Grid; (b) vector plot; (c) contours of turbulent KE (red: high values; blue: low values).

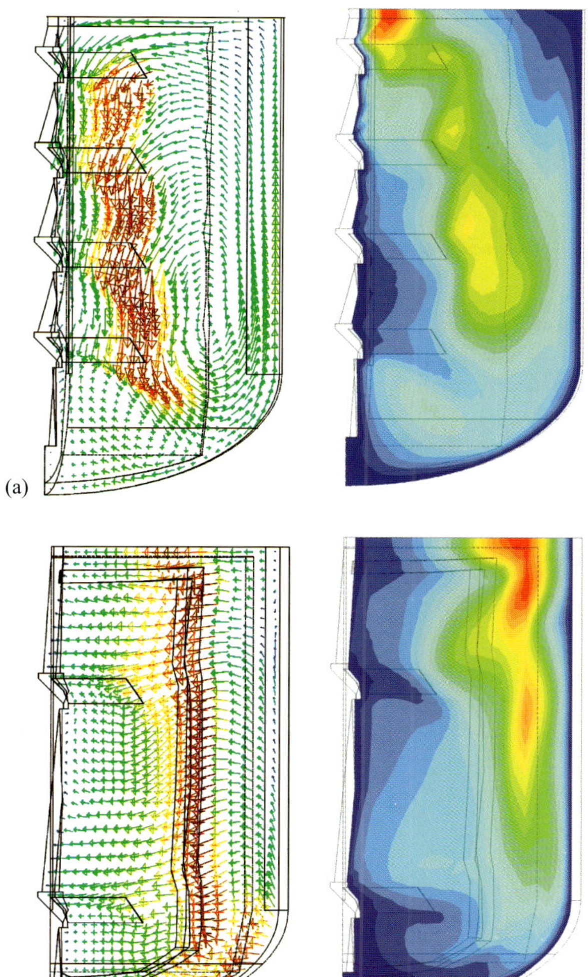

FIGURE 9.5 Simulated flow field for two alternative reactor configurations (red: high values; blue: low values; legend not shown due to confidentiality constraints). (a) Four pitched blade turbine, (b) two pitched blade turbine with cage (left: vector plots; right: contours of turbulent kinetic energy.)

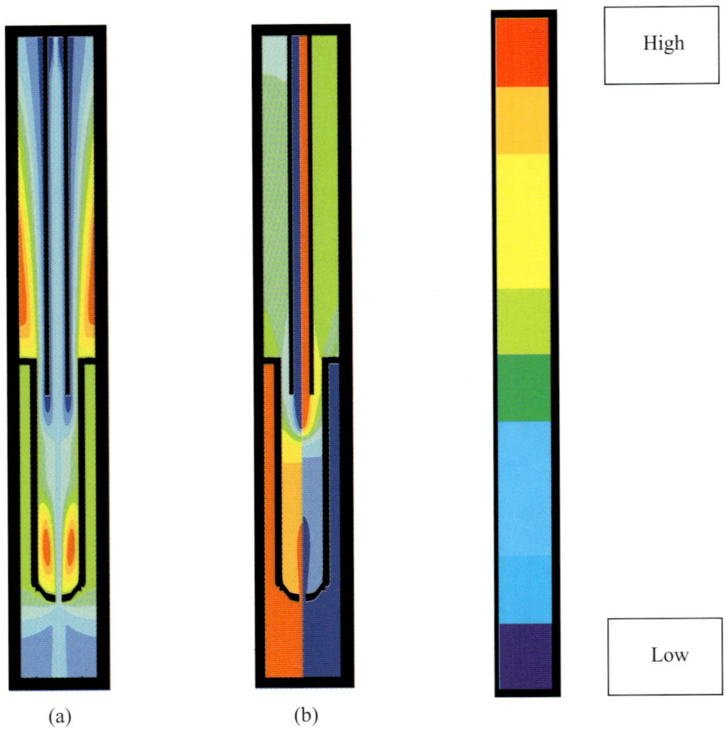

FIGURE 9.10 Flow and mixing in the mixing cup (from Ranade, 1999). (a) Contours of stream function. (b) Left side: contours of oxygen mass fraction; right side: contours of ethylene mass fraction. (Legend not shown due to confidentiality constraints).

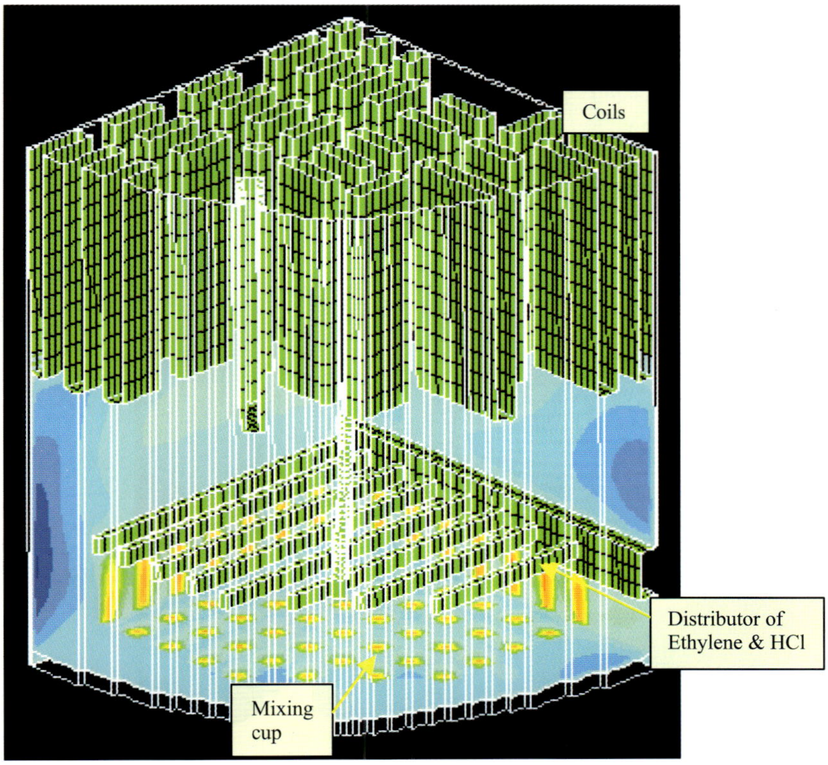

FIGURE 9.12 Contour plot of axial velocity (volume above the grid) (from Ranade, 1999b) (red: high values; blue: low values; legend not shown due to confidentiality constraints).

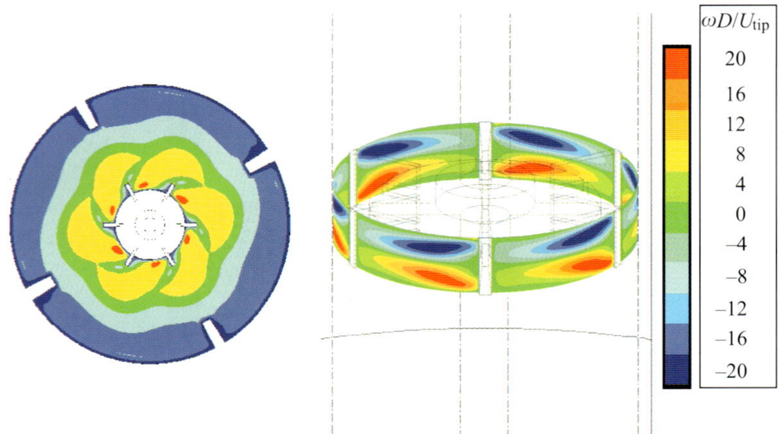

(a) (b)

FIGURE 10.10 Presence of trailing vortices (Rushton turbine). (a) Turbulent kinetic energy (impeller center plane; impeller rotation: counter-clockwise), (b) Z-vorticity ($r/T = 0.165$; impeller rotation: from left to right).

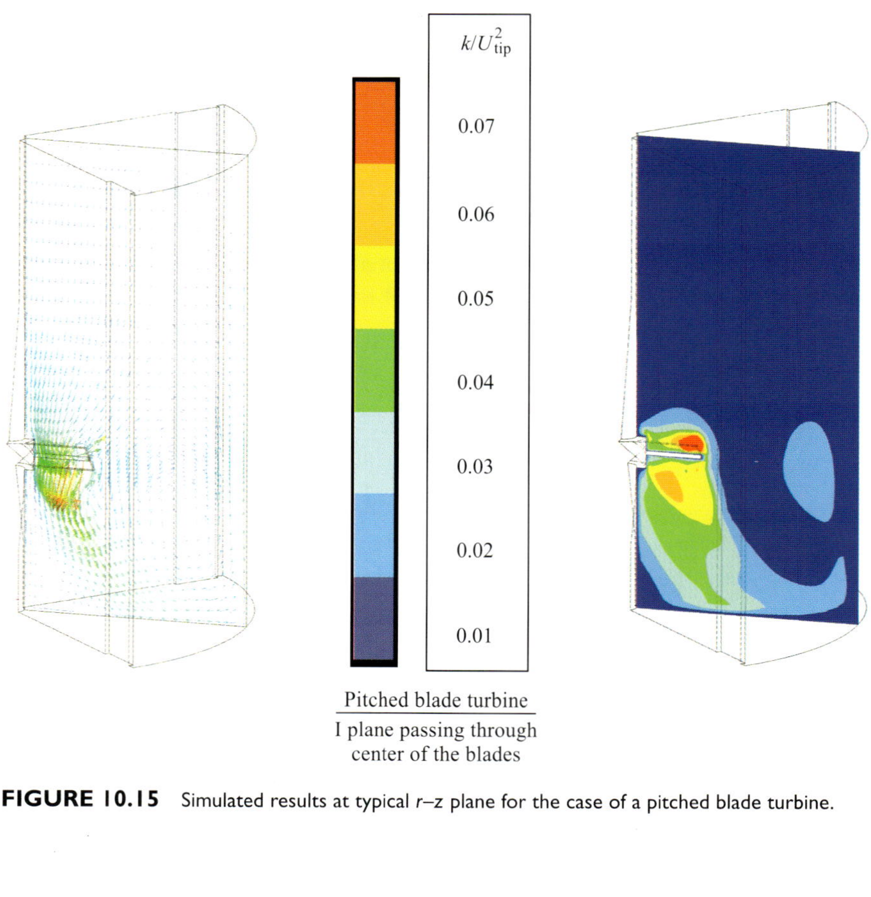

FIGURE 10.15 Simulated results at typical r–z plane for the case of a pitched blade turbine.

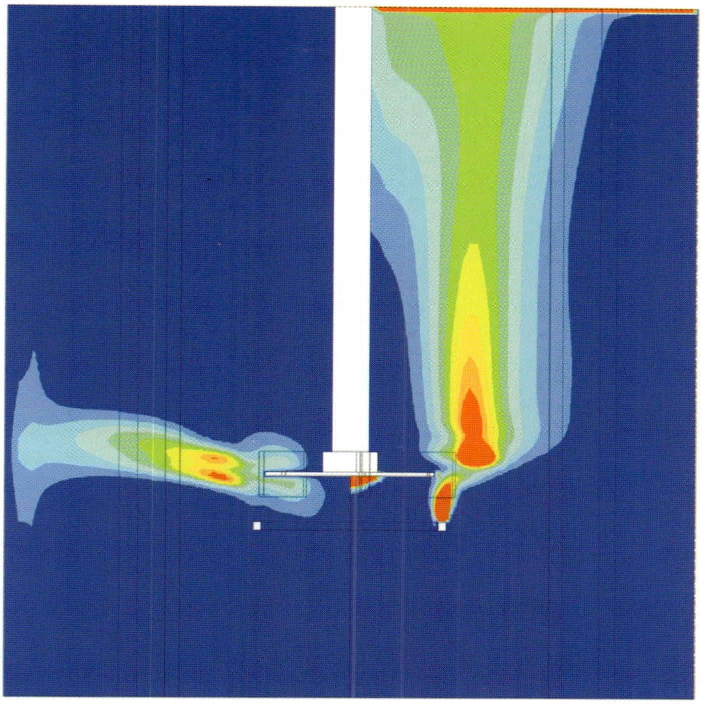

FIGURE 10.28 Typical predicted flow field. (Left: contours of dimensionless turbulent kinetic energy; Right: contours of gas hold-up). Ten uniform contours, maximum value = 0.1 (red); minimum value = 0 (blue).

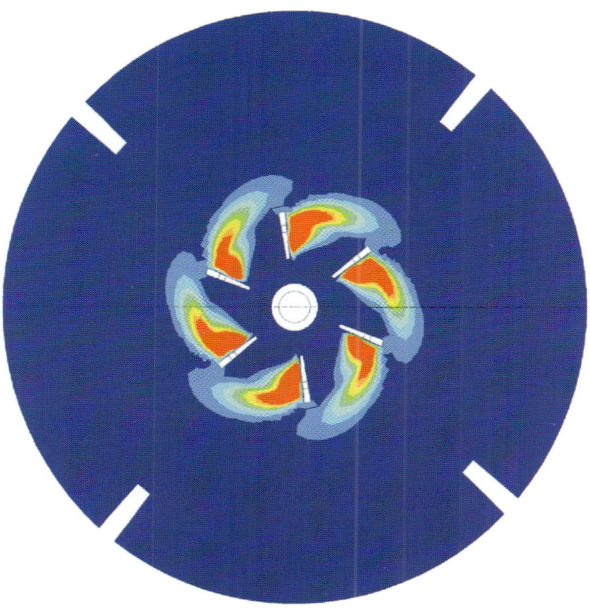

FIGURE 10.29 Contours of gas hold-up on horizontal plane located at a distance of BW/3 from impeller center plane (impeller rotation is counter-clockwise). Ten uniform contours between 0 and 0.1; Red: 0.1; Blue: 0.

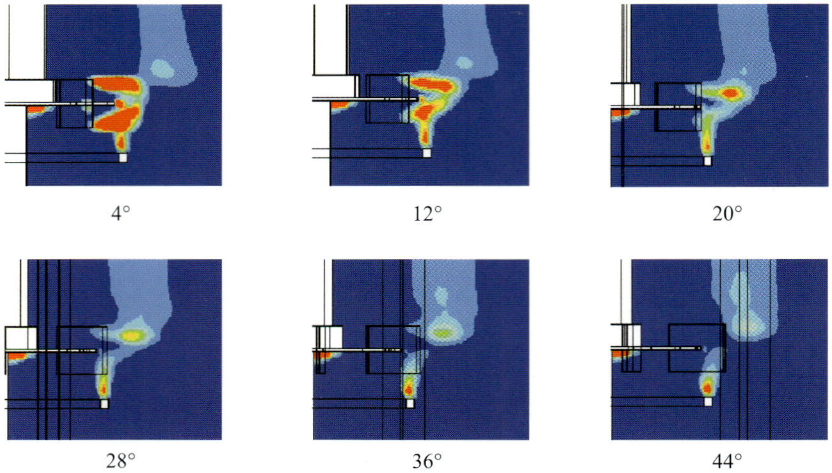

FIGURE 10.30 Computational simulation of accumulation of gas behind impeller blades (Blue: 0; Red: >0.1).

algorithm discussed in the previous chapter. It has three specific components developed for the simulation of multiphase flows, namely, derivation of pressure equations, a partial elimination algorithm (PEA) to handle tight coupling between momentum equations of two phases, and reformulation of continuity equations to calculate phase volume fractions to ensure that the sum of the volume fractions is unity.

Let us consider these three aspects in reverse order. Before we proceed, it must be emphasized that the usual interpolation rules, calculation of mean (harmonic/algebraic) and procedures to obtain finite volume discretized equations discussed in the previous chapter are applicable to multiphase flows as well. Applying the general methodology of the finite volume technique to two fluid flows, a discretized equation for any general variable ϕ can be written:

$$\sum_{\text{nb}} b_{\text{nb}}\phi_{\text{P}} = \sum_{\text{nb}} a_{\text{nb}}\phi_{\text{nb}} + S_{\text{C}} \tag{7.10}$$

The coefficients a consist of all the inflow contributions (convective as well as diffusive) while the coefficients b consist of all the outflow contributions. In the absence of any source or sink, the mass conservation equation dictates that the sum of inflow contributions is equal to the sum of outflow contributions. In the presence of linearized source terms, one can write,

$$\sum_{\text{nb}} b_{\text{nb}} = \sum_{\text{nb}} a_{\text{nb}} - S_{\text{P}} = a_{\text{P}} \tag{7.11}$$

If the flows are unsteady, the terms containing a_{P0} can be added on both sides of Eq. (7.10) (refer to Section 6.4). It must be noted that for multiphase flows, the inflow and outflow terms require considerations of interpolations of phase volume fractions in addition to the usual interpolations of velocity and the coefficient of diffusive transport. The source term linearization practices discussed in the previous chapter are also applicable to multiphase flows. It is useful to recognize that special sources for multiphase flows, for example, an interphase mass transfer, is often constituted of terms having similar significance to the a and b terms. Such discretized equations can be formulated for each variable at each computational cell. The issues related to the phase continuity equation, momentum equations and the pressure correction equation are discussed below.

(a) *Phase continuity equation*: To calculate a phase volume fraction, it is necessary to solve the phase continuity equation. There is one such equation for every phase. It is, however, useful to solve equations for all phases except one. The volume fraction of the remaining phase can then be deduced from the knowledge that the sum of volume fractions of all phases at any point (computational cell) is unity. The discretized phase continuity equation for each phase can be written in the form of Eq. (7.10). However, the as and bs appearing in this equation must be defined without the phase volume fractions, since phase volume fraction replaces the general variable ϕ in this case. Because of this, Eq. (7.11) relating inflow and outflow contributions is no longer valid for discretized phase continuity equations. This may lead to difficulties with iterative solutions of phase continuity equations. Before convergence, the values of as and bs may not be in proper balance. Direct solution of discretized equations may generate non-physical values of phase volume fractions. It is, therefore, useful to build 'traps' into the solution procedure to catch and avoid non-physical values.

To illustrate the two possible ways of avoiding non-physical values of phase volume fractions, let us consider a dispersed two-phase flow. The volume fraction of two phases can be obtained by solving the following equations:

$$\alpha_{\mathrm{P}}^{\mathrm{D}} a_{\mathrm{P}}^{\mathrm{D}} = F_{\mathrm{P}}^{\mathrm{D}} \qquad \alpha_{\mathrm{P}}^{\mathrm{C}} = 1 - \alpha_{\mathrm{P}}^{\mathrm{D}} \tag{7.12}$$

where the superscript indicates either a continuous (C) phase or a dispersed phase (D). F consists of all the inflow contributions including the sources at any grid node P and a contains all the coefficients of the outflow contributions. As mentioned earlier, straightforward solution of Eq. (7.10) may lead to non-physical values of volume fractions (less than zero or greater than one). One of the ways to avoid this is to build a constraint on the sum of two volume fractions within the solution procedure. This requires formulation of a discretized equation for the volume fraction of continuous phase and combining the two discretized equations to obtain:

$$\alpha_{\mathrm{P}}^{\mathrm{D}} = \frac{F_{\mathrm{P}}^{\mathrm{D}} a_{\mathrm{P}}^{\mathrm{C}}}{F_{\mathrm{P}}^{\mathrm{D}} a_{\mathrm{P}}^{\mathrm{C}} + F_{\mathrm{P}}^{\mathrm{C}} a_{\mathrm{P}}^{\mathrm{D}}} \tag{7.13}$$

This formulation ensures that the sum of the two volume fractions is unity. This method is very simple to implement when the volume fraction equation is solved using a point-by-point method, and is recommended by Spalding (1980). For more implicit calculations of volume fractions, further algebraic manipulations are necessary to accommodate Eq. (7.13) within the implemented numerical technique.

The other alternative is to subtract the two discretized continuity equations to obtain:

$$\alpha_{\mathrm{P}}^{\mathrm{D}} = \frac{a_{\mathrm{P}}^{\mathrm{C}} - F_{\mathrm{P}}^{\mathrm{C}} + F_{\mathrm{P}}^{\mathrm{D}}}{a_{\mathrm{P}}^{\mathrm{C}} + a_{\mathrm{P}}^{\mathrm{D}}} \tag{7.14}$$

It is also possible to subtract the original continuity equations before discretization and then apply the usual discretization procedures to derive the corresponding algebraic equations. This alternative has a special advantage when used with the pressure correction equations derived from the overall continuity equations (sum of two individual phase continuity equations). This combination then ensures that, simultaneously, both phase continuity equations are satisfied. Pressure correction enforces $D + C = 0$, while the volume fraction calculation enforces $D - C = 0$, leading to satisfaction of $D = 0$ and $C = 0$ (D and C denote dispersed phase and continuous phase continuity equations, respectively). This option is, however, restricted to two-phase flow simulations. The earlier option (Eq. (7.13)) suggested by Spalding (1980) can be extended to simulations of any number of phases in a straightforward manner.

Once the possibility of non-physical values of volume fraction is eliminated, solving phase continuity equations does not exhibit any other peculiarities, and the methods discussed in the previous chapter can be applied. One more point that must be mentioned while discussing the solution of phase continuity equations is of numerical or false diffusion. Numerical diffusion or false diffusion is not specific to multiphase flows and is related to any fixed-grid numerical solution procedure. However, it becomes very important in simulating multiphase flows. For example, suppose that in a field of uniform velocity, a 'front' exists across which phase volume fraction exhibits a discontinuity. In the absence of diffusion, such a front will move within the fluid without losing its discontinuous character. Numerical computations discussed here, however, would lead to smearing of the discontinuous front. Extra precautions are, therefore, necessary to recognize and control the extent of numerical diffusion when simulating multiphase flows.

(b) *Momentum equations*: Momentum equations differ from general transport equations because of the pressure gradient terms in the source terms. It is necessary to estimate the pressure field before solving the momentum equations. Of course this is necessary even for the simulation of single-phase flows and is discussed in the previous chapter. As discussed there, several ways of treating pressure–velocity coupling have been developed. The most widely applied are the SIMPLE family of algorithms, in which the pressure field is obtained either by solving the pressure correction equation (SIMPLE) or by solving directly the pressure equation (SIMPLER). Similar algorithms can be developed for multiphase flows. However, the presence of more phases widens the possible choices for deriving the discretized pressure correction or pressure equations. These issues are discussed later. At this stage, it may be assumed that a suitable pressure field is available to solve the multiphase momentum equations.

The other specific feature of multiphase momentum equations is the term containing interphase momentum transport (Eq. (4.16)). The interphase momentum transport terms invariably contain the velocities of all interacting phases at that grid node. Typically, the discretized momentum equation for two-phase flows (for the node P) can be written:

$$a_{\mathrm{P}}^{1} U_{\mathrm{P}}^{1} = \sum_{\mathrm{nb}} a_{\mathrm{nb}}^{1} U_{\mathrm{nb}}^{1} + S_{\mathrm{C}}^{1} + V_{\mathrm{P}}^{1} \left(\frac{\delta p}{\delta x} \right) + \beta_{12} \left(U_{\mathrm{P}}^{2} - U_{\mathrm{P}}^{1} \right) \tag{7.15}$$

Superscripts indicate phase index. All coefficients appearing in this equation can be derived by following the standard methods discussed earlier. The coefficient β_{12} represents all the relevant interphase interaction terms, which cause slow convergence, as mentioned earlier. Large interaction coefficients 'tie together' the velocities of two phases. Therefore, any iterative procedure involving one variable at a time proceeds very slowly. It is necessary to manipulate the discretized equations to eliminate the presence of the velocity of the other phase from the discretized momentum equations. This can easily be done by using an equation for U_{p}^{2} analogous to Eq. (7.15). The modified equation can be written:

$$\begin{aligned} &\left[a_{\mathrm{P}}^{1} a_{\mathrm{P}}^{2} + \beta_{12} \left(a_{\mathrm{P}}^{1} + a_{\mathrm{P}}^{2} \right) \right] U_{\mathrm{P}}^{1} \\ &\quad = \left(a_{\mathrm{P}}^{2} + \beta_{12} \right) \left(\sum_{\mathrm{nb}} a_{\mathrm{nb}}^{1} U_{\mathrm{nb}}^{1} + S_{\mathrm{C}}^{1} \right) + \beta_{12} \left(\sum_{\mathrm{nb}} a_{\mathrm{nb}}^{2} U_{\mathrm{nb}}^{2} + S_{\mathrm{C}}^{2} \right) \\ &\qquad + \left[V_{\mathrm{P}}^{1} \left(a_{\mathrm{P}}^{2} + \beta_{12} \right) + \beta_{12} V_{\mathrm{P}}^{2} \right] \frac{\delta p}{\delta x} \end{aligned} \tag{7.16}$$

This equation implicitly accounts for the interaction between the velocities of two phases and therefore, enhances convergence rate. When the interphase interaction coefficient is zero, the above equation reduces to that for single-phase flows. It is useful to note here that the coefficient of pressure gradient term also becomes modified by the presence of the second phase. These modified coefficients should be used when deriving the discretized pressure correction or pressure equations. These equations are now discussed below.

(c) *Pressure correction equation*: Following the procedures discussed in Section 6.3.2, it is possible to derive the pressure correction equation for multiphase flows. For this purpose, any one of the phase continuity equations can, in principle, be used. In general, it has been found that use of an overall continuity equation is more suitable. The overall continuity equation is obtained by adding the continuity equations of all phases. Since the phases present may have large difference in densities, it is often advantageous to normalize the phase continuity equations by phase-specific reference densities. Practical experience indicates that the density of each phase can be used as a reference density of that phase. This means that pressure correction equations or pressure equations are derived on the basis of overall volumetric (since the phase continuity equation is normalized by the density of that phase) continuity equations. It may be noted that in the overall continuity equation, the transient term as well as diffusion and mass source terms are absent. This is because the sum of volume fractions of all phases is unity and by definition, the sum of diffusion terms is zero. The sum of all interphase mass source terms is zero, because even though mass may be transferred from one phase to another, the net mass source must be zero.

Usual interpolation rules and definitions of velocity and pressure corrections, similar to single-phase flows (Eq. (6.29)), can be used to derive a pressure correction equation from the discretized form of the overall continuity (normalized) equation. The momentum equation for multiphase flows (Eq. (7.16)) can also be written in the form of Eq. (6.28) for single-phase flows. Again, following the approximation of SIMPLE, one can write an equation for velocity correction in terms of pressure correction, p':

$$u_{\mathrm{P}'}^{1} = -\frac{\left[V_{\mathrm{P}}^{1}\left(a_{\mathrm{P}}^{2}+\beta_{12}\right)+\beta_{12}V_{\mathrm{P}}^{2}\right]}{\left[a_{\mathrm{P}}^{1}a_{\mathrm{P}}^{2}+\beta_{12}\left(a_{\mathrm{P}}^{1}+a_{\mathrm{P}}^{2}\right)\right]}\left(\frac{\delta p'}{\delta x}\right) \tag{7.17}$$

A similar equation can be derived for velocity corrections for all components and for all phases. The above expression neglects velocity corrections from the right-hand side, following the single-phase flow practice. It is useful to note that in handling pressure–velocity coupling, the coefficients of the pressure gradient term appearing in Eq. (7.17) need not be very precise. The skilled numerical analyst can often enhance convergence by changing their magnitudes selectively or by further approximating them to reduce the computational demands. What is, however, important is that the coefficients have the right sign and that they properly reflect the relative sensitivities of the various phases to changes of pressure. Straightforward application of the procedure discussed here, does achieve this. Substitution of corrected velocities in the discretized overall continuity equation after using appropriate expressions of $\delta p'$ results in a pressure correction equation in the form of Eq. (6.32). The mass imbalance term in Eq. (6.32) will be replaced by an overall (normalized) imbalance term.

Having established the required discretized equations, the overall solution procedure for simulations of multiphase flows is as follows:

- Solve the volume fraction equations for all but one phase. The methods for avoiding non-physical values of volume fractions should be employed.
- Solve the momentum equations for all phases based on the guessed pressure field (or that obtained from solution of the pressure correction equation during

the previous iteration). The partial-elimination algorithm (PEA) should be used to handle the tight coupling between velocities of various phases.
- The pressure correction equation is solved based on the normalized overall continuity equation.
- The velocity and pressure fields are corrected based on the pressure correction field (for the SIMPLE algorithm).
- This cycle of adjustments is repeated several times until the errors remaining in all equations are acceptably small.

If the SIMPLER algorithm is to be used, corresponding pressure equations need to be solved following the procedures discussed in the previous chapter. The usual solution methods employed for single-phase flow simulations will be equally applicable to solving discretized equations of multiphase flows and, therefore, need not be discussed here again. When there are additional transport equations such as enthalpy or species equations (in addition to the momentum equations), PEA should be used to tackle the tight coupling between enthalpies and concentrations in various phases. When simultaneous mass and energy transfers are taking place, special manipulations may be applied to retain the applicability of PEA.

It is often useful to simulate multiphase flows by employing the techniques of unsteady flows. This provides an added under-relaxation, which is often necessary for multiphase flows with large dispersed phase volume fraction. There are several physical and numerical parameters which influence predicted results and the convergence behavior of the computational model. It is not possible to discuss all these issues here. Just to illustrate the possible results of Eulerian–Eulerian simulations, an example considered in the previous section is simulated here using the Eulerian–Eulerian approach, which allows simulation with higher gas flow rates. Therefore, the gas mass flow rate through the sparger was specified as ten times higher than that considered for the case simulated using a Eulerian–Lagrangian approach (0.1 kg s^{-1}). In these simulations, the top surface of the cavity was considered as a wall when solving the liquid phase and as an outlet while solving the gas phase. Details of the implementation of such a boundary condition are discussed in Chapter 11. The predicted results are shown in Fig. 7.18. It can be seen that strong circulatory flow generated by the impeller leads to the accumulation of gas near the eyes of circulation (Fig. 7.18c). The approach can be used to simulate complex multiphase flows as illustrated in Chapters 9

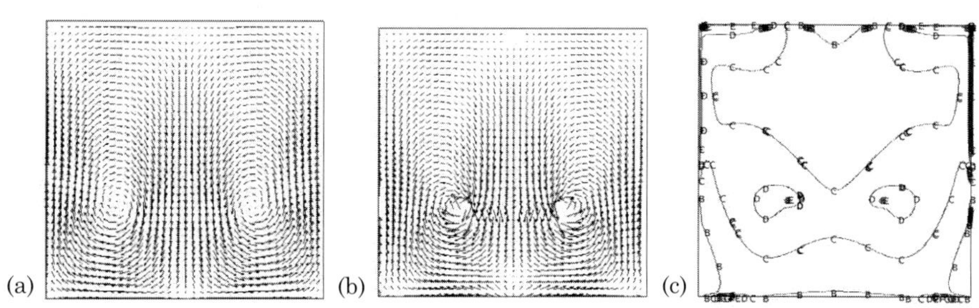

FIGURE 7.18 Results of Eulerian–Eulerian simulations. (a) Liquid flow field (maximum velocity = 6.5 m/s), (b) Gas flow field (maximum velocity = 8 ms^{-1}), (c) Contours of gas volume fraction (8 uniform contours between 0 [A] to 0.07 [G]).

to 14. The convergence behavior of multiphase flow simulations depends on several factors including selected algorithm, extent of PEA, applied under-relaxation and initial guess. In most cases, the convergence behavior of multiphase flows cannot be discussed independently of the solver employed (and programs). Some general comments are made when discussing applications of the Eulerian–Eulerian approach to simulate complex multiphase flows in later chapters (Chapters 10 to 14).

7.3. SIMULATION OF REACTIVE FLOWS

Various approaches to modeling reactive flows are discussed in Chapter 5. For most approaches, based on RANS equations, the usual finite volume method can be applied to solve the required transport equations of mean or variance of relevant quantities. However, obtaining a converged solution in a reacting flow can be difficult for a number of reasons. The chemical reactions and corresponding energy changes may have a strong impact on the basic flow patterns. This is especially true for gaseous combustion reactions, in which reactions release a large amount of energy causing significant changes in density, and large accelerations. Strong coupling between the mass/momentum transport equations and the species transport equations exists for such systems, which may lead to difficulties in convergence. Even when there is no significant coupling between momentum and species transport equations, non-linear coupling between different species equations due to chemical kinetics may make the solution task more complicated. In many cases, the reaction source term of any single species depends on concentrations of other species. Unless the solver is solving all the species equations simultaneously (which is not usually the case), this interdependence can lead to convergence difficulties. Another convergence issue in reacting flows is related to the magnitude of reaction source terms. For fast chemical reactions, the reaction source term may dominate the discretized species transport equations and it may no longer remain diagonally dominant. Such source-dominated equations may lead to rapid and unstable changes in species concentrations.

Some of the modeling approaches used for dealing with very rapid chemistry are discussed in Chapter 5. Apart from these modeling approaches, several techniques have been evolved to tackle convergence difficulties. In many cases, it is advantageous to start simulations from a simplified case. For example, it is often beneficial to first carry out cold flow simulations without considering chemical reactions. Using these results as an initial guess, complete model including chemical reactions and energy equations can be solved. For reactive flows, it is essential to carry out the time scale analysis of the processes under consideration (as discussed in Chapter 5). The relative magnitudes of characteristic time scales of convection, mixing and chemical reactions often provide guidelines for selecting suitable parameters of the numerical method. If such a time scale analysis reveals very different time scales for different processes, it may be necessary to use a fractional time step method, which uses different time steps for different processes. For example, when implementing the multi-environment model, Ranade and Bourne (1991) used two different time steps, one for simulating large-scale processes such as convection and turbulent diffusion and the other for simulating micromixing and reactions occurring within each computational cell.

When using a conserved scalar approach with the equilibrium assumption, it is necessary to carry out computations of: (1) equilibrium composition of gas from

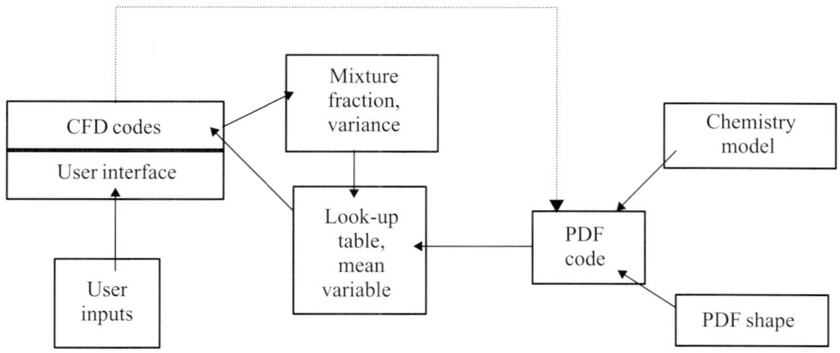

FIGURE 7.19 Generic coupling between a PDF solver and a CFD solver.

the atomic composition and the total enthalpy; and (2) mean scalar values from the instantaneous mixture fraction. Often these calculations are carried out using a separate program by executing it outside the main flow solver. The results of these computations can be stored in look-up tables. These look-up tables along with an efficient interpolation algorithm, are used by the flow solvers to estimate the required quantities. The generic coupling of such external codes with CFD solvers is shown in Fig. 7.19. Details of numerical methods required for interpolation, integration etc. are not discussed here and can be found in Press *et al.* (1992). For full PDF methods, Monte Carlo methods may be used (Pope, 1981; 1985). Roekaerts (1989) extended these methods using a Monte Carlo ensemble associated with a fixed grid, instead of using stochastic differential equations. This approach can conveniently be implemented in conventional turbulent flow solvers. The above cited papers and a recent review by Fox (1996) can be referred to for more details of full PDF methods and their relationship with other approaches to modeling reactive flows.

To simulate multiphase reactive flows, it is necessary to devise suitable partial or full elimination algorithms to treat coupling between multiple phases due to interphase mass transfer and chemical reactions. If the reactions are slow, the standard partial elimination algorithm, discussed earlier, can be applied since in such a case, the interphase mass transfer terms are linear. When chemical reactions interact with mass transfer, interphase transfer terms become non-linear and special algorithms need to be developed on a case-by-case basis. If enhancement in mass transfer rate (multiplier to the standard linear interphase mass transfer term, see Eq. (5.32)) is accounted for by developing a look-up table (following the strategy used for PDF models), the standard elimination algorithm discussed earlier can be used. Computationally, however, it is more efficient to develop a case-specific linearization to account for the functional dependence of mass transfer enhancement on species concentrations. For very complex multiphase reactive flows, it may be useful to use a multiscale modeling approach rather than developing an all-encompassing comprehensive CFD model. In the multiscale approach, complex chemistry and its interaction with mass transfer and mixing are modeled using a simpler (than CFD) modeling framework comprising fewer computational cells or sub-regions. Such a model, therefore, requires several empirical inputs regarding the underlying flow patterns, degree of mixing, phase volume fractions and so on. Detailed flow simulations using a suitably simplified (with respect to chemistry) CFD model is used to generate the necessary information.

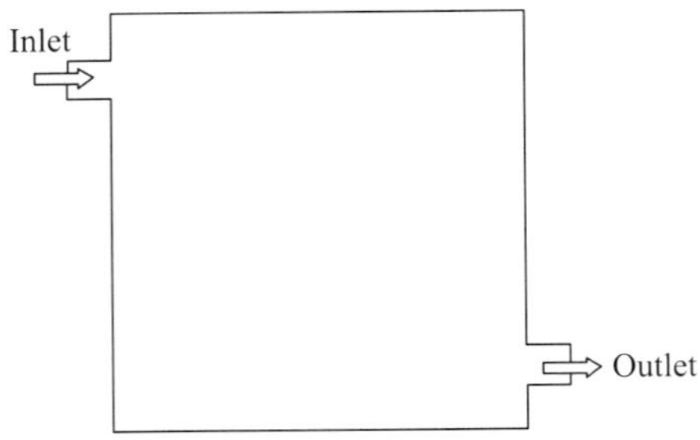

Reaction: $A \longrightarrow B$
Molecular weights of A and $B = 20$
Liquid density $= 1000\,\mathrm{kg\,m^{-3}}$
Reactor volume $= 0.01\,\mathrm{m^3}$
Residence time $= t = 10\,\mathrm{s}$
Reaction rate constant $= k = 1.0, 0.1, 0.01$ l/s
Conversion based on ideal mixing: $X_{\mathrm{mix}} = 1/1 + k\tau$
Initial conditions: mass fractions, $m_{\mathrm{A}} = 1.0, m_{\mathrm{B}} = 0.0$
Boundary conditions: at inlet, $m_{\mathrm{A}} = 1.0, m_{\mathrm{B}} = 0.0$
Sample of simulated results:

Sr. No.	Rate constant, l/s	Impeller speed, $\mathrm{m\,s^{-1}}$	$(1 - X_{\mathrm{A}})_{\mathrm{mix}}$	$1 - X_{\mathrm{A}}$
1	1.0	5.0	0.090909	0.06083
2	1.0	1.0	0.090909	0.04453
3	1.0	0.0	0.090909	0.07500
4	0.1	5.0	0.5	0.49383

FIGURE 7.20 Initial and boundary conditions for reactive flow simulations.

CFD results can provide guidelines to select an appropriate simplified model. Some examples of such an approach are discussed in Chapter 9. A simple example, which illustrates the evaluation of the often-used assumption of a completely mixed reactor, is discussed here, by continuing the case of the cubical reactor considered in earlier examples.

A simple, homogeneous (slow) first-order reaction was considered. Simulations were carried out for cases with and without impeller in the same cubical reactor. Initial and boundary conditions are shown in Fig. 7.20. It can be seen that the mean residence time of the reactor is 10 s. Three cases with different first-order reaction rate constants ($0.01\,\mathrm{s^{-1}}$, $0.1\,\mathrm{s^{-1}}$, $1.0\,\mathrm{s^{-1}}$) were simulated (samples of the results are listed with Fig. 7.20). Results of simulations with an impeller velocity of $5\,\mathrm{m\,s^{-1}}$ are discussed first. As expected, for the lowest reaction rate constant, where the characteristic reaction time scale is much higher than mean residence time, the simulated results agree quite well with the analytical solution obtained based on the assumption of a completely mixed reactor. Even for the case of characteristic reaction time scale of 10 s (which is the same as the residence time), deviation from the analytical solution (of predicted outlet concentration of reactant) is just about 1% (for the case with rate constant $0.1\,\mathrm{s^{-1}}$). As the reaction time scale becomes smaller than residence time (rate constant $1.0\,\mathrm{s^{-1}}$), deviation increases and is equal to 33%! If the reaction rate becomes even faster, one has to use special reactive mixing models discussed in Chapter 5. This simple exercise illustrates the well-known fact that the extent of deviation from ideal mixing is dependent on relative time scales of reaction and mixing. Simulations of a case with rate constant 1.0 s^{-1} for an impeller speed 1 m s^{-1} indicates an even higher deviation of 51% from the ideal mixed predictions. The case without an impeller, however, leads to 17.5% deviation. This means that the situation with impeller velocity of 1 m s^{-1} leads to the highest conversion of reactant. Deviation from ideal mixing is expected to lead to higher conversion of reactant than that predicted by the ideal model. The higher the impeller velocity, the closer the system becomes to the ideal system. Therefore, higher conversion is obtained with an impeller velocity of 1 m s^{-1} than 5 m s^{-1}. However, when there is no impeller, the inlet fluid short circuits through the reactor. This causes a decrease in the effective volume of the reactor resulting in lower conversion, although it gives a maximum deviation from the ideally mixed situation. Additional examples of using CFD models for reactor applications are discussed in later chapters. Some issues relevant to the application of CFD methods to industrial equipment are discussed in the following section.

7.4. SPECIAL TOPICS

7.4.1. Complex Geometry

Many flows relevant to chemical reactor engineering practice involve complex geometries. Although the principles of discretization and solution methods for algebraic systems described earlier may be used, some modifications are required to handle such complex geometries. The properties of the solution algorithm depend on choice of the grid and the arrangement of variables on the grid. Some of these issues are discussed in this section.

For a regular (for example, rectangular or circular) geometry, the grid lines usually follow the co-ordinate directions. In complicated geometries, the choice of grid is not trivial. The grid is subject to constraints imposed by the discretization method and solution algorithm. If the algorithm is designed for structured quadrilaterals, an unstructured grid consisting of triangles cannot be used. When the geometry is complex, some compromises have to be made to fulfill the constraints. Body-fitted non-orthogonal grids are most often used to calculate flows in complex geometries (most commercial codes use such grids). In such grids, grid lines follow the boundaries of the solution domain, which makes implementation of boundary conditions easier. The transformed equations for non-orthogonal grids, however, contain additional terms leading to difficulty in programming and increased computational costs. Despite this disadvantage, these grids are used in most applications. Grid generation for complex geometries will not be discussed here. Some relevant comments are included in Chapter 1. More details of grid generation can be found in Thompson *et al.* (1985) and Arcilla *et al.* (1991). Some general comments relevant to numerical solutions are included here.

Though complex geometry demands that the grid be non-orthogonal, it is useful to make it as orthogonal as possible. In finite volume methods, orthogonality of grid lines at corners (vertices) of computational cells (CV) is not important. The angle between the cell face normal vector and the line connecting the CV centers on either side is important. Cell topology is also important. If the midpoint rule integral approximation and linear interpolation is used, then the accuracy will be higher if CVs are quadrilaterals than if CVs are triangles (in 2D). Accuracy is also improved if one set of grid lines closely follows the streamlines of flow (especially for convective flows). This can be achieved with a structured grid (of quadrilaterals in 2D) but not with triangular grids. Complex geometries also demand non-uniform grids. A finer grid should be used in the regions where strong variations are expected to occur. When generating non-orthogonal and non-uniform grids, three measures of grid quality should be kept in mind:

- ratio of adjacent cell sizes: preferably less than two;
- aspect ratio of a computational cell (ratio of adjacent edges of a cell): preferably less than five;
- skewness of a computational cell (angle between adjacent edges of a cell): preferably greater than 45°.

When the geometry is complex, grid generation may require a significant fraction of the time necessary to complete the development and application of the computational model. Since the accuracy of the flow solution depends as much on the grid quality as on the approximations used for discretization of the equations, time spent generating a quality grid is a worthwhile investment.The basic principles of the finite volume method discussed in the previous chapter are independent of the type of grid used. There are, however, some new features, which need to be introduced to handle arbitrary non-orthogonal grids. Some of these are discussed here.

As discussed in the previous chapter, with the finite volume method, we need to approximate the surface and volume integrals to calculate fluxes and sources. Consider the two-dimensional control volume shown in Fig. 7.21. Following Eq. (6.6), the mass

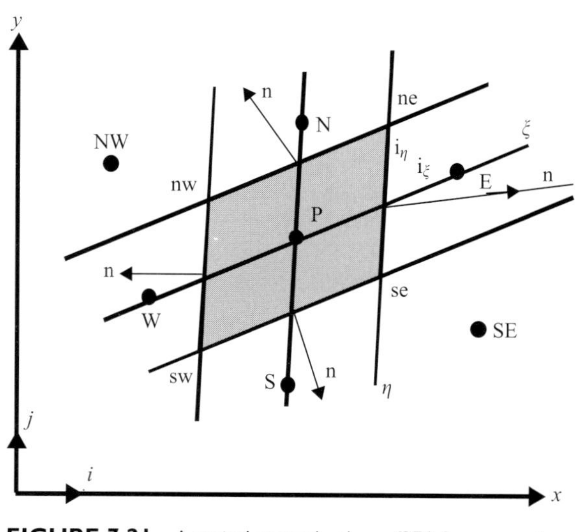

FIGURE 7.21 A typical control volume (2D) for non-orthogonal grid.

flux through face e can be written as:

$$m_e = (\rho U \mathbf{n})_e S_e \tag{7.18}$$

where **n** is a unit normal vector to the east face. Unlike with a regular grid, the surface vector has components in more than one Cartesian direction and all the velocity components contribute to the mass flux. Mass flux can be calculated by summing products of each Cartesian velocity component and the corresponding surface vector component (projection of the cell face on a Cartesian co-ordinate plane):

$$m_e = \rho_e \left(U_x S^x + U_y S^y\right)_e \tag{7.19}$$

where superscripts or subscripts indicate Cartesian co-ordinate direction. The convective flux of any transported quantity can be calculated as the product of mass flux through the face and the value of transported property at the center of the cell face. Various interpolations discussed in the previous chapter can be used to estimate the value of transported property at the center of the cell face. The integrated diffusive flux in a general coordinate system can be written:

$$D_e = (\Gamma \operatorname{grad} \phi \cdot \mathbf{n})_e S_e \tag{7.20}$$

The gradient of ϕ at the cell face center can be expressed either in terms of the derivatives with respect to global Cartesian co-ordinates or local orthogonal co-ordinates. If the local orthogonal system attached to the cell face center is used, then only the derivative in the normal (n) direction contributes to the diffusive flux:

$$D_e = \Gamma_e \left(\frac{\partial \phi}{\partial n}\right)_e S_e \tag{7.21}$$

On a Cartesian grid, $n = x$ at the e face and the usual schemes can be used to estimate gradient at e. For example, a central differencing scheme will give:

$$\left(\frac{\partial \phi}{\partial n}\right)_e = \frac{\phi_E - \phi_P}{L_{PE}} \tag{7.22}$$

where L_{PE} is the distance between nodes E and P. When the grid is non-orthogonal, the above expression must be corrected by a term containing the difference between the gradients in the ξ and n direction. Mujaferija (1994) has proposed the correction as:

$$D_e = \Gamma_e \left(\frac{\phi_E - \phi_P}{L_{PE}}\right) S_e + \Gamma_e S_e (\operatorname{grad} \phi)_e \cdot (n - i_\xi) \tag{7.23}$$

where i_ξ is the unit vector in the ξ direction (Fig. 7.21). The second term of the right-hand side is usually evaluated explicitly from previously known values.

Apart from the convective and diffusive fluxes, it is also necessary to evaluate source terms. As mentioned in the previous chapter, the volume integral can be calculated as a product of the CV center value of the integrand and the CV volume. This approximation is independent of the CV shape. For non-orthogonal grids, the calculation of the cell volume becomes more complicated. For 2D quadrilaterals, the volume of the cell can be calculated by taking the vector product of the two diagonals. The expression for cell volume of the cell shown in Fig. 7.21 becomes:

$$V_{\text{cell}} = \frac{1}{2}\left[(x_{\text{ne}} - x_{\text{sw}})(y_{\text{nw}} - y_{\text{se}}) - (x_{\text{nw}} - x_{\text{se}})(y_{\text{ne}} - y_{\text{sw}})\right] \tag{7.24}$$

In three-dimensional solution domains, the cell faces are not necessarily planar. Suitable approximations are necessary. Further details of discretization on non-orthogonal grids will not be presented here. The purpose of this section was just to highlight some of the relevant issues. Reader may refer to Ferziger and Peric (1995) and references cited therein for more details. Even if a reactor engineer is not interested in developing an in-house CFD code, familiarity with these issues is essential for developing computational models of complex flows in complex geometry. More often than not, poor quality grids lead to divergence, and suitable corrective measures need to be taken to obtain convergence. Some examples of the simulation of complex flows in industrial equipment are discussed in Chapters 9 to 14.

7.4.2. Enhancing Convergence Performance

Overall convergence performance depends on several factors. Factors such as, large number of computational cells, overly conservative under-relaxation factors, strong non-linearity and coupling between different equations, hinder convergence. Grid quality also affects the convergence rate significantly. It is often necessary to use various 'tricks' to enhance the convergence performance. Different classes of flow problems (with varying degrees of complex flow physics and complex geometry) may require different strategies. Some of the general ways of enhancing convergence are discussed here.

Supplying an initial guess for important flow variables often enhances overall convergence behavior. The process of providing an initial guess also allows the user to examine the main characteristic space and time scales. Examination of these scales is necessary to select appropriate numerical parameters such as time step and under-relaxation factors. The process is also useful to verify the adequacy of the generated grid. Another commonly used technique to enhance convergence performance of complex flow problems is to break down the overall problem into a sequence of problems with increasing complexity at each stage of the sequence. For example, when solving a non-isothermal problem, it may be a good idea to first obtain a reasonable solution (need not be completely converged) to the isothermal problem, which can act as a good initial guess for the non-isothermal problem. Solution of the simplified isothermal problem can be started by setting the initial guess to the temperature field, which will remain unchanged during the solution process. After obtaining reasonable convergence for the isothermal problem, solution of the enthalpy equation can be started. Sometimes it is advantageous (computationally) to switch off the solution of momentum and continuity equations while solving the enthalpy equations. Once the enthalpy equation starts converging, all the equations can be included in the solution process. Several examples of such a step-by-step procedure to improve the convergence of complex flow problems are discussed in Chapter 9 and later chapters.

As mentioned in the previous chapter, it is advantageous to use under-relaxation factors to improve the convergence behavior of a set of non-linear coupled equations. Under-relaxation needs to be applied not only to direct flow variables such as velocity, pressure, temperature etc. but also to indirect variables like fluid properties (density, viscosity, heat capacity), when these variables are composition or temperature dependent. It is indeed impossible to provide generalized guidelines for setting under-relaxation parameters since several factors such as the algorithm, parameters of the linear equation solver, the extent of non-linearity and coupling affect suitable values of under-relaxation factors. Usually, the solution is started with rather conservative values of under-relaxation factors. The values may be increased as the solution progresses with the help of continuous monitoring of residual history. The influence of under-relaxation factors on convergence rate is demonstrated in Fig. 6.18. Unless repeated simulations of similar cases have to be carried out, it may not be computationally economical to optimize under-relaxation factors.

Apart from the formulation of discretized governing equations and algorithms to treat various couplings, the solution method of the resulting linear algebraic equations also has a significant impact on convergence rate. In many CFD simulations of complex flows, iterative line-by-line solvers are used. Two parameters of line-by-line solvers, namely, the direction of sweeping lines in the solution domain and the number of sweeps for each equation, govern the overall convergence behavior. In general, lines which are normal to the primary flow direction, are solved in the direction of the primary flow. When there is no single dominant flow direction, it is useful to use alternating sweep directions. An increase in the number of sweeps for any equation leads to more computations per iteration; however, this may improve the local and therefore, global convergence behavior. Of course, there will be an optimum number of internal iterations or of sweeps throughout the solution domain, to minimize overall convergence time. Generally, a higher number of sweeps needs to be specified for pressure and for any equation which is difficult to converge (e.g. species equations in the presence of non-linear chemical reactions). When the flow problem involves large body forces, it is often necessary to increase the number of sweeps of the pressure equation.

In addition to these parameters of line-by-line solvers, several other techniques have been proposed to accelerate the convergence rate. Some of these methods are discussed in Section 6.2.2 and only brief comments will be added here. One-dimensional block corrections based on an additive correction philosophy (Kelkar and Patankar, 1989) reduce long wavelength errors in the direction in which they are applied. However, these methods are not suitable if very steep gradients exist in the solution. Multigrid methods are effective in reducing long wavelength errors in such situations. As mentioned earlier, choice of such parameters as number of grid levels, number of iterations on each level, the order in which various levels are visited, interpolations between various levels and so on will affect convergence behavior. The values of these parameters need to be tuned to accelerate the overall convergence performance. It is not possible to discuss all these details here, and the reader is referred to Hackbusch (1985) and Ferziger and Peric (1995).

For time-dependent flows, in addition to the factors discussed above, the values of time step and number of iterations per time step, govern the overall convergence behavior. In general, the selected time step should be at least an order of magnitude smaller than the smallest relevant time scale of the modeled flow process. If the explicit method is used to march in time, iterations within a time step are not required. However, in such a case, the value of time step is severely constrained. For an implicit method, it may be necessary to use more than one iteration per time step to obtain a converged solution at each time step. In general, the value of time step is selected in such a way that the number of iterations per time step does not increase beyond 20. For many practical transient flows, a very fast 'start-up' phase exists, which may decay rapidly. In such cases, the value of time step may be gradually increased as the calculations proceed. When the problem is being solved as a transient problem and the steady or pseudo-steady solution is of interest, it may not be necessary to obtain complete convergence for each time step at the beginning. Once the solution is developed, the internal iterations can be increased to achieve the desired accuracy of the solution. This simple technique is useful for solving complex multiphase flows, which are often solved as time-dependent flows. In addition, several problem-dependent techniques can be used to accelerate the overall convergence behavior of multiphase flows. Examples of these are discussed in Chapters 9 to 13.

7.4.3. Error Analysis of Complex Simulations

Errors in CFD simulations arise mainly from two sources:

- inherent errors in representing reality by the set of model equations (physically deficient representation); and
- errors arising from inexact solution methods (numerically deficient representation).

It is essential to identify and separate these two types of errors to avoid confusion. If numerical errors are not isolated, they may lead to undesirable spurious model calibration exercises. It is, therefore, necessary to devise systematic methods to quantify numerical errors. The basic idea behind error analysis is to obtain a quantitative measure of numerical errors, to devise corrective measures to ensure that numerical errors are within tolerable limits and the results obtained are almost independent of numerical parameters. Having established adequate control of numerical errors, the simulated results may be compared with experimental data to evaluate errors in physical modeling. The latter process is called model validation. Several examples of model validation are discussed in Chapters 10 to 14. In this section, some comments on error analysis are made.

Low-order numerical methods contribute to the robustness and computational efficiency of the CFD code. However, this same robustness and speed make it imperative that error estimates be available so that plausible looking results are not confused with accurate results. In many complex reactor-engineering applications, the reactor engineer may be interested in capturing the trends rather than absolute values. Even then, it is essential to verify that captured key flow features are independent of numerical parameters. Formal error estimates for grid-based numerical methods may be based on Taylor series expansions (Roache, 1976). These analytic approaches are valuable for development and evaluation of numerical methods but are rarely used to assess complex flow simulations. The usual method of assessing the numerical accuracy of complex flows is through grid refinement. In this approach, the computations are repeated on progressively finer grids and resolution is presumed to be adequate when results do not change significantly with grid density. Estimates of the local converged solution may be obtained by extrapolating solutions obtained on two or more grids to an infinitely dense grid (zero grid spacing). An example of such a method is discussed in Chapter 6. It must, however, be remembered that routine application of grid refinement to complex flow simulations (with complex flow physics and complex geometry) is problematic for several reasons. Most flow simulations relevant to industrial reactor engineering routinely use a few hundred thousand computational cells (see examples in Chapter 9 to 14). Moreover, for complex geometric configurations, numerical errors resulting from non-uniform distribution of grids, and from departures from grid orthogonality further complicate the quantification of numerical errors. In such cases, systematic assessment of grid sensitivity requires variation in both grid density as well as grid distribution and topology. More often than not, difficulties in grid generation and the magnitude of computational resources required for such complex flow simulations preclude the routine use of grid sensitivity tests.

When systematic grid refinement is not possible to assess numerical errors, global balances of numerically non-conserved quantities (quantities that are not conserved at the control volume level in the construction of the numerical scheme) can be used. Haworth *et al.* (1993) described this approach in detail. The method is based on volume-integrated partial differential equations for primary or derived physical quantities of interest. Balances can be applied to the full computational domain or to any sub-domain down to the single-cell level. Comparison of relative magnitudes of terms in the balances provides insight into the physics of the flow being computed. For quantities that are not conserved on a computational cell level, the imbalance provides a direct measure of numerical inaccuracy using a single grid simulation. Haworth *et al.* (1993) recommended imbalance in mean kinetic energy, which they show to be a good measure of low-order spatial discretization error. For more details, the original paper may be consulted. Such an approach, combined with grid refinement studies (wherever possible), can provide a useful measure of numerical errors.

For multiphase flows, the analysis of numerical errors becomes more difficult but even more important. In many practical multiphase flows, it may not be possible to obtain grid-independent solutions. More often than not, the reactor engineer has to rely on CFD simulations, which may show grid dependence, when making important practical design decisions. In such cases, it is essential to ensure that grid dependence is not affecting key conclusions on which the engineering decision is being based (even though the overall flow field may show grid dependence). Some examples of developing useful engineering decisions based on flow simulations obtained with modest grid requirements are discussed in Chapters 9 to 14.

7.5. SUMMARY

Modifications and enhancements in the basic finite volume method, necessary for simulations of complex multiphase or reactive flows, are discussed in this chapter. Approximations invoked in linearization of source terms and interpolation practices need to be examined carefully in light of their implications on convergence and accuracy. For most of the multiphase flow simulation methods, suitable modifications need to be incorporated in the discretized equations to avoid non-physical results. Some such modifications are discussed in this chapter. Complex geometry of the considered solution domain often poses severe challenges to convergence behavior and accuracy of the simulation method. Some suggestions with respect to these aspects are included. Aspects of error analysis to identify various sources of errors appearing in the construction of the overall numerical solution method are also discussed. Once an adequate control on numerical errors is established, evaluation or validation of the underlying physical model may be carried out. Even though the user is not interested in writing an in-house code, the issues discussed in this chapter will be useful for carrying out simulations of complex flows using ready-to-use commercial CFD codes.

REFERENCES

Arcilla, A.S., Hauser, J., Eiseman, P.R. and Thompson, J.F. (eds) (1991), "Numerical Grid Generation in Computational Fluid Dynamics and Related Fields", North Holland, Amsterdam.

Brackbill, J.U., Kothe, D.B. and Zemach, C. (1992), A continuum method for modeling surface tension, *J. Computat. Phys.*, **100**, 335–354.

Carver, M.B. (1984), Numerical computation of phase separation in two fluid flow, *J. Fluids Eng.*, **106**, 147–153.

Delnoij, E. (1999), Fluid dynamics of gas liquid bubble columns, PhD thesis, University of Twente, Enschede, The Netherlands.

Delnoij, E., Kuipers, J.A.M. and van Swaaij, W.P.M. (1999), A three dimensional CFD model for gas–liquid bubble columns, *Chem. Eng. Sci.*, **54**, 2217–2226.

Ferziger, J.H. and Peric, M. (1995), "Computational Methods For Fluid Dynamics", Springer Verlag, Berlin.

Fox, R.O. (1996), Computational methods for turbulent reacting flows in the chemical process industry, *Rev. Inst. Francois du Petrole*, **52**, 215.

Hackbusch, W. (1985), "Multi-grid Methods and Applications", Springer, Berlin.

Haworth, D.C., El Tahry, S.H. and Huebler, M.S. (1993), A global approach to error estimation and physical diagnostics in multidimensional CFD, *Int. J. Num. Meth. Fluids*, **17**, 75–97.

Hirt, C.W. and Nichols, B.D. (1981), Volume of fluid method for the dynamics of three boundaries, *J. Comput. Phys.*, **39**, 201.

Hoomans, B.P.B., Kuipers, J.A.M., Briels, W.J. and van Swaij, W.P.M. (1996), Discrete particle simulation of bubble and slug formation in a two dimensional gas fluidized bed: a hard approach, *Chem. Eng. Sci.*, **51**, 99.

Kelkar, K.M. and Patankar, S.V. (1989), Development of generalized block correction procedure for the solution of discretized Navier–Stokes equation, *Comput. Phys. Commun.*, **53**, 329–336.

Kothe, D.B., Mjolsness, R.C. and Torry, M.D. (1991), RIPPLE: a computer program for the incompressible flows with free surfaces, Los Alamos National Laboratory, Report LA – 12007 – MS.

Krishna, R. and Van Baten, J.M. (1999), Simulating the motion of gas bubbles in a liquid, *Nature*, **398**, 208.

Mujaferija, S. (1994), Adaptive finite volume method for flow predictions using unstructured meshes and multigrid approach, PhD thesis, University of London.

Pope, S.B. (1981), Monte Carlo method for the PDF equations of turbulent reactive flow, *Combust. Sci. Technol.*, **25**, 159–174.

Pope, S.B. (1985), PDF methods for turbulent reactive flows, *Prog. Energy Combust. Sci.*, **11**, 119–192.

Press, W.H., Teukolsky, S.A., Vellarling, W.T. and Flannery, B.P. (1992), "Numerical Recipes", Cambridge University Press.

Ranade, V.V. (1992), Flow in bubble column: some numerical experiments, *Chem. Eng. Sci.*, **47**, 1857.

Ranade, V.V. (1997), Modeling of turbulent flow in a bubble column reactor, *Chem. Eng. Res. Des.*, **75**, 14–23.

Ranade, V.V. and Bourne, J.R. (1991), Fluid mechanics and blending in agitated tanks, *Chem. Eng. Sci.*, **46**, 1883.

Ranade, V.V. and van den Akkar, H.E.A. (1994), A computational snapshot of gas liquid flow in baffled stirred reactors, *Chem. Eng. Sci.*, **49**, 5175–5192.

Rider, W.J. and Kothe, D.B. (1995), Stretching and rearing interface tracking methods, Los Alamos National Laboratory (http://www.c3.lanl.gov/~wjr/pubs.html).

Roache, P.J. (1976), "Computational Fluid Dynamics", Hermosa, Albuquerque.

Roekaerts, D. (1989), Monte-Carlo composition PDF method for turbulent reactive flow in a jet stirred reactor, in "Numerical Methods in Laminar and Turbulent Flows", Vol. 6, Part 2.

Rudman, M. (1997), Volume tracking methods for interfacial flow calculations, *Int. J. Num. Methods Fluids*, **24**, 671.

Spalding, D.B. (1980), Numerical computation of multi-phase fluid flow and heat transfer in, "Recent Advances in Numerical Methods in Fluids", Pineridge Press, pp. 139–197.

Thompson, J.F., Warsi, Z.U.A and Mastin, C.W. (1985), "Numerical Grid Generation-foundations and Applications, Elsevier, New York.

Tsuji, Y., Tanaka, T. and Yonemura, S. (1993), Discrete particle simulation of two dimensional fluidized bed, *Powder Technol.*, **77**, 79.

Youngs, D.L. (1982), Time dependent multi-material flow with large fluid distortion, In "Numerical Methods for Fluid Dynamics", K.W. Morton and M.J. Bianes (Eds), Academic Press, New York, pp. 273.

8 COMPUTATIONAL TOOLS FOR SIMULATING FLOW PROCESSES

Basic mathematical models governing flow processes are discussed in Chapters 2 to 5. These model equations are usually partial differential equations, which need to be solved using numerical methods. Some of the relevant numerical methods are discussed in Chapters 6 and 7. It must be mentioned here that knowledge of fluid dynamics (for model development) and numerical methods to solve the model equations can be useful only if appropriate computational tools are available to apply these to solving the problem at hand. In this chapter, process of mapping model equations and numerical methods on digital computers is discussed. The tasks and desired characteristics of computational tools (programs) required for such mapping and for carrying out numerical simulations of flow processes of practical interests are also discussed. Use of these computational flow-modeling tools for reactor-engineering applications is discussed in the subsequent chapters.

8.1. MAPPING A COMPUTATIONAL FLOW MODEL ON A COMPUTER

The overall process of any computational flow-modeling project was discussed in Section 1.2 (see Fig. 1.11 for key steps). It will be instructive to re-examine such a process with the background of Chapters 2 to 7. The first step of any flow-modeling project is to identify key controlling processes and relate these controlling processes to underlying fluid dynamics. This analysis will allow one to formulate clear objectives for the flow-modeling exercise. It must be mentioned here that, usually, the potential

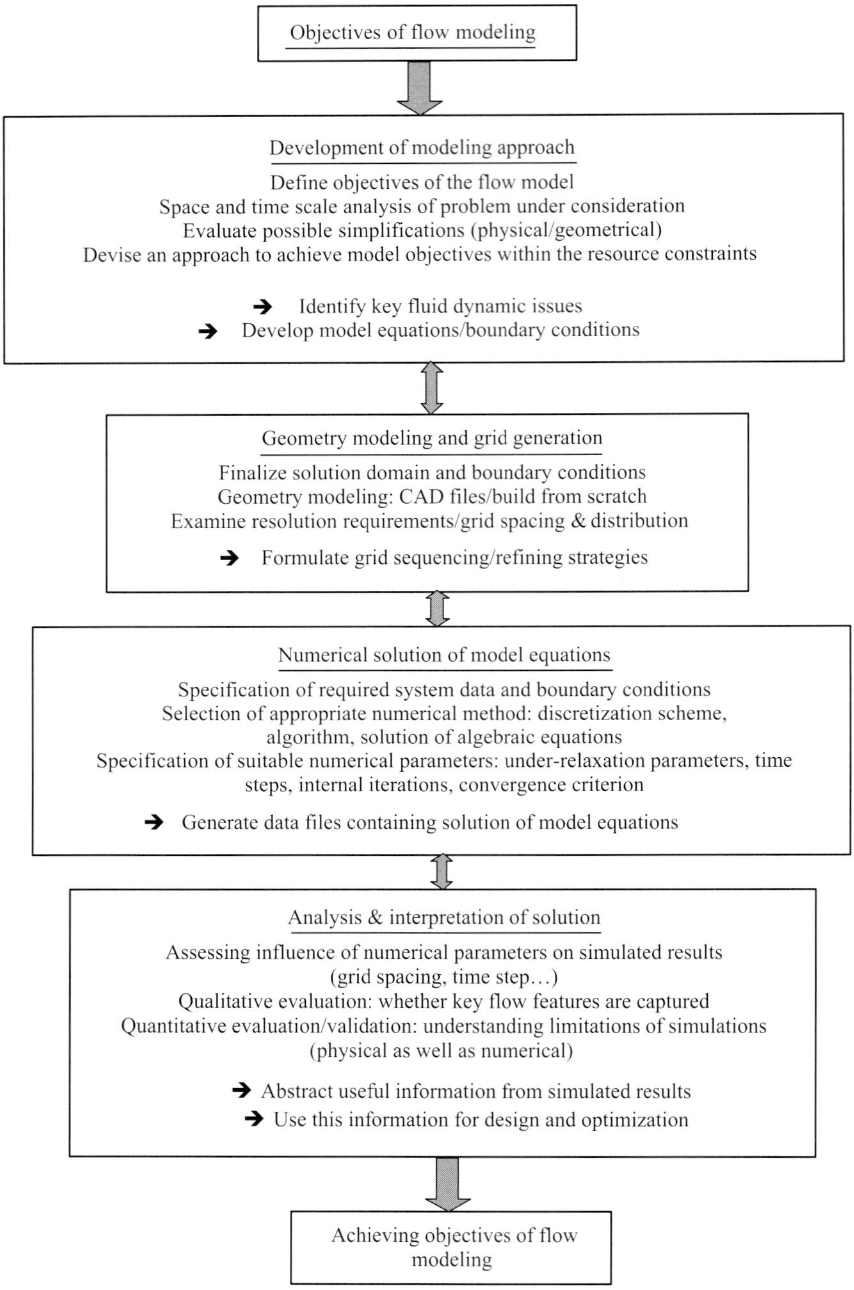

FIGURE 8.1 Mapping computational models onto CFD tools.

benefit of undertaking a flow-modeling exercise will determine the extent of resources made available to the project. Clear understanding of the role of fluid dynamic modeling in the overall project is essential. Detailed knowledge of fluid dynamics, analysis of space and time scales of the specific problem at hand and analysis of the available resources (computing resources, time, expertise and so on), are required to develop an appropriate modeling approach. The modeling approach devises ways of dividing the complex problems into tractable sub-problems and ways of achieving the project objectives within the allocated resources. A thorough knowledge of computer implementation of flow models is essential to evolve a suitable modeling approach. Steps in the implementation of a computational flow model on a computer are discussed below.

The basic elements of mapping a computational flow model on a computer are shown in Fig. 8.1. Some comments on developing a modeling approach were made in Chapter 1. Ways of devising a suitable modeling approach are discussed further in Chapter 9 with the help of practical examples. In this chapter, we essentially restrict the discussion to the basic elements which are necessary to generate simulated results from the flow model.

- *Geometry modeling of the reactor under study.* It is first necessary to select an appropriate solution domain to decouple the system under investigation from the surrounding environment. While finalizing the extent of the solution domain, care must be taken to understand and eliminate the influence of domain boundaries on the predicted flow results. Once the domain is finalized, it is important to decide what geometrical features are essential to model to capture the influence of equipment hardware on flow processes of interest. For example, if the near wall region is an important concern (say to estimate wall heat transfer coefficient), it is necessary to consider the geometry and shape of the wall accurately. If the interest is only in understanding global flow patterns, the complex shape of the wall may be approximated, without jeopardizing the utility of the simulations.
- *Grid generation.* To implement the finite volume method, it is necessary to divide the solution domain into a number of computational cells, this process being called 'grid generation'. As briefly mentioned in Chapter 1, either structured or unstructured grids may be employed. Prior knowledge of various relevant scales and likely regions of steep gradients helps in generating a suitable grid for the problem at hand. While generating the grids, care should be taken to avoid extremes of aspect ratios and skewness. It is also necessary to formulate grid sequencing and refinement strategies to understand the influence of grid spacing/distribution on simulated results. More often than not, it will be difficult to obtain a truly grid-independent solution for complex flows in industrial reactors. Systematic grid sequencing studies may help to derive maximum benefit from the simulated results, despite the non-availability of a truly grid-independent solution.
- *Specification of necessary information/data related to flow process under consideration.* Once a suitable grid is generated, the user has to specify the necessary information concerning the physicochemical properties of fluids such as molecular viscosity, density, conductivity etc. for the solution of model equations. If the process under consideration involves chemical reactions, all the other necessary data about reaction kinetics (and stoichiometry, heat of reaction etc.) need to be supplied. In addition to system-specific data, specification of boundary conditions on the edges/external surfaces of the solution domain is a further crucial aspect of the solution process. It is also necessary to provide all the information related to the numerical method selected

to solve the model equations (under-relaxation parameters, time step, internal iterations and so on). It may sometimes be necessary to provide an initial guess to start the iterative solution procedure.

- *Solution of model equations for the generated grid.* Once the grid is generated and the required data are available, the main task of implementing a numerical method to solve the model equations can be initiated. The numerical solution involves formulation of algebraic equations by discretizing model equations on the generated grid, and solution of these algebraic equations until convergence using a suitable algorithm. Relevant details of numerical methods are discussed in Chapters 6 and 7. It is necessary to strike a balance between efficient implementation of numerical methods (which may be better if programs are developed for specific cases) and its general applicability.
- *Analysis of simulated flow results.* The solution process generates huge amounts of data about the simulated flow process (flow, species and temperature fields within the solution domain). With large numerical simulations, one may become lost in the sea of numbers in the absence of appropriate tools to analyze the simulation results. Appropriate analysis strategies and tools to implement these strategies must be developed to draw useful conclusions about the flow process under consideration. Some ways of identifying key flow features, such as vortices, are also useful for qualitative evaluation of simulation results. Methods and tools for error analysis and for validation are also essential to derive maximum information from the simulation results and to plan further studies.

The necessary computational tools required to carry out these steps are generally classified into three categories: pre-processors, solvers and post-processors. The temptation to give a brief review of some of the major available commercial CFD codes is resisted here since all these codes are fast evolving and the information available today may not be relevant even in the near future. The relevant CFD products of some of the leading vendors are listed in Table 8.1. The web sites mentioned in this table may be visited to get up-to-date information about these codes. Links to other available CFD codes may be found at www.cfd-online.com. Instead of comparing different CFD codes at their present stage, which may not be relevant for long, here we discuss some of the key issues which will be useful when evaluating CFD codes.

Although in many commercially available CFD codes, some capabilities of pre- and post-processors are bundled up with the solver, it will be useful to discuss the CFD tools by classifying them in the stated three categories. It is important to mention here that it is more useful to compare CFD codes based on underlying technological issues rather than based on their 'features'. The main technological issues in pre-processors, solvers and post-processors are listed in Table 8.2, and are discussed in the following sub-sections.

8.2. PRE-PROCESSORS

This category usually includes geometry modeling and grid generation tools. In some cases, specification of the required information about the system under consideration and the numerical technique used can also be specified using pre-processors. Some

TABLE 8.1 Some Leading CFD Codes

Vendor	Products
General Purpose CFD Codes	
FLUENT	Pre-processors: preBFC, GAMBIT, Tgrid Main codes: Fluent4.5, Fluent5, FIDAP, Rampant, Nekton, MixSim Post-processors: in-built in above codes, Flpost www.fluent.com
AEA Technology	Pre-processors: CFX-Build Main codes: CFX4, CFX5, CFX-ProMixus Post-processors: CFX-Visualize www.aeat.com/cfx
CHAM	Main code: PHOENICS Post-processor: PHOTON www.cham.co.uk
STAR-CD	Pre- and post processor: PROSTAR Main code: STAR-CD www.cd.co.uk
AVL	Pre-processor: FAME Main codes: FIRE, SWIFT Post-processor: in-built in above codes www.avl.com
CFDRC	Pre-processor: CFD-GEOM Main code: CFD-ACE6, CFD-ACE (U) Post-processors: CFD-VIEW www.cfdrc.com
Stand-alone Pre-processors	
Pointwise	Gridgen www.pointwise.com
ICEM-CFD	ICEM-CFD Tetra, ICEM-CFD Hexa www.icemcfd.com
Stand-alone Post-processors	
AVS	AVS/ AVS Express www.avs.com
CEI	Ensight, EnsightGold www.ceintl.com

of the major tasks of any CFD pre-processor are:

- to enable the user to model the geometry of the problem under consideration;
- to generate a suitable computational grid for the modeled geometry;
- to compile all the necessary data and information about the grid in a form suitable to the CFD solver;
- to accept relevant input data from the user;
- to check the consistency of the input data (as far as possible);
- to store all this information in a form suitable for reading into CFD solvers for further processing.

Geometry modeling and grid generation are the major elements of CFD pre-processors. For simple geometry conforming to a standard co-ordinate system (for example, Cartesian or cylindrical-polar co-ordinates), geometry modeling and grid

TABLE 8.2 Key Issues for Evaluating CFD Pre-processors, Solvers and Post-processors

Pre-processor	Solver			Post-processor
Geometry modeling approach: solid modeler/surface modeler; top-down/bottom-up Geometry import facilities: CAD packages, general formats like IGES Geometry repair facilities: gaps/trimmed surfaces, removal of coincident entities	Grid types: import from different pre-processors; co-located/ staggered; (un) structured Automatic grid refinement tools, addition of grid elements Geometry modifications (change scale/cell type etc.) without re-meshing	Porous media models: isotropic/non-isotropic; pressure drop model; UD? Rheological models: non-Newtonian fluids/UD? Algorithm? Reactive-flows: Phenomenological models-EB, ESCIMO, multigroup E model	Algorithms: pressure-correction/density based; multiple pressure corrections? Multiphase flows: partial/full elimination? Pressure correction? Multiphase flows: calculation of volume fractions/internal traps	Ease of analysis during simulation: coupling with solver/local integral quantities Error analysis: residue reduction, distribution within domain Basic presentation capabilities: vectors, contours, streak-lines, iso-surfaces
Visualization: internal grids, multiple views Grid types: single/multi-block; structured/unstructured/mixed	Memory: 1 million cell problem:~ 0.35–1 GB Compressible/incompressible; primary variables/stream function	PDF-based models: presumed/ full PDF algorithm? Surface reactions: options for rate controlling steps/UD? Multiphase reactive flows: mass transfer/reactions in all phases?	Segregated/coupled solver? Option? Source-dominated flows: handling of user-defined sources/scalars	Computation of fluxes, sub-domain balances Automatic feature detection: trailing vortices/re-attachment
Grid generation tools: automatic/parametric generation, recovery from error (UNDO facilities)	Transient simulations: automatic control on time steps/efficient storage		Convergence behavior: sensitivity to under-relaxation parameters	Presentation of user-defined derived quantities: constraints/ flexibility
Boundary layer capability Mesh control: clustering, aspect ratios, skewness	Turbulence models: user-defined model (UD)? Wall functions: constraints on near wall cells	Boundary conditions: profile/transient/UD? Special/user-defined BCs for multiphase flows?	Algebraic equation solvers: conjugate gradient? Acceleration tools: multigrid/block correction	Visualizing results on arbitrary surfaces Overlay capabilities/lighting/ shading
Tools for assessment of grid quality	Simulation of rotating flows: sliding mesh/multiple reference frames	Consistency checks for BCs/input data	Parallelization: technology? speed-up efficiency	Importing tabular data for validation/comparisons
Grid refinement: smooth-ing/orthagonality/clustering	User-defined scalar equations: constraints on form/algorithm	Importing physical property and kinetics data from external databases	On-line convergence monitoring tools	XY plots, Function calculators to compare global results
Setting fluid properties/input data: databases/consistency checks	Multiphase flows: Eulerian–Eulerian (EE) capabilities: closure/drag laws/additional forces	Discretization schemes: space/time; higher order/user defined?	Data storage/Exporting data to different post-processors	Post-processing of transient simulations/multiple datasets
Setting boundary conditions/defining cell types Exporting information to different solvers	EE-granular flows: model options/Eulerian–Lagrangian (EL): true/psuedo? particle models/UD?	Limiter functions to avoid non-physical results/UD? Special discretization procedures for multiphase flows	Access to the source code/internal flow Overall computational performance/bench mark cases	Animation/video facilities/different formats Exporting results to other presentation tools (RGB, BMP, MPEG, PS, EPS)
Future developments: new technologies	VOF: surface forces/ adhesion/contact angle; UD?	Facility to provide internal traps/limits	Future developments: algorithms/algebraic solvers	Future developments: better integration

generation is fairly straightforward and can be executed by accepting relevant data from the user. However, most industrial reactors have complex configurations and therefore require advanced geometry modeling tools. Complex geometries may be developed either by using a bottom to top approach (defining points, lines, faces and so on to construct higher order objects) or by using a top to bottom approach (starting with solid volumes and carrying out Boolean operations on them to arrive at the desired geometry). With the advent of widespread applications of computer aided design (CAD) and solid mechanics analysis, several geometry modeling tools are now available. Most of these tools allow use of a top to bottom approach to define the desired geometry. Most pre-processors of the commercially available CFD codes allow one to import geometry from these design tools. In addition to importing geometry information from these design tools, most CFD pre-processors also have in-built geometry modeling tools. Some tools are also provided to repair 'dirty' geometry (gaps, trimmed surfaces and so on). These capabilities are essential and must be critically evaluated during the selection process.

Meshing or generating a suitable computational grid for the modeled geometry is one of the most important pre-processor tasks. Quite sophisticated algorithms and tools are required to divide the modeled geometry into computational cells based on either a structured or unstructured grid. A structured grid requires that all interior nodes have an equal number of adjacent elements (typically all elements are quadrilateral or hexahedral). This restriction is relaxed in an unstructured grid (triangular or tetrahedral elements may be used). The type of grid is subject to constraints imposed by the discretization method selected and the solution algorithm. Once the type of grid is selected (structured or unstructured), several methods are available to generate the desired grids. Details of these methods will not be discussed here. More information on grid generation may be found in Thompson (1996) and at an excellent website on grid generation maintained by Steven Owen: http://www.andrew.cmu.edu/user/sowen/mesh.html.

It must be mentioned here that geometry modeling and grid generation may account for a substantial percentage of the time required to carry out the total flow modeling task. For example, in aerospace engineering applications, the time spent on geometry modeling and grid generation may account for more than 50% of the total project time. Even for reactor engineering applications, where model development may require most of the time, the time spent on grid generation is not insignificant. It is, therefore, important to evaluate various facilities made available in any grid generation tool, to reduce the time spent on grid generation. Most commercial grid generation tools allow parametric grid generation to facilitate faster grid generation for similar geometries. Facilities to recover from errors, while building the geometry or while generating the grids, are also very useful (e.g. customizable UNDO features). A boundary layer capability to ensure adequate resolution near walls and corners is also useful. Appropriate tools to provide control of clustering, cell aspect ratio and cell skewness, are essential to generate good quality grids. More often than not, some refining operations are needed to make the generated grid better suited to flow simulations. Such refining operations may be classified into (1) smoothing (includes operations which adjust node locations while maintaining the element connectivity), and (2) clean-up (operations which change element connectivity). Capabilities for grid refinement and tools to assess the quality of the generated grid are very important and need to be examined critically.

Although boundary conditions and fluid properties may be set in pre-processors, most commercial codes allow these to be set in CFD solvers.

8.3. SOLVERS

Solver tools implement the numerical methods discussed earlier (Chapters 6 and 7) to solve the model equations. It is important to give appropriate importance to (1) general applicability, (2) ease of use, (3) economy of computations, (4) maintainability, and (5) expandability. These five requirements may have contradictory demands on the way computer programs are generally written and developed. Most computer programs developed by academic research groups focus on including more complex physical models and may tolerate deficiencies in other requirements, such as ease of use and maintainability. The capability to handle complex grids is also, generally, moderate in such academic codes. Most commercial codes try to provide ease of use and maintainability along with the capability to handle complex grids. Such codes may, however, have to trade some of the recent advances in understanding of the physics of complex flow processes (e.g. multiphase and reactive flows), to provide general applicability and robustness. The provisions to include new mathematical models may, therefore, become one of the important criteria in the selection of commercial CFD code, especially for reactor engineering applications. Before reviewing key issues in evaluating commercial CFD codes, some comments on in-house CFD code are relevant.

Although commercial CFD tools are being increasingly used to address complex, industrial reactor engineering problems, the experience and insight gained through the use of in-house CFD codes is often very useful. It is always beneficial to develop some CFD tools in-house, to get a first hand feel. Patankar (1980) listed several suggestions for the development of such in-house CFD codes. It is beneficial to adopt a modular approach to construct the required CFD tools. Cross *et al.* (1989) discussed some of the guidelines and trends in CFD software engineering, which may also be useful for the new code developer. Ferziger and Peric (1995), in their excellent book, discussed various numerical methods and their computer implementation. Corresponding FORTRAN programs are available from their website (ftp.springer.de/technik/pub/peric). The process of development of a CFD code, its de-bugging and validation can provide much needed insight into the behavior of flow processes, as well as their numerical simulation. This process and experience may significantly enhance the ability to use and to modify various commercially available CFD tools. In-house code may also serve the purpose of testing new models by simulating relatively simple validation problems. The validated model can then be incorporated in a commercial CFD code to carry out numerical simulations of industrial process equipment. With the advent of the world wide web (WWW), it is now easy to download the necessary components and construct an in-house CFD tool kit. A good source to find useful CFD resources is http://www.cfd-online.com. Free and shareware CFD programs as well as several general purpose numerical programs are listed on this site.

Industrial reactor engineering applications are generally carried out using commercial CFD tools to ensure enhanced maintainability and useful life of the developed models. Key characteristics of CFD solvers and tools are summarized in Table 8.2. For reactor engineering applications, one of the most important features of CFD codes is the ability to extend the in-built models via user-written modules. No matter how general the CFD code is, it will always be necessary to develop specific sub-models (see e.g. case studies discussed in Chapter 9) to simulate specific reactors. It is important to understand the power and limitations of such user-defined capabilities of any CFD code before one commits to use it for reactor engineering applications. Documentation and tools to assist the incorporation of new models into commercial CFD code also play an important role in determining the effort and resources required to extend commercial CFD code to include specific model equations. Every commercial CFD code vendor offers different ways and facilities to incorporate new models. Many commercial CFD codes impose constraints (form of the equations, algorithm used for the user defined equations and so on) on user-defined equations, which need to be evaluated carefully. In many situations, it is necessary to replace some of the terms in the default model equations. In such situations, a facility to select terms in the default model equations is very useful. If such a facility is not present, the user has to develop programs to subtract the unwanted terms in the default equations and include the new ones. This may lead to some inconsistencies if the discretization methods used by the user and those used in the default code are not the same. Many of the leading commercial CFD vendors organize 'User Group Meetings' to promote exchange of expertise and exchange of user-defined enhancements. Archives of 'user-defined routines' are also maintained by some vendors. Such archives and proceedings of user group meetings are very useful sources of information related to the use of a particular CFD code in reactor-engineering applications.

Apart from the available mathematical models and facilities for adding new mathematical models, there are several other issues of concern when selecting an appropriate CFD code. The facility to import grids from a variety of grid generation tools/pre-processors is obviously needed. A facility for scaling an entire geometry without the need for re-meshing will be useful for studying scale-up or scale-down (geometrically similar) behavior. An ability to introduce minor modifications in the geometry (e.g. introducing or removing baffles), without re-meshing, will be useful for evaluating different reactor configurations. An ability to handle grids of high aspect ratio and high skewness is important since most industrial reactors have complex geometry. It is difficult to identify upper limits of grid aspect ratio or skewness which these codes can handle since these values are strongly problem dependent. A facility for automatic grid refinement according to user-defined criteria will also be useful. Automatic grid refinement and appropriate data interpolation tools greatly facilitate grid sequencing studies and the generation of grid-independent results. Not all commercial codes provide these facilities. In addition to grid refinement, higher order discretization schemes play an important role in enhancing the accuracy of simulation results. An ability to incorporate a user-defined discretization scheme will, therefore, be a useful facility (which is not provided by most currently available commercial CFD codes).

To simulate turbulent flows, Reynolds-averaged Navier–Stokes (RANS) equations form the basis for most codes. Several turbulence models are usually provided. A new turbulence model may also usually be incorporated via user-defined routines. Recently, many of the commercial CFD codes have announced the inclusion of large eddy simulation (LES) capabilities. Considering the importance of rotating equipment used in reactor engineering applications, the ability to handle multiple reference frames or sliding meshes is important. Most leading commercial CFD codes provide similar facilities to simulate single-phase flows. Capabilities to simulate multiphase flows may, however, differ considerably from code to code. The same is true for reactive mixing or combustion models. This is expected to be so as both of these fields are still evolving at a fast pace. The same comments are also applicable to porous media models, complex rheological models and surface reaction models. The user-defined capabilities of CFD codes mentioned above become even more important in these areas and need to be evaluated based on the intended reactor engineering applications. Available options for boundary conditions also must be examined, especially for multiphase flows. Some sort of consistency checks on input data and on permissible combinations of boundary conditions are always useful. A facility to import physicochemical data from available databases is useful when simulating flow systems with large numbers of components.

The SIMPLE or PISO family of algorithms (SIMPLE, SIMPLER, SIMPLEC, SIMPLEST, PISO, SIMPISO) are usually used to treat pressure–velocity coupling. Most commercial codes provide options to use state of the art multigrid techniques and block correction methods to accelerate the solution of algebraic equations. Often, for single-phase flows, the solver performance of most codes is similar, but may, however, differ significantly for multiphase flows, depending on algorithms and traps used to handle the interphase coupling (partial elimination or full elimination, calculation of volume fractions and so on). Unfortunately, information on how the multiphase flow equations are discretized and what in-built traps are included to avoid non-physical results, is usually not disclosed by commercial CFD vendors. The availability of various options for interpolation and trajectory calculations when carrying out Eulerian–Lagrangian simulations of dispersed multiphase flows may also differentiate the available codes. Several versions (and different implementations) of VOF models also make direct comparisons difficult. It may be useful to formulate a few benchmark problems (related to the intended reactor engineering applications) to evaluate the performance of different CFD codes. On-line convergence monitoring tools are often useful and are needed to carry out complex simulations. The ability to run the CFD solver on multi-CPU machines is also important to reduce the turn-round time of complex reactor engineering problems. The speed-up ratios achieved for specific parallel hardware should be examined before selecting the CFD solver (or the hardware).

Although it is important to compare the underlying technologies of different CFD codes, it should be noted that the ability to carry out the desired simulation using a given CFD code depends more on the expertise of the user rather than on the CFD code itself. The skilled CFD user can obtain the desired results from any available commercial CFD code by suitably exploiting user-defined routines. The tools required to analyze the results obtained by CFD codes are discussed below.

8.4. POST-PROCESSORS

Numerical solutions of model equations generate large sets of numbers. Appropriate post-processing tools are essential to analyze and to interpret these simulation results. Many commercial CFD codes provide in-built post-processing facilities or allow results to be exported to other post-processing packages. The key issues in evaluating CFD post-processors are briefly summarized in Table 8.2.

The first component in the analysis of simulation results is usually checking the degree of convergence and estimating numerical errors. These facilities are usually incorporated in solvers rather than in separate post-processors. Most CFD codes report normalized residuals. It is important to evolve criteria to judge the adequacy of residual reduction suitable for the application under consideration: different variables often need different residual reduction criteria. The progress of residual reduction and the distribution of residuals often indicate whether the numerical solution is adequate. A facility to report sub-domain or global balances is also useful for examining the adequacy of the numerical solution. Once adequate convergence (more often than not, multiple criteria are needed to ensure adequate convergence) has been confirmed, the simulation results may be studied in several ways.

Two of the most common ways of examining simulation results are: (1) vector plots, in which the length of every arrow indicates the magnitude of the local velocity, and the direction of the arrow indicates the direction of the local velocity; and (2) contour plots, which represent the predicted field in the form of constant value contours. Superimposing a vector plot of two components of velocity on the contours of the remaining component of velocity is often done to provide information about the three velocity components in a plane. Most post-processors allow such vector or contour plots on any arbitrarily defined planes or surfaces within the solution domain. Other options to visualize simulation results, such as three-dimensional iso-surfaces, particle streak lines, and particle tracks can reveal important features of the predicted flow field. Automatic feature detection facilities are offered by some of the advanced visualization tools, which may be able to automatically detect 'trailing vortices' behind impeller blades and are, therefore, useful for verifying whether the simulation results have captured essential features of the flow or not. Additional facilities such as different options for coloring vectors or iso-surfaces, perspective views, overlaying different views and so on, are often useful to clearly understand interactions between different variables of interest and to enhance the quality of the results presented.

For quantitative validation of simulation results, it is often necessary to compare predicted profiles (of velocity or other variable of interest) with experimental data: X–Y plotting facilities are useful for this purpose. Most post-processors allow the user to import tabulated data for comparison with simulation results. Facilities to calculate the usual global quantities of interest to reactor engineers, such as overall pressure drop, dispersed phase volume fraction, heat or mass transfer rates and so on, are necessary to address reactor engineering concerns. Most codes allow use of user-defined routines to evaluate different quantities of interest, which may then be displayed using the standard tools discussed above.

It is often necessary to evolve problem-specific post-processing strategies in order to extract as much information as possible from the generated numbers. The need for good post-processing tools is even greater when detailed post-processing studies indicate that the agreement between simulation results and experimental data is not satisfactory. Under such circumstances the user needs to understand the simulation results to identify possible causes for the observed discrepancies. Rather than blindly blaming the underlying model, careful post-processing of simulation results may reveal a wealth of information which will be useful for further development of a mathematical model. When the simulated flow results look satisfactory, the reactor engineer has to extract useful information for further use. Generally, different models are used to address different practical reactor-engineering projects (refer to discussion in Chapter 1). More often than not, flow models are used to obtain the desired information for the other intermediate reactor models such as mixing cell models. Some such examples are discussed in the next chapter (Chapter 9). Post-processing tools should allow easy exchange of information among different levels of models. Such an exchange, until recently, used to be manual or via a case-specific in-house interface. However, there is an increasing trend to automate the information exchange so that flow information from the CFD model can be exported to intermediate reactor models, and reaction information may be imported to CFD code from such reactor models. Development of these interfaces is still in the early stages and more up-to-date information may be found on different web sites (for example, see www.pfd.ie).

8.5. SUMMARY

The basic elements involved when using a computational flow model for reactor engineering or any other application, are: (1) geometry modeling and grid generation; (2) specification of system data and selection of mathematical models and boundary conditions; (3) solution of model equations; and (4) analysis and interpretation of simulation results. The tools required to carry out these elements are generally classified into three groups: pre-processors, solvers and post-processors. Some of the leading commercial tools are listed in Table 8.1. Rather than comparing these commercial tools, key issues in evaluating any CFD code are discussed briefly in this chapter (Table 8.2). Some comments on the importance of using an in-house CFD code and resources to construct such an in-house code are also included. In principle, the skilled CFD user can obtain the desired results from any reasonable commercial CFD code by suitably exploiting user-defined routines. It is important to critically examine the capabilities of user-defined routines and constraints imposed on the use of these routines.

Knowledge of underlying physics and its mathematical representation (Chapters 2 to 5), of numerical methods to solve such mathematical representations (Chapters 6 and 7) and of computational tools to implement these numerical methods (this chapter), equip the reader to harness the potential of computational flow modeling for reactor engineering. It is essential to develop an appropriate modeling approach to suit the reactor-engineering objectives at hand. Development of such approaches is discussed in Chapter 9 with the help of practical examples.

REFERENCES

Cross, M., Richards, C.W., Ierotheou, C. and Leggett, P. (1989), In Flow Modelling of Industrial Processes, Eds. Bush, A.W., Lewis, B.A. and Warren, M.D., Ellis Harwood, Chichester.

Ferziger, J.H. and Peric, M. (1995), "Computational Methods for Fluid Dynamics", Springer-Verlag, Berlin.

Patankar, S.V. (1980), "Numerical Heat Transfer and Fluid Flow", Hemisphere, Taylor & Francis Group, New York.

Thompson, J.F. (1996), A reflection on grid generation in the 90s: trends, needs and influences, 5th International Conference on Numerical Grid Generation in Computational Field Simulations, Mississippi State University, April, pp. 1029–1110.

PART III
CFM FOR CRE

9 FLOW MODELING FOR REACTOR ENGINEERING

Basic tasks of reaction and reactor engineering are discussed in the first chapter. A general methodology for applying computational flow modeling tools to reactor engineering is also briefly discussed in Section 1.3. Basic information about the elements of computational flow modeling (CFM) is given in Section 1.2 and Chapters 2–8. Applications of CFM to reactor engineering are now discussed here in detail.

A variety of chemical reactors are being used in industrial practice: some typical reactors are shown in Fig. 1.2. Pertinent design issues for each of these reactor types are different and are impossible to discuss in a single chapter. A general methodology can, however, be discussed without going into details of each reactor type. Before we proceed, it should be noted that most industrial chemical reactors present severe challenges to the mathematical modeler. A reactor engineer needs to be familiar with the basic concepts of the mathematical modeling of physical processes (see, for example, Denn, 1986; Aris, 1978; Polya, 1962). The relative importance and roles of governing equations, constitutive equations, boundary conditions and input data need to be clearly understood while interpreting results and drawing engineering conclusions based on simulation results.

Adequate mathematical representation of any complex physical process may require many different mathematical models, perhaps a continuum of models, each having different capabilities, appropriate to its specific objectives. Reactor engineers must recognize the possibility of employing a hierarchy of models to develop the necessary understanding and to obtain the required information to achieve complex reactor engineering objectives. Perhaps an analogy with the variety of vehicles available for transport may make the point clear. Various alternative vehicles, from a bicycle, scooter, car and helicopter to aircraft are available for a person who wants to travel. Each of these vehicles has unique features and a corresponding range of applications. Availability of powerful alternatives for transport has not made other less powerful modes obsolete. More often than not, the best way to travel the desired distance is based on using different vehicles for different parts of the journey. Similarly, there will be a hierarchy of mathematical models, each having some unique features and corresponding range of application, which may be used to construct as complete a picture of the physical process as possible. Computational flow modeling is certainly a very powerful tool and in principle, a self-consistent, comprehensive mathematical model can be constructed to simulate the behavior of industrial reactors within a CFM framework. However, it would be inefficient to use such a complex model to obtain information which might be obtained by relatively simple models. The reactor engineer has, therefore, to match the available modeling tools and reactor engineering objectives at hand. It is often difficult to develop a mathematical model which addresses the practical reactor engineering problem directly. Instead, it is necessary to use different models to develop the required understanding and information, and combining this with engineering judgement to propose an appropriate reactor engineering solution. CFM certainly enhances the capability of a reactor engineer to make deeper journeys into the underlying physics for a better understanding. It should, however, be used along with other models with different capabilities to construct an overall picture. The necessity of using a hierarchy of modeling tools and establishing a clear relationship between the reactor engineering objectives and computational flow modeling, is illustrated here with the help of some examples.

9.1. REACTOR ENGINEERING METHODOLOGY

A general reactor engineering methodology is shown in Fig. 1.10. Based on available information concerning the chemistry and catalysis of the process under consideration, the first step in reactor engineering is to select a suitable reactor type. Krishna (1994) discussed a systems approach for reactor selection. He advocates setting up a 'wish list' for reactor selection. The subject of reactor selection is not discussed further here, and interested readers may refer to the original paper (Krishna, 1994). It must, however, be emphasized that setting up of such a 'wish list' is one of the most important steps not only for the selection of reactor type but also for any reactor engineering or mathematical modeling activity. The success of the application of mathematical (or otherwise) modeling to any reactor engineering project depends on setting up such 'wish lists' which act as maps or guides for the selection and application of relevant tools. The results obtained by these various tools and the 'wish lists' are used to evolve a suitable reactor engineering solution.

For the development of a new reactor technology, a typical 'wish list' could be (from Krishna, 1994):

- operability within technologically feasible region;
- intrinsically safe operations;
- environmentally acceptable;
- maximum possible conversion of feed stocks;
- maximum selectivity of reaction to the desired products;

- acceptable impurity profiles;
- lowest capital and operating costs.

To enhance the performance of an existing reactor technology/hardware, a typical wish list could be:

- more throughput per unit volume;
- improved selectivity and better quality product;
- safer operation;
- reduced energy consumption;
- more environment friendly operation.

The next step is to translate the wish list into a quantitative form and establish a relationship between items in the wish list and reactor hardware and operating protocols. The reactor engineer's task is to design and tailor the reactor hardware and operating protocols to realize the wish list. Several activities are involved in this process. It may often turn out that some of the items in the wish list require contradictory options of hardware and operation. In such cases, a careful analysis of different items in the wish list must be made to assign priorities. Operability, stability and environmental constraints often receive precedence over throughput and energy consumption when such conflicting requirements arise.

Some of the tasks of the reactor engineer when establishing the relationship between reactor configuration/operation and performance are shown in Fig. 1.10. Examination of these tasks emphasizes the need for developing a multilayer modeling strategy. Some of the tasks, such as examining the influence of reactant flow rate and operating temperature on the performance of the reactor (conversion, selectivity, stability and so on), can be answered by developing conventional reaction engineering models. In these models, some assumptions are made regarding the flow and mixing of various species in the reactor, instead of solving the fluid dynamics equations. Thus, although these models cannot directly relate the reactor hardware with performance, these models are computationally much less demanding than CFD-based models and can give a quick understanding of the overall behavior of the reactor. These models can be used to identify the important parameters/issues, which may require further study. Of course, the class of conventional chemical reaction engineering models itself contains a variety of models. It will be useful to distinguish between 'learning' models and 'design' models at this stage.

'Learning' models are developed to help to understand basic concepts and to obtain specific information about unknown processes. The results obtainable from such models may not lead directly to design information but are generally useful to take appropriate engineering decisions. 'Design' models, on the other hand, yield information or results, which can be used directly for reactor design and engineering. It is first necessary to develop design models to estimate reactor sizing and to evolve a preliminary reactor configuration. Several 'learning' models can then be developed to help understand various reactor engineering issues, such as:

- start-up and shut-down dynamics;
- multiplicity and stability of thermo-chemical processes occurring in the reactor;
- sensitivity of reactor performance with respect to mixing and residence time distributions;
- selectivity and by-product formations.

The understanding gained by development and application of these 'learning' models is helpful in identifying the needs for developing more sophisticated simulation models to establish the desired reactor design. These models are also useful in identifying the likely impact of reactor fluid dynamics on reactor performance. The results allow the reactor engineer to identify gaps between available knowledge and that required to fulfill the 'wish list'. The identified gaps can then be bridged by carrying out experiments in the laboratory and/or pilot plant(s), and by developing more comprehensive fluid dynamic models.

Computational flow modeling enters the reactor engineering activity at this point. Despite the advantages, conventional chemical reaction engineering models will not be directly useful for understanding the influence of reactor hardware on reactor performance. For example, how the design of the distributor for dispersed phase affects the radial distribution of dispersed phase and thereby the reactor performance, will be difficult to predict without developing a detailed fluid dynamic model (CFM) of the reactor or without carrying out experiments on a scale model. The CFM-based approach will make valuable contributions at this stage by providing the required insight, by helping to devise the right kind of experiments and by allowing the screening of alternative configurations and by providing tools for extrapolations and scale-up. Of course, the whole process of reactor engineering is not sequential! All steps interact with and influence each other. The results obtained in laboratory experiments on hydrodynamics and residence time distribution (RTD) or from the computational flow model may demand changes and revisions in the earlier analysis and the whole process is iterated until a satisfactory solution emerges. In this book, we are particularly concerned with the application of computational flow modeling to obtain the relevant information about reactor engineering. Translating reactor engineering requirements to formulate suitable flow models and the use of such flow models for reactor engineering is illustrated here with the help of a few examples.

Before we discuss the examples, some general comments on CFM for reactor engineering will be useful. Computational flow models can be built either as 'learning' models or 'design' models. For 'design' models, which are expected to yield directly applicable design results, relating reactor engineering objectives to computational flow modeling objectives is relatively simple and straightforward. Some special types of reactors, such as chemical vapor deposition reactors, are designed directly based on a comprehensive computational flow model. Such comprehensive CFD models enable the reactor engineer to directly relate reactor hardware (and operating protocols) to reactor performance. In several other cases, however, it may be necessary to use computational flow models to assist the process of reactor engineering decision-making. In such cases, correct formulation of the flow problem plays a crucial role. Developing computational models to obtain the required information about the behavior of industrial chemical reactors is a complex task and requires specialized knowledge and approach. Previous chapters have provided basic information about the elements of computational flow modeling. Part IV of this book contains separate chapters on three major reactor types, namely stirred reactors, bubble column reactors and fluidized bed reactors. One chapter is included to cover miscellaneous reactors, along with fixed and trickle bed reactors. These chapters are designed to provide specialized knowledge pertinent to different reactor types, which will assist the reactor engineer wishing to develop reactor flow models. In this chapter, examples are discussed to illustrate the basic methodology and to relate results obtained from computational flow modeling to reactor engineering objectives.

9.2. EXAMPLE I – SUSPENSION POLYMERIZATION REACTOR

Suspension polymerization is an old and relatively simple process to produce polymers and copolymers for various applications. It is mainly used to produce specialty copolymers which have high value but low volume demand. Because of the operational problems associated with the transport of highly viscous droplets in suspension, continuous operation of suspension polymerization process is difficult: polymerization is carried out in a stirred reactor operated in batch mode. Controlling the particle size distribution (PSD) is one of the major reactor engineering objectives apart from high conversion and selectivity. Although the process has been widely studied, the understanding of factors that affect the PSD and several other physical phenomena that occur inside the vessel is still limited. Most suspension polymerization reactors are designed and operated based on wisdom accumulated from prior experience. In this example, the potential of using computational flow modeling to enhance our understanding and, thereby, enhance control of the performance of a suspension polymerization reactor is discussed.

Let us consider a typical suspension polymerization process for manufacturing polymer beads (for example, polystyrene beads for ion-exchange resins). For such a process, control of particle size distribution is crucial as it determines the usable yield from the process. Different applications demand different ranges of particle sizes. Typical ion-exchange applications may require polymer bead diameters within the range 250 to 1000 μm. Any polymer particles falling outside this range are a waste of raw materials. For specialty applications, demands on particle size distribution are even more stringent. A typical suspension polymerization reactor is shown schematically in Fig. 9.1. While many operating protocols are used, it is common to disperse catalyzed monomer into aqueous phase containing a suspending or stabilizing agent (Leng and Quarderer, 1982). A certain time period is allowed for drops to attain a stable size distribution, after which the batch is heated to polymerization temperature. It is important that coalescence or agglomeration is prevented during polymerization. Failure to achieve adequate stabilization may lead to mass polymerization and reactor shutdown. Of course, avoiding such a possibility is no longer a problem, but enhancing the yield of polymer beads within the usable range is still a challenge for a reactor engineer.

Despite several studies spanning five decades, the understanding of factors which control PSD and the several phenomena that occur inside the stirred reactor is still limited. Several (design and operating) parameters affect the PSD. Some of the more important parameters include:

- Impeller
  - type of impeller (shape and number of blades),
  - number of impellers and their locations,
  - impeller diameter,
  - impeller speed;
- reactor geometry (shape, height to diameter ratio);
- water to monomer ratio;

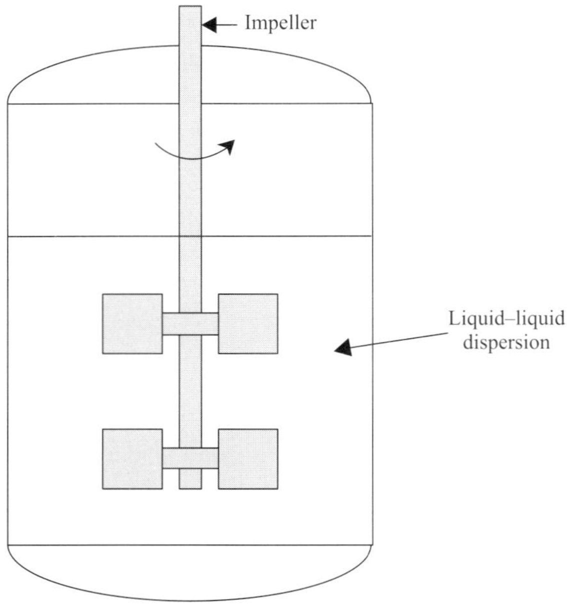

FIGURE 9.1 Suspension polymerization reactor.

- chemical recipe (type and concentration of initiator, stabilizer, surfactant, catalyst and so on).

It is not possible (and also not necessary) to review all the available information on suspension polymerization here. Some recent reviews may be referred to for more information (Vivaldo-Lima *et al.*, 1997, 1998). Most of the answers to the questions related to chemical recipe may have to be obtained by conducting specific experiments. Other questions, such as selection of operating temperature, batch time etc., can be answered by developing a conventional reaction engineering model (a single-drop polymerization reactor model, by assuming complete mixing, will give information about the progress of polymerization with time). The need for a detailed understanding of fluid dynamics is, however, essential to an understanding of the liquid–liquid dispersion process occurring in the reactor. The breakage of monomer liquid phase into individual droplets and their dispersion within the reactor ultimately controls the particle size distribution. This is where computational flow modeling can make significant contributions.

The literature on drop breakage is extensive (see the recent review by Zhou and Kresta, 1998). Grossly approximating, one may state that the main drop breakage and coalescence events occur at the impeller at intervals defined by the mean circulation time. Different drop size distributions arise due to equilibrium between drop break-up and coalescence. For the case of stabilized dispersion (such as used in suspension polymerization reactors), the extent of coalescence is significantly reduced. For such systems, it is necessary to understand the relationship between fluid dynamics and drop breakage as well as between reactor hardware and the resulting fluid dynamics to evolve suitable reactor design. Several models have been developed to describe drop breakage in turbulent flows (see, for example, Kumar *et al.*, 1998). A suitable drop breakage model (and a coalescence model if necessary) can be combined with a population balance model to simulate drop size distribution and thereby bead size distribution of a batch suspension polymerization reactor.

These models require information about mean velocity and the turbulence field within the stirred vessels. Computational flow models can be developed to provide such fluid dynamic information required by the reactor models. Although in principle, it is possible to solve the population balance model equations within the CFM framework, a simplified compartment-mixing model may be adequate to simulate an industrial reactor. In this approach, a CFD model is developed to establish the relationship between reactor hardware and the resulting fluid dynamics. This information is used by a relatively simple, compartment-mixing model coupled with a population balance model (Vivaldo-Lima *et al.*, 1998). The approach is shown schematically in Fig. 9.2. Detailed polymerization kinetics can be included. Vivaldo-Lima *et al.* (1998) have successfully used such an approach to predict particle size distribution (PSD) of the product polymer. Their two-compartment model was able to capture the bi-modal behavior observed in the experimental PSD data. After adequate validation, such a computational model can be used to optimize reactor configuration and operation to enhance reactor performance.

It is also possible to use computational flow models without explicitly linking them with models predicting the particle size distribution. In such an approach, one can use insight gained from the results of the CFD model by implicitly combining it with an understanding of drop breakage phenomena and polymerization reaction, to evolve the desired reactor engineering solution. Recently, Ranade (1999a) demonstrated such an application to enhance the performance of an industrial suspension polymerization reactor. Ranade (1999a) considered the case of an existing industrial polymerization reactor agitated with two pitched blade impellers. The reactor was designed based on laboratory-scale experiments carried out in a 5 liter reactor and a few experiments on a pilot scale reactor (700 liter). The plant scale reactor was operated in batch mode. The yield of usable polymer beads (particles) was about 65%, which clearly indicated scope for enhancing the reactor performance. The approach of Ranade (1999a) is discussed below.

As mentioned earlier, both chemical (catalyst, surfactants, stabilizers) and physical (fluid dynamics, energy dissipation rates, circulation time and so on) factors control the performance of the suspension polymerization reactor. It is first necessary to examine the available experimental data to clearly understand the role of these chemical and physical factors. The available data indicates that the yield of usable polymer beads in laboratory scale reactor is more than 85%. Laboratory experiments were then planned to examine the sensitivity of the yield to various parameters of the polymerization recipe under the same hydrodynamic conditions. These experiments showed that the yield is relatively insensitive to small deviations in the chemical recipe. Analysis of the available data on pilot and plant scale indicated a progressive decrease in the yield of usable polymer beads from laboratory to pilot to plant scale. This analysis and some indirect evidence suggested that it may be possible to re-design the plant-scale reactor hardware to generate better fluid dynamics and mixing to increase the yield of particles in the desired size range.

One may use an approach discussed earlier in which a comprehensive mathematical model is developed, which relates the reactor hardware to fluid dynamics and polymerization reactions in one framework. However, it is extremely difficult

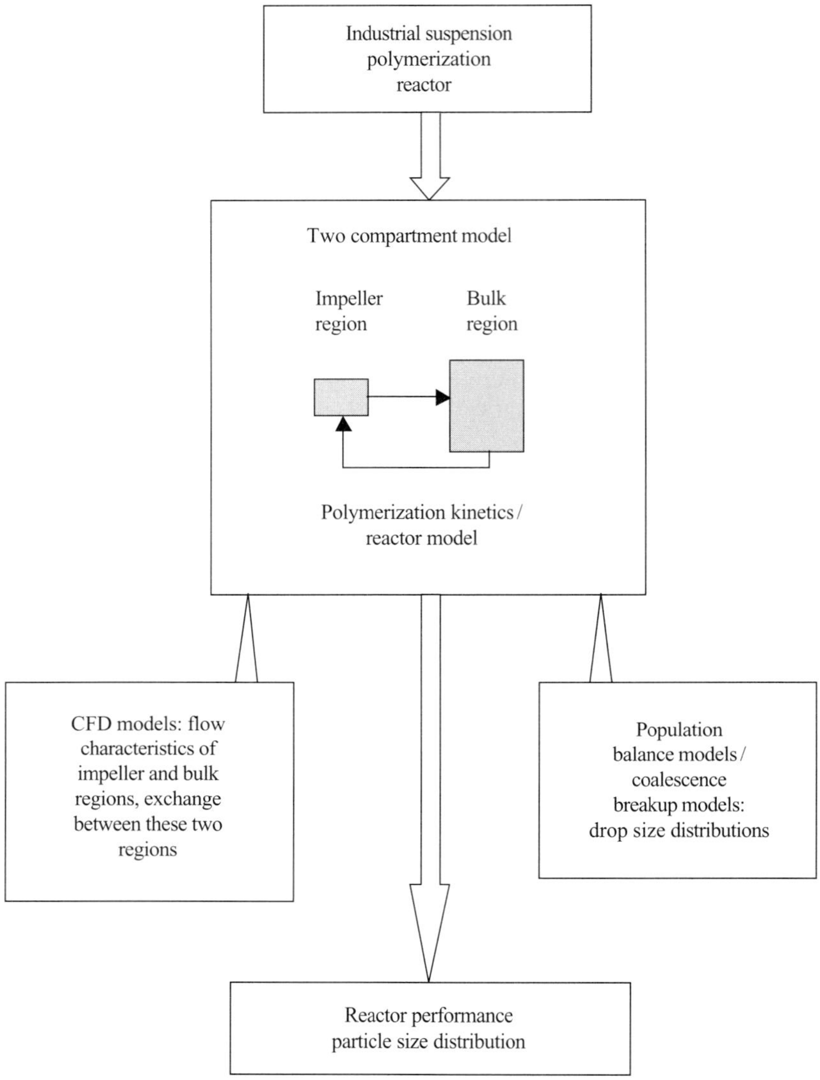

FIGURE 9.2 Modeling a suspension polymerization reactor (approach of Vivaldo-Lima *et al.*, 1998).

and time consuming to develop such an approach for an industrial polymerization reactor. The uncertainties in kinetics and physicochemical properties coupled with the complexities of coalescence-break-up models may raise doubts about the direct correspondence between model predictions and plant performance. Ranade (1999a) therefore used an approximate approach, in which the first step is to understand the role of fluid dynamics in controlling the PSD without mathematically relating them. It is first necessary to identify the controlling drop breakage mechanism (shear, elongation, turbulence and so on). Without going into specific details of any particular application, it can be said that:

- Wide distribution of shear strain rates within the reactor will result in a wider PSD. This means impeller rotational speed should be kept small enough to ensure narrower strain rate distribution. It should, of course, be able to provide the necessary bulk flow and should be able to keep the monomer droplets well dispersed within the reactor. Adequate dispersion of monomer droplets ensures that they all experience the same environment and leads to narrower PSD.

- Impeller size, shape and speed should ensure that the turbulence energy dissipation rates within the impeller zone are not excessive so as to avoid unwanted finer particles.

Several other qualitative requirements may be added. These may, however, be sufficient to illustrate the possible application of CFM. These fluid dynamical requirements form the 'wish list' of the reactor engineer, who has to evolve a suitable reactor configuration (height to diameter ratio, impeller type, size, location, number and so on) to satisfy this wish list. The conventional way is to modify some standard configuration, test it in pilot scale and then scale it up for the full-scale plant. Unfortunately, because of the costs and time involved in testing new configurations at pilot scale, usually new concepts/designs are sidelined in favor of known configurations. In such cases, CFD-based models can make substantial contributions. CFD models can be used to select an appropriate impeller, number of impellers, location of feed pipes, to satisfy the fluid dynamical 'wish list'. If the fluid dynamical 'wish list' is evolved carefully, the CFD-based model will be useful in optimizing the polymerization reactor without explicitly developing the detailed reaction and particle size distribution model. It may be necessary to modify the 'wish list' based on the understanding gained via CFD models. In most cases, however, the whole process converges to an appropriate solution in a couple of iterations.

After establishing the fluid dynamical requirement, the first step is to analyze the fluid dynamics of the existing industrial reactor. Details of the computational modeling of flow generated in a stirred reactor are discussed in Chapter 10. Without discussing those details, results reported by Ranade (1999a) are discussed here. A typical computational grid and predicted results for the flow generated by two pitched blade turbines are shown in Fig. 9.3. The simulated flow field was used to predict

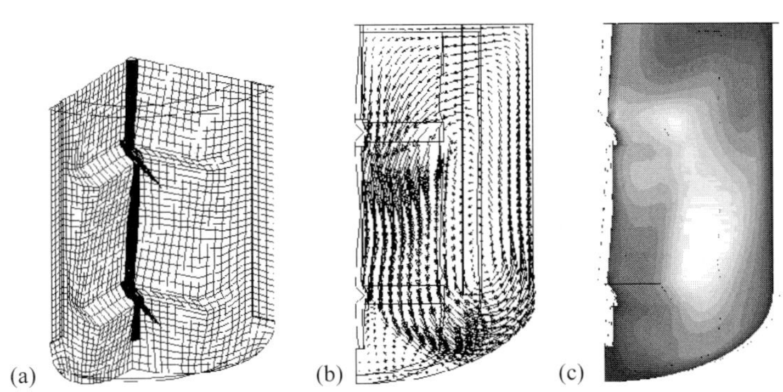

FIGURE 9.3 Sample of simulation results for a two pitched blade turbine (legend not shown due to confidentiality constraints). (a) Grid; (b) vector plot; (c) contours of turbulent KE (white: highest value; black: lowest value). Reproduced in colour plate section between pages 210 and 211.

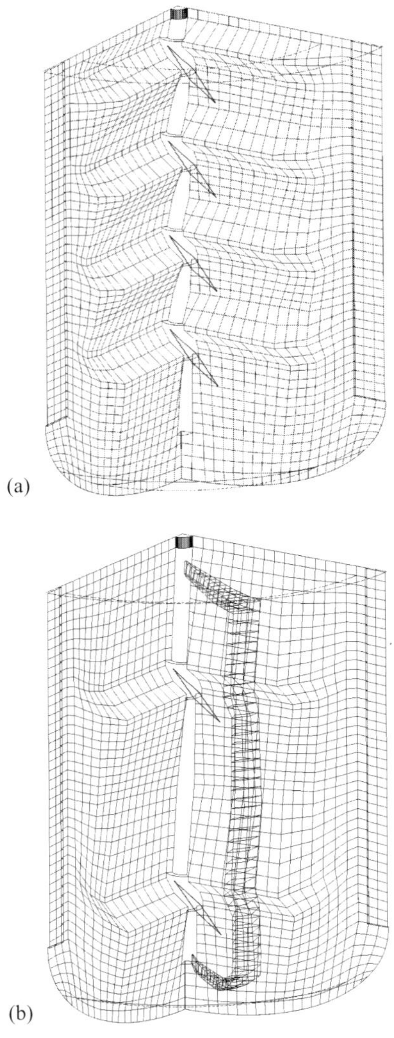

FIGURE 9.4 Two alternatives to enhance reactor performance. (a) Four pitched blade turbine, (b) two pitched blade turbine with cage.

circulation time distributions, volume averaged velocity and other relevant flow characteristics. The average as well as maximum and minimum shear rates and energy dissipation rates were examined. Evaluation of these simulation results by combining the available information/understanding of drop breakage and the performance of a working reactor in the plant, indicated that it may be beneficial to reduce the impeller rotational speed without reducing the volume-averaged velocity to ensure the required bulk flow. One way to achieve this is to use more impellers and/or use larger diameter impellers. Another alternative is to combine the two pitched blade impellers with a cage to facilitate dispersion at lower speeds. To narrow the circulation time distribution, a draft tube could be used, however, in view of the possibility of polymer deposition on a draft tube and the subsequent cleaning problems, the option of a draft tube was not considered further. Various alternative reactor configurations

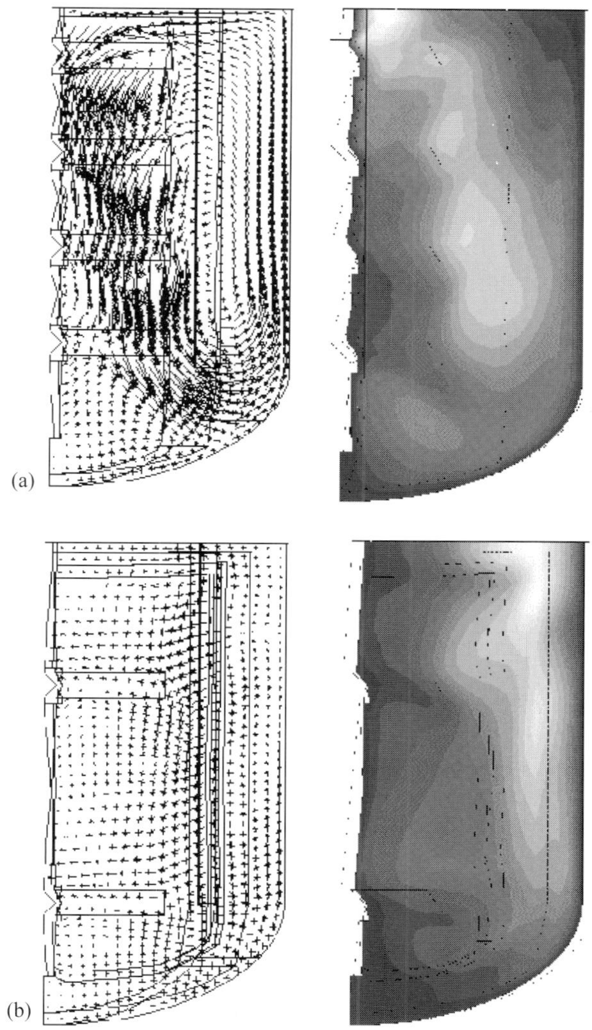

FIGURE 9.5 Simulated flow field for two alternative reactor configurations (white: highest value; black: lowest value; legend not shown due to confidentiality constraints). (a) Four pitched blade turbine, (b) two pitched blade turbine with cage (left: vector plots; right: contours of turbulent kinetic energy.) Reproduced in colour plate section between pages 210 and 211.

were evolved and screened heuristically to check whether they satisfied the 'wish list'. Shortlisted configurations were then studied using the computational model. The two alternative reactor configurations are shown in Fig. 9.4. Flows generated by these configurations were then simulated. The simulated flow field indicated that the volume-averaged velocity within the reactor is adequate (see Fig. 9.5 for sample results). The four-impeller configuration was found to be more effective in reducing the heterogeneity within the vessel. The pitched blade impellers, however, generate strong velocity gradients just below the impellers, which may widen the resulting PSD. The shape of the blade was, therefore, modified to generate as uniform a velocity as possible across the blade length. To achieve this, a simple phenomenological model which approximately relates the axial flow generated by the blade with blade angle and blade width was used:

$$\text{Flow} \propto (B_W r \Delta r \sin\theta) \tag{9.1}$$

This proportionality was used to determine suitable blade width (B_W) and blade angle (θ) profiles along its length. The flow generated by these hydrofoil impellers was then simulated. Critical evaluation and comparison of the flow generated by hydrofoil impellers with that generated by PTD indicated that with four hydrofoil impellers, the polymerization reactor may be operated at an impeller speed which gives minimum variation in circulation time and much less heterogeneous distribution of turbulent energy dissipation rates, without affecting the bulk flow within the vessel. Plant trials with the new hydrofoil impellers resulted in 15–20% increase in the yield of usable polymer beads (Ranade, 1999a). Thus, in this case, even without combining the PSD model and CFD framework, it was possible to enhance reactor performance by judicious application of computational flow modeling. In many practical industrial reactor engineering problems, such an approach may have to be adopted.

9.3. EXAMPLE 2 – OXY REACTOR FOR EDC

Ethylene dichloride (EDC) is used to manufacture vinyl chloride monomer (VCM), which is one of the largest commodity chemicals produced in the world. EDC may be produced by the direct chlorination of ethylene or oxychlorination of ethylene in the presence of oxygen and hydrogen chloride. Pyrolysis of EDC produces VCM and an equal amount of hydrogen chloride as a co-product. This hydrogen chloride produced in the pyrolysis reactor is utilized by the oxychlorination process as one of the reactants. Therefore, the component processes of direct chlorination, EDC pyrolysis and oxychlorination are combined to develop a balanced process for the production of VCM with no net consumption or production of hydrogen chloride:

$$C_2H_4 + 2\ HCl + \tfrac{1}{2}\ O_2 \xrightarrow{\text{Catalyst}} C_2H_4Cl_2 + H_2O \tag{9.2}$$

The development of oxychlorination technology in the late 1950s encouraged new growth in the vinyl chloride industry. Here, we will be considering an oxychlorination (OXY) reactor to illustrate the application of computational flow modeling to reactor engineering.

In the oxychlorination process ethylene reacts with dry hydrogen chloride and oxygen to produce EDC and water. Though commercial processes for oxychlorination differ somewhat, the reaction, in general, is carried out in the vapor phase in either a fixed bed or a fluidized bed reactor. The reaction is carried out at a temperature of about 200°C and at a pressure of about 500 kPa (Ullmann, 1986). At these operating conditions, the reactants are in gaseous form. Air, oxygen-enriched air or pure oxygen is used to supply the oxygen necessary for the reaction. Oxychlorination catalysts contain copper (II) chloride as the main active ingredient along with numerous additives. The catalyst used in the reaction is solid at the operating conditions. It is a highly exothermic reaction and, therefore, an efficient means of heat removal is essential for temperature control. Higher reactor temperatures result in increased by-product formation and catalyst deactivation. Most modern, large-capacity EDC plants therefore use fluidized bed reactors to carry out this process (Ullmann, 1986).

In fluidized bed reactors the gaseous reactants are introduced below the bed of solid catalyst particles. The upward flowing gas fluidizes the solid catalyst particles (under fluidized conditions the gravity force acting on the solid particles is compensated by the drag force exerted by the gas flow and particles behave like a fluid). The high mobility of the solids ensures excellent heat transfer characteristics, which makes fluidized bed reactors an appropriate choice for highly exothermic gas–solid reactions, especially for large-capacity plants (Kunii and Levenspiel, 1991). A schematic of a fluidized bed OXY reactor is shown in Fig. 9.6. Manufacturing companies have developed different versions of fluidized bed reactor technology, and despite its widespread use in practice, the technology of fluidized bed OXY reactors is still very complicated and details are closely guarded. The complexity of the technology originates in the extremely complex fluid dynamics of these reactors. Depending on particle characteristics (size, shape, density, restitution coefficient, etc.), geometry of the equipment (diameter, height, gas distributor, etc.) and operating conditions (gas and solid flow rates, pressure, temperature), fluidized bed reactors may exhibit different regimes of gas–solid flows. Small changes in reactor configuration or any of the operating conditions may change the underlying fluid dynamics and, therefore, may change the performance significantly.

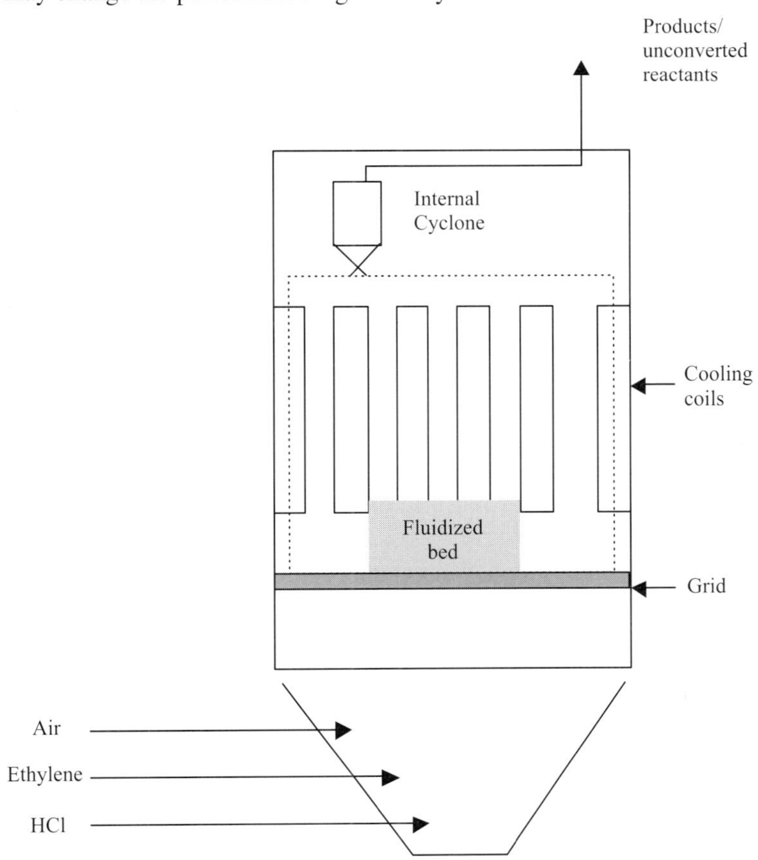

FIGURE 9.6 Schematic diagram of OXY reactor (from Ranade, 1999b).

Major reaction engineering issues in fluidized bed reactors are discussed in several excellent textbooks (see, for example, Kunii and Levenspiel, 1991). The conventional reaction engineering models (discussed in these textbooks) along with the knowledge of reaction chemistry, kinetics and thermodynamics may allow the reactor engineer to establish a relationship between reactor volume (amount of catalyst), feed flow rates and yield and selectivity obtainable under specific operating conditions. Several issues related to catalyst (activity, high temperature stability, ageing, etc.) need to be known. Of course, even at this stage, some assumptions about the underlying flow processes need to be invoked to estimate rates of backmixing, mass and heat transfer processes. Computational fluid dynamic models can help the reactor engineer to obtain the required information about the fluid dynamics. It is also possible to couple simulations of reactions within the CFD framework (see, for example, Samuelsberg, 1994). Details of the modeling of fluidized bed reactors are discussed in Chapter 12. In this section, use of a computational flow model to enhance the performance (capacity) of an existing industrial OXY reactor is discussed.

9.3.1. Capacity Enhancement of an Existing OXY Reactor

In order to explore the possibility of enhancing the capacity of an existing OXY reactor, several issues need to be carefully examined. Due to the sensitivity of fluidized bed reactors to operating flow rates, the strategy of forcing more feed through the reactor to enhance the capacity has a rather restricted applicability. The increased feed rate may cause such problems as increased catalyst carry-over etc. The other alternative to enhance capacity is to use oxygen-enriched air or pure oxygen as the oxidation medium instead of ordinary air. This will allow a higher feed rate of reactants without increasing the total gas flow rate through the reactor. Processes operated with oxygen-enriched air or pure oxygen may also lead to significant reductions in gas treatment problems. Before converting the existing process/reactor operating with air, either to an oxygen-enriched or pure oxygen process/reactor, it is essential to ensure that the existing reactor hardware is able to handle such a change. It must be ensured that the local concentrations of oxygen and flammable compounds (such as ethylene) are within safe limits. Considering the extreme corrosiveness of the system, likely scenarios such as malfunctioning of the gas distributor, and the effect on reactor performance and safety of operations need to be carefully evaluated. Computational flow models can be used to achieve this.

In an industrial OXY reactor, air is introduced in the bottom conical portion of the reactor (below the grid). The air stream is mixed with other reactants (ethylene and HCl) in specially designed mixing elements attached to the grid to ensure fast and adequate mixing. Various proprietary and elaborate designs are used to ensure proper mixing of ethylene- and oxygen-containing streams and to restrict the volume of fluid containing a flammable mixture. Without disclosing any proprietary information, one of the simplest and effective mixing elements, a so-called 'mixing cup' is schematically shown in Fig. 9.7. This mixing element is designed in such a way that the composition of mixture exiting these cups is outside the flammability envelope. Air enters mixing elements attached to the grid through the bottom orifice. Ethylene and HCl streams are supplied to each element via a suitable distributor. The grid of the OXY reactor may contain several mixing elements. The reactor engineer has to ensure that air is fed to these various mixing elements uniformly. Non-uniform distribution

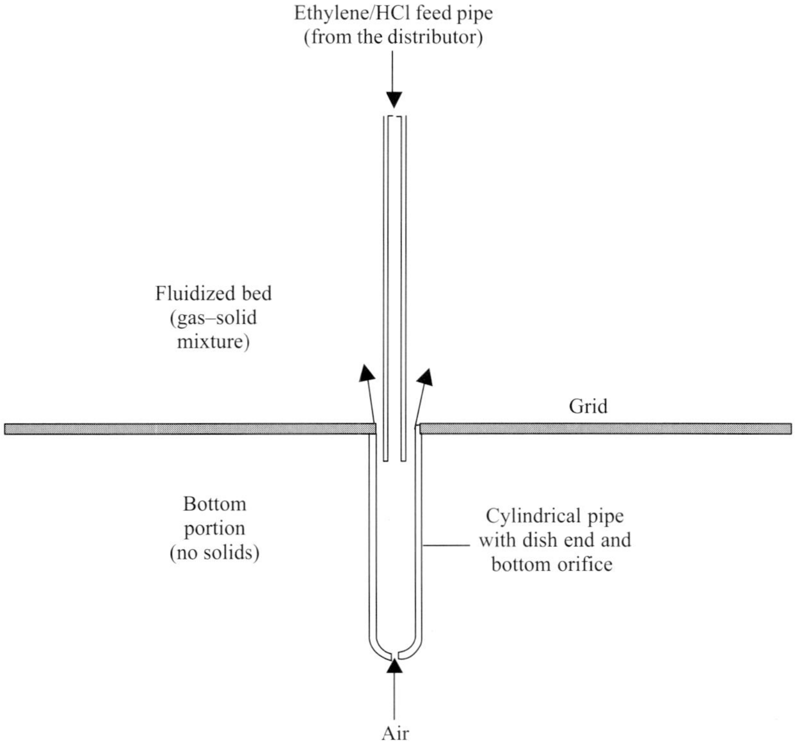

FIGURE 9.7 Schematic of mixing cup (from Ranade, 1999b).

of air to these elements will lead to mal-distribution of oxygen in the fluidized bed. The layout of these elements on the grid will have an influence on gas distribution within the fluidized bed reactors.

These issues indicate that it is crucial to obtain quantitative information about fluid dynamics and mixing in mixing elements as well as in the overall reactor in order to evaluate the possibility of capacity enhancement using oxygen-enriched air. One of the concerns is to examine the scenario of malfunctioning of a mixing element and to evaluate and compare the consequences for ordinary and enriched air feed. Prior experience and knowledge about the catalyst and kinetics of the reaction suggested that catalyst and process conditions were adequate to convert additional feed, provided the reactor is operated in the same flow regime. Due to this fact and the limited time available, it was decided that it is sufficient to develop a computational model to simulate gas flow and mixing within the industrial fluidized bed reactor without considering any reactions. This decision facilitated rapid development and application of the computational model. Possible consequences must, however, be kept in mind when interpreting and applying the results obtained from the computational flow model. When developing a computational flow model for OXY reactors, several demands imposed by the set objectives should be kept in mind. It is necessary to consider the overall configuration of OXY reactor to evaluate possible mal-distributions. The construction of an industrial OXY reactor is extremely complex. It is normally fitted with internal cooling coils to remove and recover the heat of reactions. The presence of internal cooling coils may also lead to mal-distribution. The bottom conical portion, grid containing mixing elements, feed distributors, internal supports, etc. makes the task of modeling the geometry of an industrial reactor quite complex. To restrict the computational demands, an appropriate modeling methodology needs to be evolved. Here we discuss the methodology used by Ranade (1999b) to simulate flow in a complex industrial OXY reactor by developing different modeling layers and some of his results. The methodology will be useful for identifying and enhancing the capacity limits of existing reactor hardware.

9.3.2. Methodology to Simulate Flow in an OXY Reactor

Construction of a large-scale industrial OXY reactor is extremely complex. A wide range of length scales, ranging from a few meters (reactor diameter and length) to a few millimeters (orifice of mixing element), appears to be important. There is a corresponding two to three orders of magnitude difference between gas velocities in the various elements of an OXY reactor. Resolving these widely different length and velocity scales (typically in the range, 0.01 to 4 m and 0.2 to 100 m s^{-1}) simultaneously may stretch the limits of computational resources. It is, therefore, necessary to evolve a suitable modeling strategy. It must be emphasized that at every stage, the reactor engineer must be aware of the underlying assumptions (explicit and implicit) and their consequences, when interpreting and using the results.

The overall problem of modeling the fluid dynamics of an industrial OXY reactor was first divided into several small components (mixing element, bottom conical portion of the reactor, portion above the grid). Each of these components was studied using a separate model. The understanding gained through these studies was then combined to construct the model for the whole reactor (the methodology is shown pictographically in Fig. 9.8). From the discussion of Section 9.3.1, it is clear that it is essential to resolve all the fine-scale flow characteristics of the mixing element. It may not be necessary (or possible) to resolve such fine scales when simulating flow in the bottom portion or upper portion of the OXY reactor. Therefore, in the present work, a three-layer modeling strategy was used. A computational model was first developed to understand the fluid dynamics of the mixing elements. Apart from the mixing, it was also used to characterize the pressure drop across the mixing elements under different operating conditions. In the second layer, gas flow in the bottom portion of the reactor was modeled to examine possible mal-distribution of feed air. Flow in the top portion above the grid was modeled to examine the influence of layout of mixing elements on the grid. In the third layer, gas flow in the complete reactor (excluding the internal cyclones) was simulated. The grid plate supporting the fluidized bed was modeled as a porous plate with pressure drop characteristics obtained from results of the first modeling layer. An attempt was made to evaluate and synthesize information obtained from all three modeling layers, validate these whenever possible (either directly or indirectly) and then use the information to evaluate various scenarios.

Suitable computational models for each of the layers discussed above were developed on the basis of available information and a time scale analysis of flow in OXY reactors (see Ranade, 1999b for more details). Because of the magnitude of pressure drop across the grid, it was found necessary to employ compressible flow equations. An ideal gas assumption was used to calculate the density of gas at any point (as a

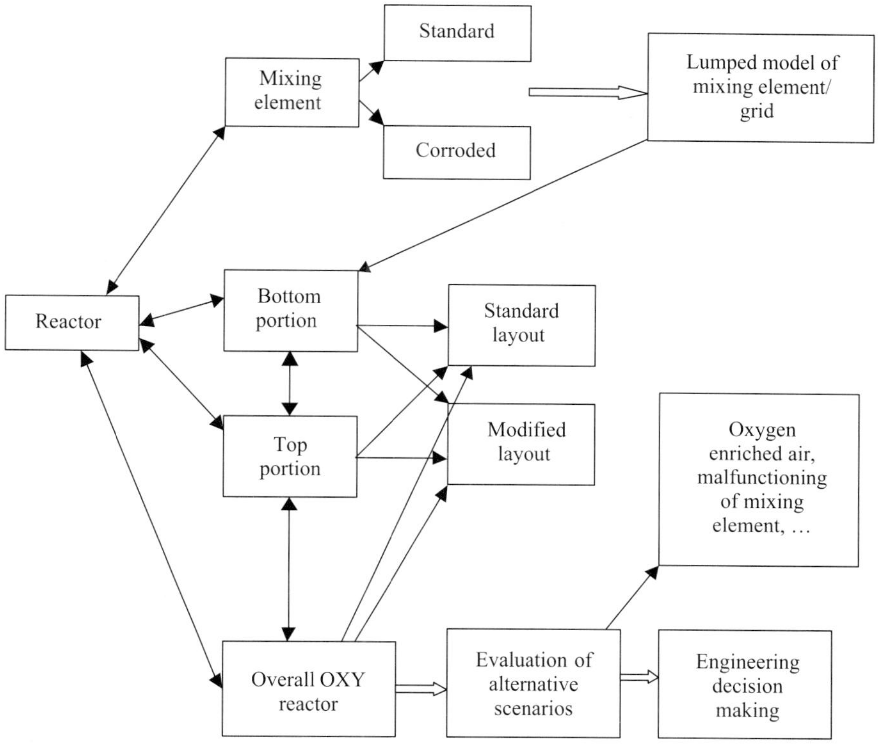

FIGURE 9.8 Modeling methodology (from Ranade, 1999b).

function of local pressure, temperature and effective molecular weight of the gas). Under normal operating conditions, the flow was found to be turbulent. Turbulent stresses were modeled using a suitable two-equation turbulence model (see Chapter 3). In order to capture the influence of the shape of the mixing cup, it was modeled using a body-fitted grid. Suitable boundary conditions were developed. The bottom part of the OXY reactor containing the bottom conical portion, the grid and the top portion up to the cooling coils was modeled using body fitted grids. Air feed was modeled by prescribing appropriate mass and momentum sources to the cells located just below the air feed pipe. The open area of the grid plate was modeled as a porous media. Appropriate sources of ethylene and HCl were specified at grid porous cells to simulate feed pipes. The characteristic resistance of these porous media was prescribed from results obtained for a single mixing element. The coil bundle inside the reactor was modeled as porous media and the top surface of the solution domain was modeled as a constant pressure surface. Six species namely, oxygen, nitrogen, inert, water, ethylene and HCl were considered for these simulations. The computational model was mapped on to a commercial CFD code, FLUENT (Fluent Inc., USA) with the help of user-defined subroutines.

9.3.3. Fluid Dynamics of OXY Reactor

(a) Mixing element: Flow in a mixing element (cup) is governed mainly by the pressure drop across the grid plate. Pressure outside a mixing cup is higher than that

prevailing over the annular open space of the cup. This pressure difference causes airflow from the surrounding space into the cup through the bottom orifice. This high velocity air jet impinges on the jet of ethylene and HCl mixture, generating intense turbulence and leading to complete mixing of the two streams, which escape from the annular opening of the cup.

Simulations were first carried out to examine the relationship between pressure drop across the grid and the resulting airflow through the cup. For all these simulations, the flow rates of ethylene and HCl were set to pre-determined values corresponding to reactor loading. The pressure drop across the cup was then adjusted to get the right amount of airflow through the cup. These simulations were carried out for three reactor loadings. After verifying the model predictions, by comparing these with plant data (see Fig. 9.9), the computational model was used to gain an insight into the fluid dynamics of the mixing elements. Predicted contours of stream function in the mixing cup are shown in Fig. 9.10a. It can be seen that the two impinging jets (air jet from the bottom orifice and mixture of ethylene and HCl from the pipe) generate a complex re-circulating flow within the mixing cup. The incoming, high velocity jet of air through the bottom orifice causes formation of two re-circulating loops near the walls of the mixing cup. There is relatively little exchange between these recirculating loops and the high velocity upward flow. Predicted contours of oxygen mass fraction and ethylene mass fraction within the mixing cup are shown in Fig. 9.10b.

The stagnation point formed by the two impinging jets is located near the end of ethylene and HCl feed pipe. Particle streak lines calculated based on the predicted flow results (not shown in the figure) clearly indicate the location of the stagnation point,

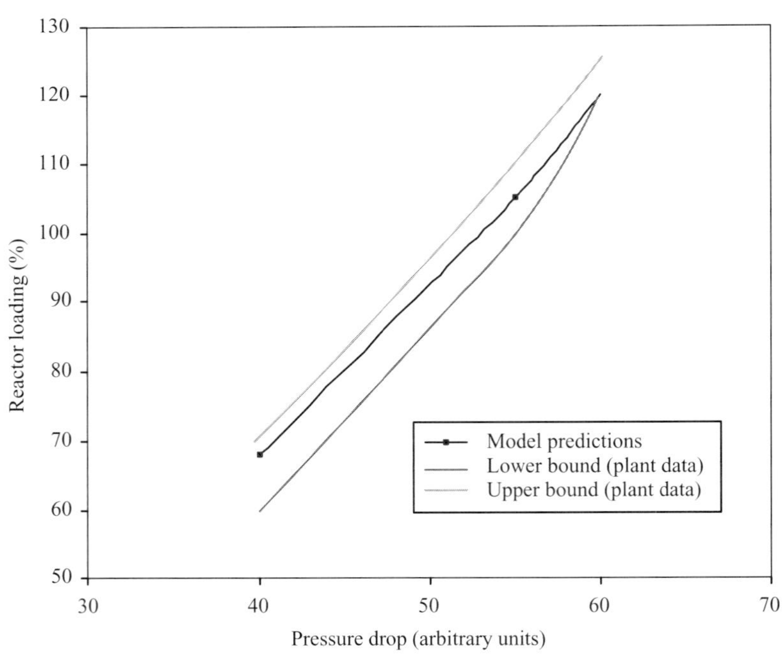

FIGURE 9.9 Comparison of predicted pressure drop with plant data (from Ranade, 1999b).

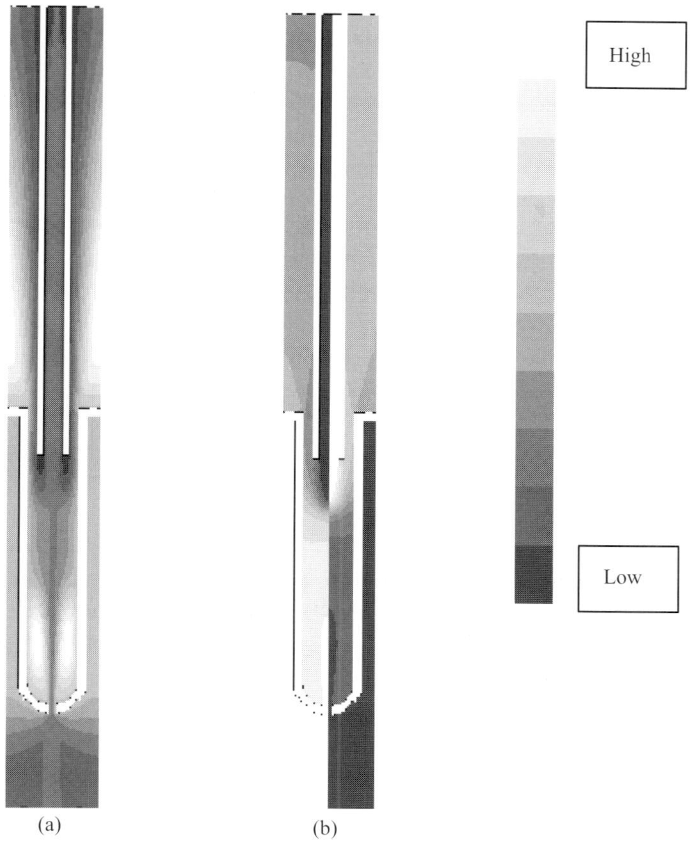

FIGURE 9.10 Flow and mixing in the mixing cup (from Ranade, 1999b). (a) Contours of stream function. (b) Left side: contours of oxygen mass fraction; right side: contours of ethylene mass fraction. (Legend not shown due to confidentiality constraints). Reproduced in colour plate section between pages 210 and 211.

which of course depends on the relative flow rates of air and the mixture of ethylene and HCl. It can be seen that (Fig. 9.10) the fluid escaping through the annular open space travels almost vertically upward. The maximum turbulent kinetic energy is located near the bottom orifice. The region of highest turbulent viscosity (and, therefore, of highest mixing rates) is, however, somewhat away from the bottom orifice (near the top of the two recirculating loops at the bottom of the mixing cup). The maximum value of turbulent viscosity is almost 5000 times the value of molecular viscosity. These detailed flow and composition results were analyzed to identify regions containing mixtures within the flammability envelope and variations with design and operating parameters. The possible accumulation of ethylene and HCl in the re-circulation loops near the bottom of the cup was also examined quantitatively.

The validated model for the mixing cup was then used to examine the possibilities of operation at higher flow rates and with higher oxygen concentrations. At higher oxygen concentrations, the flow rate of the ethylene stream becomes higher than that of the air stream and the stagnation point moves downwards. Two important design concerns (the possibility of an enlarged bottom orifice due to corrosion, and the possibility of a non-symmetric distributor pipe in the mixing cup), were examined using the computational model with both ordinary and oxygen-enriched air. The influence of an asymmetric feed pipe for the ethylene/HCl stream on flow and mixing within the mixing cup was also quantitatively examined. These results were useful in understanding the fluid dynamics and the limits of the existing configuration of mixing element and distributor for the ethylene/HCl stream.

(b) OXY reactor: When simulating overall flow in the OXY reactor, it is computationally intractable to resolve scales of the order of the bottom orifice of the mixing cup. Therefore, the resistance offered by such small openings and associated abrupt direction changes within the mixing cup were represented by a sub-model (based on the concepts of flow through porous media). Simulation results of throughput versus pressure drop across the mixing element were used to adjust the inertial resistance coefficient of the porous media (assuming that the contribution of laminar resistance is negligible). The value of this inertial resistance coefficient naturally depends on the diameter of the bottom orifice of the mixing element (for a corroded bottom, the value will be lower) and other construction details.

Overall flow simulations of the reactor were carried out to simulate normal operation as well as operation with malfunctioning mixing elements. Typical predicted flow results are shown in Fig. 9.11 in the form of contour and iso-surface plots. The flow simulations give an insight into operation of the OXY reactor. Air fed to the reactor first flows in a downward direction. After impinging on the reactor bottom, air is distributed evenly in the bottom portion below the grid and enters the mixing elements. It mixes with ethylene and HCl and escapes from the annular openings (with a velocity of the order of $5\,\mathrm{m\,s^{-1}}$) of the mixing cup. It can be seen that the jets from the annular opening reach up to the ethylene and HCl stream distributor (see Fig. 9.11b). In order to examine the influence of reactor internals and the layout of mixing elements on gas flow above the grid plate, a volume above the grid plate was modeled separately. It must be noted that flow above the grid plate may be significantly influenced by the presence of solid particles. The model used in the present work can be extended to simulate gas–solid flows using recent advances in the understanding of the kinetic theory of granular flows. However, here, the scope was restricted to understanding the role of layout of mixing elements on the grid in distributing gas in the reactor. The high velocity jets emanating from the mixing elements dominate the immediate region above the grid plate. Typical predicted results of simulations of gas flow above the grid plate using single-phase flow equations are shown in Fig. 9.12. These predicted results were then used to calculate particle trajectories to obtain useful information about particle impingement on reactor internals and possible implications for the erosion of internals. The model and results were used to examine alternative layouts of mixing cups on the grid plate to minimize mal-distribution and re-circulating regions above the grid plate. The results were also used to understand and to evaluate possible de-fluidization of catalyst particles near the wall region.

The model of the overall reactor was used to examine various scenarios, such as a cup with enlarged bottom orifice or the total absence of a cup. This type of malfunctioning mixing element (enlarged orifice or absent mixing cup) offers a point of

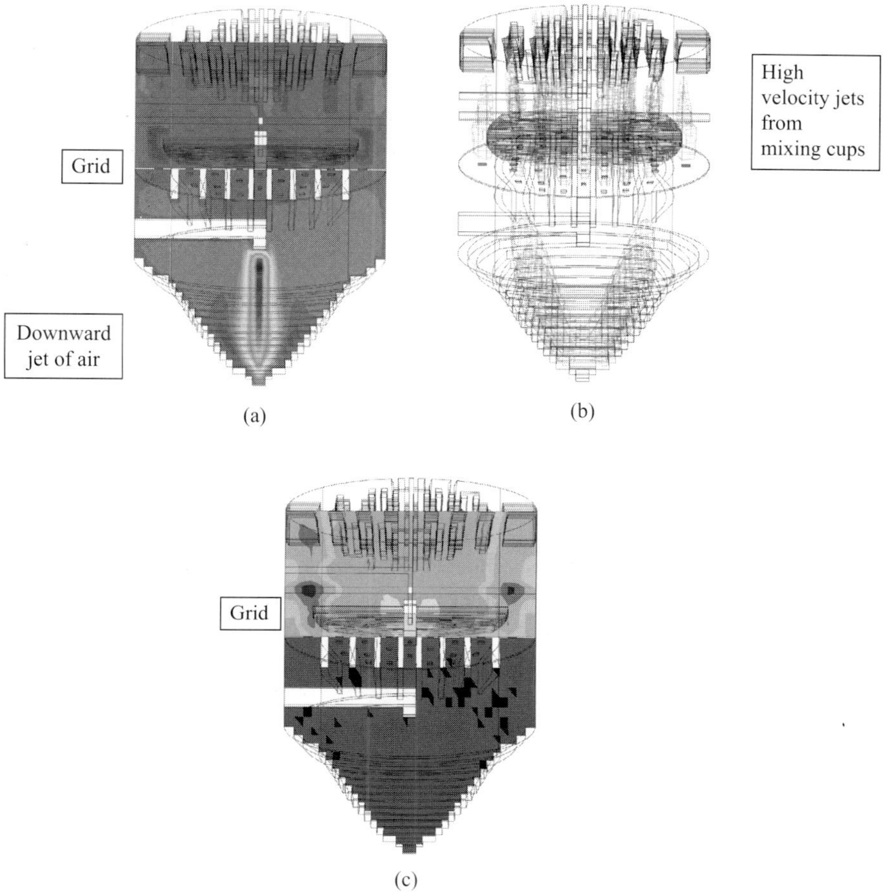

FIGURE 9.11 Flow characteristics of oxyhydrochlorination reactor (from Ranade, 1999b). (a) Contours of axial velocity, (b) iso-surfaces axial velocity (0.75 $m s^{-1}$), (c) contours of oxygen mass fraction (legend not shown due to confidentiality constraints).

least resistance to the airflow. This leads to substantially higher velocity jets escaping the grid plate (with velocities up to 80 $m s^{-1}$). Such high velocity jets may lead to significant mal-distribution and erosion within the OXY reactor. Such localized high velocity flow provides significantly more oxygen in that region, which may be of concern from safety and selectivity (reactor performance) point of views. The computational flow model presented here provided much more quantitative information about the gas flow in the OXY reactor. Not all the quantitative results can be discussed here for reasons of brevity and confidentiality. The results presented here may, however, give an essence of what kind of analysis can be carried out using the detailed computational flow model to evaluate the influence of various operating parameters on flow, and therefore on reactor operation. The computational model allowed not only quantitative estimation of the limits of existing reactor hardware, it also allowed evaluation of alternative configurations (mixing element/layout) to improve these limits. Despite certain limitations (since reactions and some other aspects were not included in the model), the computational model was found to be quite helpful in engineering decision making to realize performance enhancement of an existing

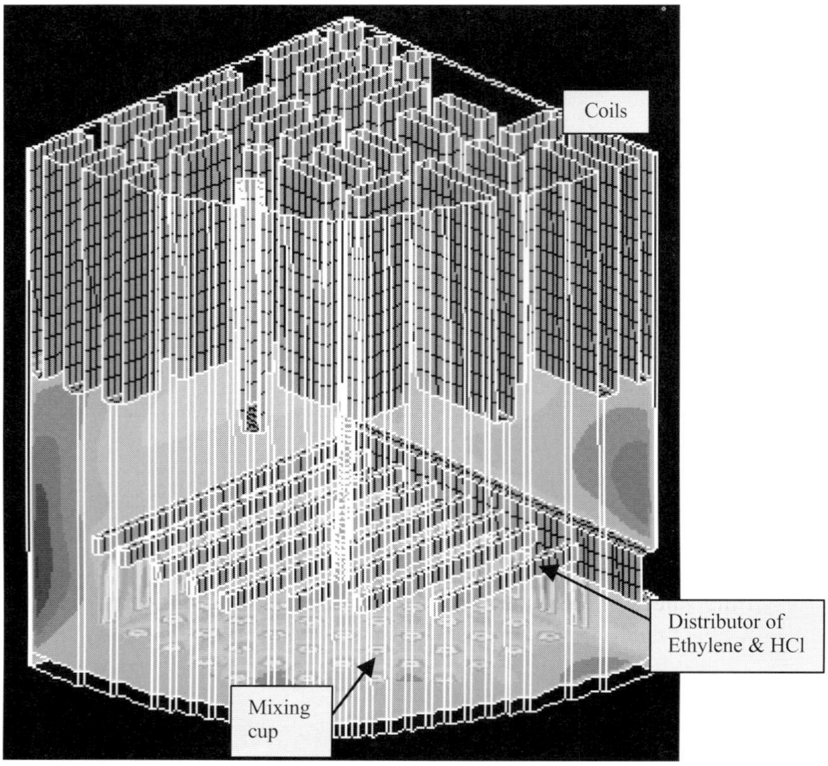

FIGURE 9.12 Contour plot of axial velocity (volume above the grid) (from Ranade, 1999b) (legend not shown due to confidentiality constraints). Reproduced in colour plate section between pages 210 and 211.

OXY reactor. The results obtained and the flow model form a sound basis for further work on the modeling of gas–solid flows in fluidized reactors. It may be possible to include reactions in such a model to develop a comprehensive tool to enhance OXY reactor technology. The methodology can be used to enhance both existing and new reactor technologies.

9.4. EXAMPLE 3: BUBBLE COLUMN REACTOR

Bubble column reactors, in which sparged gas provides the necessary mixing, offer an attractive way to carry out gas–liquid processes. Because of their simple construction and operation, bubble columns are widely used in process industries. However, the simple construction also has the drawback of having fewer degrees of freedom available to a reactor engineer to tailor performance. The performance of bubble columns is controlled by several physical and chemical phenomena with different spatial and temporal scales. Gas–liquid fluid dynamics is determined by local gas volume fraction (hold-up) but extends over the whole reactor. Gas–liquid mass transfer and chemical reactions depend on local concentrations and on local gas–liquid interfacial areas. Interfacial area depend on local gas hold-up and bubble size distribution. Bubble size distribution depends on a variety of parameters, including type and location of sparger, local and global mean and turbulence fields properties of liquid phase and so on. Although much progress has been made in gaining a better understanding of each of the phenomena mentioned, a comprehensive computational model, which is able to simulate all of the above interactions simultaneously, is still too difficult to develop and use for industrial applications. As mentioned in the case of the polymerization reactor, uncertainties in estimating the parameters of sub-models describing various phenomena make the task of developing a comprehensive model less justifiable. On the other hand, conventional reaction engineering models, which include detailed descriptions of reaction and mass transfer from bubbles, normally consider ideally mixed systems or one-dimensional models (see for example, Fleischer *et al.*, 1995). Both the assumptions often do not hold true for bubble column reactors. Under these circumstances, it may be more efficient and may be necessary to use a multilayer or multiscale modeling strategy. Recently Bauer and Eigenberger (1999) proposed such a multiscale modeling strategy based on the fact that the influence of mass transfer and reaction on fluid dynamics can be represented by three variables:

- interphase drag coefficient or interphase momentum exchange terms;
- interfacial area; and
- local gas flux due to mass transfer and reaction from gas bubbles.

If the values of local mean bubble diameter and local gas flux are available, a fluid dynamic model can estimate the required influence of mass transfer and reactions on the fluid dynamics of bubble columns. Fortunately, for most reactions, conversion and selectivity do not depend on details of the inherently unsteady fluid dynamics of bubble column reactors. Despite the complex, unsteady fluid dynamics, conversion and selectivity attain sufficiently constant steady state values in most industrial operations of bubble column reactors. Accurate knowledge of fluid dynamics, which controls the local as well as global mixing, is however, essential to predict reactor performance with a sufficient degree of accuracy. Based on this, Bauer and Eigenberger (1999) proposed a multiscale approach, which is shown schematically in Fig. 9.13.

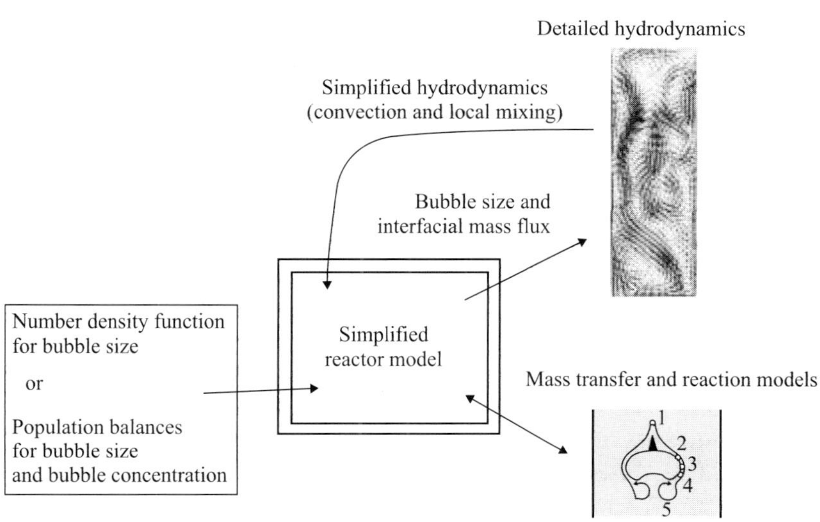

FIGURE 9.13 Concept of multiscale modeling of bubble column reactors (from Bauer and Eigenberger, 1999).

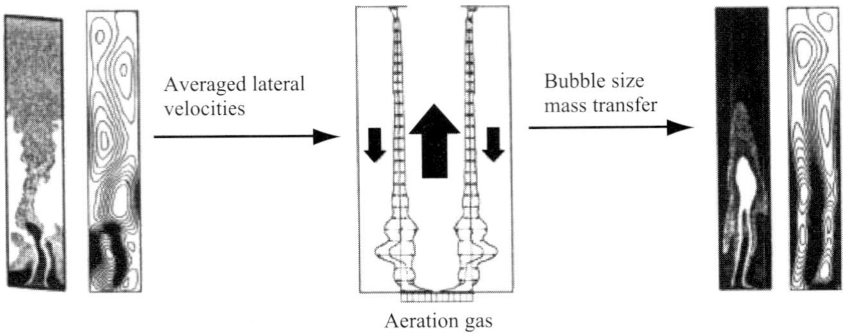

FIGURE 9.14 Iterative process used in multiscale modeling (from Bauer and Eigenberger, 1999).

In this approach, a simplified reactor model acts as a hub. Instead of invoking conventional simplifying assumptions to develop the model, this approach uses information obtained from detailed fluid dynamic models and detailed bubble–bubble interaction (population balance) models. Such a basic reactor model provides the local mean bubble diameter and the interfacial mass flux to the hydrodynamic model. The details of modeling approaches to simulate the fluid dynamics of bubble column reactors are discussed in Chapter 11. We restrict the scope here to discussing the overall approach. The whole reactor behavior is simulated by employing an iterative procedure over these different modeling layers as shown in Fig. 9.14. Some results obtained by Bauer and Eigenberger (1999) using this approach to simulate a pseudo-first-order reaction in a two-dimensional bubble column are shown in Figs 9.15 to 9.17. Four iterations were required to obtain the converged results. Gas sparged at the bottom disappears rapidly due to the reactive consumption and does not extend over the entire column. This changes the flow field of the liquid phase, and mixing significantly. The influence of changes in mixing in the reactor can be clearly seen from the mass fraction profiles within the reactor (Fig. 9.17). The approach can be extended to simulate more complex industrial bubble column reactors.

Recently Ranade (2000) used a similar multiscale approach to simulate a complex industrial loop reactor. The objective of the project was to develop a comprehensive understanding of the fluid dynamics of the operating loop reactor and to develop appropriate scale-up guidelines based on such an understanding. The schematic of the industrial loop reactor considered is shown in Fig. 9.18 (in 2D). The reactor was designed to carry out a pre-polymerization (condensation polymerization) reaction. The low molecular weight products of the condensation reaction and solvent are vaporized in the heater section. These vapors lead to gas-lift action and generate the circulation within the loop reactor, which ensures the desired mixing in the reactor. Generally, the circulation rate is orders of magnitude greater than the net flow through the reactor. The vapors generated are removed from the top after separating from the liquid in the vapor separator. Vapor bubbles erupting at the gas–liquid interface throw some liquid droplets into the vapor space and a fraction of these liquid droplets may be carried over with the removed vapor. Such a carry-over of liquid often imposes limits on enhancing reactor capacity. One of the objectives of the project was, therefore,

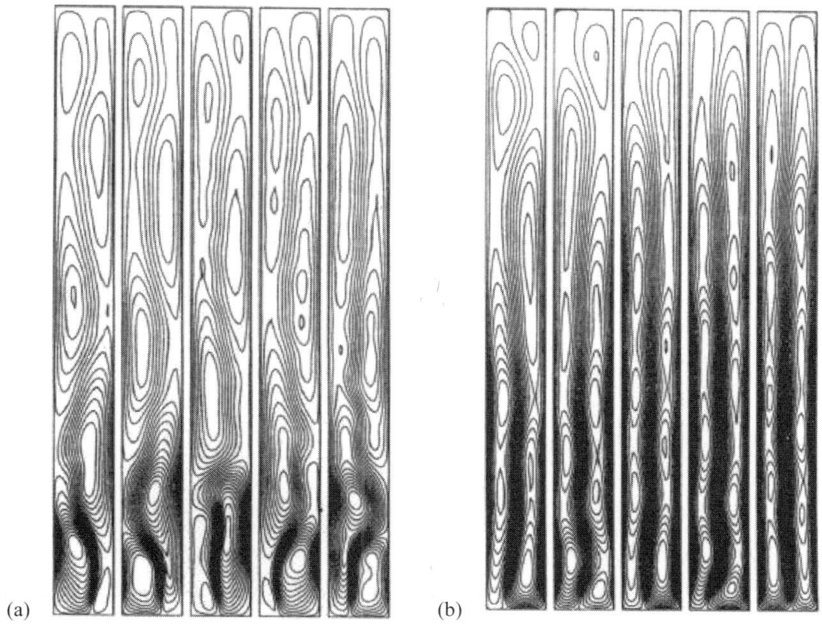

FIGURE 9.15 Predicted streamlines of liquid flow (from Bauer and Eigenberger, 1999). (a) Neglecting mass transfer, (b) accounting for mass transfer.

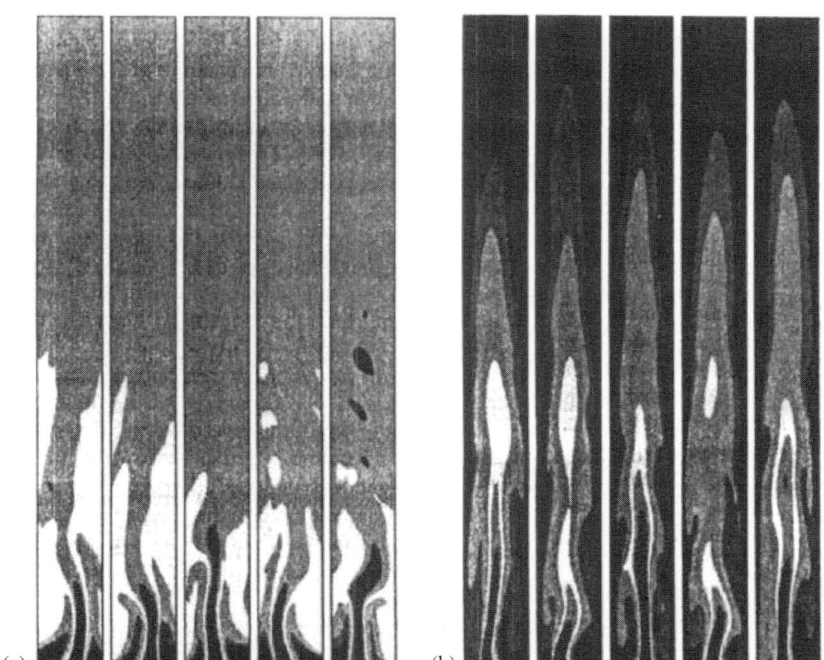

FIGURE 9.16 Predicted contours of gas hold-up (from Bauer and Eigenberger, 1999). (a) Neglecting mass transfer, (b) accounting for mass transfer.

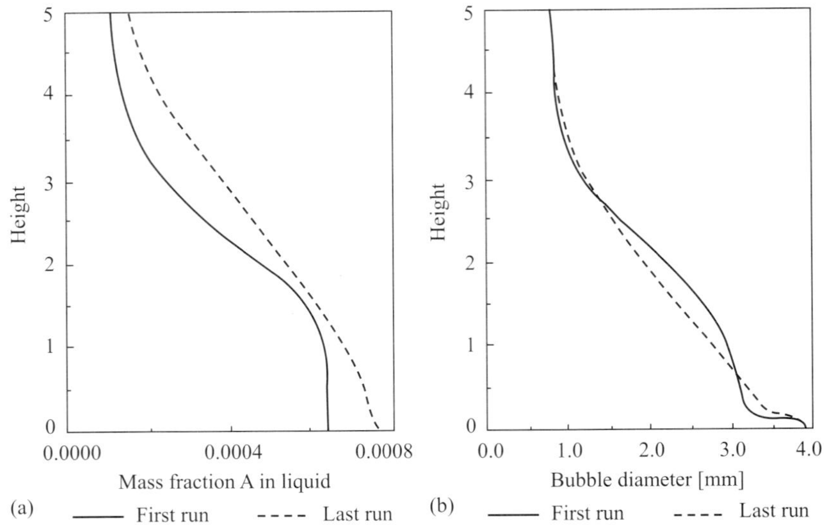

FIGURE 9.17 Predicted concentration and bubble diameter profiles within the column (from Bauer and Eigenberger, 1999).

to understand liquid carry-over in the loop reactor. An accurate understanding of the factors controlling the circulation rate and mixing within the reactor is essential for scaling up the reactor.

From this brief description it is clear that the fluid dynamics of the loop reactor is intimately connected to the reaction. The reaction generates volatiles, which ultimately drive the circulation. However, it was found that it is possible, and may be more efficient, to decouple the reaction part from the flow. The overall problem was tackled by dividing it into several sub-problems. The methodology is shown in Fig. 9.19. In the first sub-problem, using the available empirical information about the operating plant, the fluid mechanics and mixing was approximated to develop a reactor model (plug flow for the loop and complete mixing for the vapor–liquid separator). The reactor model was calibrated and validated by comprehensive comparisons of predicted results with plant data. Such a model was used to predict profiles of concentration, temperature and vapor generation. This information, combined with additional information about the flow regimes in the heater section, was supplied to the flow model.

Computational fluid dynamics based flow models were then developed to simulate flow and mixing in the loop reactor. Even here, instead of developing a single CFD model to simulate complex flows in the loop reactor (gas dispersed in liquid phase in the heater section and liquid dispersed in gas phase in the vapor space of the vapor–liquid separator), four separate flow models were developed. In the first, the bottom portion of the reactor, in which liquid is a continuous phase, was modeled using a Eulerian–Eulerian approach. Instead of actually simulating reactions in the CFD model, results obtained from the simplified reactor model were used to specify vapor generation rate along the heater. Initially some preliminary simulations were carried out for the whole reactor. However, it was noticed that the presence of the gas–liquid interface within the solution domain and inversion of the continuous phase,

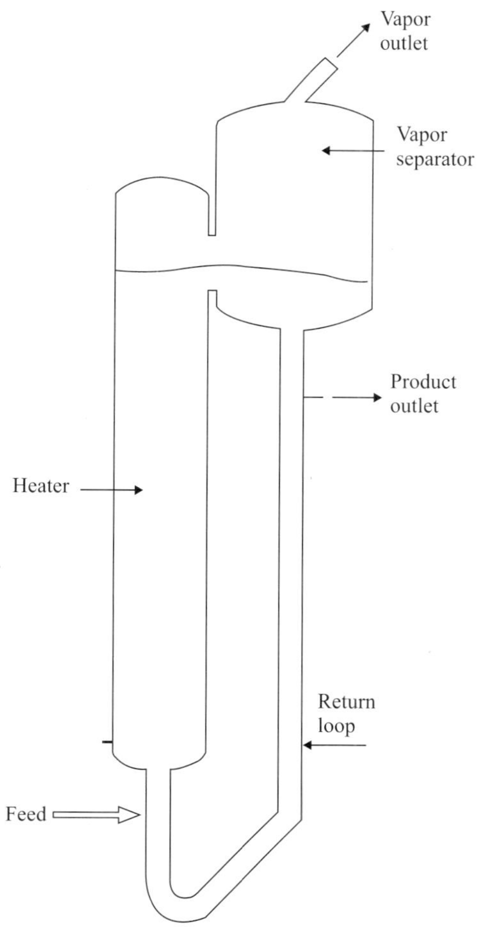

FIGURE 9.18 Schematic of industrial loop reactor.

presented severe challenges to numerical methods, leading to difficulties in obtaining converged results. The exact shape of the gas–liquid interface does not significantly affect the flow and mixing in the vapor–liquid separator. The shape of the gas–liquid interface was, therefore, assumed. A typical grid used for flow simulation is shown in Fig. 9.20. A sample of the simulated flow field in the bottom portion of the loop reactor is shown in Fig. 9.21.

In the second part, flow in the vapor space of the separator, where the gas phase is a continuous phase, was modeled. An Eulerian–Lagrangian approach was used to simulate trajectories of the liquid droplets since the volume fraction of the dispersed liquid phase is quite small. The grid used for the vapor space is shown in Fig. 9.20. The simulated gas volume fraction distribution near the gas–liquid interface and corresponding gas flow in the vapor space are shown in Fig. 9.22. The gas volume fraction distribution and the gas velocity obtained from the model of the bottom portion of the loop reactor were used to specify boundary conditions for the vapor space model. In addition to the gas escaping from the gas–liquid interface, it is necessary to estimate the amount of liquid thrown into the vapor space by the vapor bubbles erupting at the

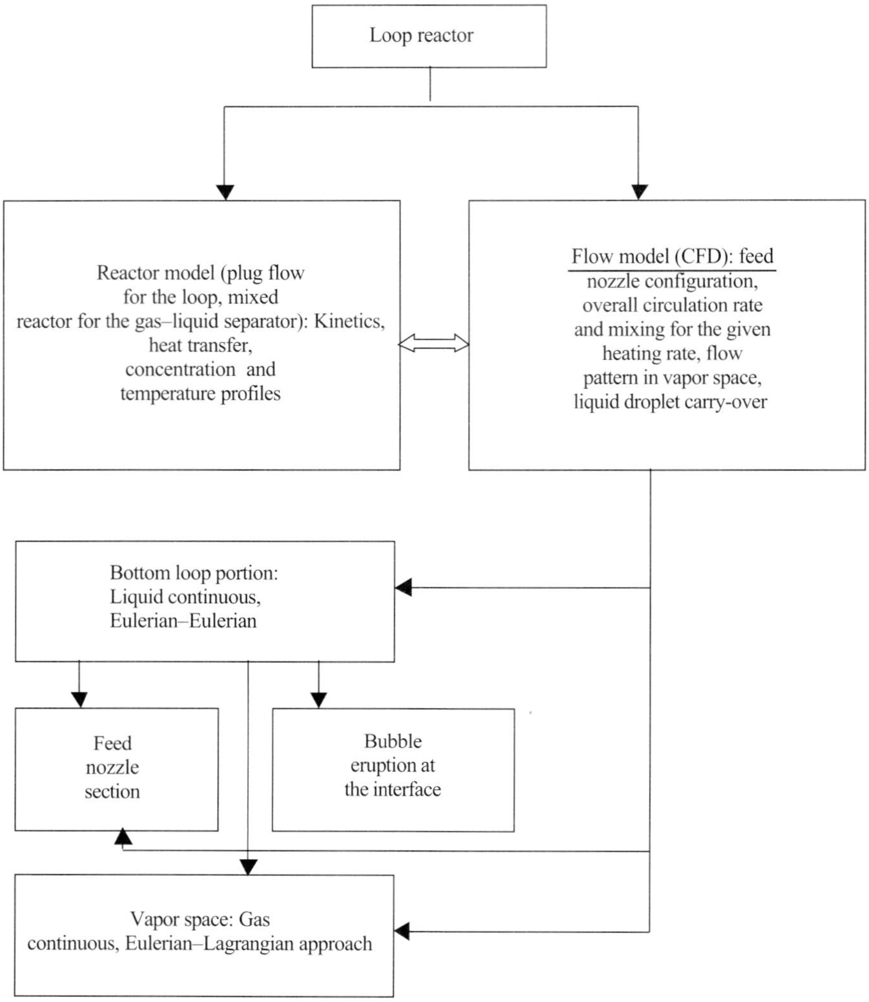

FIGURE 9.19 Methodology used for model loop reactor.

gas–liquid interface. A separate volume of fluid (VOF) based model was developed to understand bubble eruption processes and to estimate the amount of liquid thrown into the vapor space. It was, however, found that the predicted results of amount of liquid thrown per bubble were significantly different than the available data. An expression for estimating the amount of liquid thrown per bubble based on a phenomenological model of Azbel (1981) was, therefore, used to couple the loop part with the vapor space part. In addition, a separate flow model to simulate details of mixing near the feed nozzle (interaction of feed flow with re-circulating flow) was developed. An attempt was made to validate various sub-components of the computational models using the available data. The models were then used to carry out various numerical experiments on computer. These results were used to construct detailed information about the loop reactor and to evolve appropriate scale-up guidelines.

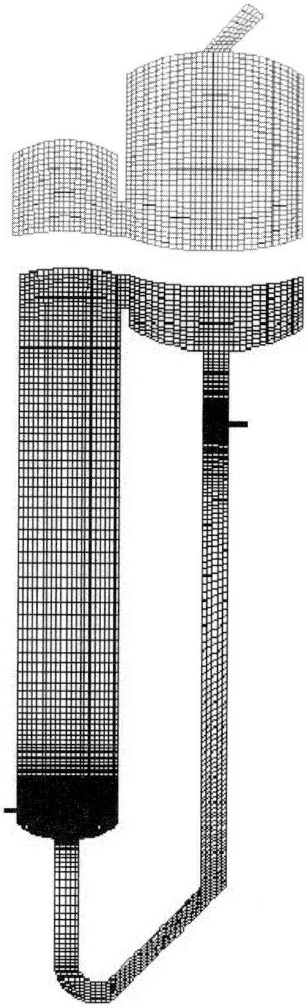

FIGURE 9.20 Computational grid.

9.5. EXAMPLE 4: FCC REGENERATOR

Fluidized catalytic cracking (FCC), which converts heavy oil to value added low boiling point products is an important process in refineries around the world. During cracking reactions, catalyst is deactivated rapidly owing to coke deposition. In industrial FCC units, the deactivated catalyst is continuously regenerated by employing a regenerator connected to the cracking reactor. Besides regenerating the catalyst (by contacting it with air), the FCC regenerator also provides the heat required for the endothermic cracking reactions.

A schematic diagram of a typical industrial FCC regenerator is shown in Fig. 9.23. The spent catalyst particles are circulated through the regenerator. The orientation, size and location of the spent catalyst distributor are important parameters controlling solids mixing. The regenerated catalyst is withdrawn from the outlet located at the

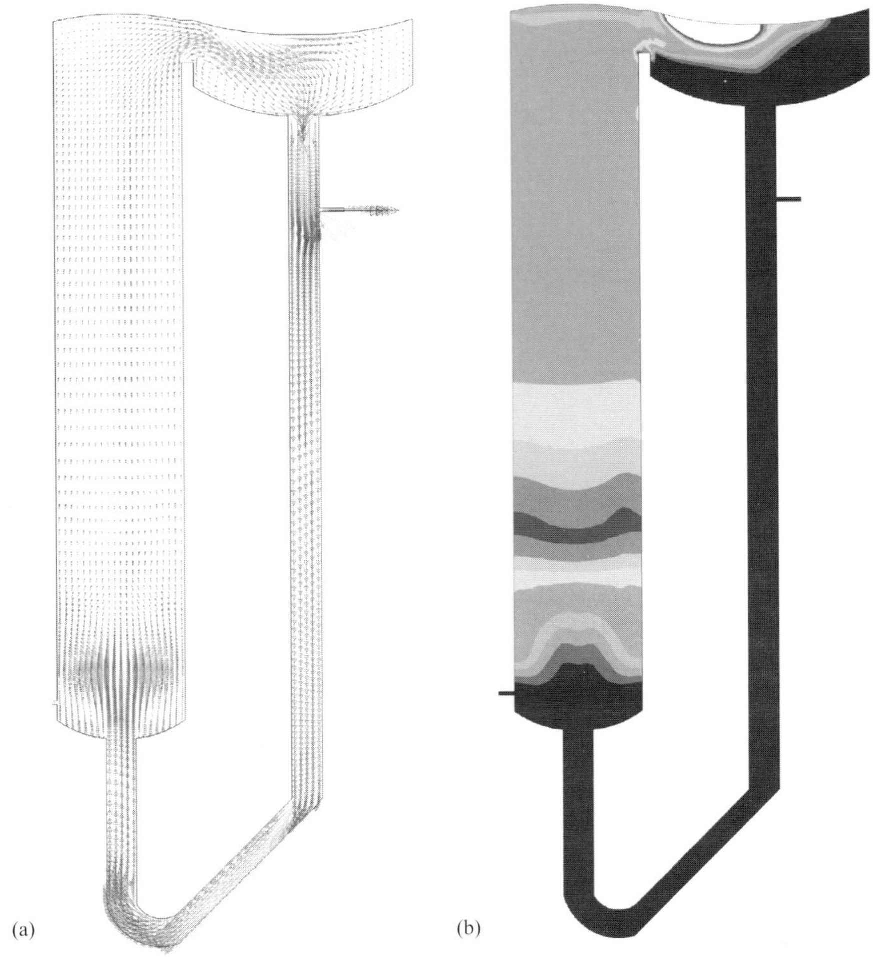

FIGURE 9.21 Typical predicted results for the loop reactor (excluding vapor space). (a) Vector plots (liquid phase), (b) contours of gas volume fraction (legend not shown due to confidentiality constraints). Reproduced in colour plate section between pages 210 and 211.

bottom conical portion. Air is introduced in the regenerator through a distributor located just above the bottom conical part of the reactor. The regenerator is operated in a dense bed (or turbulent bed) regime (superficial gas velocity is much higher than the minimum fluidization velocity). The extent of regeneration of catalyst particles depends on effective contacting between supplied air and catalyst particles. Most of the supplied air passes through the regenerator in the form of large gas bubbles (voids). These voids interact with each other and may coalesce or break up within the dense bed. As these voids rise through the dense bed, a macroscopic circulation of catalyst particles is set-up within the dense bed. When these voids break up at the top surface of the dense bed, solid particles are thrown into the free board region (dilute bed). Reaction of coke on these solid particles with un-reacted oxygen in the dilute bed region may cause excessive temperature excursions (called after-burning, which has a detrimental effect on throughput as well as catalyst and equipment life). Some of

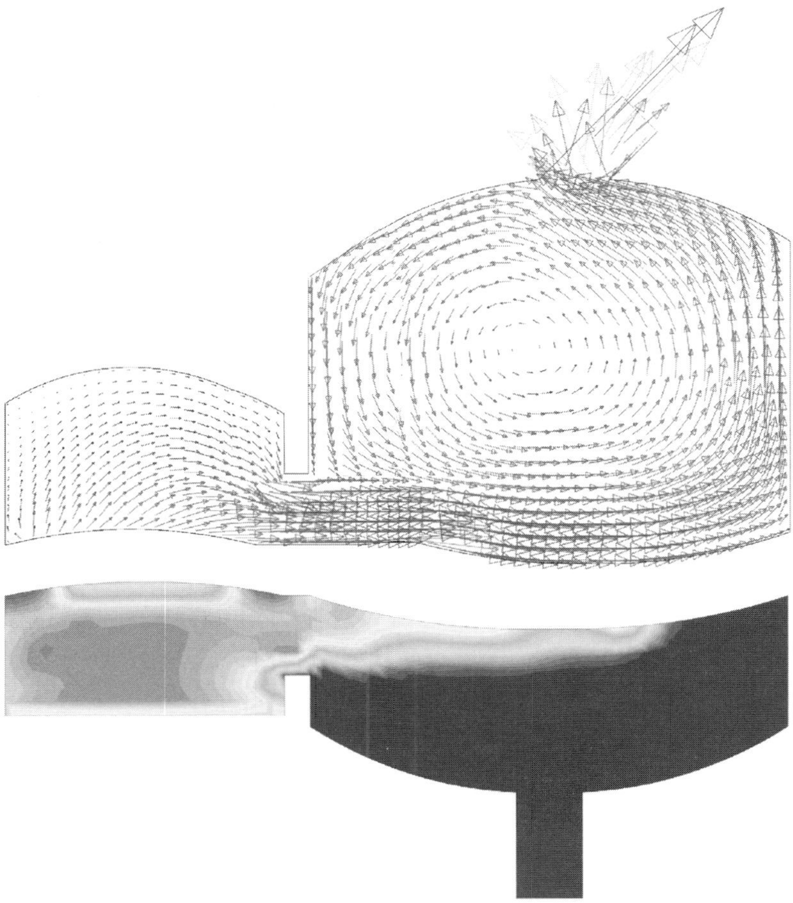

FIGURE 9.22 Typical predicted results for the loop reactor (top: vector plot and vapour space; bottom: contours of gas volume fraction) (legend not shown due to confidentiality constraints). Reproduced in colour plate section between pages 210 and 211.

the main requirement in the reactor engineering of FCC regenerators are therefore, to limit the extent of after-burning and to ensure adequate regeneration of spent catalyst. Use of computational flow modeling within the framework of a multilayer modeling strategy to address these issues is discussed below.

9.5.1. Modeling Approach

Gas–solid flow and reactions occurring in an industrial FCC regenerator present severe challenges to flow modelers and reactor engineers. Several attempts have been made to model gas–solid flows based on an analogy with the kinetic theory of gases. A detailed review of these attempts is given in Chapter 12. It is sufficient to state here that none of the available models for simulating dense bubbling beds, were able to predict the continuous bubbling with corresponding satisfactory estimations of bubble volume fractions. Ranade (1996) reported that in many cases Eulerian–Eulerian computational models predicted eventual carry-over of all solids from the regenerator

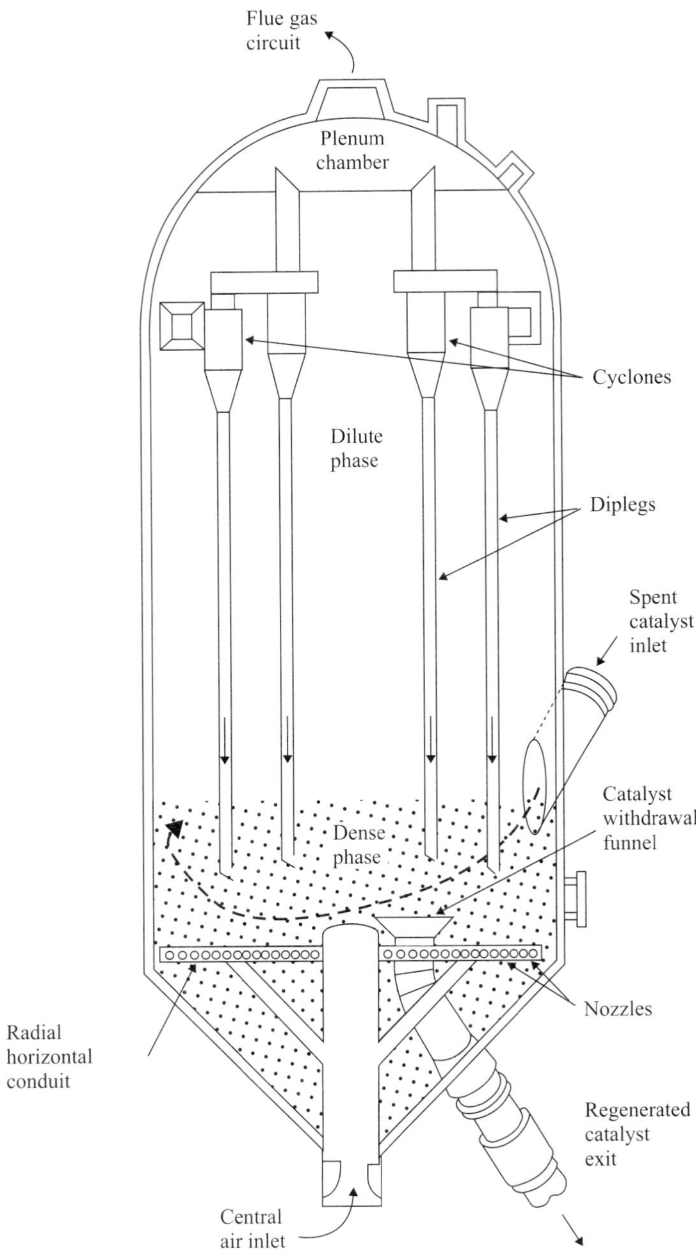

FIGURE 9.23 Schematic diagram of typical industrial FCC regenerator.

at high superficial gas velocities. Though there has been some progress in simulating bubbling fluidized beds (see, for example, van Wachem *et al.*, 1999), it may be necessary to use a multilayer modeling strategy to simulate industrial bubbling fluidized bed reactors. Ranade (1998) used a three-layer approach, which is shown schematically in Fig. 9.24.

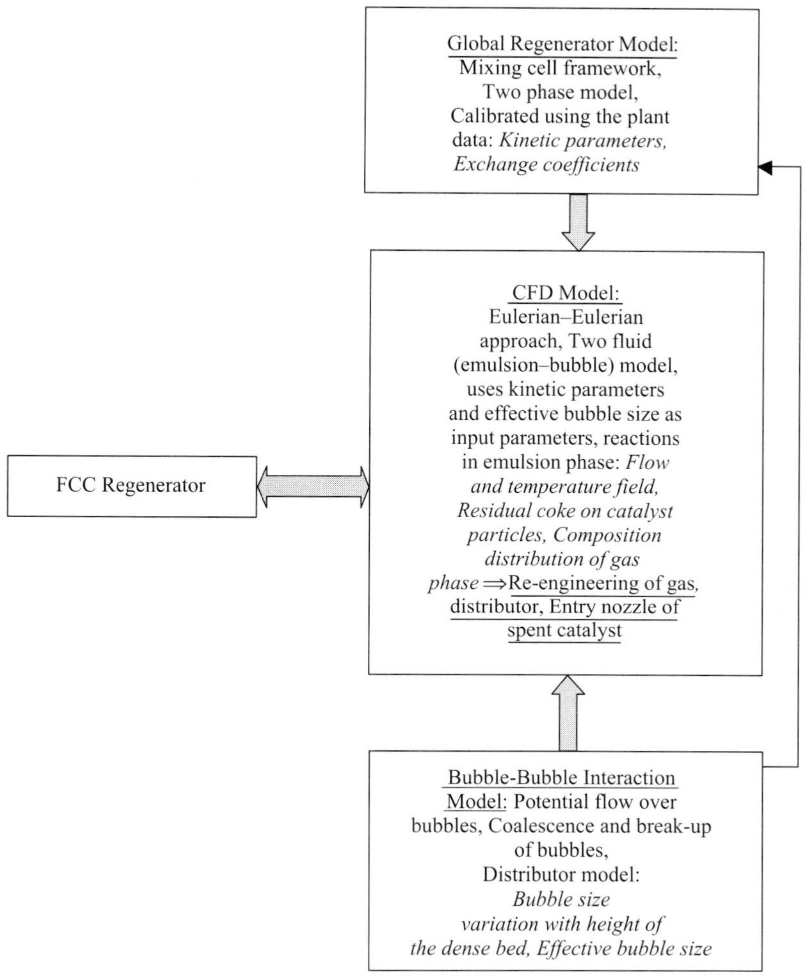

FIGURE 9.24 Multilayer modeling of FCC regenerator.

A regenerator performance model based on a mixing cell framework is used as a first layer. The model is used to gain an understanding of the overall behavior of the FCC regenerator. The sensitivity of the regenerator performance to a variety of operating conditions was studied. The model was used to fit some of the kinetic constants by comparing model predictions with plant data. A second modeling layer comprised a bubble–bubble interaction model to track bubble trajectories. This Lagrangian model was used to understand the coalescence of bubbles and to estimate the bubble size distribution within the dense bed. A third, CFD-based modeling layer was developed to simulate complex macroscopic flow and reactions in a FCC regenerator. The flow of information between these layers is not unidirectional. There has to be significant interaction and exchange of information during the development and application of these three modeling layers to obtain as much information about the FCC regenerator as possible. The application of these three modeling layers to develop a comprehensive understanding of a FCC regenerator is described below.

9.5.2. Regenerator Performance Model

In view of the possibility of limiting mass transfer from the voids phase, a heterogeneous model (comprising two phases: emulsion and voids (or bubbles)) was used to simulate the dense bed. The homogeneous model was used for the dilute bed region. The generalized mixing cell framework used in the model is shown in Fig. 9.25. It can be seen that the framework allows the flexibility of independent selection of appropriate mixing in the dense phase, voids phase and dilute bed. Mass balances were written for bubble (void), emulsion and dilute bed regions of the regenerator (Utikar and Ranade, 1997). Model equations were incorporated into a user-friendly code called **MoBB** (**Mo**del for **B**ubbling **B**eds), to simulate regenerator performance.

Preliminary numerical experiments were carried out to select an appropriate value of time step. To illustrate the typical results obtained using **MoBB**, a sample of results is shown in Fig. 9.26. It was observed that the regenerator attained steady state in approximately 30 min. The coke on regenerated catalyst reduced from 1% initially to about 0.35% at steady state. The emulsion temperature increased from 723 to 932 K. The oxygen mole fraction at the outlet was about 0.003 and that of carbon dioxide was 0.146. In addition to the prediction of these outlet parameters, the simulation model also provided information about the variation of concentrations and temperatures within the regenerator. The influence of air flow rate and coke on spent catalyst (CSC) on oxygen breakthrough from the dense bed is shown in Fig. 9.26. It is interesting to note that exit oxygen concentration (from the dense bed) does not

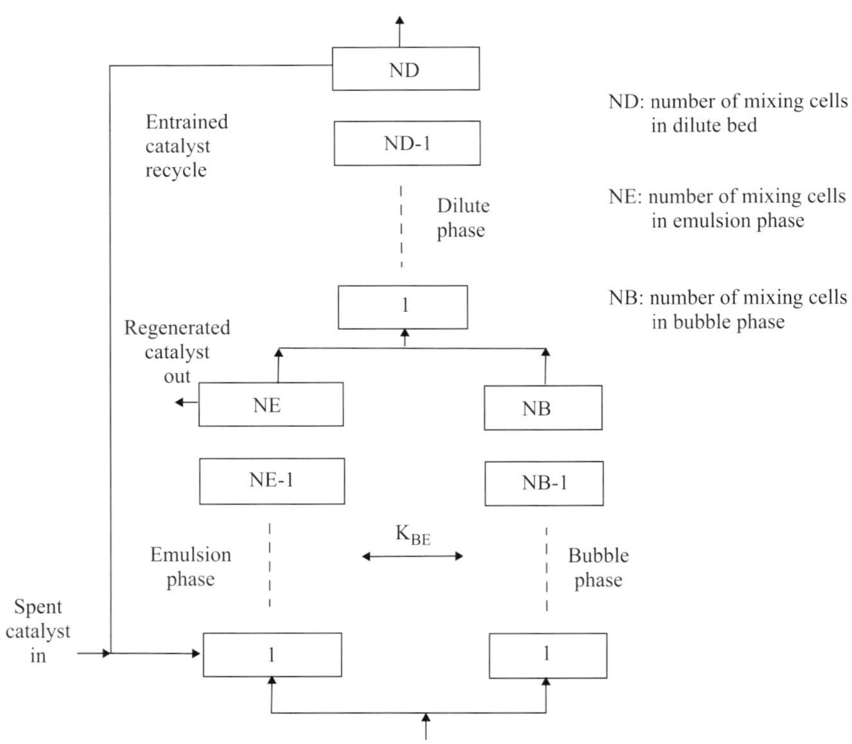

FIGURE 9.25 Mixing cell model (from Ranade, 1998).

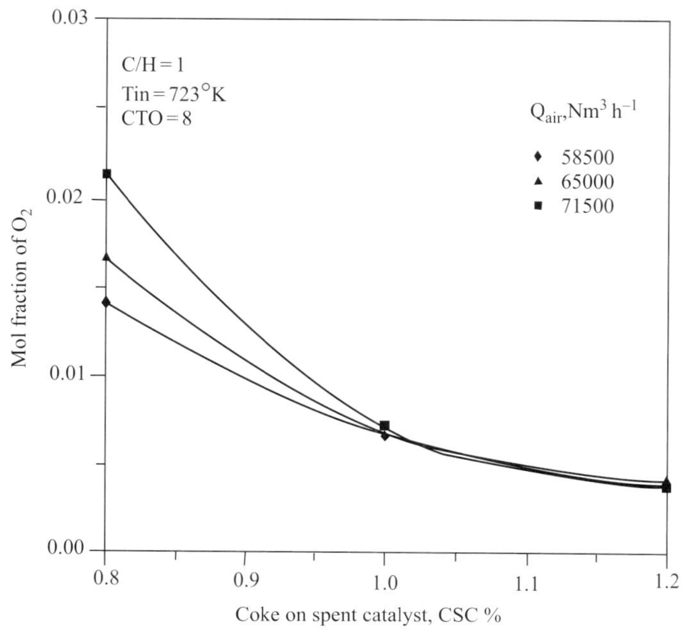

FIGURE 9.26 Typical results obtained from mixing cell model (from Ranade, 1998).

increase with increase in gas flow rate, if CSC is equal or greater than 1% (within the range studied here). As expected, as airflow rate increases, emulsion temperature increases and the amount of coke on the regenerated catalyst decreases. The model parameters (kinetic and transport parameters) were calibrated by comparing model predictions with available plant data.

9.5.3. Bubble–Bubble Interaction Model

In a gas–solid fluidized bed, where gas velocity is equal to the minimum fluidization velocity, the solid particles are suspended and this suspension behaves as a fluid. When gas flows at a higher rate than required for minimum fluidization, it results in the formation of voids or bubbles (regions devoid of solids). Most of the gas supplied in excess of the minimum fluidization velocity flows through the bed in the form of bubbles. The gas velocity, orifice diameter and minimum fluidization velocity control bubble formation at the gas distributor. For a specific reactor configuration and gas–solid system, the latter two variables are well defined. If the gas distributor consists of multiple orifices, it will be necessary to estimate the non-uniform gas flow through these multiple orifices. The gas flow through each orifice is controlled by the pressure drop across the distributor (difference between pressure below the distributor orifice and the static head above that orifice). The static head at any point above the distributor plate is in turn controlled by the bubble voidage distribution within the whole dense bed. These phenomena were modeled in a second layer to estimate the bubble size distribution and effective bubble size within the dense bed of a regenerator.

A bubble–bubble interaction model based on potential flow over bluff bodies was developed and incorporated in a code called, **BuDY** (for **Bu**bble **DY**namics). The model is based on an assumption that the instantaneous velocity of an individual bubble in a fluidized bed can be obtained by adding to its rise velocity in isolation, the velocity which the emulsion phase would have had at the nose of the bubble, if the bubble was absent. The details of model development, model equations and solution procedures are described in Ranade (1997a). Appropriate representation of bubble formation, coalescence and exit of bubbles from the dense bed were included in the model. With the knowledge of initial bubble positions and bubble size, subsequent bubble positions can be tracked to predict instantaneous velocities and bubble positions within the dense bed.

The bubble-tracking model is capable of giving the number of bubbles present in the dense bed, their positions, diameter and velocity at any instant of time. Using these data, time variation of average bubble holdup as a function of time can be found. It can be used to examine the radial distribution of bubbles at various desired axial locations. A separate program was developed to calculate time-averaged voidage distribution (in a Eulerian framework) within the dense bed from the computed bubble trajectories. The model was also used to understand the role of bubble–bubble interactions and coalescence on the bubble dynamics of dense beds. Several numerical experiments were carried out to understand the influence of bubble diameter, orifice spacing etc. on bubble dynamics. The predicted bubble dynamics from the model reproduces the main dynamical characteristics observed in experiments. This model was used to simulate bubble distribution for the industrial gas distributor comprising 648 orifices. It was found that the number of bubbles decreased drastically as bubbles rise through the dense bed. The total number of bubbles and bubble volume fraction within the dense bed fluctuated quite significantly (the predicted fluctuations were found to be chaotic, Ranade, 1997a). The attractor reconstructed from the predicted voidage fluctuations showed remarkable similarity with that reconstructed from the experimental data. The model was used to obtain an effective bubble size within the dense bed of a FCC regenerator.

9.5.4. CFD Model

In order to understand the macroscopic circulation within the dense bed, it is necessary to develop a CFD-based model. Such a model will also be necessary to simulate radial non-uniformity in oxygen and temperature distributions. The validated CFD model can be used to evaluate various configurations of air distributor and spent catalyst distributor. As mentioned earlier, it was not possible to use the kinetic theory of granular flows to simulate flow and reactions in the dense bed of a regenerator. Ranade (1998) alternatively used the analogy of bubbles in fluidized beds with bubbles in viscous liquids to simulate macroscopic flow patterns in a bubbling FCC regenerator. The flow in the dense bed of the FCC regenerator was modeled as a two-phase flow comprising an emulsion phase (representing gas–solid mixture with minimum fluidization voidage) and a void phase (representing almost solids-free gas regions within the bed). The two-fluid model of Ranade (1997b) was used for this purpose. The available design and operating information, published correlations and results of the first two modeling layers were used to estimate various relevant scales such as bubble diameter, entrainment, catalyst circulation rate and so on. A wide range of space and velocity scales co-exists in a FCC regenerator. The diameter of the regenerator ($\sim$ 5 m) is larger by a few orders of magnitude than the holes of a gas distributor or cyclone standpipes (a few centimeters). It is therefore impractical to resolve all these scales in a single computational model. Appropriate sub-models representing the small-scale internals were developed to make the problem computationally tractable. The results obtained using other modeling layers (kinetic and transport parameters, effective bubble size within the dense bed and so on) were used as input parameters to the CFD model.

The detailed model equations were described by Ranade (1998). In applying two-fluid theory to the bubbling dense bed of a regenerator, it must be noted that the continuous phase density needs to be calculated from the voidage in the dense phase (emulsion phase) and from the density of the catalyst particles. The molecular viscosity of the emulsion phase was specified to be 1 Pa.s based on empirical evidence. The average bubble diameter was specified based on the results obtained using **BuDY**. The reactions occurring in the dense bed of the FCC regenerator were simulated using species conservation equations (and enthalpy) for the emulsion and bubble phase. Only the principal coke burning reaction (to form carbon dioxide) was considered. Terms representing heat generated due to the combustion of coke and heat transfer from bubble to emulsion phase were adequately modeled. As mentioned earlier, all parameters appearing in the above set of equations were estimated using available data and the results of the first two modeling layers. The governing equations described above were solved using a commercial CFD code, FLUENT (Fluent Inc., USA). Details of the mapping of these model equations onto FLUENT and solution strategies are discussed in Ranade (1998).

The model was used to simulate the macroscopic flow and reactions occurring in a FCC regenerator. A typical grid and predicted velocity field for emulsion phase are shown in Fig. 9.27a and 9.27b, respectively. It can be seen that, except in the region near the regenerator walls, the emulsion phase flows in an upward direction. The predicted velocities in the horizontal planes are much smaller than those in the vertical plane. Fig. 9.27c shows void phase distribution at a typical vertical plane in the dense bed. These flow results were used to simulate coke burning in the dense bed of the regenerator. As expected, higher values of oxygen mass fractions are predicted near the air distributor. The oxygen mass fraction in the void phase quickly drops down as one goes away from the distributor. The knowledge of oxygen breakthrough from the top surface (Fig. 9.28) of the dense bed is important for estimating the extent of after-burning and possible locations of hotspots. The results presented here constitute only a small fraction of the information obtained from the model. The simulation results were analyzed in detail to extract useful information about the behavior of the FCC regenerator. The predicted results were compared with proprietary, plant and experimental data. The predicted extent of solids mixing was found to be less than that indicated by the data. With appropriate tuning of model parameters, however, adequate agreement was obtained between predicted results and available data. The tuned CFD-based model was then used to aid understanding of the macroscopic flow and its influence on reactions occurring in the dense bed of a FCC regenerator. Some results obtained using the model are discussed below.

It is important to develop the capability to simulate the influence of changes in the air distributor on regenerator performance. During the operating life of a regenerator,

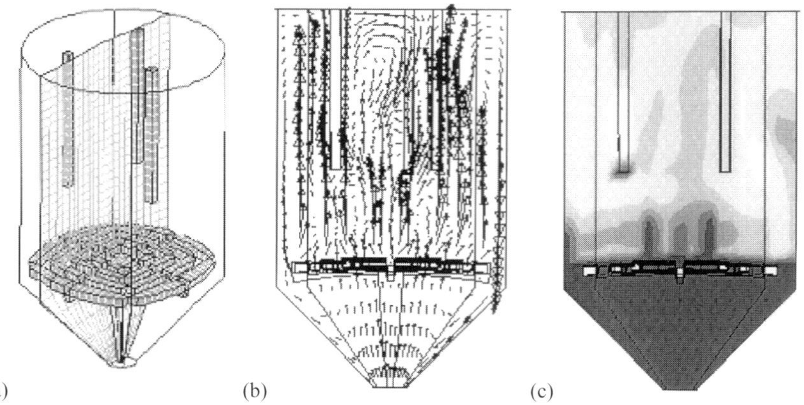

(a) (b) (c)

FIGURE 9.27 Computational grid and typical predicted results for the FCC regenerator (from Ranade, 1998). (a) Grid, (b) vector plot, (c) contours of gas volume fraction. (Light: high values; dark: low values; legend not shown due to confidentiality constraints.)

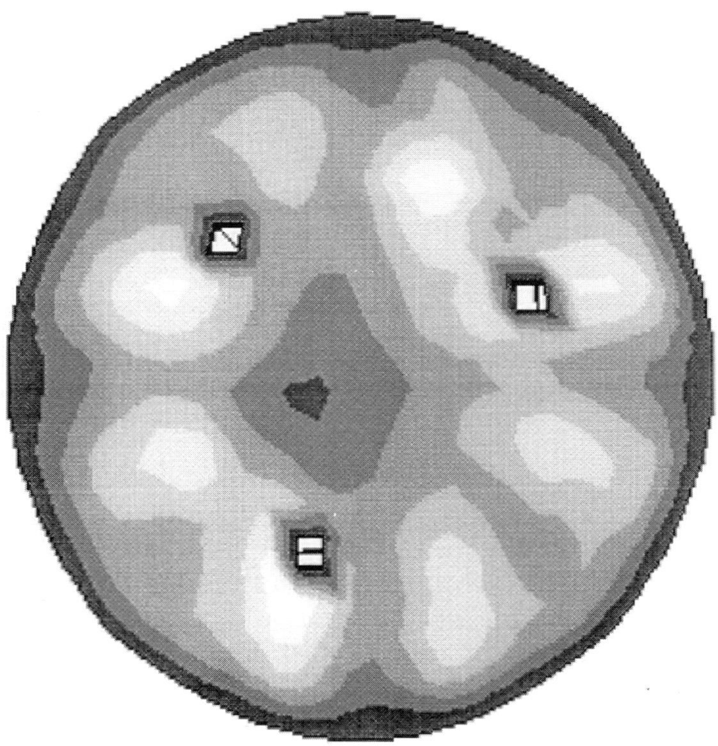

FIGURE 9.28 Oxygen breakthrough from the top surface of the dense bed (contours of oxygen mass fraction) (from Ranade, 1998). (Light: high values; dark: low values; legend not shown due to confidentiality constraints.)

the distribution of sparger orifices may change several times owing to either mechanical or operational considerations. The bubble–bubble interaction model (BuDY) was used to simulate the influence of distributor design on bubble formation, coalescence and effective bubble sizes. The CFD-based model was used to examine the influence of distributor design on time-averaged void distribution and macroscopic circulation within the dense bed. The results were useful in understanding the sensitivity of the generated flow to changes in distributor configuration. Examination of the simulation results for the emulsion phase indicates the possibility of short-circuiting spent catalyst particles. To avoid this, several techniques are used in practice, one of the simplest being to install a ski jump type platform near the entry of the spent catalyst. Such a ski jump throws the spent catalyst particles inside the dense bed (instead of releasing them at the regenerator wall), such that the particles enter the upward flowing region of the dense bed. The CFD model was used to evaluate various configurations of spent catalyst entry. Although these results are not included here, it is sufficient to state that the CFD model, along with the other two models (MoBB and BuDY), was used successfully to characterize quantitatively the performance of the industrial FCC regenerator. Results obtained using these models proved quite useful when making engineering decisions regarding gas distributor and spent catalyst entry configurations.

9.6. SUMMARY

The examples discussed in this chapter illustrate that the multilayer approach is not only useful but may also be necessary to develop useful and tractable simulation models of industrial reactors. Computational flow (CFD) models play a crucial role in linking actual reactor hardware to reactor performance. Their ability to extrapolate cold flow results to high temperature and pressure is especially valuable. Judicious use of these computational flow models (1) to understand basic phenomena and (2) for simulation of complex reactors with the help of other modeling layers, will lead to better reactor engineering practices. Details of developing computational flow models for reactors of different types are discussed in the following chapters. The approach illustrated in this chapter may then be adapted to understand the behavior of industrial reactors, in order to (1) enhance the performance of existing reactor hardware or (2) evolve better reactor technologies.

REFERENCES

Aris, R. (1978), "Mathematical Modeling Techniques", Pitman Publishing, Southport.

Azbel, D. (1981), "Two Phase Flows in Chemical Engineering", Cambridge University Press, Cambridge.

Bauer, M. and Eigenberger, G. (1999), A concept for multi-scale modeling of bubble columns and loop reactors, *Chem. Eng. Sci.*, **54**, 5109–5117.

Denn, M.M. (1986), "Process Modeling", Longman Scientific & Technical, Harlow, Essex.

Fleischer, C., Becker, S. and Eigenberger, G. (1995), Transient hydrodynamics, mass transfer and reaction in bubble columns, *Chem. Eng. Res. Des.*, **73A**, 649–653.

Krishna, R. (1994), A system approach to multiphase reactor selection, *Adv. Chem. Eng.*, **19**, 201–249.

Kumar, S., Ganvir, V., Satyanand, C., Kumar, R. and Gandhi, K.S. (1998), Alternative mechanisms of drop breakage in stirred vessels, *Chem. Eng. Sci.*, **53**, 3269–3280.

Kunii, D. and Levenspiel, O. (1991), "Fluidization Engineering", second edition, Butterworth-Heinemann.
Leng, D.E. and Quarderer, G.J. (1982), Drop dispersion in suspension polymerisation, *Chem. Eng. Commun.*, **14**, 177–201.
Polya, G. (1962), "Mathematical Discovery", Vol. 1, John Wiley & Sons, New York.
Ranade, V.V. (1996), Modeling of a FCC regenerator: Preliminary Results, NCL Internal Report, IOCL/NCL/1/96.
Ranade, V.V. (1997a), Modeling of a FCC regenerator, NCL Internal Report, IOCL/NCL/2/97.
Ranade, V.V. (1997b), Modeling of turbulent flow in a bubble column reactor, *Chem. Eng. Res. Des.*, **75**, 14.
Ranade, V.V. (1998), Multiphase reactor engineering, *Speed Up J.*, **12**, 26–33.
Ranade, V.V. (1999a), Calibre Conference on Industrial Mixing, September 1999.
Ranade, V.V. (1999b), Pushing the limits of existing reactor hardware using CFD, *Current Sci.*, **77**, 1303–1310.
Ranade, V.V. (2000), CPCFD User Group Meeting, Cincinnati, May.
Samuelsberg, A.E. (1994), Modeling and simulation of fluidized bed reactors, PhD Thesis, University of Trondheim, Norway.
Ullmann's Encyclopedia (1986), Volume A6, VSH Publishers.
Utikar, R.P. and Ranade, V.V. (1997), MoBB: Model for bubbling fluidized bed reactors, CHEMCON.
Van Wachem, B.G.M., Schouten, J.C., Krishna, R. and van den Bleek, C.M. (1999), Validation of the Eulerian simulated dynamic behaviour of gas-solid fluidised beds, *Chem. Eng. Sci.*, **54**, 2141–2149.
Vivaldo-Lima, E., Wood, P.E., Hamielec, A.E. and Penlidis, A. (1997), *Ind. Eng. Chem. Res.*, **36**, 939.
Vivaldo-Lima, E., Wood, P.E., Hamielec, A.E. and Penlidis, A. (1998), Calculation of the particle size distribution in suspension polymerisation using a compartment mixing model, *Can. J. Chem. Eng.*, **76**, 495–505.
Zhou, G. and Kresta, S. (1998), Correlation of mean drop size and minimum drop size with the turbulence energy dissipation and the flow in an agitated tank, *Chem. Eng. Sci.*, **53**, 2063–2079.

PART IV
APPLICATIONS

10 STIRRED REACTORS

Stirred reactors, in which one or more impellers are used to generate flow and mixing within the reactor, are among the most widely used reactors in chemical and allied industries. Stirred reactors offer unmatched flexibility and control over transport processes occurring within the reactor. A skilled reactor engineer can tailor the fluid dynamics and, therefore, performance of a stirred reactor by appropriate adjustments to reactor hardware and operating parameters. Parameters such as reactor shape, aspect ratio, number, type, location and size of impellers and degree of baffling provide effective handles to control the performance of stirred reactors. However, the availability of such a large number of parameters also makes the job of selecting the most suitable configuration for the stirred reactor quite difficult. It is essential to first translate the 'wish list' of reactor performance into a 'wish list' of desired fluid dynamics of stirred reactors. Once the desired flow characteristics are identified, it is then necessary to use or to develop appropriate tools to relate reactor hardware and operating procedures to resulting flow within the reactor. In this chapter, applications of computational flow modeling tools to simulate flow within stirred reactors are discussed in detail. Emphasis is on providing adequate information to the readers to enable them to initiate simulations of industrial stirred reactors. Before that, we discuss some reactor engineering issues related to stirred reactors.

10.1. ENGINEERING OF STIRRED REACTORS

Several types of stirred reactor are used in practice and several ways of classifying these exist. Some of the widely used types of stirred reactors are shown in Fig. 10.1. The stirred reactor shown in Fig. 10.1(a) is a typical multiphase reactor used for carrying out exothermic reactions such as hydrogenations and oxidations. Stirred reactors provide excellent heat and mass transfer characteristics and can handle multiphase systems effectively. Most industrial reactors of this type use more than one impeller and have one or more set of cooling coils. Alternatively, the contents of the reactor are circulated through an external heat exchanger if the geometrical constraints restrict the provision of heat transfer area within the reactor. When per pass conversion of gas is low, gas is recirculated using an external compressor. To avoid the need for external circulation of unreacted gas, gas-inducing type impellers may be used (shown in Fig. 10.1b). It typically comprises a hollow shaft impeller with a stator arrangement to enhance gas induction rate. Numerous variations of these typical configurations are possible and are used in practice. For highly viscous systems, helical ribbon or screw impellers are used either with or without a draft tube (Fig. 10.1c). As mentioned earlier, the reactor engineer has to select the best possible hardware configuration to suit the process under consideration. Some of the industrial processes carried out in stirred reactors are listed in Table 10.1. These processes are classified on the basis of phases handled in the stirred reactor.

Engineering of stirred reactors (see Fig. 1.10 for a general methodology of reactor engineering) begins with the analysis of process requirements and evolving a preliminary configuration of the reactor. This step is based on laboratory study and on reactor models based on idealized fluid dynamics and mixing. In most industrial cases, this step itself may involve several iterations, especially for multiphase systems. It is often necessary to carry out reactor sizing for different values of relevant transport rates (heat transfer, mass transfer) or operating parameters (rotational speed, solid loading and so on). The process of evolving preliminary configuration helps to firm up performance targets for the reactor. Transformation of a preliminary reactor configuration to an industrial reactor proceeds through several steps, some of which

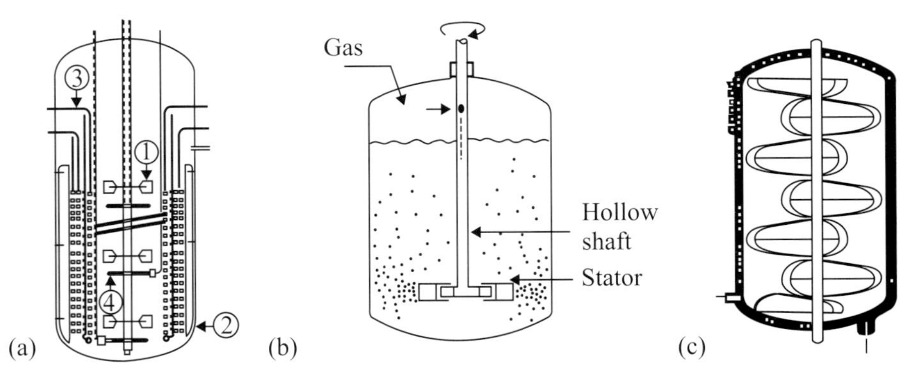

FIGURE 10.1 Types of stirred tank reactor. (a) Multiphase stirred reactor. 1: impeller, 2: baffles, 3: cooling coils, 4: gas sparger. (b) Stirred reactor with gas-inducing impeller (dead-end type). (c) Stirred reactor with helical ribbon impeller (used with or without a draft tube).

TABLE 10.1 Some Industrial Applications of Stirred Reactors

Phases handled	Applications
Liquid	Alkylations, Sulfonations, Esterifications, Bulk and solution polymerizations (styrene, acrilonitrile, ethylene, propylene) and so on
Gas–liquid	Oxidations (ethylene, paraffins), Chlorinations (acetic acid, dodecane), Carbonylations (methanol, propanol), Esterifications, manufacture of sulfuric acid, adipic acid, oxamide and so on
Gas–liquid–solid	Hydrogenations (olefins, edible oils, several chloro and nitro aromatics), Oxidations (p-xylene), Fermentations (alcohol, single cell proteins, antibiotics), Waste water treatment and so on
Liquid–liquid	Suspension and emulsion polymerizations (styrene, vinyl-chloride), Oximations, Extractions
Liquid–solid	Calcium hydroxide (from calcium oxide), Regeneration of ion-exchange resins, Anaerobic fermentations
Gas–liquid–liquid	Bi-phasic hydroformylations, Carbonylations
Gas–solid	Stirred fluidized beds (poly-ethylene, poly-propylene)

are listed below. Computational flow modeling can make substantial contributions to each of these steps.

(1) *Reaction engineering models for simulating reactor performance*: Reaction engineering models are used to examine the 'sensitivity' of reactor performance to various fluid dynamics related issues such as residence time distributions, short-circuiting and by-pass. These models are also a useful aid to understanding issues related to reactor dynamics and start-up/shutdown operations. If the performance is found to be sensitive to fluid dynamics related issues, computational flow models can be used to obtain accurate information about the desired processes. Some examples of combining information from detailed flow models with reaction engineering models based on a mixing cell framework are discussed in Chapter 1. Such combined reaction engineering models are useful to interpret and extrapolate laboratory- and pilot-scale experiments. Detailed simulations of reaction engineering models at different values of transport parameters (mass transfer coefficient, heat transfer coefficient, mixing and so on) are carried out to identify operable windows and to evolve quantitative demands on reactor hardware.

(2) *Resolving conflicting process requirements*: For most industrial situations, a reactor has to carry out several functions simultaneously. It is quite common to find that the requirements of these different functions of the reactor may be quite different or sometimes may even conflict with each other. For example, the desired fluid dynamic characteristics for blending and heat transfer are quite different (they require more bulk flow and less shear) from those for gas–liquid dispersion and mass transfer (which require more shear). Such conflicting requirements make the task of evolving a 'wish list' for the desired fluid dynamics difficult. The reactor engineer has to achieve a compromise between conflicting process requirements to achieve the best results. Not much progress can be made without a good understanding of the underlying

fluid dynamics of stirred reactors and its relation with design parameters on the one hand and with the processes of interest, on the other. Experimental investigations have contributed significantly to a better understanding of the complex hydrodynamics of stirred vessels in recent years. However, computational models offer unique advantages for understanding the conflicting requirements of different processes and their subsequent prioritization. Using a computation model, one can switch on and off various processes, which is not possible when carrying out experiments. Such numerical experiments can give useful insight into interactions between different processes and can help to resolve the challenges posed by conflicting requirements.

(3) *Translating batch data for continuous reactors*: In most cases, laboratory- and bench-scale experiments required to validate the reactor concept are carried out in batch mode. It is then necessary to translate (or to use) the data obtained in these experiments to design continuous reactors. The location of feed pipes, outlets and their influence on mixing and performance needs to be understood. Computational flow models can be of great help in this regard.

(4) *Scale-down/scale-up analysis*: It is essential to analyze the possible influence of the scale of the reactor on its fluid dynamics and performance. It should be noted that a small-scale reactor would invariably have higher shear and more rapid circulation than a large-scale reactor. Multiphase processes, therefore, are often dispersion controlled in small-scale reactors and are coalescence controlled in large-scale reactors. The interfacial area per unit volume of reactor normally reduces as the scale of the reactor increases. Scale-up/scale-down analysis is useful when planning laboratory and pilot plant tests. It may often be necessary to use a pilot reactor configuration which is not geometrically similar to the large-scale reactor in order to maintain similarity of the desired process. Conventionally, such an analysis is carried out based on certain empirical scaling rules and prior experience. Computational flow modeling can make substantial contributions to this step by providing quantitative information about the fluid dynamics.

(5) *Testing new reactor concepts*: More often than not, development of reactor technologies relies on prior experience. New reactor concepts are often sidelined due to lack of resources (experimental facilities, time, funding etc.) to test them. Experimental studies have obvious limitations regarding the extent of parameter space that can be studied and regarding extrapolation beyond the studied parameter space. A wide variety of impellers with different shapes are used in practice. Different practices relating to impeller clearance etc. are followed for different impellers and for different applications. Computational flow models, which allow *a priori* predictions of the flow generated in a stirred reactor of any configuration (impellers of any shape) with just a knowledge of geometry and operating parameters, can make valuable contributions to developing new reactor technologies.

This brief review of steps in the engineering of stirred reactors indicates that the availability of large degrees of freedom regarding reactor configuration and impellers can be effectively exploited to evolve better reactor technologies. This, however, requires detailed knowledge and understanding of the fluid dynamics of stirred reactors. For example, in a recent US patent, Roby (1997) claims development of an

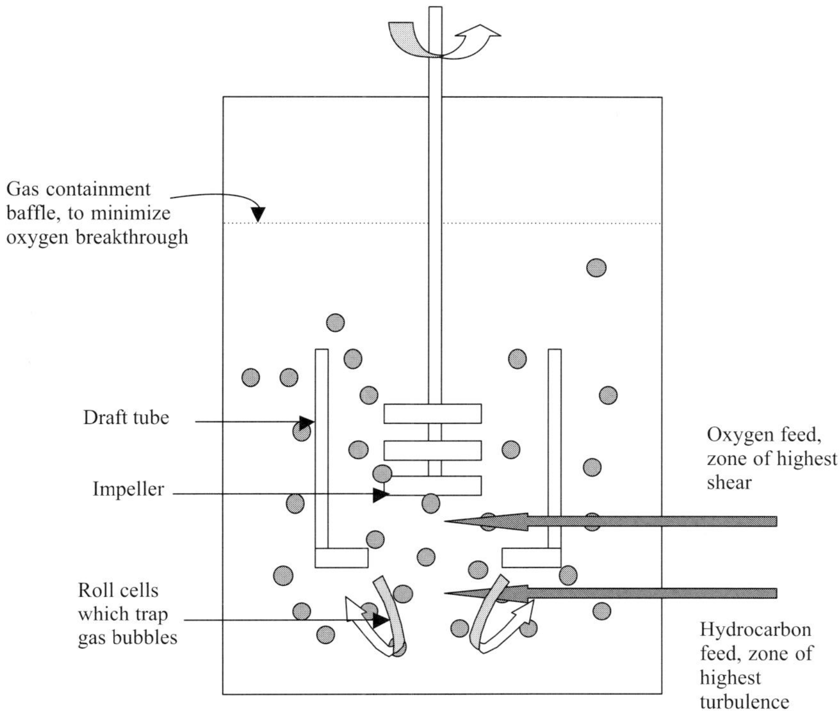

FIGURE 10.2 Schematic of liquid phase oxidation reactor patented by Roby (1997).

improved reactor for the oxidation of p-xylene to manufacture terephthalic acid. The schematic diagram of the proposed reactor hardware is shown in Fig. 10.2. A brief analysis of the methods claimed to achieve better performance in stirred oxidation reactors, may help one to understand the role and demands on CFD-based flow modeling for engineering stirred reactors. The major contribution of the claimed invention is very high efficiency of oxygen utilization in a single pass. Oxygen is introduced in a draft tube. Gas–liquid mixture is pumped downward at high velocities inside the draft tube. Pumping leads to formation of a jet below the draft tube, which entrains fluid outside the draft tube and impacts the bottom of the reactor vessel, setting up roll cells in the process. These roll cells trap gas bubbles resulting in very high efficiency of oxygen use. The formation of these roll cells is intimately related to details of hardware configuration (design of downward pumping impeller, draft tube construction, jet velocity, clearance between draft tube and reactor bottom, shape of reactor bottom and so on) and operating conditions (impeller speed, gas flow rate and so on). A computational flow model can play a very useful role here in understanding the formation of roll cells and establishing a relationship between the roll cells and reactor hardware. Apart from the formation of roll cells, the inventor emphasized the relationship between reactor performance and fluid dynamics by insisting on the following:

- oxygen should be fed into the reactor at the point of highest shear;
- reactant hydrocarbon should be fed into the reactor at the point of highest turbulence.

Identifying the locations of zones of highest shear and turbulence and how these locations change with scale and configuration of the reactor can best be carried out with the help of a computational flow model. Such a computational model can also be used to evaluate the patented concept of gas containment baffles. The purpose of such a gas containment baffle is again to increase oxygen utilization efficiency and to minimize the oxygen break-through in the vapor space in the reactor. In fact, the computational flow model can be used to evolve new hardware configurations to achieve the desired process objectives provided it can *a priori* simulate the flow in stirred reactors. Thus, a computational flow model can be used as a powerful reactor-engineering tool, provided it meets the following requirements:

- it can be applied to impellers of any shape;
- it can account for interactions between multiple impellers/reactor internals;
- it can be extended to multiphase systems.

In the following sub-section, state of the art CFD modeling of stirred reactors is reviewed with reference to these requirements.

10.2. CFD-BASED MODELING OF STIRRED REACTORS

Flow in baffled stirred reactors has been modeled by employing several different approaches which can be classified into four types, and are shown schematically in Fig. 10.3. Most flow simulations of stirred vessels published before 1995 were based on steady-state analyses (reviewed by Ranade, 1995) using the black box approach. This approach requires boundary conditions (mean velocity and turbulence characteristics) on the impeller swept surface, which need to be determined experimentally. Although this approach is reasonably successful in predicting the flow characteristics in the bulk of the vessel, its usefulness is inherently limited by the availability of data. Extension of such an approach to multiphase flows and to industrial-scale reactors is not feasible because it is virtually impossible to obtain (from experiments) accurate

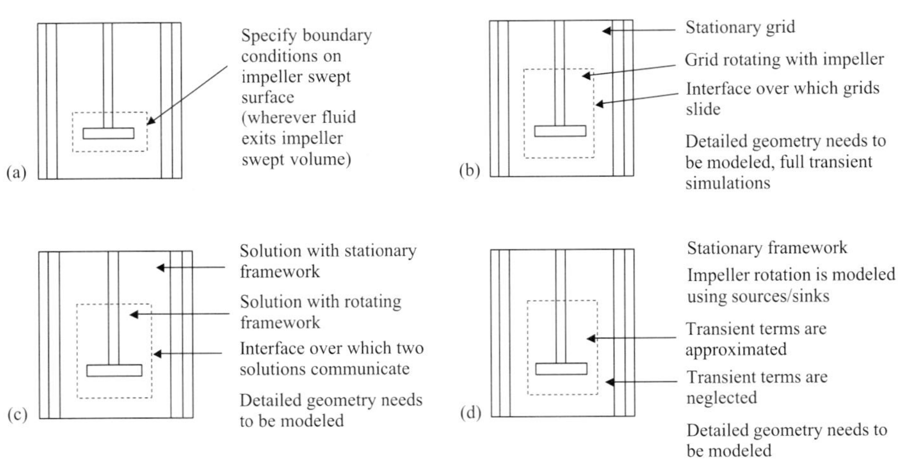

FIGURE 10.3 Approaches to modeling flow in stirred reactors. (a) Black box approach, (b) sliding mesh approach, (c) multiple reference frame or inner-outer approach, (d) snapshot approach.

boundary conditions for such systems. More importantly, this approach cannot be used to make *a priori* simulations. It cannot, therefore, be used as a design tool; hence, studies based on this approach are not discussed in this chapter.

To eliminate some of the limitations described above, recently attempts have been made to simulate flow within and outside the impeller region either with a combination of moving and deforming or with a sliding mesh (Harris *et al.*, 1996; Ranade *et al.*, 1997). In the sliding mesh approach, full transient simulations are carried out using the two grid zones (Fig. 10.3b). One grid zone is attached to the stationary baffles and reactor wall while the other is attached to the rotating impeller. Obviously, the boundary between these two zones should have a radius more than that of the impeller blade tips and less than that of the inner edges of the baffles. The detailed geometry of the impeller needs to be modeled: impeller blades are modeled as solid rotating walls. Flow within the impeller blades is solved using the usual transport equations unlike the black box approach described earlier. The sliding mesh approach has the potential to generate *a priori* predictions without requiring any experimental input. It can therefore be used as a design tool to screen different configurations, however, the following considerations make the sliding mesh approach less attractive as a reactor-engineering tool:

- As it relies on the solution of full time varying flow in a stirred vessel, its computational requirements are greater by an order of magnitude than those required by steady state simulations.
- Because of the excessive computational requirements, there are restrictions on the number of computational cells that can be used for the simulations. Such a limitation may make *a priori* predictions of the desired flow characteristics such as energy dissipation rates, shear rates near impeller blades etc. less accurate.
- The results obtained using this approach are not yet sufficiently validated for turbulent regime.

For most engineering applications, knowledge of the full time varying flow field (which becomes cyclically repeating after a number of impeller rotations) may not be necessary. It may, therefore, be desirable to develop an approach which allows *a priori* simulations of the flow generated by an impeller of any shape with the same computational requirements as required for steady state simulations. Such an approach can be used as a design tool for screening different alternative mixer configurations. There are two main approaches for approximating unsteady flow in stirred vessels. In both approaches, a fictitious cylindrical zone with a radius more than that of the impeller blade tips and less than that of the inner edges of the baffles and height sufficient to include an entire impeller is defined (Fig. 10.3c and 10.3d). The full geometry needs to be modeled and in these approaches also, impeller blades are modeled as walls.

- The first approach is called the 'multiple reference frame' (MRF) or 'inner-outer' approach (inner-outer approach in fact defines inner and outer zones with a finite overlap whereas in the MRF approach there is no overlap between inner and outer regions). In this approach, flow characteristics of the inner region are solved using a rotating framework. These results are used to provide boundary conditions for the outer region (after azimuthal averaging), flow in which is solved using a stationary framework. Solution of the outer region is used to provide boundary conditions for the inner region. A few iterations over inner and outer regions may lead to a converged solution. Brucato *et al.* (1994) and Harris *et al.* (1996) applied the inner-outer method to simulate flow in stirred vessels whereas Marshall *et al.* (1996) used a 'multiple reference frame' approach. The multiple reference frame approach (MRF) is computationally less intensive than the inner-outer method. This approach is available with several commercially available CFD codes.

- The second approach is based on taking a snapshot of flow in stirred vessels with a fixed relative position of blades and baffles. Ranade and Dommeti (1996a) proposed such a computational snapshot approach, in which impeller blades are modeled as solid walls and flow is simulated using a stationary framework for a specific blade position. Appropriate sources are specified to simulate impeller rotation. If necessary, simulations are carried out at different blade positions to obtain ensemble-averaged results over different blade positions. In this approach also, the whole solution domain is divided into two regions, similar to the MRF approach. In the inner region surrounding the impeller, time derivative terms are approximated in terms of spatial derivatives. In the outer region, time derivative terms are usually quite small in magnitude in comparison with the other terms in the governing equations and are neglected.

Recently, attempts have also been made to employ large eddy simulation (LES) models (Derksen and van den Akker, 1999) to simulate flow in stirred vessels. However, computational requirements of these models are much higher than even the sliding mesh approach, and therefore, application of this approach will be restricted to relatively simple impeller shapes. The results obtained by this approach are not yet sufficiently validated. Although sliding mesh and LES approaches look unattractive as design tools, these approaches are important as learning tools to help understand details of fluid dynamics near the impeller blades. MRF or the computational snapshot approach look promising as design tools since these can be extended to impellers of any shape, to any number of impellers and to multiphase flows, without excessive demands on computational resources. Approximations employed with both MRF and computational snapshot methods are of the same level and therefore lead to almost the same results. The computational snapshot approach can be implemented in any stationary frame CFD program without requiring any substantial modifications. Since information about MRF can be found in the manuals of most commercial CFD programs, we restrict our discussion here to the computational snapshot approach.

10.3. COMPUTATIONAL SNAPSHOT APPROACH

The flow generated by an impeller of any shape is governed mainly by pressure and centrifugal forces generated by impeller rotation and the corresponding rotating flows. The shape of the impeller blade controls the direction and characteristics of the impeller discharge stream via the generated pressure and centrifugal forces. Blade rotation causes suction of fluid at the rear side of the blades and equivalent ejection of fluid from the front side of the blades. This phenomenon of ejection and suction needs to be modeled correctly to simulate impeller rotation in the steady framework proposed in the computational snapshot approach. In the sliding mesh approach, the suction and ejection of fluid from the back and front sides of impeller blades is represented naturally, since movement of the blade is accounted for in full time varying simulations. In the computational snapshot approach, impeller blades are considered to be fixed at one particular position (similar to taking a snapshot of the rotating impeller). It is then necessary to model the suction and ejection phenomenon mentioned here using suitable means. The development of an appropriate representation of a rotating impeller in a steady framework is discussed below. It is assumed that the flow is fully developed. This means that in a frame rotating with the blades, profiles within impeller blades do not change with time.

Consider a finite volume representation of a basic conservation equation for a general variable ϕ:

$$\frac{\partial}{\partial t}(V_{\text{cell}}\rho\phi)+(\text{area}\ \rho U\phi)_{\text{e}}-(\text{area}\ \rho U\phi)_{\text{w}}+\cdots=(\text{area}\ \Gamma_{\phi}\frac{\partial\phi}{\partial x})_{\text{e}}-\cdots+S_{\phi} \qquad (10.1)$$

All the terms appearing in Eq. (10.1) are formulated following the usual finite volume method discussed in Chapter 6, except the first term containing the time derivative. Usually, the computational cell volume, V_{cell}, is considered constant and is written outside the time derivative. For the computational snapshot approach, it is useful to consider the above form. In the sliding mesh approach, the above equation needs to be modified to account for grid movement. In the snapshot approach, instead of considering a moving grid, the time derivative term in the above equation is approximated and a steady framework is used to solve Eq. (10.1).

Consider evaluation of Eq. (10.1) in a steady framework by assuming the cyclically repetitive flow between the impeller blades. As mentioned earlier, in a snapshot approach, blades are considered stationary at one position. For an instant, when the blades of the rotating impeller coincide with the position of the blades considered in the snapshot simulation, the following equation is solved in a steady framework:

$$(\text{area}\ \rho U\phi)_{\text{e}}-(\text{area}\ \rho U\phi)_{\text{w}}+\cdots=\left(\text{area}\ \Gamma_{\phi}\frac{\partial\phi}{\partial x}\right)_{\text{e}}-\cdots+S_{\phi}-\frac{\partial}{\partial t}(V_{\text{cell}}\rho\phi) \qquad (10.2)$$

It is necessary to approximate the time derivative terms appearing in this equation. By separating the variables, one can write the time derivative term as (for constant density fluid)

$$\frac{\partial}{\partial t}(V_{\text{cell}}\rho\phi)=V_{\text{cell}}\rho\frac{\partial}{\partial t}(\phi)+\rho\phi\frac{\partial}{\partial t}(V_{\text{cell}}) \qquad (10.3)$$

Generally in a fixed grid simulation, the volume of any computational cell remains constant. This can be applied to all computational cells used in the snapshot approach except those directly attached to the front and rear sides of blades. As the impeller rotates, the volume of cells attached to the front side of the blade decreases. Correspondingly, the volume of computational cells attached to the rear side of the impeller blade increases (Fig. 10.4). The rate of increase or decrease can be calculated directly from the area of the interface between computational cells and impeller blade and the velocity with which the impeller is rotating. Thus, for the computational cells attached to the front and rear sides of impeller blades, the second term of the right-hand side

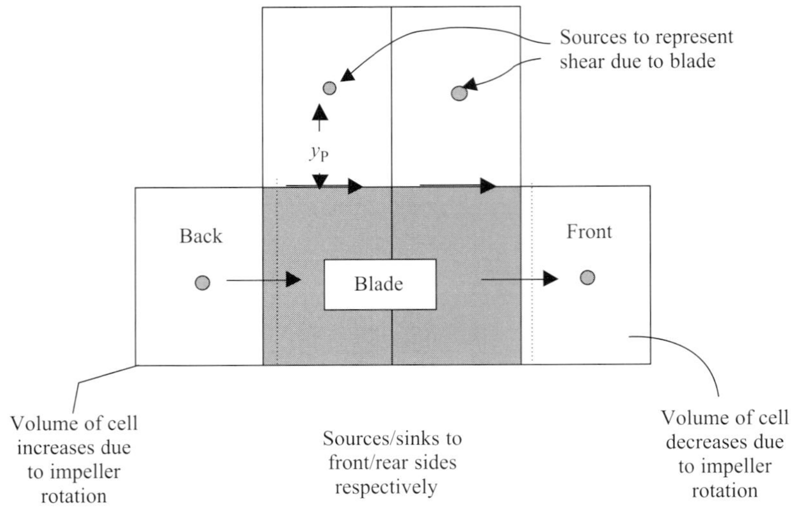

FIGURE 10.4 Computational snapshot approach.

of Eq. (10.3) can be written:

$$\rho\phi\frac{\partial}{\partial t}(V_{\text{cell}}) = \rho\phi(2\pi Nr)A_{\text{bc}} \tag{10.4}$$

where N is impeller rotational speed in revolutions per unit time. The bracketed quantity on the right-hand side is the tangential velocity of the impeller blades at radial location, r, and A_{bc}, is the projection of the area of the interface between computational cell and impeller blade on a plane normal to the tangential velocity. Please note that for the computational cells attached to the front side, volume decreases with time and therefore, there will be a negative sign on the right-hand side of Eq. (10.4). For the mass continuity equation, that is, when ϕ is unity, Eq. (10.4) represents the mass source and sink at the front and rear sides respectively.

Using the assumption of cyclically repetitive flow within the impeller region, the first term on the right-hand side of Eq. (10.3) can be approximated as

$$V_{\text{cell}}\rho\frac{\partial}{\partial t}(\phi) = -V_{\text{cell}}\rho(2\pi N)\frac{\partial}{\partial\theta}(\phi) \tag{10.5}$$

This cyclically repetitive flow will occur only in certain region around the rotating impeller; baffles at the walls destroy such cyclically repetitive flow. Fortunately, for the region where cyclically repetitive flow does not exist, the magnitude of time derivative terms is quite small compared to other terms in Eq. (10.1) and therefore, the time derivative terms may be neglected. As there is no way to find in which region flow will be cyclically repetitive without solving the full time varying equations, this region has to be specified based on available empirical information. Simulations carried out with this approach, however, indicate that the predicted results are not very sensitive to choice of the assumed region of cyclically repetitive flow. Eqs (10.4) and (10.5) can be used to simulate the flow generated by a rotating impeller in a steady state framework.

In addition, since the impeller blades are modeled as stationary walls, it is also necessary to include additional source terms to computational cells attached to the edges of impeller blades, representing the shear caused by the rotating impeller blades (Fig. 10.4). For all the computational cells attached to the four thin edges of the impeller blade, a momentum source needs to be added when solving for the tangential velocity. Though the standard wall function formulation is not strictly applicable to very thin walls, it may be used in the absence of better information to define the momentum source:

$$S_{\mathrm{W}} = \left[\frac{\kappa y^+}{\ln(Ey^+)}\right] \mu \frac{W_{\mathrm{BLD}}}{y_{\mathrm{P}}} (A_{\mathrm{B}}) \tag{10.6}$$

where W_{BLD} is the tangential velocity of the blade averaged over A_{B}, which is the contact area between the computational cell and impeller blade. y^+ is the dimensionless distance from the wall, defined by:

$$y^+ = \frac{C_{\mathrm{D}}^{1/4} \rho k^{1/2} y_{\mathrm{P}}}{\mu} \tag{10.7}$$

If the calculated value of y^+ is less than 11.225, the near wall cell center lies in the viscous sub-layer and therefore the factor in the square bracket of Eq. (10.6) is set to unity.

Ranade and Tayalia (2000) validated the snapshot approach by considering a two-dimensional case of rotating flows. Application of this approach to simulating complex, three-dimensional flows in stirred tank reactors is discussed below. The next section will discuss application of this approach to cases relevant to reactor engineering.

10.3.1. Simulation of Flow Generated by a Disc (Rushton) Turbine

Recently Ranade *et al.* (2001a, 2001b) used a computational snapshot approach to simulate the flow generated by a disc (Rushton) turbine in a fully baffled vessel. The predictions were compared with the comprehensive data available in the open literature. Computations were carried out for the stirred vessel configuration used in the experimental studies by Schafer *et al.* (1997) and Perrard *et al.* (2000). Standard wall functions were used to specify boundary conditions at all the stationary walls (Launder and Spalding, 1974). The top surface of the liquid was also modeled as a wall, since Schafer *et al.* (1997) used a closed vessel in their experiments. For the impeller shaft, disc and hub, an angular velocity corresponding to the impeller rotational speed was specified as boundary condition. Half of the vessel was considered as the solution domain. Cyclic boundary conditions were imposed at the open surfaces of the solution domain. Based on available experimental information, a region surrounding impeller blades was selected in which time derivative terms were included in the governing equations (using the approximation given by Eq. 10.5). Beyond this region, surrounding the impeller blades, time derivative terms were assumed to be negligible. The solution domains and boundary conditions used in their work are shown in Fig. 10.5.

Turbulence was modeled using the standard k–ε model. All the governing equations were discretized using a QUICK discretization scheme with SUPERBEE limiter function (Fluent User Guide, 1997). The SIMPLE algorithm (Patankar, 1980) was

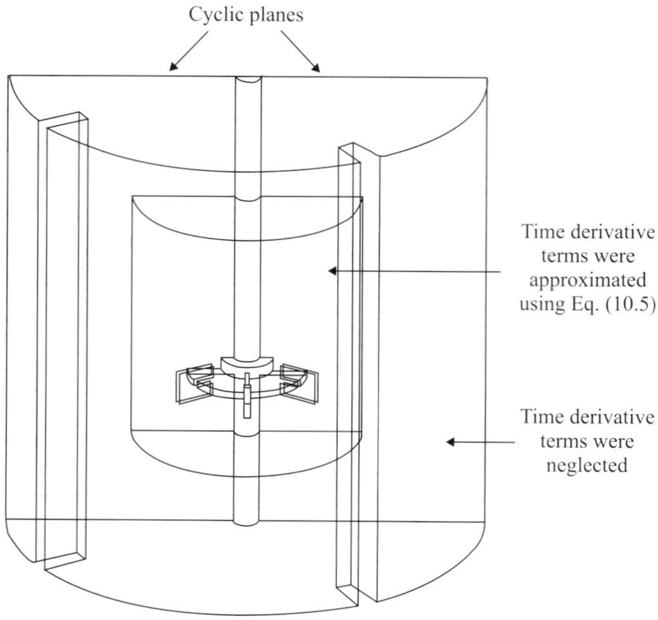

FIGURE 10.5 Solution domain and boundary conditions for simulations of a disc turbine.

used to iteratively solve discretized equations. Preliminary numerical experiments were carried out to examine the influence of grid size on predicted results. The findings of these preliminary simulations were in line with those reported by Ng *et al.* (1998). These studies indicated that in order to capture trailing vortices, it is necessary to use more than 100 cells to cover the impeller blades. Results of Ranade *et al.* (2001a) obtained with the 630 800 grids ($80 \times 83 \times 95 : : r \times \theta \times z$) are discussed below. A blade of a Rushton turbine was discretized with $29 \times 3 \times 25$ cells ($r \times \theta \times z$). Typical grids used are shown in Fig. 10.6. Iterations were continued until the sum of normalized residues fall below 1×10^{-3} and none of the local as well as volume integrated variables of interest showed any appreciable change with further iterations.

Numerical simulations carried out with the computational snapshot approach show the well-known flow patterns generated by the Rushton turbine. Predicted flow fields for typical r–z planes are shown in Fig. 10.7 (vector plot and contours of turbulent kinetic energy). Simulations indicate the upward inclination of the radial jet issuing from the impeller, which is in agreement with published experimental evidence (for example, Ranade and Joshi, 1990). The predicted turbulent kinetic energy contours show the high turbulence region in the impeller stream. Apart from the qualitative agreement, the predicted results in the bulk region also show satisfactory agreement with the experimental data of Ranade and Joshi (1990). The predicted pumping number for the Rushton turbine (calculated at $r/T = 0.18$) is 0.6, which is lower than the generally accepted value. It is, however, within the range reported in the published literature (0.75 ± 0.15). Recent angle-resolved velocity measurements also indicate a pumping number value of about 0.61 (Perrard *et al.*, 2000). The snapshot approach may underpredict the radial velocities in the immediate vicinity of the blades, since the blades are modeled as stationary walls. This leads to lower

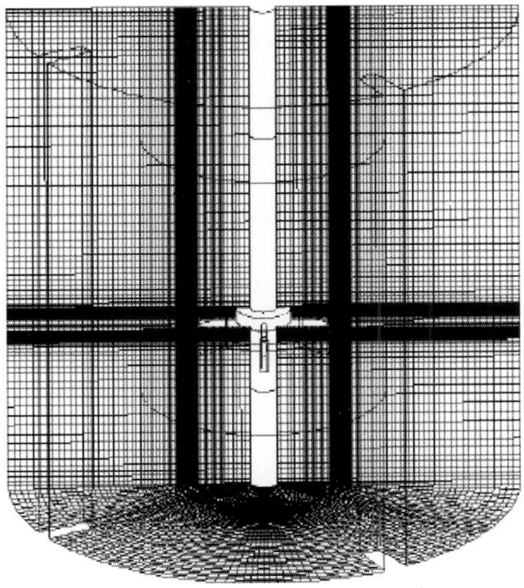

Rushton Turbine		
$r \times \theta \times z$	:	$80 \times 83 \times 95$
Blade	:	$29 \times 3 \times 25$
Region d/dt	:	$14 < K < 77$
		$J < 55$

FIGURE 10.6 Computational grid for simulations of a disc turbine.

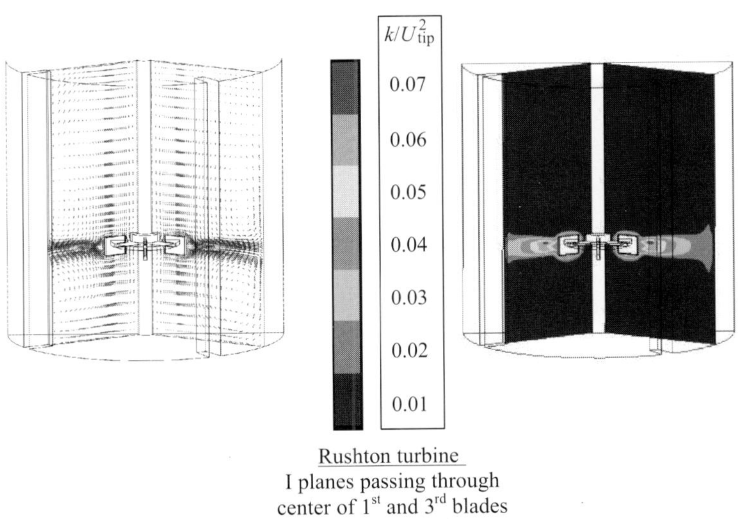

FIGURE 10.7 Predicted flow field at typical r–z planes (from Ranade *et al.*, 2001a).

tangential velocities in the immediate vicinity and therefore lower radial velocities. In general, the overall predicted results showed satisfactory agreement with experimental data. Black box approaches used in the previous decade (Ranade and Joshi, 1990; Ranade *et al.*, 1991) have shown that if the flow characteristics near the impeller swept surfaces are known, flow characteristics in the bulk region of the tank can be predicted with an accuracy adequate for most engineering applications. The crucial test of any *a priori* predictive model is therefore, whether it can predict flow near impeller blades accurately. The predicted (using a computational snapshot approach) results in the near impeller region were, therefore, examined in detail.

The predicted profiles of mean radial and tangential velocities at the impeller center plane are compared with the experimental data measured by PIV and LDA in Fig. 10.8. A similar comparison for turbulent kinetic energy is shown in Fig. 10.9.

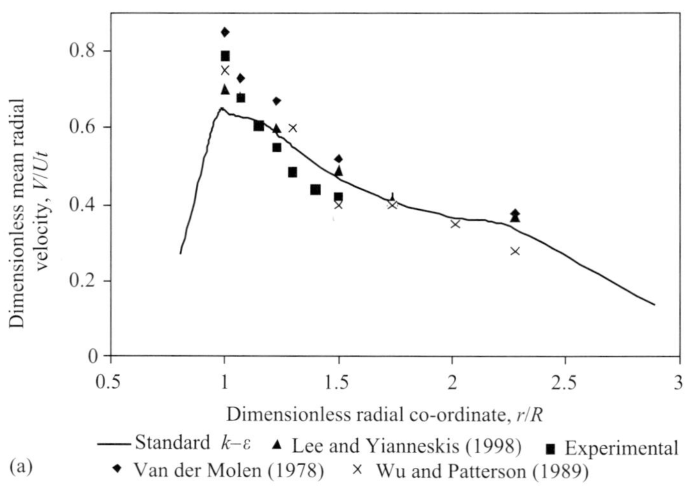

(a)

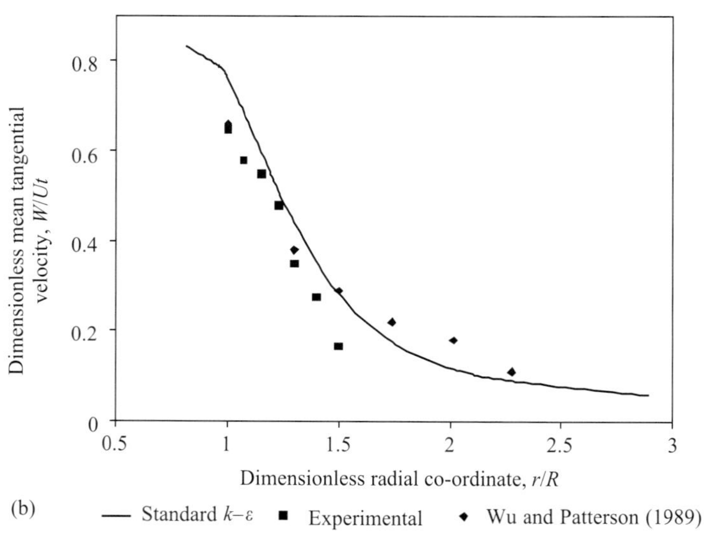

(b)

FIGURE 10.8 Comparison of predicted mean velocity field with angle-averaged PIV data (impeller center plane) (from Ranade *et al.*, 2001b). (a) Radial mean velocity (b) Tangential mean velocity.

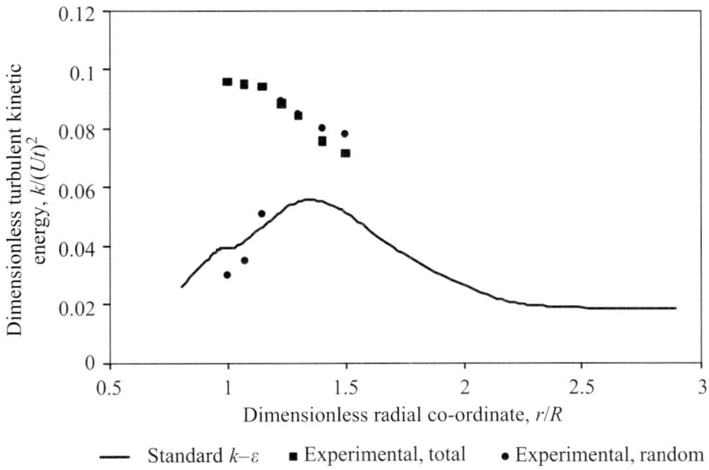

FIGURE 10.9 Comparison of predicted turbulent kinetic energy with angle-averaged PIV data (impeller center plane) (from Ranade *et al.*, 2001b).

It can be seen that agreement between predicted and experimental profiles of mean velocity is satisfactory. It must be noted that when the experimental data contain contributions due to the periodic motion of the impeller blades, the highest values of turbulent kinetic energy are obtained at the vicinity of the impeller tip, due to the apparent turbulence generated by the periodic motion. When the random turbulent kinetic energy is calculated by considering the mean value of five sets of angle-resolved data, the agreement between experiments and CFD results is improved in the vicinity of the impeller. The difference between the predicted turbulent kinetic energy and experimentally measured turbulent kinetic energy after removing the periodic component is reasonable for the standard k–ε model. The contours of predicted turbulent kinetic energy at the impeller center plane of the Rushton turbine are shown in Fig. 10.10a (impeller rotation direction is counter clockwise). It can be seen that snapshot simulations clearly show the presence of higher turbulent kinetic energy at the locations of trailing vortices behind the impeller blades. Z-vorticity contours at the z–θ plane ($r/T = 0.165$) are shown in Fig. 10.10b. This figure also clearly shows the presence of a pair of trailing vortices behind the rotating impeller blades. The trailing vortices move radially outwards and axially towards the impeller center plane, which is in agreement with experimental observations. To examine the flow structure around impeller blades, the predicted mean velocity field behind the impeller blades of the Rushton turbine at three different angles from the blade (8°, 15°, 30°) are shown in Fig. 10.11. The presence of trailing vortices and their movement within the impeller stream are clearly evident from this figure. Comparison of these predicted results with the experimental data of Schafer *et al.* (1997) shows good qualitative agreement. The predicted strengths of the trailing vortices are found to be somewhat lower than the experimental values, which leads to relatively early dissipation of trailing vortices in the simulations.

In order to assess the computational snapshot approach in more detail, predicted normalized mean velocity components and normalized turbulent kinetic energy were directly compared with the available data of Schafer *et al.* (1997). In the case of

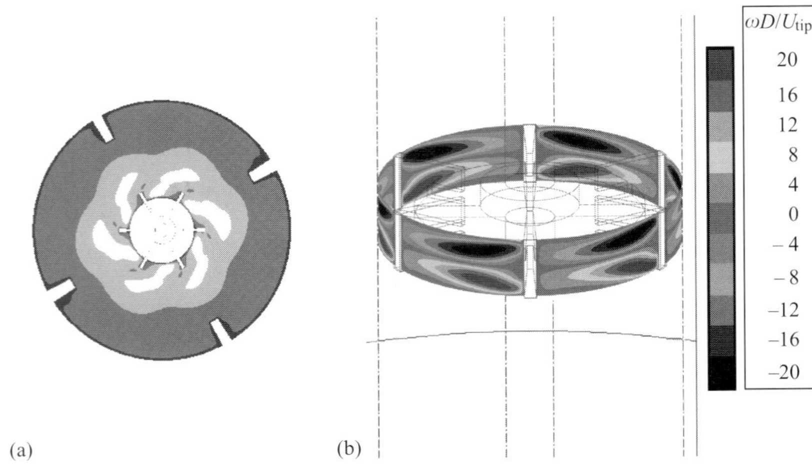

FIGURE 10.10 Presence of trailing vortices (Rushton turbine). (a) Turbulent kinetic energy (impeller center plane; impeller rotation: counter-clockwise), white: highest level, black: lowest level, (b) Z-vorticity ($r/T = 0.165$; impeller rotation: from left to right) (from Ranade *et al.*, 2001a). Reproduced in colour plate section between pages 210 and 211.

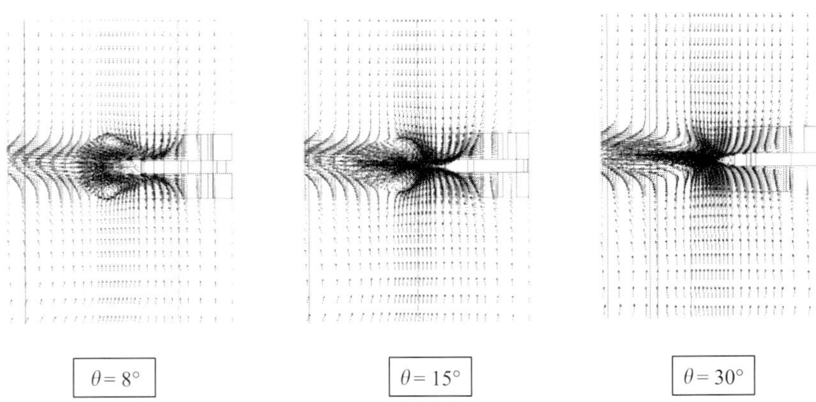

FIGURE 10.11 Flow field behind impeller blades (Rushton turbine) (from Ranade *et al.*, 2001a).

the Rushton turbine, predicted circumferential profiles at $r/T = 0.171$ and $z/T = 0.329$ were compared with the experimental data in Fig. 10.12. Fig. 10.12a shows good agreement between the predicted radial mean velocities and the experimental data. The three curves show the predicted results between the three blades of the Rushton turbine considered in the simulations. It can be seen that these three predicted profiles between the blades are quite similar. Comparison of the predicted tangential mean velocity with the experimental data is shown in Fig. 10.12b. Although overall agreement is reasonable, significant discrepancies were observed in certain areas. For the axial component (Fig. 10.12c), the predicted profiles show significantly less variation than the experimental data. It must, however, be noted that predicted profiles of axial mean velocity in the impeller stream are very sensitive to location. At a slightly different axial location at the same radial location, predicted profiles show similar behavior to that observed in the experimental data. In the case of turbulent kinetic energy (Fig. 10.12d), the agreement between predicted and experimental data is good

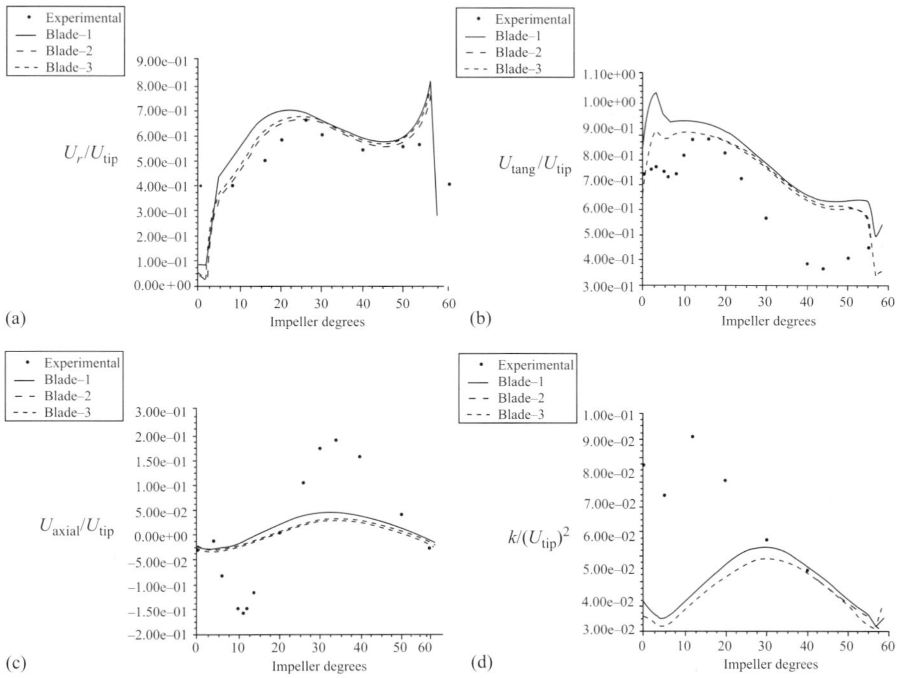

FIGURE 10.12 Comparison of simulated and experimental results for Rushton turbine ($r/T = 0.171$; $z/T = 0.329$). Traces; simulation results; • Schafer *et al.* (1997) data (from Ranade *et al.*, 2001a).

for the region near the trailing blade. In the immediate vicinity of the leading blade, predicted turbulent kinetic energy values are much lower than the experimental data. Reasons for this disagreement are not immediately obvious. A recent study using a different turbulence model (Jenne and Reuss, 1999) indicates that different time scales or anisotropy considerations (Reynolds stress models) are of minor importance and do not lead to significant improvements in the observed agreement. Further studies which combine experimental and computational investigations are needed to evaluate the influence of turbulence models (and grid refinement near the blades) on the predicted characteristics of trailing vortices and on the flow field within the blades. Despite some of the observed discrepancies, predictions using a computational snapshot are very encouraging. The snapshot approach could become a promising tool to design mixing processes in stirred vessels if it can be extended to impellers of any shape, to multiple impellers and to multiphase flows.

10.3.2. Simulation of Flow Generated by an Impeller of Different Shape

In order to examine application of the snapshot approach to simulating flow generated by an impeller of any shape, the case of a pitched blade turbine was considered. The geometry of the stirred vessel agitated by a 45°, four bladed, pitched blade turbine as used by Schafer *et al.* (1998) was modeled using structured grids. The computational grid was generated using the geometry-modeling tool, GAMBIT (Fluent Inc., USA). In view of the symmetry, only one quarter of the vessel was considered as the solution domain. Solution domains and boundary conditions used in the present work are shown in Fig. 10.13. For these simulations, 269 667 grids were used ($57 \times 57 \times 83 :: r \times \theta \times z$). The blade of the pitched blade turbine was discretized with $22 \times 3 \times 15$ cells ($r \times \theta \times z$). Typical grids used are shown in Fig. 10.14. Other boundary conditions and numerical parameters were kept the same as used for the disc turbine. For this case also, turbulence was modeled using the standard k–ε model. All the governing equations were discretized using a QUICK discretization scheme with SUPERBEE limiter function (Fluent User Guide, 1997).

Numerical simulations carried out with the computational snapshot approach show the well-known flow patterns generated by a pitched blade turbine. Predicted flow fields for typical r–z planes are shown in Fig. 10.15 (vector plot and contours of turbulent kinetic energy). Simulations of the pitched blade turbine clearly show the presence of a reverse loop directly below the impeller. This is also in agreement with experimental observations (Ranade and Joshi, 1989). The predicted pumping number for the pitched blade turbine (calculated at the K plane just below the impeller) is 1.0, which is in good agreement with published data (Ranade and Joshi, 1989). The predicted results also show good overall agreement with experimental data in the bulk region of the tank. As mentioned in the previous section, it is important to examine the quality of simulations in the region near the impeller since this controls the overall quality. Flow near the impeller blades is, therefore, examined in detail. A single trailing vortex is detected behind the blades of the pitched blade turbine. An iso-surface of predicted Z-vorticity (ω) for the pitched blade turbine is shown in Fig. 10.16 (the impeller blade is moving inside the plane of the paper). It can be seen that the trailing vortex is attached to the rear side of the blade and flows

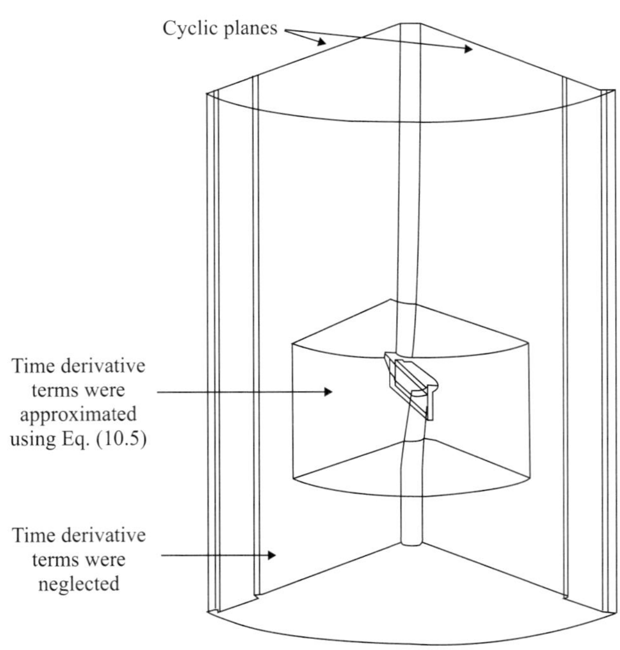

FIGURE 10.13 Solution domain and boundary conditions for pitched blade turbine simulation.

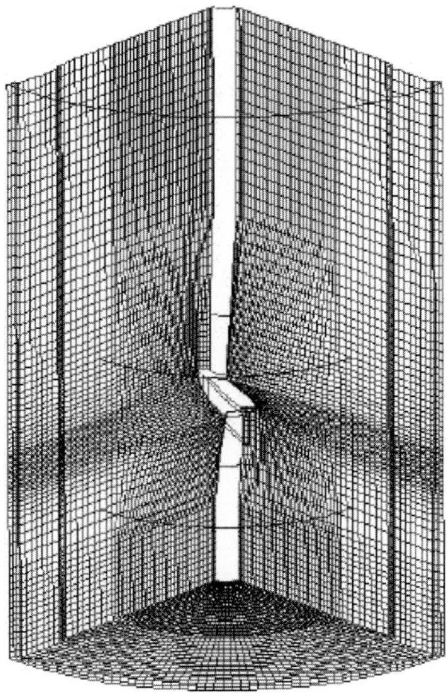

Pitched blade turbine		
$r \times \theta \times z$	:	$57 \times 57 \times 83$
Blade	:	$22 \times 3 \times 15$
Region *d/dt*	:	$17 < K < 54$
		$J < 40$

FIGURE 10.14 Computational grid for pitched blade turbine simulation.

downwards as it moves away from the leading blade. To examine the flow structure around the impeller blades, predicted mean velocity fields behind the impeller blades of the pitched blade turbine at four different angles from the blade (1°, 8°, 15°, 30°) are shown in Fig. 10.17. The presence of the trailing vortex and its movement within the impeller stream is clearly evident from these figures. Comparison of these predicted results with the experimental data of Schafer *et al.* (1997, 1998) shows good qualitative as well as quantitative agreement.

The predicted circumferential profiles at three different radial locations at $z/T = 0.329$ were compared with experimental data. Figs 10.18–10.20 show the results of normalized axial and radial velocity components, and normalized turbulent kinetic energy, respectively for the pitched blade turbine. It can be seen that the predicted results of axial velocity show good agreement with experimental data (Fig. 10.18). In the region near the trailing blade, predicted results show a sharp peak in the downward velocity, which was not observed in the experimental data. It may, however, be noted that experimental data measured using LDA generally has a large scatter in the region near the rotating blades. Outside the impeller swept region, the agreement between predicted and experimental data looks quite satisfactory. Similar

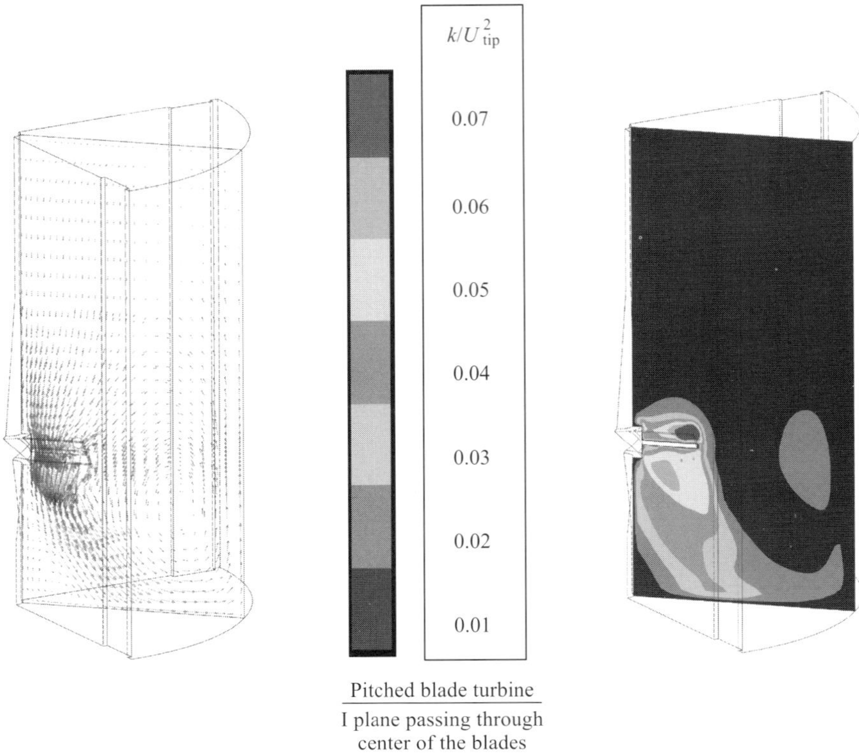

FIGURE 10.15 Simulated results at typical r–z plane for a pitched blade turbine (from Ranade *et al.*, 2001a). Reproduced in colour plate section between pages 210 and 211.

conclusions can be drawn from the comparisons of normalized radial velocity shown in Figs 10.19a–c. For the case of turbulent kinetic energy, Fig. 10.20a indicates that predicted turbulent kinetic energy values are much higher than those observed in experimental data obtained within the impeller swept region. Outside the impeller swept region, however, agreement between predicted and experimental data is much better. The snapshot approach was also shown to be capable of capturing the influence of blade angle and blade width of a pitched blade turbine on generated flow (Ranade and Dommeti, 1996b). Thus, the snapshot approach can be used to simulate flow generated by impellers with complex blade shapes. It can be used to evaluate the influence of impeller blade shape and size on the generated flow field.

10.3.3. Simulation of Flow Generated by Multiple Impellers

Results described so far suggest that the snapshot approach can be used to make *a priori* predictions of the complex flow generated in stirred vessels for impellers of any shape. A number of industrial stirred tank reactors make use of two or more impellers mounted on the same shaft. When more than one impeller is used, the flow complexity is greatly increased, especially when there is interaction between the flow generated by the two impellers. The extent of interaction depends on relative distances between the two impellers (and clearance from the vessel bottom). In order to examine whether the computational snapshot approach can be used to simulate

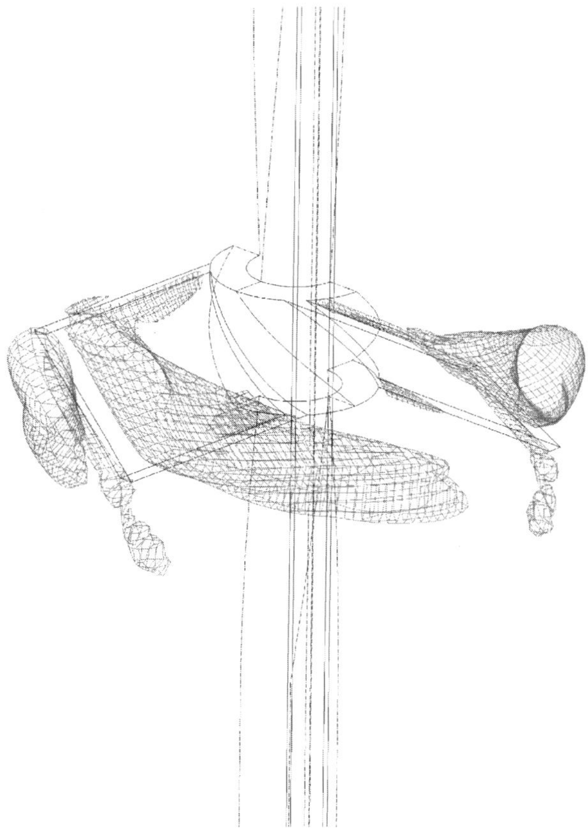

Iso-surface of Z-vorticity ($\omega D/U_{tip}=-7$)
Impeller rotation: from right to left

FIGURE 10.16 Presence of trailing vortices (pitched blade turbine) (from Ranade *et al.*, 2001a).

interaction between multiple impellers, the case of a dual Rushton turbine, studied by Rutherford *et al.* (1996), was considered.

The flow structure in vessels agitated by dual impellers is determined mainly by the flow characteristics of the impellers and interactions between them. When the clearance between the two impellers is sufficiently high, they are likely to act independently of each other. For smaller clearances, the two impeller streams may interact, resulting in complicated and often unstable flow patterns. Rutherford *et al.* (1996) experimentally studied the flow generated by dual Rushton turbines in cylindrical baffled vessels. They report three stable flow patterns observed with different values of lower impeller clearance ($C1$), impeller separation ($C2$) and upper impeller submergence ($C3$). These three patterns are qualitatively shown in Fig. 10.21. The parallel flow pattern shown in Fig. 10.21a was observed when two impellers were well separated ($C1 = C3 = 0.25T$, $C2 = 0.5T$). In this pattern, each impeller generated its own characteristic upper and lower ring vortex leading to formation of four stable ring vortices. When impeller separation was decreased ($C1 = C2 = C3 = T/3$), the flow pattern shown in Fig. 10.21b was observed. It was termed 'merging flow'

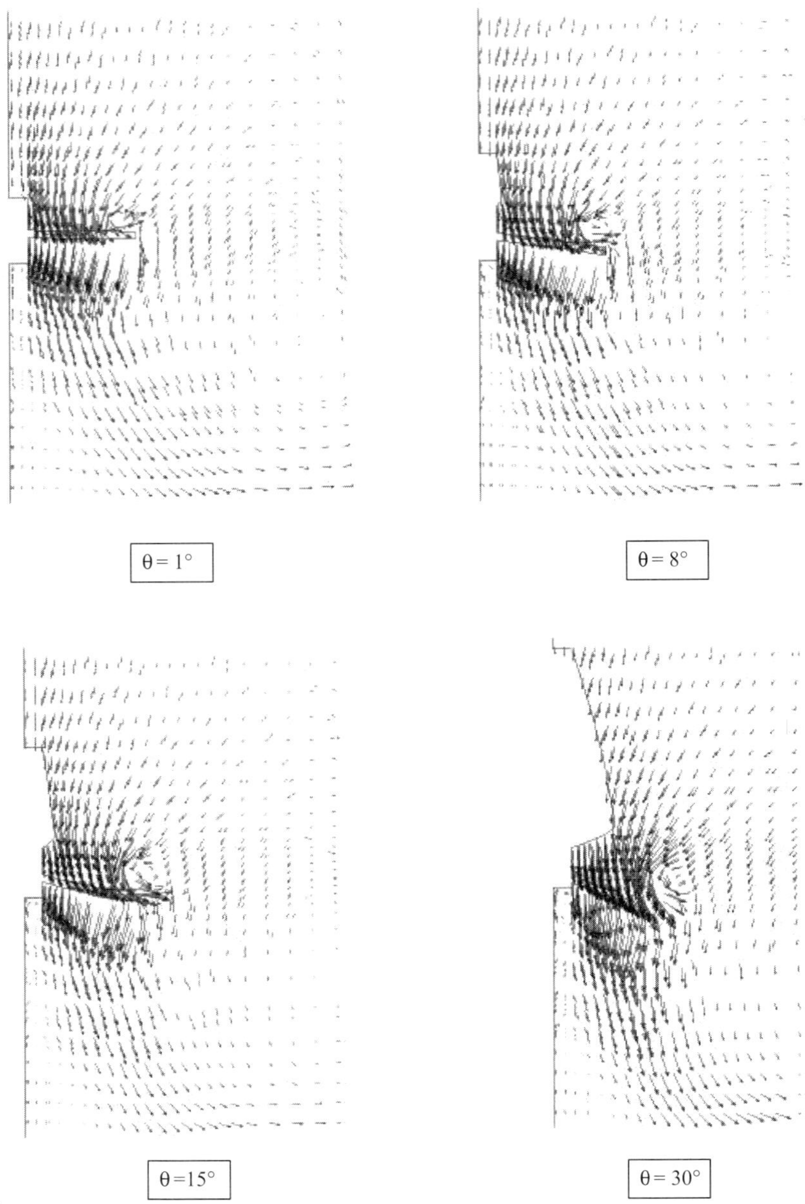

FIGURE 10.17 Flow field behind impeller blades (pitched blade turbine) (from Ranade *et al.*, 2001a).

since two impeller streams merge and form two large ring vortices. The third stable flow pattern was named 'diverging flow' (Fig. 10.21c) and was observed for smaller bottom clearance at the lower impeller ($C1 = 0.15T$, $C2 = 0.5T$, $C3 = 0.35T$). In this case, the lower impeller stream is directed towards the vessel bottom. This results in the lower impeller producing one large ring vortex while the upper impeller generates the usual well-defined two ring vortices.

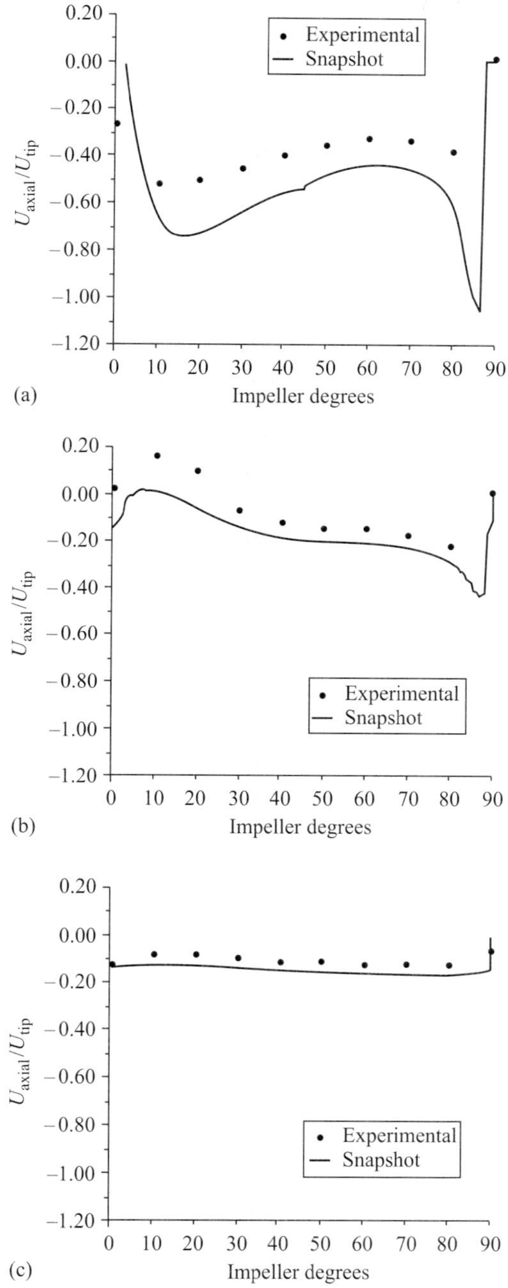

FIGURE 10.18 Comparison of simulated and experimental results for pitched blade turbine (normalized axial velocity, U_{axial}/U_{tip}). $r/T =$ (a) 0.118; (b) 0.171; (c) 0.197. Traces; simulation results; • Schafer *et al.* (1998) data (from Ranade *et al.*, 2001a).

The computational snapshot approach was used to simulate flow generated in these three impeller configurations (for more details, see Deshpande and Ranade, 2001). The predicted velocity vectors in the r–z plane located midway between the two baffles for parallel, merging and diverging flow configurations are shown in

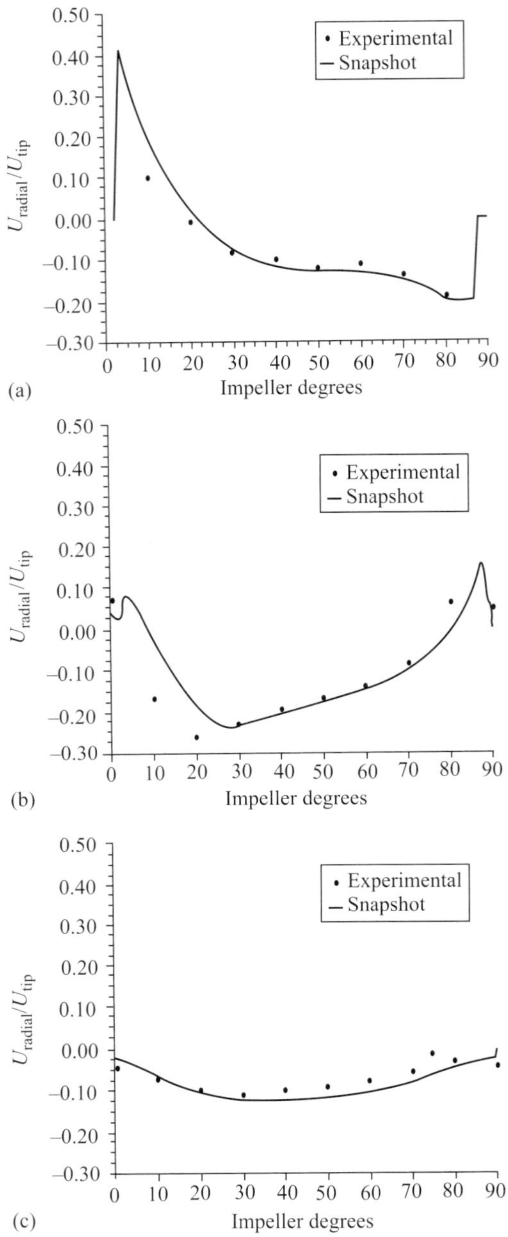

FIGURE 10.19 Comparison of simulated and experimental results for pitched blade turbine (normalized radial velocity, U_{radial}/U_{tip}). $r/T =$ (a) 0.118; (b) 0.171; (c) 0.197. Traces; simulation results; • Schafer *et al.* (1998) data (from Ranade *et al.*, 2001a).

Figs 10.22–10.24 respectively. Experimental results corresponding to these flow patterns are also shown in the respective figures. It can be seen that agreement between predicted and experimental results is satisfactory. Good agreement for the parallel flow, where there is almost no interaction between impeller streams, can be anticipated from the good agreement found in the single impeller case. For small impeller

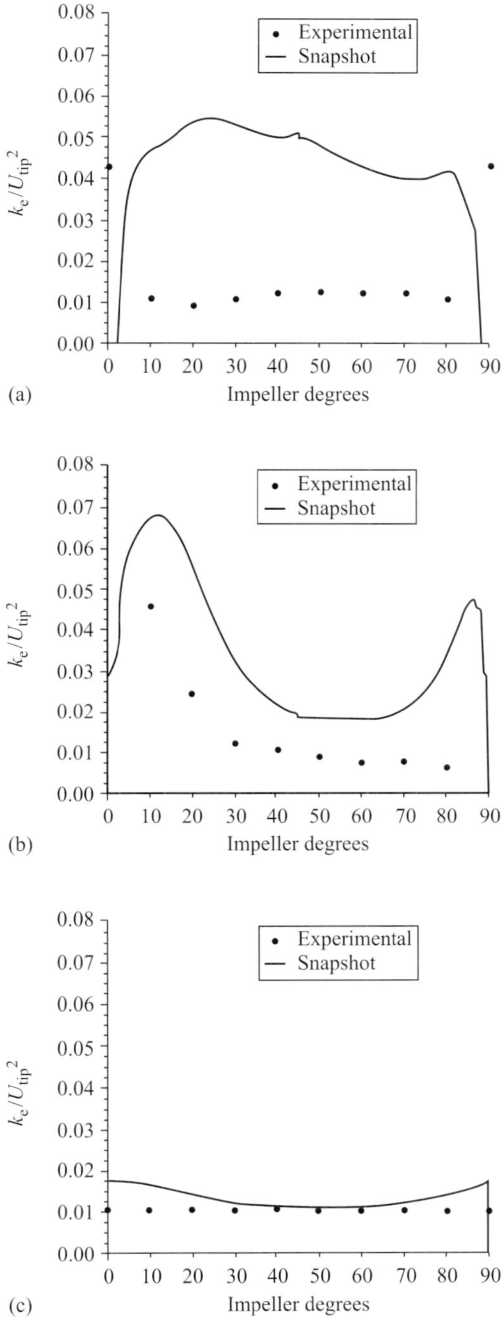

FIGURE 10.20 Comparison of simulated and experimental results for pitched blade turbine (normalized turbulent kinetic energy, k/U_{tip}) $r/T =$ (a) 0.118; (b) 0.171; (c) 0.197. Traces; simulation results; • Schafer *et al.* (1998) data (from Ranade *et al.*, 2001a).

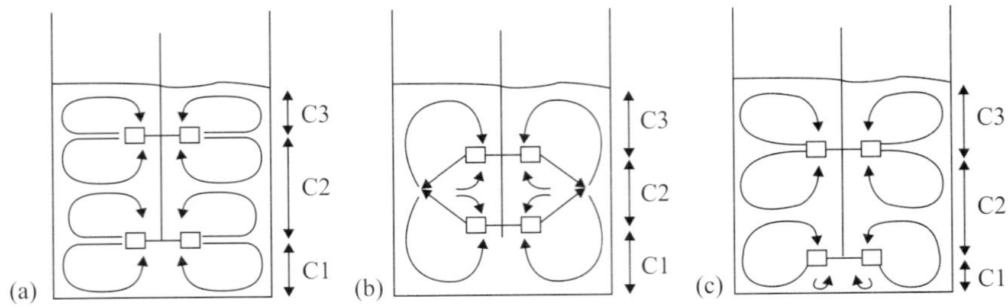

FIGURE 10.21 Schematic of stable flow patterns observed with dual Rushton turbines (from Rutherford *et al.*, 1996). (a) Parallel flow, (b) merging flow, (c) diverging flow.

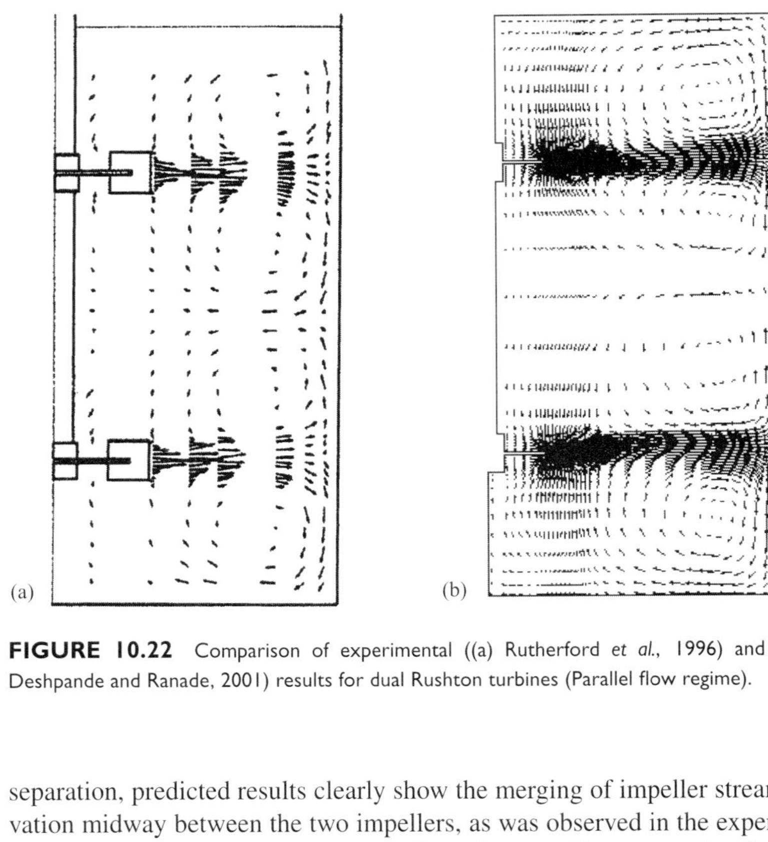

FIGURE 10.22 Comparison of experimental ((a) Rutherford *et al.*, 1996) and predicted ((b) Deshpande and Ranade, 2001) results for dual Rushton turbines (Parallel flow regime).

separation, predicted results clearly show the merging of impeller streams at an elevation midway between the two impellers, as was observed in the experiments. The influence of lower impeller clearance from the vessel bottom on the direction of the impeller stream was also predicted quite well, leading to the diverging flow pattern. Similar interaction between impeller streams was also evident from the contours of the predicted turbulence kinetic energy (not shown here). Qualitatively, these results agree fairly well with the experimental results reported by Rutherford *et al.* (1996). However, the predicted values of turbulent kinetic energy are slightly lower than the experimental data. Quantitative comparison of predicted mean velocity and experimental data is shown in Figs 10.25 and 10.26 for two different values of radial positions. These results indicate that the computational snapshot approach could adequately simulate the three different flow patterns having varying degrees of interaction

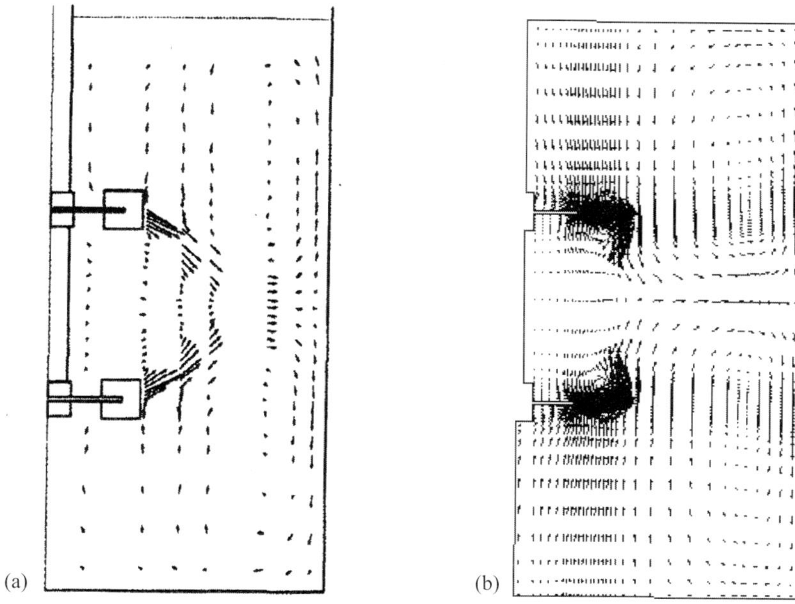

FIGURE 10.23 Comparison of experimental ((a) Rutherford *et al.*, 1996) and predicted ((b) Deshpande and Ranade, 2001) results for dual Rushton turbines (merging flow regime).

between two impellers without requiring any adjustable parameter or any empirical input. Similar predictions can also be obtained from other quasi-steady-state approaches such as MRF and inner-outer, or full transient approaches such as sliding mesh. For example, predicted results reported by Micale *et al.* (1999) for the corresponding dual impeller cases are also shown in Figs 10.25 and 10.26, which more or less agree with the predictions of the snapshot approach. One reason for the observed differences in predictions of the different approaches is the difference in the number of grids used when carrying out the simulations. In general, it can be said that either snapshot or other state of the art approaches (MRF or sliding mesh) may be used to make *a priori* predictions of the flow field generated by multiple impellers. An absence of rotating framework or moving grids makes the computational snapshot approach easier to implement, especially with higher order discretization schemes and multiphase flows, which are discussed in the following section.

10.3.4. Simulation of Multiphase Flows

Many of the situations encountered by reactor engineers involve (refer to Table 10.1) contact with more than one phase in a stirred tank. It is, therefore, essential to examine whether CFD models can simulate complex multiphase flows in stirred tanks. Here the case of gas–liquid flows in a stirred tank is considered. Similar methodology can be applied to simulate other two-phase or multiphase flows in stirred vessels. The computational snapshot approach discussed previously has been extended to simulate gas–liquid flows (see Ranade *et al.*, 2001c for more details). A two-fluid model was used to simulate gas–liquid flow in a stirred vessel: the model equations and boundary conditions are listed below.

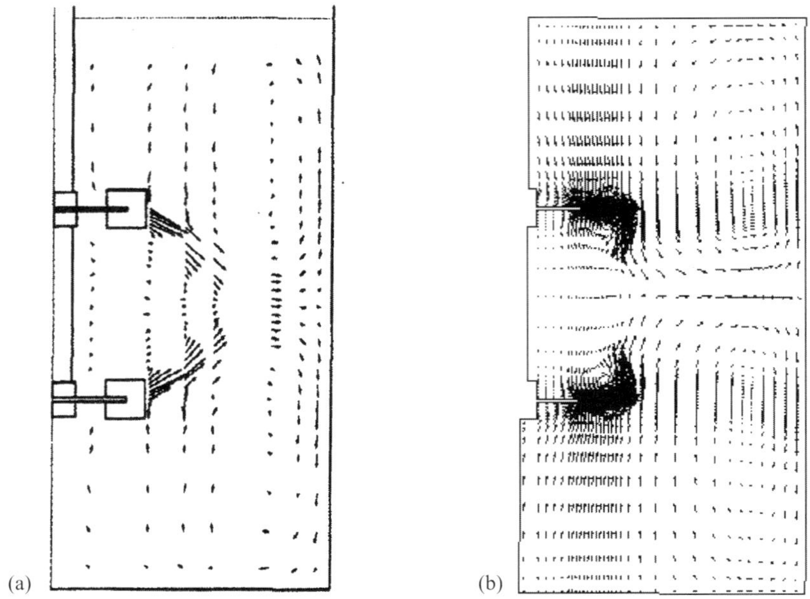

FIGURE 10.24 Comparison of experimental ((a) Rutherford *et al.*, 1996) and predicted ((b) Deshpande and Ranade, 2001) results for dual Rushton turbines (diverging flow regime).

Mass balance equations:

$$\frac{\partial}{\partial t}(\rho_k \alpha_k) + \frac{\partial}{\partial x_j}(\rho_k \alpha_k V_{ki}) = 0 \tag{10.8}$$

Momentum balance equations:

$$\begin{aligned} &\frac{\partial}{\partial t}(\rho_k \alpha_k V_{ki}) + \frac{\partial}{\partial x_j}(\rho_k \alpha_k V_{ki} V_{kj}) \\ &\quad = -\alpha_k \frac{\partial p}{\partial x_i} + \rho_k \alpha_k g_i + F_{ki} + \frac{\partial}{\partial x_j}\left(\alpha_k \mu_k \left(\frac{\partial V_{ki}}{\partial x_j} + \frac{\partial V_{kj}}{\partial x_j}\right)\right) \\ &\quad - \frac{2}{3}\frac{\partial}{\partial x_i}\left(\alpha_k \mu_k \frac{\partial V_{km}}{\partial x_m}\right) \end{aligned} \tag{10.9}$$

where F_{ki} is interphase momentum exchange term:

$$F_{2i} = -\frac{3\alpha_L \alpha_G C_D |V_{2i} - V_{1i}|(V_{2i} - V_{1i})}{4\, d_B} \tag{10.10}$$

Balance equations listed here are before time averaging. For more details of time-averaged two-phase balance equations, the reader is referred to Ranade and van den Akker (1994) and the FLUENT manual. Turbulence was modeled using a standard k–ε turbulence model. Governing equations for turbulent kinetic energy, k and

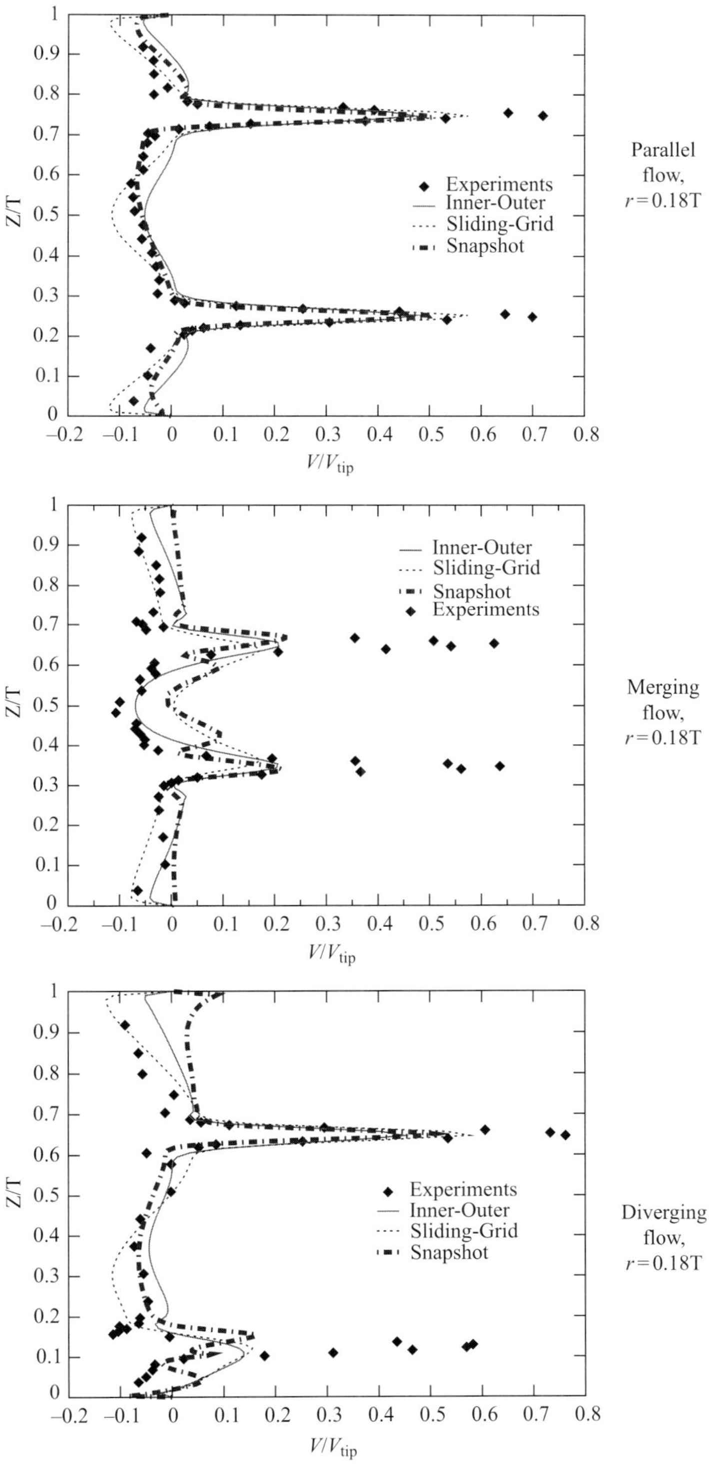

FIGURE 10.25 Comparison of experimental and predicted results for dual Rushton turbines (from Deshpande and Ranade, 2001).

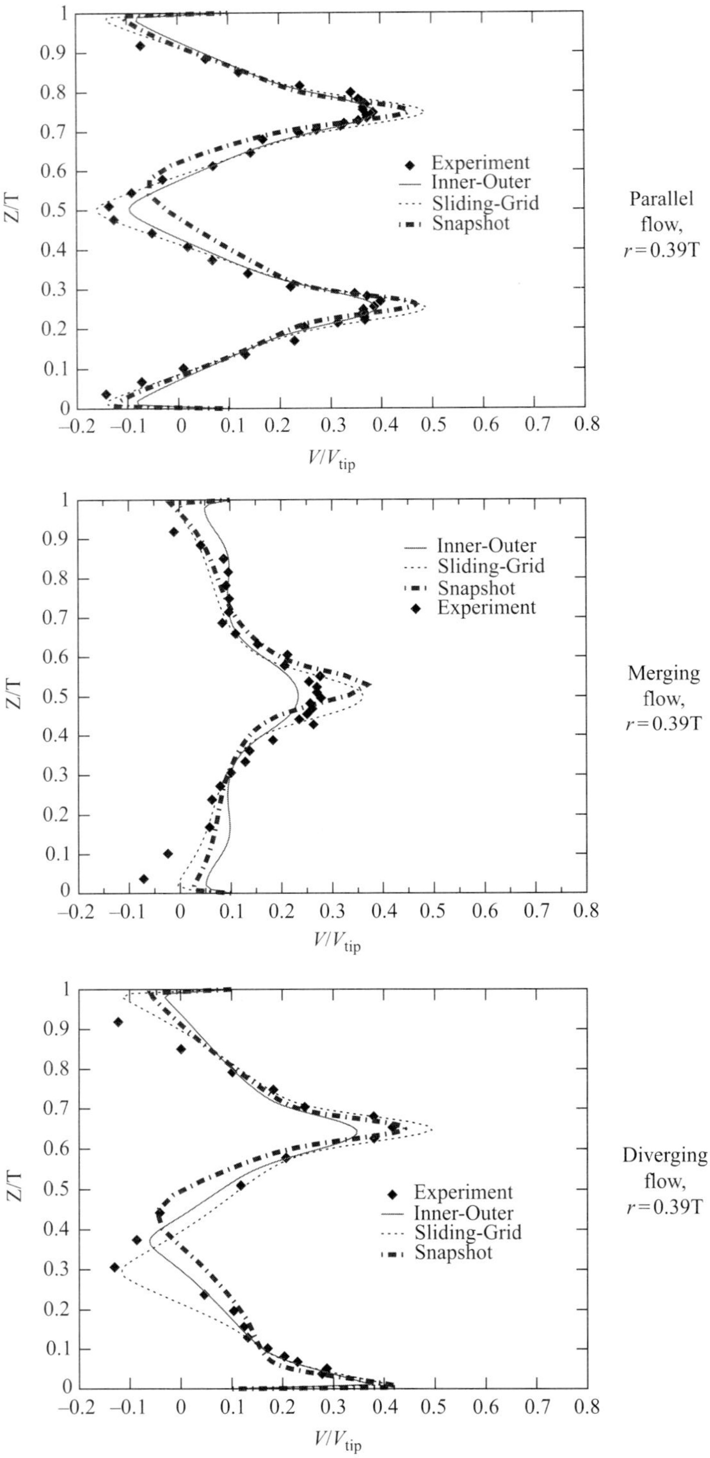

FIGURE 10.26 Comparison of experimental and predicted results for dual Rushton turbines (from Deshpande and Ranade, 2001).

turbulent energy dissipation rates, ε are listed below:

$$\frac{\partial}{\partial t}(\rho_L \alpha_L k) + \frac{\partial}{\partial x_j}(\rho_L \alpha_L V_{Li} k) = \frac{\partial}{\partial x_j}\left(\alpha_L \frac{\mu_t}{\sigma_k}\frac{\partial k}{\partial x_j}\right) + \alpha_L(G - \rho_L \varepsilon) \tag{10.11}$$

$$\frac{\partial}{\partial t}(\rho_L \alpha_L \varepsilon) + \frac{\partial}{\partial x_j}(\rho_L \alpha_L V_{Li} \varepsilon) = \frac{\partial}{\partial x_j}\left(\alpha_L \frac{\mu_t}{\sigma_\varepsilon}\frac{\partial \varepsilon}{\partial x_j}\right) + \alpha_L \frac{\varepsilon}{k}(C_1 G - C_2 \rho_L \varepsilon) \tag{10.12}$$

where G is turbulence generation rate and μ_t is turbulent viscosity, which are given by:

$$G = \mu_t\left(\frac{\partial V_j}{\partial x_i} + \frac{\partial V_i}{\partial x_j}\right)\frac{\partial V_i}{\partial V_i} \qquad \mu_t = \frac{\rho_L C_\mu k^2}{\varepsilon} \tag{10.13}$$

In the absence of better knowledge, standard values of k–ε model parameters are generally used in these multiphase simulations. Wall functions were used to specify wall boundary conditions. Gas was introduced at the sparger by defining an appropriate source of gas at the sparger cells. The top surface of the dispersion was assumed to be flat and was modeled as a free slip wall. Bubbles escaping from the vessel were simulated by specifying an appropriate sink at the top row of computational cells (see Chapter 11 for detailed discussion on boundary conditions used for simulating dispersed gas–liquid flows).

The snapshot approach for gas–liquid flows was implemented using a commercial CFD code, FLUENT (Fluent Inc., USA). User-defined subroutines were used for this purpose. Half of the vessel was considered as a solution domain. The solution domain and details of the finite volume grid used was similar to those used for single-phase flows discussed earlier (however, the number of cells in the θ direction were half of that used in single-phase simulations). A QUICK discretization scheme with SUPERBEE limiter function was used to integrate all the equations (Fluent User Guide, 1997). Simulations were carried out for three values of dimensionless gas flow rates (Q_G/ND^3), 0.01, 0.02 and 0.03.

Predicted gas–liquid flow fields for a dimensionless gas flow number 0.01 at the typical r–z planes are shown in Figs 10.27 and 10.28. The simulations indicate significant upward inclination of the radial jet issuing from the impeller in the presence of gas, which is in agreement with the published experimental evidence. It can be seen that even at such a low gas flow rate, simulations indicate that gas bubbles are not dispersed in the lower circulation loop (left side of Fig. 10.27). Significant upward inclination in the presence of gas is also obvious from the contours of turbulent kinetic energy shown in Fig. 10.28. Contours of gas hold-up confirm that the impeller is unable to re-circulate gas bubbles in the lower loop. Contours of predicted gas hold-up on horizontal plane passing through the impeller are shown in Fig. 10.29 (impeller rotation direction is counterclockwise). It can be seen that snapshot simulations of gas–liquid flows clearly show the presence of gas accumulation at the locations of trailing vortices behind the impeller blades. The gas hold-up just behind the blade is orders of magnitude larger than the average gas hold-up. Such gas accumulation significantly modifies the flow around impeller blades. Predicted contours of gas hold-up at different r–z planes near the impeller region are shown in Fig. 10.30. It can be seen that just behind the leading blade, gas accumulates in the core of two trailing vortices. In the present computational model, coalescence was not modeled

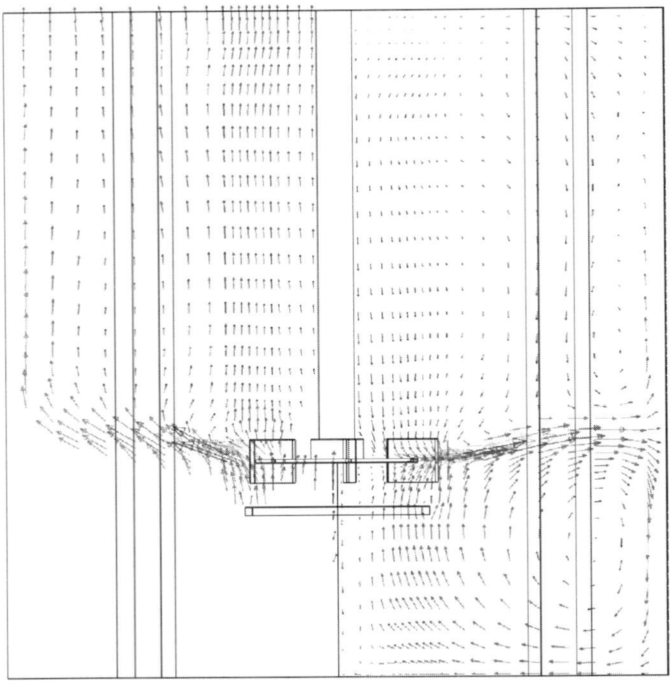

FIGURE 10.27 Typical predicted flow field. Left: vectors of gas phase; Right: vectors of liquid phase (from Ranade *et al.*, 2001c).

and hence the model is not able to simulate the formation of gas cavities behind impeller blades. However, even in the absence of a coalescence model, computations could capture significant gas accumulation in the region of the trailing vortices. As one moves away from the leading blade, the lower region of gas accumulation shifts upwards and eventually merges with the upper region as observed in the experimental data. Thus, it can be said that the computational snapshot approach can capture the essential features of gas accumulation behind the impeller blades. If a suitable coalescence model is combined with the present computational model, formation of gas cavities may be simulated. Coalescence and break-up models, which may be used to simulate the evolution of bubble size distribution in dispersed gas–liquid flows, are discussed in Chapter 11. Similar models can be used to estimate bubble size distributions and interfacial area in gas–liquid stirred reactors. It is, however, necessary to obtain detailed experimental data for gas–liquid flows in stirred vessels to quantitatively validate these computational models. Even in the absence of such quantitative validation, these models may be used to qualitatively evaluate different configurations of gas–liquid stirred reactors. Simulated results may be used to identify regions of high mass transfer coefficient and high interfacial area within the reactor to guide locations of feed pipes etc.

Two-fluid or multifluid models can be extended to simulate not only gas–liquid flows but also any combinations of different phases present in stirred reactors. To simulate gas–liquid–solid, slurry reactors, liquid and solid phases are often lumped together and treated as a slurry phase with effective properties. This approximation is reasonable as long as the solid volume fraction is low ($\sim 1\%$). For higher solid loading,

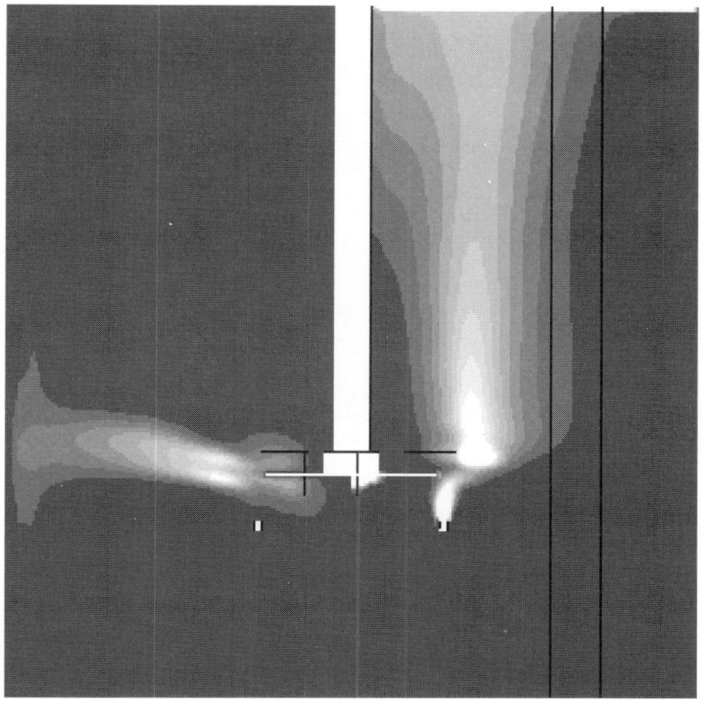

FIGURE 10.28 Typical predicted flow field. (Left: contours of dimensionless turbulent kinetic energy; Right: contours of gas hold-up). Ten uniform contours, maximum value = 0.1 (white); minimum value = 0 (black) (from Ranade *et al.*, 2001c). Reproduced in colour plate section between pages 210 and 211.

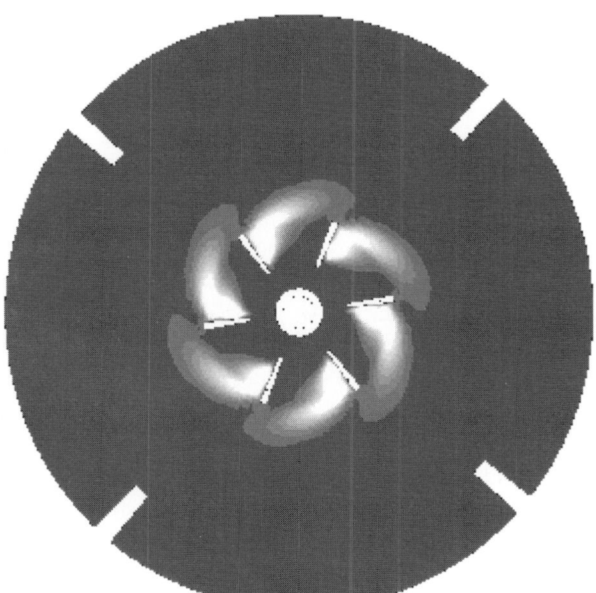

FIGURE 10.29 Contours of gas hold-up on horizontal plane located at a distance of BW/3 from impeller center plane (impeller rotation is counter-clockwise). Ten uniform contours between 0 and 0.1; white: 0.1; black: 0 (from Ranade *et al.*, 2001c). Reproduced in colour plate section between pages 210 and 211.

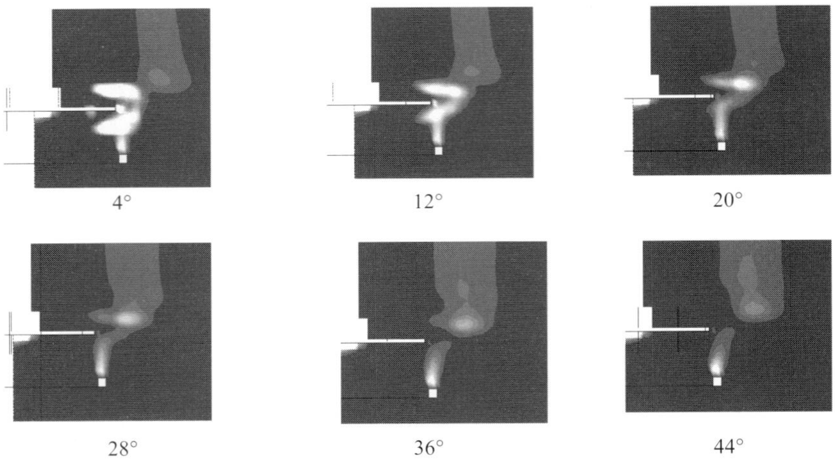

FIGURE 10.30 Computational simulation of accumulation of gas behind impeller blades (black: 0; white: >0.1) (from Ranade *et al.*, 2001c). Reproduced in colour plate section between pages 210 and 211.

it may be necessary to treat the three phases separately. For such systems, it is often necessary to model the motion of solid particles using models based on the kinetic theory of granular flows. Some aspects of this are discussed in Chapter 4. Application of granular flow models to simulate the motion of dispersed solids is discussed in more detail in Chapter 12 for fluidized bed reactors. Dispersion of solid particles in liquid can be simulated using the two-fluid models discussed above (Gosman *et al.*, 1992; Micale *et al.*, 2000). Coalescence break-up models, discussed with reference to gas–liquid flows in Chapter 11, can also be applied to simulate coalescence and break-up processes in gas–liquid and liquid–liquid dispersions (Lane *et al.*, 1999).

In general, it may be concluded that the computational snapshot approach or other equivalent, state of the art CFD models can capture the key features of flow in stirred tank reactors and can be used to make either quantitative (for single-phase or pseudo-homogeneous applications) or semi-quantitative (for complex, multiphase applications) predictions. Possible applications to reactor engineering are discussed below.

10.4. APPLICATION TO REACTOR ENGINEERING

The possibility of using CFD models to screen configurations of industrial reactors will allow reactor engineers to spend more time evolving creative and innovative reactor designs. For example, the configuration proposed for a liquid phase oxidation reactor (LOR) can be studied using a computational flow model to help understand the relation between reactor configuration and claimed performance enhancement. Ranade (1998) discussed the use of CFD models to aid understanding of the formation of roll cells and the region of high turbulence just below the draft tube in the proposed LOR. Detailed analysis (using post-processing and visualization tools) of results predicted by such CFD models will be useful in tailoring LOR configurations to suit different process requirements. At this point, it is essential to re-emphasize the importance of understanding the limitations and assumptions involved in setting up the computational model when interpreting the predicted results. As discussed earlier, predictions of CFD models can go wrong for two main reasons (other than human error and machine malfunction): they may be based upon a physically incorrect mathematical representation or upon numerically deficient representation. Inadequacies of the second kind can be and should be eliminated or minimized by using careful numerical experimentation with grid distributions, discretization schemes etc. (refer to Chapters 6 and 7 for more discussion on these issues). Inadequacies of the first kind will almost always be present for the tractable simulation of complex industrial reactors. Reactor engineers therefore have to identify the most important aspects of the flow which are relevant to reactor performance, and to accurately represent those aspects in the mathematical model. In most cases, one has to break up the problem into several sub-problems and employ a hierarchy of modeling tools with appropriate degrees of sophistication.

Considering again the example of LOR, one of the most important functions of LOR hardware is to set up roll cells below the draft tube, which can capture gas bubbles to enhance the efficiency of oxygen use. As shown by Ranade (1998), it is possible to use CFD models to obtain qualitative as well as quantitative understanding of such roll cells. However, from the reactor engineering point of view, a major objective is to examine whether the roll cells formed provide adequate residence time for gas bubbles to achieve the desired oxygen consumption. It is therefore necessary to understand the phenomenon of bubble capture within these roll cells and its influence on mass transfer (with chemical reaction) from a single gas bubble. Before setting up the computational model to simulate turbulent gas–liquid flow in a complicated geometry, it may be worthwhile to develop a bubble-tracking model employing a Eulerian (for liquid phase)–Lagrangian (for bubbles) framework. Such a model will allow one to undertake a preliminary screening of alternative configurations without developing the complete model. It is possible to represent detailed mass transfer with reaction (based on validated reaction kinetics) by such a computational model. Apart from preliminary screening, results of such a model will also provide the basis for developing a realistic but tractable model in a Eulerian–Eulerian framework.

Development of a detailed model based on a Eulerian–Eulerian framework may be necessary to make realistic estimations of bubble size distribution, bubble flow, its influence on impeller power dissipation and flow field. Ranade and van den Akker (1994) have shown that gas–liquid flow in the bulk region of stirred reactors can be reasonably predicted using the computational snapshot approach. However, unless details of flow near the impeller blades are simulated adequately, it is not possible to determine the desired characteristics of gas–liquid flow (and their variation with configuration, scale and operating parameters). Recent work (Ranade *et al.*, 2001c) shows that it is possible to simulate trailing vortices and gas accumulated in these vortices using a two-fluid model. However, these models are not able to predict the cavity formation behind blades without becoming computationally too demanding. In order to address the reactor engineering issues of interest, it may be necessary to break the overall problem into sub-problems and again use an appropriate modeling approach for each sub-problem. For example, the complex problem of trailing vortices behind impeller blades and their interaction with bubbles may be simplified by studying vortices behind a single blade. Ranade and Deshpande (1999) modeled and simulated gas–liquid flow over a single impeller blade. They were able to predict the details of trailing vortices and the capture of gas bubbles within these vortices.

Rigby *et al.* (1997) also applied a CFD-based model to understand bubble break-up from ventilated cavities in gas–liquid reactors. Ranade *et al.* (2001d) used a volume of fluid (VOF) approach to understand cavity formation behind blades. Observations and insight gained through such studies may be used to develop appropriate sub-models, which can then be incorporated in a detailed reactor-engineering model.

With appropriate validation (direct and indirect), detailed reactor engineering models can be used to screen and optimize reactor hardware. For most practical reactor engineering applications, validation of a computational model can be carried out only via indirect means. For single-phase, homogeneous flow applications it is often possible to use CFD models to optimize reactor hardware. For such applications, it is necessary to include species conservation equations in the mathematical model. The influence of species concentrations on fluid properties can easily be accounted for in such models. When reactions are slow compared to mixing, extension to include species conservation equations is straightforward. In such cases, CFD models can be used directly to simulate reactor performance and to evaluate the influence of design and operating parameters on reactor performance (Middleton *et al.*, 1986; Brucato *et al.*, 2000). When reactions are fast compared to mixing, special models to account for microscale segregation need to be developed (see Chapter 4 for more discussion on the modeling of mixing with fast reactions). Ranade (1993) described an example of the application of a CFD model (with a multi-environment micromixing model) to evaluate the influence of design and operating parameters of a stirred reactor on its performance. Some of his results are discussed here.

Ranade (1993) considered the case of a semi-batch stirred reactor to carry out diazotization reactions. The underlying chemistry can be represented by classical series-parallel reactions:

$$A + B \rightarrow R \qquad B + R \rightarrow S \tag{10.14}$$

The first reaction is extremely fast compared to the second reaction and compared to the expected mixing rate in stirred reactors. Reactions are carried out in a semi-batch mode with reactant B fed over a time t_{feed} to a reactor containing pure component A. Thus, if the added reactant B mixes instantaneously with A, a second reaction cannot take place. All the added B will be consumed in the first reaction (since B is a limiting reactant). If the mixing is not fast enough, all the added B will not be in contact with A and will have the opportunity to undergo a second reaction to produce component S. The yield of component S can therefore be considered as a measure of mixing: the more the yield of S, the poorer will be the mixing. The objectives of Ranade's (1993) study were to establish relationships between reactor configuration (feed pipe location, scale) and operating parameters (impeller speed, feed flow rate) and reactor performance, that is, the yield of desired product, R. Since the physical properties of liquids were not strong functions of species concentrations and operation was practically isothermal, it was possible to decouple the flow and reactive mixing models. In the first phase, a computational model was developed to predict detailed mean and turbulence characteristics of the stirred reactor equipped with a standard Rushton turbine. Since the feed pipes were located in such a way that most of the reaction zone lies outside impeller swept volume, a black box approach was conveniently used to generate the desired results quickly. The predicted results were verified by comparing with the published data on flow generated by Rushton turbines. These results were then used to simulate reactive mixing in stirred reactors. The multi-environment model of Ranade and Bourne (1991), which is discussed in Chapter 4, was used. Comparison of the predicted influence of feed location, impeller speed and reactant concentrations with experimental observations is shown in Fig. 10.31. It can be seen that the computational model correctly captures the influence of all of these parameters. The validated model was then used to select an appropriate feed location and other operating conditions. It was further used to evaluate the possibility of using multiple feed inlets to enhance reactor capacity without reducing the yield of desired product R.

Even if the feed location is near the impeller stream, higher feed flow rate leads to reduction in the yield of the desired product as shown in Fig. 10.31 (feed rate and therefore reactor capacity will be inversely proportional to the feed time, t_{feed} shown in this figure). A possible alternative to increase reactor capacity is to use multiple feed pipes at the same radial and axial locations to ensure the same levels of turbulence at all feed pipes. If multiple feed pipes can be used, reactor capacity can be enhanced without changing the feed rate through each feed pipe. However, it must be noted that feed introduction via multiple inlets may lead to deterioration of selectivity of the desired product if the reaction plumes emanating from different feed inlets interact with each other. The computational model was used to evaluate the idea of introducing feed through multiple inlets. The predicted results are shown in Fig. 10.32. It can be seen that, for feed location A, selectivity remains unaffected by an increase in the number of inlets, up to eight feed inlets. This means it is possible to reduce feed time or increase capacity by a factor of eight without affecting selectivity towards the desired product! Thus, the computational model can be applied to optimize reactor configurations if the necessary cost data is available.

Computational models can be used for reactor engineering applications in a variety of other ways. Even for multiphase reactors, where direct verification of models is difficult, CFD-based models can be used to evaluate alternative reactor configurations and to characterize existing reactor hardware. Such characterizations or fluid dynamic audits of existing reactor hardware will be useful to identify the scope for potential improvement and ways of realizing this potential by evolving retrofit designs. Bakker and coworkers (Bakker *et al.*, 1994a; 1994b; Fasano *et al.*, 1994) cited several examples of using CFD models to enhance the performance of

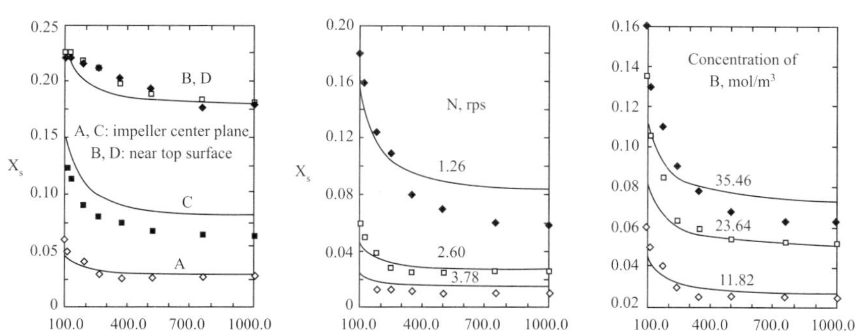

FIGURE 10.31 Comparison of predictions of CFD model with experimental data (from Ranade, 1993). Influence of (a) feed locations (denoted by A, B, C and D), (b) impeller speed, (c) reactant concentration.

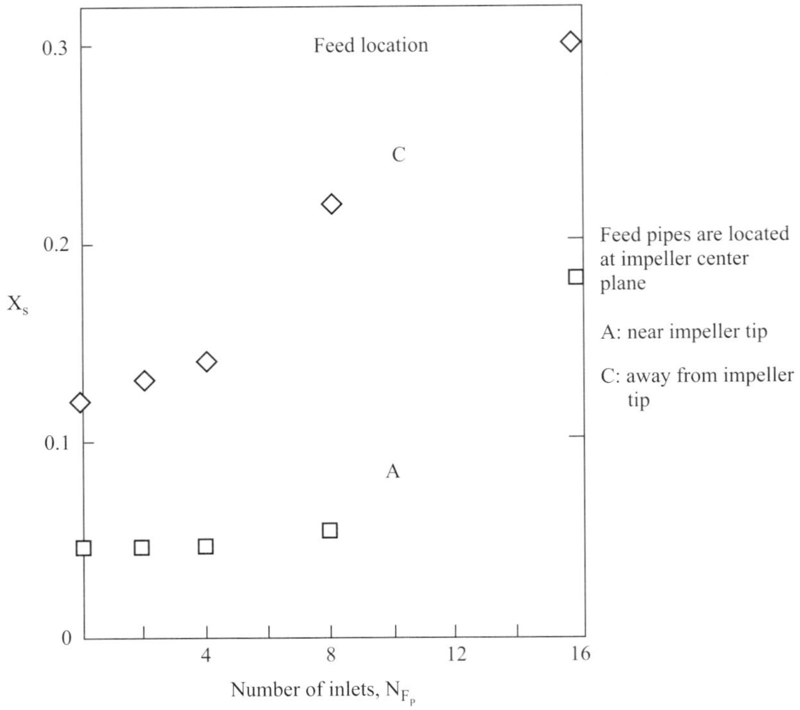

FIGURE 10.32 Influence of the number of feed inlets on selectivity (from Ranade, 1993).

stirred reactors. For example, maps of volumetric mass transfer coefficients ($k_L a$) for gas–liquid stirred reactors can be generated based on information about turbulence characteristics predicted using CFD models and empirical relationships between these characteristics and bubble diameters. Such maps are used to identify regions of high mass transfer rates and regions of high driving (for mass transfer) force (near feed pipe). It makes sense to provide the highest mass transfer rates in the region where concentration-driving force is also highest. Such a provision will be much more productive than the case where high mass transfer rates exist in a region of low concentration-driving force. Such models can therefore be used to select or to devise the best-suited reactor configuration to achieve the best mass transfer performance.

CFD models will also be used to carry out scale-up and scale-down analysis, especially for non-geometric scale-up. In many reactor-engineering applications, it is necessary to carry out laboratory-scale or bench-scale experiments to understand the behavior of large-scale reactors. It is essential to undertake systematic scale-down analysis to ensure that small-scale experiments mimic key features of the large-scale system. More often than not, it is necessary to use a geometrically dissimilar system in order to mimic key features of a large-scale system. Scale-down and scale-up analysis using CFD models may prove to be very valuable in such an endeavor and will help to derive maximum benefit from the small-scale experiments. CFD models also allow extrapolation of cold flow results to actual operating conditions (high temperature and pressure) and provide tools to interpret and extrapolate small-scale experimental data.

Detailed characterization of flow generated by various impellers also leads to extremely useful information about the sensitivity of the impeller fluid dynamics to fabrication details, providing evidence for the well-known saying that 'impellers, which look alike may not perform alike'. The insight gained via computational models will lead to better reactor and process engineering. Creative analysis of CFD simulations may lead to new impeller designs. Ultimately, it may be possible to create 'designer' flow fields to ensure better reactor performance. In many situations, CFD models may be used to generate information which will be used by other sets of models. Compartment models or zones-in-loops models mentioned in Chapter 1 fall into such a category. With a combination of two or more different modeling tools, it is possible to derive useful engineering information. For example, recently Vivaldo-lima *et al.* (1998) developed combined CFD and compartment models to simulate a suspension polymerization reactor. They showed that the combined model could capture the key features of complex interactions of coalescence and break-up processes with polymerization reactions. Thus, judicious combinations of CFD models with other modeling tools may lead to realistic simulations of complex multiphase reactors. Use of computational flow models to understand basic phenomena and to simulate complex industrial reactors (using a hierarchy of modeling tools) establishes a link between reactor hardware (and operating protocols) and reactor performance and eventually leads to better reactor engineering.

10.5. SUMMARY

State of the art CFD models can be used to make *a priori* predictions of flow in stirred reactors, at least for homogeneous systems. Quasi-steady approaches (MRF or computational snapshot approach) look promising, in view of their *a priori* nature and low computational requirements. They can predict the flow generated by impellers of arbitrary shape and can predict interaction between multiple impellers. They can be extended to simulate multiphase flows as well. In general, predicted results show good agreement with experimental data. Important characteristic flow features around impeller blades are captured adequately. Careful numerical experiments using these CFD models can be used to better understand the characteristics of existing reactor hardware and to enhance performance. Even in the case of multiphase flows, where accurate quantitative predictions are difficult, computational models will be for qualitative grading of different configurations, and can greatly assist engineering decision making process.

REFERENCES

Bakker, A., Fasano, J.B. and Leng, D.E. (1994a), Pinpoint mixing problems with lasers and simulation software, *Chem. Eng.*, **101**(1), 94–100.

Bakker, A., Smith, J.M. and Myers, K.J. (1994b), How to disperse gases in liquids, *Chem. Eng.*, **101**(12), 98–104.

Brucato, A., Ciofalo, M., Grisafi, F. and Micale, G. (1994), Complete numerical simulations of flow fields in baffled stirred vessels: the inner-outer approach, *I ChemE Symposium Series no.* **136**, 155.

Brucato, A., Ciofalo, M., Grisafi, F. and Tocco, R. (2000), On the simulation of stirred tank reactors via computational fluid dynamics, *Chem. Eng. Sci.*, **55**, 291–302.

11 BUBBLE COLUMN REACTORS

The processes involving reactions between liquid and gas phases are technologically important in many industries. In a bubble column reactor, reactant gas itself (along with an inert gas, if present) provides the required stirring action. It offers an attractive way to carry out gas–liquid and gas–liquid–solid reactions because of its simple construction and operation. However, because of the simple construction, bubble column reactors also have an inherent limitation of having fewer degrees of freedom available to tailor performance characteristics. In a bubble column reactor, local flow, turbulence and gas hold-up distribution are interrelated in a complex way with the operating and design variables. Fluid dynamics of bubble columns may change considerably with variations in physicochemical properties and scale of operation. This causes problems in efficient design and scale-up of bubble column reactors and often results in oversizing of these reactors. Oversizing does not always reduce unreliability and may often cause additional problems concerning product quality and stable reactor operation at varying loads. Development of a detailed fluid dynamic model is therefore essential to understand of the complex interaction between multiphase fluid dynamics and the design and operating variables. Such a model can be used to reduce the number of experiments and to interpret the experimental results with more confidence. The detailed predicted flow field can give an accurate insight and may sometimes give information that cannot be obtained from experiments. This chapter reviews and discusses the application of computational fluid dynamics based models to bubble column reactors.

11.1. ENGINEERING OF BUBBLE COLUMN REACTORS

Several types of bubble column reactor are used in practice, some of which are shown in Fig. 11.1. As can be seen from this figure, several different modes of

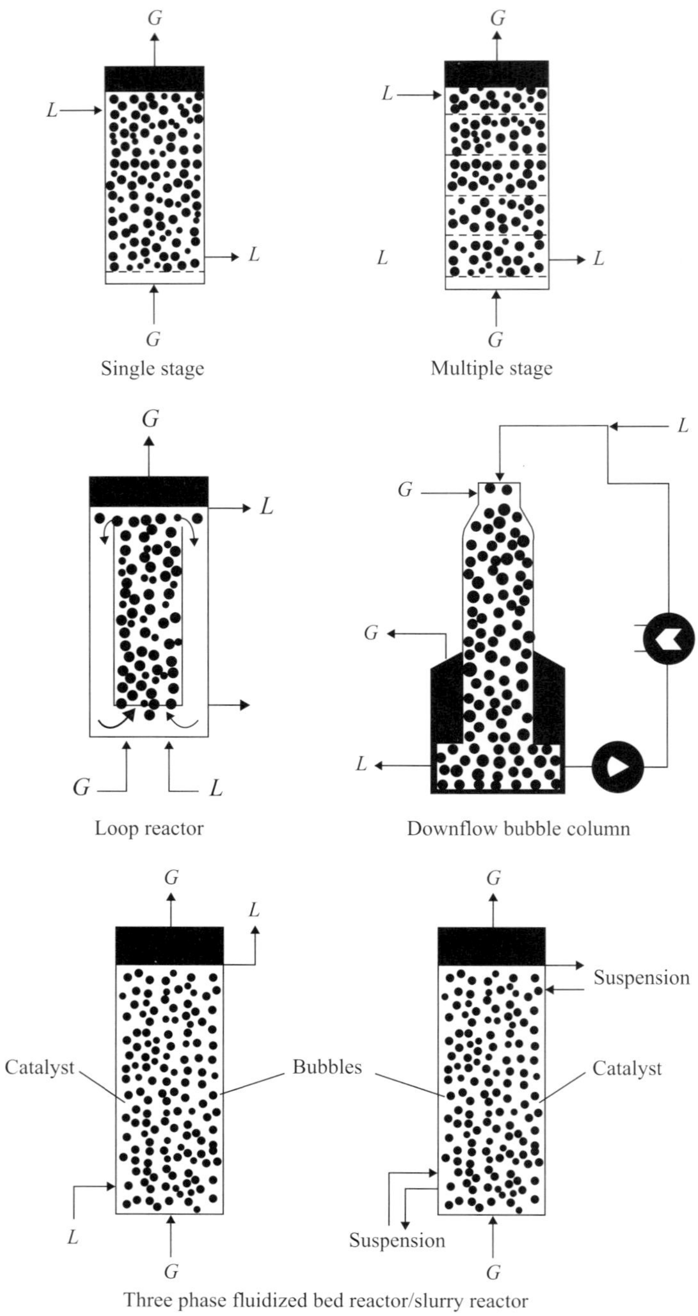

FIGURE 11.1 Types of bubble column reactors (from Lee and Tsui, 1999).

TABLE 11.1 Some Applications of Bubble Column Reactors

Process	Reactants	Main Products
Oxidation	ethylene, cumene, butane, toluene, xylene, ethylbenzene, acetaldehyde, cyclohexane, cyclohexene, n-paraffins, glucose	vinyl acetate, phenol, acetone, methyl ethyl ketone, benzoic acid, phthalic acid, acetophenone, acetic acid, acetic anhydride cyclohexanol and cyclohexanone, adipic acid, sec-alcohols, glutonic acid
Chlorinations	aliphatic hydrocarbons, aromatic hydrocarbons	chloroparaffins, chlorinated aromatics
Alkylation	ethanol, propylene, benzene, tolune	ethyl benzene, cumene, iso-butyl benzene
Hydroformylation	olefins	aldehydes, alcohols
Carbonylations	methanol, ethanol	acetic acid, acetic anhydride, propionic acid
Hydrogenation	benzene, adipic acid dinitrile, nitroaromatics, glucose, ammonium nitrate, unsaturated fatty acids	cyclohexane, hexamethylene diamine, amines, sorbitol, hydroxyl amines
Gas to Liquid Fuels	F-T synthesis, methanol from syngas	liquid fuels
Coal Liquification	coal	liquid fuels
Desulferization	petroleum fractions	desulferized fractions
Aerobic Bio-Chemical Processes	molasses	ethanol

operation are possible for bubble column reactors. These bubble column reactors are also extensively used for gas–liquid–solid processes. Bubble column reactors provide excellent heat and mass transfer characteristics. Some of the important industrial applications are listed in Table 11.1. Similar to any reactor type, the engineering of bubble column reactors begins with the analysis of process requirements and evolving a preliminary configuration for the reactor. Before relating the process requirements and design of bubble column reactors, it will be useful to give a brief overview of the complex fluid dynamics of bubble columns. This will facilitate an appreciation of various design issues and the role of rigorous flow modeling in the design and scale-up of bubble column reactors.

In a bubble column reactor, gas is sparged at the bottom of the liquid pool contained by the column. The net liquid flow may be co-current or counter-current to the gas flow direction or may be zero. Large varieties of spargers or gas distributors are used in industrial practice to introduce gas in bubble columns. Sparger design controls bubble size distribution in the bottom portion of the bubble columns. Spargers, like porous plates, generate uniform size bubbles and distribute the gas uniformly at the bottom of the liquid pool. For such spargers, when gas superficial velocity is small (less than 2 cm s^{-1}), all the bubbles formed at the sparger rise almost vertically. Larger (>0.2 cm diameter) bubbles may rise with inherent oscillations. This flow regime is called homogeneous. In this flow regime, macroscopic internal liquid circulation does not exist. The presence of bubbles may generate turbulence and affect the transport characteristics as described by Ranade and Joshi (1987). However, such an operating regime is unstable and even small perturbations can cause transition to a heterogeneous regime.

In a heterogeneous regime, significant bubble–bubble interactions occur and coalescence sets in to generate a wider bubble size distribution. Long-time averaging indicates that gas bubbles move towards the column center while rising upwards. Experimental data reported by Yao *et al.* (1991), measured using an ultrasonic Doppler technique, clearly show radially inward motion of gas bubbles (in a time-averaged sense). Such an inward motion and strong interphase coupling results in non-uniform gas hold-up profile, with maximum at the column center. This leads to strong macroscopic internal liquid circulation in the column with upflow in the central region and downflow in the near-wall region. Such internal re-circulation results in increased backmixing, which is one of the major drawbacks of bubble column reactors. Several internal designs like draft tubes, radial baffles etc. have been proposed to control the degree of backmixing in bubble column reactors. In recent years, inherently unsteady characteristics of gas-liquid flows in bubble columns have been studied (Chen *et al.*, 1994; Delnoij, 1999). These studies indicate that capturing the unsteady flow structures may be essential for accurate description of mixing in bubble columns. Various factors such as type of sparger, column diameter, height to diameter ratio, physico-chemical properties, solid volume fraction (and other properties such as size and settling velocity) and operating conditions (pressure, temperature, and superficial velocities) affect the unsteady flow and mixing in bubble column reactors (Ranade and Utikar, 1999; Ranade and Tayalia, 2001). The presence of solid particles may further complicate the fluid dynamics of bubble columns. The fluid dynamic influence of solid particles depends on mean particle size, size distribution, particle density and solids volume fraction. The superficial gas velocity, resulting internal circulation, and solid particles interact in a complex way. In most design applications, empirical correlations and pilot-scale experiments on two or more scales are used to establish the relationship between these adjustable design and operating parameters and self-adjusting fluid dynamics and mixing in various phases.

A general procedure for the design and scale-up of reactors is discussed in Chapter 1. As discussed there, preliminary configurations are evolved on the basis of laboratory study and reactor models, which assume idealized fluid dynamics and mixing. Using idealized reactor models, various configurations and modes of operation are evaluated. In most industrial cases, this step itself may involve several iterations. The process of evolving a preliminary configuration helps to firm up performance targets for the reactor. Transformation of such a preliminary reactor configuration to an industrial reactor proceeds through several steps. Some of the relevant reactor engineering issues for bubble column reactors are summarized in Fig. 11.2. Some of these issues are discussed later, in Section 11.3. As discussed in Chapter 1, basic reaction engineering models based on approximations of the underlying fluid mechanics allow estimates of reactor size and reactor performance for different operating modes. Such studies are often used to select the type of reactor configuration and mode of operation (co-current/counter-current, upflow/downflow and so on). The influence of operating conditions on conversion and selectivity of the desired products can be examined using these reaction engineering models. These models are used to select feasible operating windows, and also to understand the sensitivity of reactor performance with a degree of backmixing, mass transfer coefficient, interfacial area, heat

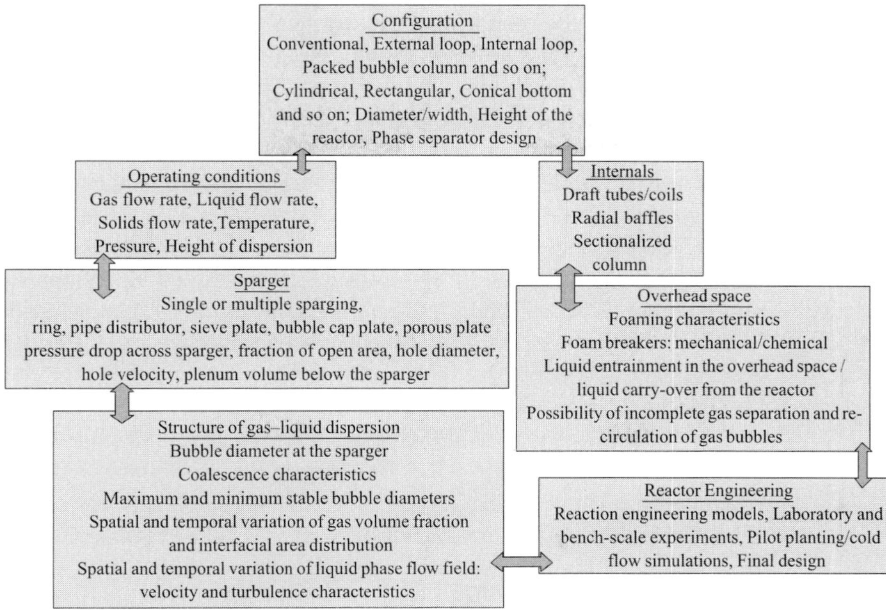

FIGURE 11.2 Reactor engineering of bubble column reactors: relevant issues.

transfer, operating regime and so on. Such studies are useful to quantify key desired fluid dynamic characteristics of the reactor. These models are, however, unable to predict the influence of actual hardware details, as all the fluid dynamic information used in these models is usually based on empirical correlations.

Studies from reaction engineering models and basic process economics set the 'wish list' of the reactor, which may read something like the following: reactor hardware should (1) operate in a churn-turbulent regime over the specific gas flow rate range; (2) provide a certain minimum volumetric mass transfer coefficient and certain minimum heat transfer coefficient; (3) provide a certain minimum heat transfer area; (4) provide radially and axially uniform gas distribution; (5) provide adequate mixing to ensure that mixing time is less than the specified time; (6) entrainment of liquid droplets with the escaping gas phase should be less than the specified mass flow rate; and so on. In order to address these issues, it is necessary to develop comprehensive fluid dynamic models. If it turns out that some of the demands cannot be met with realistic reactor hardware, new iterations of studies with reaction engineering models are carried out, based on the information provided by the detailed fluid dynamics model of realistic reactor hardware. In some cases, it is possible to include detailed reaction engineering models within the CFD framework to develop a combined model. In some cases, for example, those involving very fast reactions, such combined models are mandatory for realistic simulations. However, even in other cases where it is usually more efficient to keep reaction engineering models and detailed fluid dynamic models separate, significant exchange of information takes place between these two types of model (see examples discussed in Chapter 9).

CFD-based models allow identification and quantification of the extent of non-idealities (such as bypass and channeling). These models also allow reliable extrapolation of results obtained on experimental and pilot scales. Apart from providing inputs to reaction engineering models, detailed CFD models establish relationships between hardware configurations such as sparger, internal baffles or draft tubes and resulting fluid dynamics and, therefore, with reactor performance. More often than not, the development of reactor technologies relies on prior experience. New reactor concepts are often sidelined due to lack of resources (experimental facilities, time, funding etc) to test them. Experimental studies have obvious limitations regarding the extent of parameter space that can be studied and regarding extrapolation beyond the studied parameter space. Computational flow models, which allow *a priori* predictions of the flow generated in a bubble column reactor of any configuration (different mode, spargers, internals) with just a knowledge of geometry and operating parameters, can make valuable contributions to developing new reactor technologies.

The fluid dynamics of bubble column reactors is very complex and several different CFD models may have to be used to address critical reactor engineering issues. The application of various approaches to modeling dispersed multiphase flows, namely, Eulerian–Eulerian, Eulerian–Lagrangian and VOF approaches to simulate flow in a loop reactor, is discussed in Chapter 9 (Section 9.4). In this chapter, some examples of the application of these three approaches to simulating gas–liquid flow bubble columns are discussed. Before that, basic equations and boundary conditions used to simulate flow in bubble columns are briefly discussed.

11.2. CFD-BASED MODELING OF BUBBLE COLUMN REACTORS

Most flow models published before 1990 to predict the flow characteristics of the heterogeneous regime in a bubble column reactor were restricted to one-dimensional approximations (reviewed by Ranade, 1992). These models require experimental information about the radial gas hold-up profile and turbulent viscosity and, therefore, lack generality (Kumar *et al.*, 1994). Application of a computational fluid dynamics (CFD) based approach is being increasingly adopted to predict the detailed fluid mechanics of bubble columns. In a bubble column reactor, gas is sparged at the bottom of the liquid pool, through which gas bubbles rise upwards. While rising, these gas bubbles may interact with each other and may generate complex, re-circulating turbulent flow. The resulting flow is characterized by many distinct flow structures of various length scales (from tiny vortices shed by the bubble to macroscopic circulation covering the whole reactor).

Depending on the required resolution, various approaches to modeling dispersed multiphase flows have been developed. For example, when it is essential to resolve small-scale fluid dynamics around individual bubbles, it is necessary to use a volume of fluid (VOF) approach. With VOF, it is possible to resolve small-scale vortices behind bubbles, bubble–bubble interactions (coalescence/breakup) and mass and heat transfer between bubbles and surrounding liquid. These simulations can, therefore, be used to predict mass transfer coefficients and other interphase exchange terms. However, application of VOF is usually restricted to simulations of a few bubbles due to the huge computational requirements. If it is reasonable to model the small-scale flow around individual bubbles using lumped parameters such as drag coefficient or mass transfer coefficient, but it is necessary to simulate trajectories of individual bubbles, a Eulerian–Lagrangian approach needs to be used. This approach allows one to simulate bubble-scale phenomena accurately. However, it becomes computationally too demanding if millions of bubbles (which may exist in any typical industrial bubble column reactor) need to be simulated over a long period of time. For such cases, it is necessary to use a Eulerian–Eulerian approach, which invokes extensive modeling to simulate the behavior of gas–liquid dispersions with high gas volume fractions. As in most industrial applications of bubble column reactors, dispersed phase hold-up is not small (and often the dispersed phase is introduced through a distributed sparger rather than a single nozzle), a Eulerian–Eulerian approach will be most suitable and, therefore, it is discussed in more detail here.

11.2.1. Eulerian–Eulerian Approach

Most earlier attempts at understanding and modeling the fluid dynamics of bubble columns were aimed at characterizing the flow with the help of one or two characteristic parameters (circulation velocity and/or average turbulent intensity) (see, for example, the widely cited paper of Joshi and Sharma, 1979). Recent advances in computational fluid dynamics encouraged vigorous application of CFD to modeling flow in bubble columns. Professor Svendsen and coworkers (Torvik and Svendsen, 1990; Svendsen *et al.*, 1992) and Professor Hofmann and coworkers (Grienberger and Hofmann, 1992; Hillmer *et al.*, 1994) published initial results of such CFD approaches, apart from Ranade (1992; 1993a). Jakobsen *et al.* (1997) and Delnoij (1999), among others, have reviewed some of the recent modeling attempts. Model equations, their application to the simulation of flow in bubble columns and a brief review of recent simulations of bubble columns using a Eulerian–Eulerian approach are discussed in this section.

Model equations

Generally a two-fluid approach is used to derive governing continuity and momentum transport equations (discussed in Chapter 4) for dispersed multiphase flows. Invariably, some kind of averaging method needs to be employed to derive these governing equations. Several different averaging methods are used (Drew, 1983; Ahmadi, 1987; Besnard and Harlow, 1988; Lahey and Drew, 1989). Because a variety of flow structures co-exist in bubble columns, it will be useful to make some comments on the relationship between the averaging method, governing equations, fluid dynamics of bubble columns and possible simulated results. The starting point for the derivation of governing equations is definition of a control volume. To simulate dispersed multiphase flows, careful definition of the control volume will provide guidance for the interpretation of simulated results.

If the considered control volume size is smaller than the dispersed phase particle, it will be necessary to track the gas–liquid interface as is done in the VOF approach. In the Eulerian–Eulerian approach, control volume is assumed to be large enough to define local phase volume fractions. For a meaningful definition of phase volume fractions in a control volume, control volume should be large enough to contain a sufficiently large number of dispersed phase particles. In bubble columns, when there is a wide bubble size distribution, control volume should be large enough to contain a sufficiently large number of the biggest size bubbles. The mean values of different variables of interest are then defined on the basis of such a control volume.

Obviously, approximations employed for the terms comprising deviations from mean values and the resulting equations will depend on the assumed size of the control volume. When developing model equations by considering such a large (with respect to bubble size) control volume, all the small-scale (of the order of bubble size) flow structures need to be modeled. The small-scale flow around individual bubbles and its effects are generally modeled by introducing interphase coupling terms in the governing equations, defined in terms of flow properties averaged over control volume (and its faces). Small-scale turbulence is also modeled using an appropriate turbulence model. It is important to note here, that there is no relationship between size of control volume assumed when deriving the governing equations and size of computational cells used to solve these governing equations numerically. Size of the assumed control volume affects the terms appearing in the governing equations. Once the governing equations are derived (modeled), their numerical solution can be carried out using a computational grid of any size to ensure grid independence.

In bubble columns, the flow is inherently unsteady. Significant flow structures, which are larger than the typical bubble size but smaller than column diameter, exist in the column. Such structures are clearly evident in visualizations of flow in bubble columns (Chen *et al.*, 1994). If it is intended to resolve these unsteady structures, model equations should be based on a control volume larger than the bubbles but smaller than the characteristic scale of such internal flow structures. If it is sufficient to simulate only the long-time averaged flow, even larger control volumes (larger than the characteristic scales of internal flow structures) may be used. In such a case, additional terms, representing the influence of transient internal structures, will appear in the model equations. Two recent modeling studies based on these two options are discussed briefly below.

Recently, Pfleger *et al.* (1999) simulated gas–liquid flow in an apparent two-dimensional bubble column. The expected bubble size in the system investigated by these authors is 2 to 5 mm. The governing equations were derived by assuming control volumes larger than gas bubbles but smaller than the expected size of the internal circulation cells. The local flow around individual bubbles was modeled using appropriate interphase coupling terms. The resulting model equations were solved using different sizes of computational cells. Small-scale turbulence was modeled using a standard k–ε turbulence model (with and without dispersion). Their results indicate that results obtained with a computational cell volume of about 0.1 cm^3 (which is of the same order as bubble volume) are almost grid independent and agree quite well with experimental data. Samples of their results are shown in Fig. 11.3a (time averaged) and 11.3b (transients). Long-term averaging of these simulated results shows the well-known flow pattern with upward motion at the column center. In addition to correct prediction of time-averaged results, their model was also able to adequately capture inherently transient oscillations of the bubble plume. The standard k–ε turbulence model was found to capture the inherent dynamics of gas–liquid flows in bubble columns.

While deriving the time-averaged governing equations, if the characteristic time scale is defined to be larger than the characteristic time scales of local circulation cells, additional terms representing the influence of inherently unsteady circulation cells on the long-time averaged flow pattern will appear in the governing equations. For example, Ranade (1997) introduced two additional terms in the momentum transport equations to simulate long-time-averaged effects: one to account for the effect of

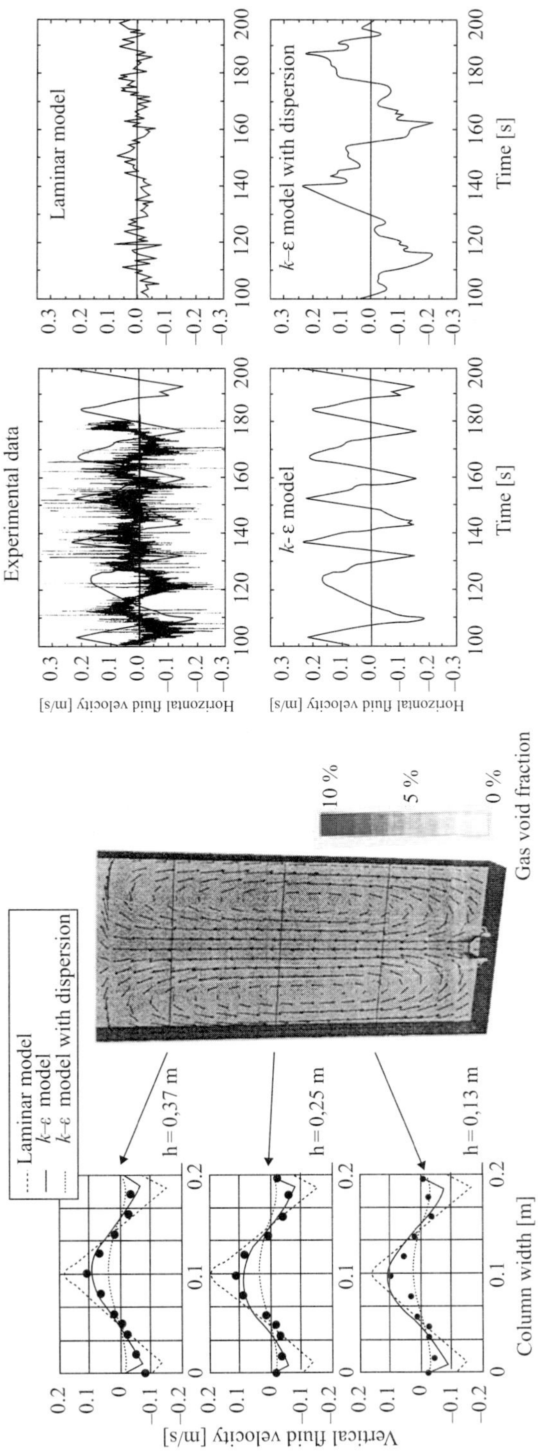

FIGURE 11.3 Simulated results for rectangular 2D bubble column (from Pfleger *et al.*, 1999) (a) Time-averaged results, (b) transient results.

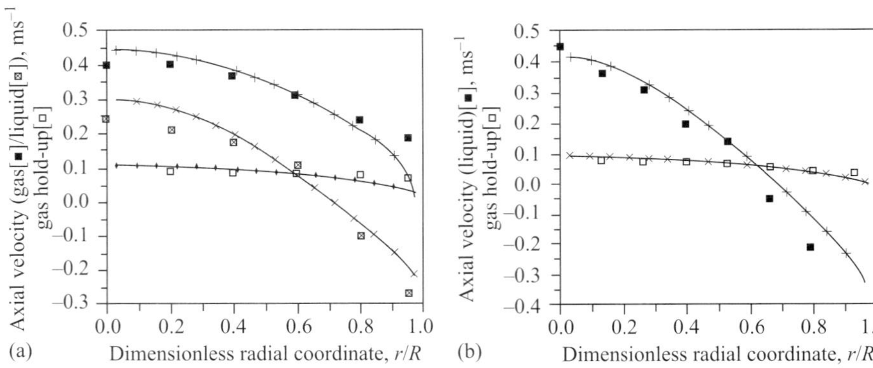

FIGURE 11.4 Simulations of time-averaged flow in bubble columns (from Ranade, 1997). Comparison with experimental data of (a) Grienberger and Hofmann (1992): $V_G = 0.02\,\mathrm{ms}^{-1}$, and (b) Menzel *et al.* (1990): $V_G = 0.024\,\mathrm{ms}^{-1}$.

column wall and the other to account for the effect of bubble wakes. If the influence of local circulation cells is appropriately included in the model equations, no matter how small the computational cells used to solve the resulting equations, local circulation cells will not appear in the simulation results and the solution will directly predict the long-time-averaged flow pattern. Some results reported by Ranade (1997) are shown in Fig. 11.4, and show good agreement between experimentally measured time-averaged flow characteristics and simulated results. Whether it is necessary to capture inherently unsteady local circulation cells, or it is sufficient to predict long-time-averaged results, depends on the objective at hand. Care must be taken to use appropriate assumptions and derive appropriate model equations to suit the objectives under consideration. Once the model equations are derived, the user must ensure that simulated results are not grid dependent. With these comments, we describe here governing equations for turbulent gas–liquid flows, derived using a control volume larger than the bubbles, which are able to capture inherently unsteady local circulation cells.

The time-averaged mass conservation equation can be written:

$$\frac{\partial}{\partial t}(\rho_k \alpha_k) + \frac{\partial}{\partial x_j}(\rho_k \alpha_k V_{ki} + \rho_k \overline{\alpha_k v_{ki}}) = 0 \tag{11.1}$$

where ρ_k is the density of phase k, α_k is the volume fraction of phase k and V_{ki} is the mean velocity of phase k in direction i. The second term and third term represent the convective mass transport and the turbulent diffusive mass transport, respectively. The time-averaged momentum equation can be written:

$$\begin{aligned}\frac{\partial}{\partial t}(\rho_k \alpha_k V_{ki}) + \frac{\partial}{\partial x_j}(\rho_k \alpha_k V_{ki} V_{kj}) = -\alpha_k \frac{\partial p}{\partial x_i} - \overline{\alpha_k \frac{\partial p'}{\partial x_i}} + \rho_k \alpha_k g_i + \overline{F_{ki}} \\ - \rho_k \frac{\partial}{\partial x_j}\left(\alpha_k \overline{v_{ki} v_{kj}} + V_{ki} \overline{v_{kj} \alpha'_k} + V_{kj} \overline{v_{ki} \alpha'_k}\right) \\ + (\text{viscous shear terms})\end{aligned} \tag{11.2}$$

where $\overline{F_{ki}}$ represents all the interphase coupling terms except pressure. v_{ki}, p' and α' indicate fluctuating components of velocity, pressure and volume fraction, respectively. It should be noted that pressure, p, is regarded as being 'shared' by both phases and therefore it appears in the transport equations of both phases. Formulation of the pressure term has occasioned some uncertainty (Spalding, 1978) and it is sometimes thought that different pressures 'ought' to be provided for each phase. Pressure inside an individual bubble is related to the pressure of the continuous phase via surface tension and bubble radius. However, this pressure inside the bubble has no relation to the flow of dispersed phase particles and is, therefore, irrelevant for the description of flow equations (Rietema and van den Akker, 1983). Pressure at the gas–liquid interface can be assumed to be equal to the liquid phase pressure since equations are spatially averaged over a control volume larger than individual bubbles (Johansen, 1988). For most reactor engineering situations, where speed of sound in each phase is large compared to velocities of interest, an assumption of microscopic pressure equilibration is adequate (Spalding, 1978; Drew, 1983).

Interphase coupling terms make two-phase flows fundamentally different from single-phase flows. Formulation of these terms, F_{ki}, must proceed carefully, with attention being paid to force balance for a single bubble and to any possible inconsistencies. Interphase coupling terms must satisfy the following relation:

$$F_{1i} = -F_{2i} \tag{11.3}$$

where subscript 1 and 2 denote liquid and gas (dispersed) phase, respectively. For dispersed two-phase flows, there are at least two transient forces acting at the interface in addition to the standard drag force, namely virtual mass force arising from the inertia effect (Ishii and Zuber, 1979; Auton, 1983; Cook and Harlow, 1986) and Basset force due to the development of a boundary layer around a bubble (Basset, 1888). In addition to this, transversal lift force, created by gradients in relative velocity across the bubble diameter, may also act on the bubble (Thomas *et al.*, 1983). Time averaging of interphase coupling terms is tedious and involves several unknown correlations, which need to be modeled. Neglecting all third-order correlations and all correlations involving gradients of a fluctuating quantity, Johansen (1988) derived an expression for the time-averaged interphase coupling term (with an assumption of low volume fraction for the dispersed phase), which is given below:

$$\begin{aligned}\overline{F_{1i}} = {} & \frac{3}{4}\frac{\rho_2 C_{\mathrm{DB}}}{d_{\mathrm{B}}}\left\{\left[\alpha_1|V_{2i}-V_{1i}| + 2\overline{\alpha_1'(v_{2i}-v_{1i})}\right](V_{2i}-V_{1i})\right.\\ & \left.+\alpha_1 \times \overline{v_{1i}^2 - 2v_{1i}v_{2i} + v_{2i}^2}\right\} + f_V\rho_2\left[\alpha_1\left(V_{2j}\frac{\partial V_{2i}}{\partial x_j} - V_{1j}\frac{\partial V_{1i}}{\partial x_j}\right) + \langle\rangle_i\right]\\ & + f_{\mathrm{B}}\frac{6\mu}{d_{\mathrm{B}}}\int_0^t\left\{V_{2j}\frac{\partial V_{2i}}{\partial x_j} - V_{1j}\frac{\partial V_{1i}}{\partial x_j} + \frac{\langle\rangle_i}{[\pi\nu(t-t')]^{1/2}}\right\}dt'\\ & + f_{\mathrm{L}}\rho_2\varepsilon_{mli}\varepsilon_{rsl}\left[\alpha_1(V_{2m}-V_{1m}) + \overline{\alpha_1'(v_{2m}-v_{1m})}\right]\frac{\partial V_{2s}}{\partial x_r}\end{aligned} \tag{11.4}$$

Where ε_{rsl} is the Levi-Cevita tensor and

$$\langle\rangle_i = \overline{\alpha_1' v_{2j}}\left(\frac{\partial V_{2i}}{\partial x_i} - \frac{\partial V_{1i}}{\partial x_j}\right) \tag{11.5}$$

The terms on the right-hand side of Eq. (11.4) correspond to interphase drag force, virtual mass force, Basset force and lift force, respectively. f_{L} is a transversal lift coefficient and is about 0.5 for potential flows and spherical particles (Drew *et al.*, 1979). f_B is a Basset force coefficient. For low volume fractions of dispersed phase, its value is about 1.5. f_V is a virtual mass coefficient. The numerical value of f_V is generally shape dependent: for rigid, spherical solid particles, it is reported as 0.5 (Maxey and Riley, 1983). For bubbles in water, Cook and Harlow (1986) used a value of $f_V = 0.25$. C_{DB} is a drag coefficient, which will be a function of bubble Reynolds number, which should be based on the resultant slip velocity between two phases.

It must be noted that the Basset history term will be significant only for the simulation of unsteady flows. An order of magnitude analysis presented by Hunt *et al.* (1987) suggests that, for large bubble columns ($D > 0.15$ m), where square of the terminal rise velocity of the bubble would be smaller than the product of the gravitational constant and the characteristics length scale, the interphase coupling term will be dominated by the drag force term. Various correlations are available to estimate the value of drag coefficient for the dispersed phase particles (Clift *et al.*, 1978; Ranade and Joshi, 1987). For the commonly encountered range of bubble Reynolds numbers, that is, $500 < \mathrm{Re}_B < 5000$, the following correlation may be used to estimate the drag coefficient (Clift *et al.*, 1978):

$$C_{DB} = \frac{0.622}{0.235 + (1/Eo)} \quad \because \quad Eo = \frac{g \Delta \rho d_B^2}{\sigma} \tag{11.6}$$

For an air–water system, terminal rise velocity of bubbles is not very sensitive to bubble diameter. Therefore, for bubbles with diameters in the range 3 to 8 mm, the ratio of drag coefficient to the bubble diameter (C_{DB}/d_B) can be considered as approximately constant. Ranade (1997) carried out simulations by setting the ratio of drag coefficient to bubble diameter (C_{DB}/d_B) equal to 290 m^{-1}.

For the swarm of bubbles, it is necessary to modify this equation to account for the interaction between bubbles and bubble wakes. Measurements by Tsuji *et al.* (1984) for two spheres in the Reynolds number range 100 to 200 can be expressed as

$$C_{DB} = C_{DB0} \left[1 - \left(\frac{d_B}{L_B} \right)^2 \right] \tag{11.7}$$

where L_B is the distance between centers' of two moving spheres (which can be related to the volume fraction of dispersed phase) and C_{DB0} is the drag coefficient of an isolated bubble. In many cases, it is difficult to estimate the influence of the presence of other bubbles on the interphase drag coefficient under operating conditions. In such cases, it is often beneficial to use empirical information about the velocity of bubble swarms to back-calculate the interphase drag coefficient:

$$C_D = \frac{4 \Delta \rho g d_B}{3 \rho_L V_b^2} \tag{11.8}$$

where V_b is effective bubble velocity in a swarm. For the swarm of large bubbles, Krishna *et al.* (1999) measured rise velocity and proposed the following correlation:

$$V_b = V_{b\infty}(2.25 + 4.09 U_G) \tag{11.9}$$

where U_G is superficial gas velocity (ms^{-1}) and $V_{b\infty}$ is the rise velocity of a single bubble. This expression is recommended to estimate the drag coefficient of large bubbles in swarms.

It must be noted that although Eq. (11.4) describes the time-averaged form of interphase coupling terms, how turbulence (and dispersed phase volume fraction) affect several empirical coefficients appearing in this expression, is seldom known. (Note that, fortunately, influences of higher turbulence and higher volume fraction of dispersed phase on interphase drag coefficient are opposite to each other.) In the absence of quantitative information, it is not really meaningful to rigorously include various terms appearing in the interphase coupling forces due to time averaging. In most cases, therefore, only those terms containing mean values of variables are retained and all other effects are lumped by suitably modifying values of empirical coefficients appearing in this equation. Unfortunately, no systematic data or study is available to independently validate values of empirical coefficients used in practice. Such an effort is essential to make further progress in modeling interphase coupling terms. When turbulence effects are neglected and interphase drag force dominates the overall interphase coupling terms, the interphase coupling term can be written (for multidimensional flows):

$$F_{D2i} = -\frac{3\alpha_1\alpha_2\rho_1 C_{DB}\left(\sum(V_{2j}-V_{2i})^2\right)^{1/2}(V_{2i}-V_{1i})}{4d_B} \tag{11.10}$$

It also must be kept in mind that all consistent two-phase momentum equations should reduce to single-phase equations if there is no slip between the two phases or the volume fraction of dispersed phase is zero.

Apart from interphase coupling terms, time-averaged transport equations demonstrate the effects of turbulence via various higher order and unknown terms. The viscous shear terms normally can be neglected in comparison with the turbulent shear terms. For closure of time-averaged transport equations, the concept of eddy viscosity is generally employed. Velocity correlations (Reynolds stresses) are generally modeled following the practice of single-phase flows:

$$\overline{v_{ki}v_{kj}} = -\nu_t\left(\frac{\partial V_{ki}}{\partial x_j}+\frac{\partial V_{kj}}{\partial x_i}\right)+\frac{2}{3}\delta_{ij}\left(k+\nu_t\frac{\partial V_{kl}}{dx_l}\right) \tag{11.11}$$

where δ_{ij} is the Kronecker delta and ν_t is the kinematic turbulent viscosity. Johansen (1988) reported an alternative route to anisotropic modeling of these velocity correlations. The form reported in Eq. (11.11), however, is most commonly used. Several authors proposed empirical formulae to estimate effective turbulent viscosity (Sato *et al.*, 1981; Salcudean *et al.*, 1985; Clark *et al.*, 1987). Most of these formulae, however, prescribe a unique value of turbulent viscosity for the entire reactor and, therefore, fail to account for its spatial variation. To account for this variation, the desired turbulence model should be able to predict turbulence length and velocity scale correctly. Two-equation turbulence models are the simplest models that promise success for flows in which length scale cannot be prescribed empirically. Among the various two-equation turbulence models, the k–ε model is the most widely tested and used. With this model, turbulence viscosity is related to local values of turbulent kinetic energy, k and the rate of turbulent energy dissipation, ε in that phase:

$$\nu_t = \frac{C_\mu k^2}{\varepsilon} \tag{11.12}$$

The above equation has been proposed for single-phase flows. The interaction of various turbulence length scales may affect the validity of this equation or values of parameters for two-phase flows. Lahey (1987) proposed a correlation of C_μ in terms of gas hold-up. However, his correlation is valid only for small diameter tubes with large liquid throughput. For large diameter columns, with low liquid throughput, no systematic study is available. Therefore, following general practice, the same value of C_μ may be used as that for single-phase flows (0.09).

The correlation between fluctuating velocity and hold-up is modeled using a gradient transport approximation as:

$$\overline{v_{ki}\alpha'_{ki}} = -\frac{\nu_t}{\sigma_G}\left(\frac{\partial \alpha'_k}{\partial x_i}\right) \tag{11.13}$$

where σ_G is the turbulent Schmidt number for the gas bubbles. Simple gradient transport is strictly valid only when the size of energy-containing eddies is much smaller than the distance over which the volume fraction gradient varies appreciably. More general formulations are available (Lumley, 1975; Elghobashi and Abou-Arab, 1983), when this condition is not satisfied. The value of turbulent Schmidt number for bubbles will, in principle, depend on bubble size and scale of turbulence. Turbulent eddies smaller than bubble size will not contribute to the bubble dispersion. However, no systematic data or theory is available to quantitatively estimate the values of turbulent Schmidt number for gas bubbles. Recently, Ranade and Mashelkar (1993) attempted to subtract the effect of eddies from a particular range of length scales from the overall turbulent transport. A similar model may be able to predict the value of Schmidt number for a given bubble size. At this stage, however, the general practice is to set the value of turbulent Schmidt number to unity.

The pressure coupling term has the same magnitude but opposite sign in continuous and dispersed phase momentum equations. This term, therefore, implies a transfer of momentum between the two phases. Elghobashi and Abou-Arab (1983) developed a closure approximation for the correlation of fluctuating volume fraction and fluctuating pressure. However, values of the constants appearing in their model are known only approximately due to lack of relevant experimental data. In this situation, an approximation derived by Johansen (1988) may be used to represent pressure coupling term:

$$\overline{\alpha'_k \frac{\partial p'}{\partial x_i}} = -\rho_k \overline{\alpha'_k v_{kj}} \frac{\partial V_{ki}}{\partial x_j} - \rho_k V_{kj} \frac{\partial}{\partial x_j} \overline{\alpha'_k v_{ki}} \tag{11.14}$$

Modeling of correlations of fluctuating volume fraction and fluctuating velocity appearing in this equation have already been discussed.

In order to close the set of modeled transport equations, it is necessary to estimate turbulent viscosity or if the k–ε model is used, the turbulent kinetic energy, k and turbulent energy dissipation rate, ε. The modeled forms of the liquid phase k and ε transport equations can be written in the following general format (subscript 1 denotes the continuous phase):

$$\frac{\partial}{\partial t}(\alpha_1 \phi) + \frac{\partial}{\partial x_i}(\alpha_1 V_{ki} \phi) = \frac{\partial}{\partial x_i}\left(\alpha_1 \frac{\nu_t}{\sigma_\phi} \frac{\partial \phi}{\partial x_i}\right) + S_\phi \quad (11.15)$$

where ϕ can be either k or ε, and σ_ϕ is the model parameter describing turbulence dispersion of ϕ. The corresponding source terms for k and ε can be written as:

$$S_k = \alpha_1[(G + G_e) - \varepsilon] \quad (11.16)$$

$$S_\varepsilon = \alpha_1 \frac{\varepsilon}{k}[C_1(G + G_e) - C_2 \varepsilon] \quad (11.17)$$

where C_1 and C_2 are model parameters of the k–ε model. The general practice is to use the same values of these parameters as proposed for single-phase flows (Launder and Spalding, 1972) used to estimate turbulence in two-phase flows (these values are listed in Table 3.1). G is turbulence generation based on the single-phase mechanism and G_e is an extra turbulence generation due to the presence of dispersed phase. The turbulent generation term, G, is given by:

$$G = -\overline{v_{1i} v_{1j}} \frac{\partial V_{1i}}{\partial x_j} \quad (11.18)$$

Correlation of fluctuating velocities appearing in this expression is modeled using Eq. (11.11). Extra turbulence generation G_e can be modeled in different ways. Johansen (1988) modeled it as

$$G_e = -\rho_2 \overline{\alpha_1 v_{2i}} g_i - f_V \rho_2 \alpha_1 \overline{v_{2i} v_{2j}} \left(\frac{\partial V_{2i}}{\partial x_j}\right) \quad (11.19)$$

where f_V is a virtual mass coefficient. Svendsen *et al.* (1992) related the extra turbulence generation with the interphase drag force:

$$G_e = C_b F_{\text{Dres}} \left(\sum (V_{2i} - V_{1i})^2\right)^{1/2} \quad (11.20)$$

where C_b is an empirical constant. Kataoka *et al.* (1992) carried out a detailed analysis of these extra terms in the source of turbulent kinetic energy. Their analysis suggests that the extra generation of turbulence due to large bubbles (represented by Eq. 11.20) is almost compensated by the extra dissipation due to the small-scale interfacial structures. Based on comparison of predicted turbulent kinetic energy with experimental data, published computational studies also indicate that the value of parameter C_b is almost zero (Ranade, 1997), which indirectly confirms the analysis of Kataoka *et al.* (1992). Before we discuss some published results, it is essential to discuss special boundary conditions required to simulate flow in bubble columns.

Application of model equations to simulate flow in bubble columns

The first step in the application of model equations to simulate flow in a bubble column is to select an appropriate solution domain and formulate corresponding boundary conditions. Consider a typical bubble column configuration, where gas is introduced in a plenum below the sparger (Fig. 11.5). Figure 11.5 shows semi-batch

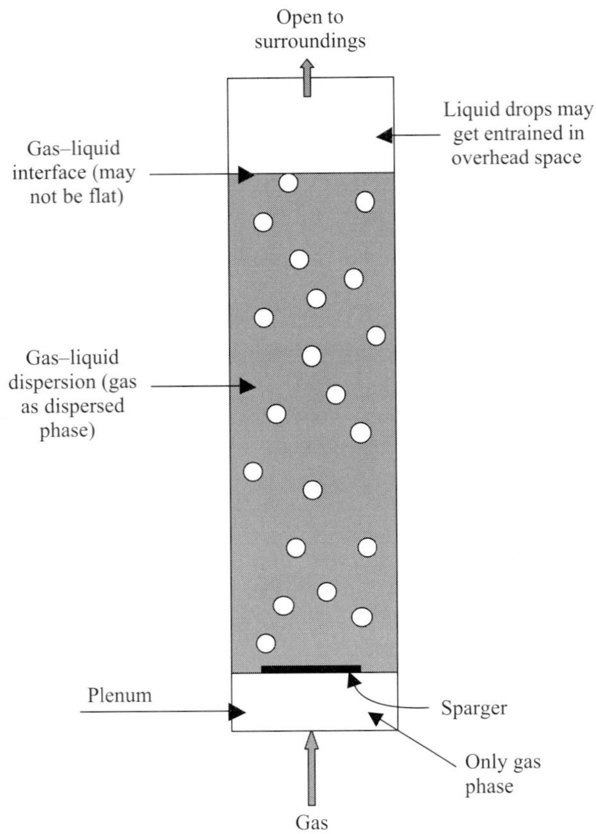

FIGURE 11.5 Outline of two-dimensional bubble column.

operation. The gas pressure in the plenum is sufficient to support the liquid head above the sparger and to maintain the required gas flow through the pool of liquid. Higher plenum pressure prevents liquid from weeping through the sparger. As gas is introduced in the column, gas bubbles rise through the liquid pool and raise the liquid level in the column. Gas bubbles burst at the gas–liquid interface, and is shown schematically in Fig. 11.6. Bursting bubbles may throw some liquid droplets into the overhead space. Depending on the gas flow rate, droplet size (settling velocity) and overhead space, these droplets may or may not escape the column from the top opening. If there is a net liquid flow, a gas–liquid separator needs to be configured at the top region of the column. One has now to select a suitable solution domain and formulate appropriate boundary conditions to translate this physical picture into a mathematical framework.

Generally, the gas pressure in the plenum is assumed to be uniform and plenum is not considered in the solution domain. The region above the sparger is considered to be within the solution domain. In most published simulations, the sparger is assumed to distribute the gas uniformly through the sparger region and was modeled as an inlet. To model the sparger as a velocity inlet, it is necessary to specify the velocity and volume fraction at the inlet boundary. Since the gas volume fraction below the sparger is unity, it is tempting to specify gas volume fraction at the sparger boundary as unity,

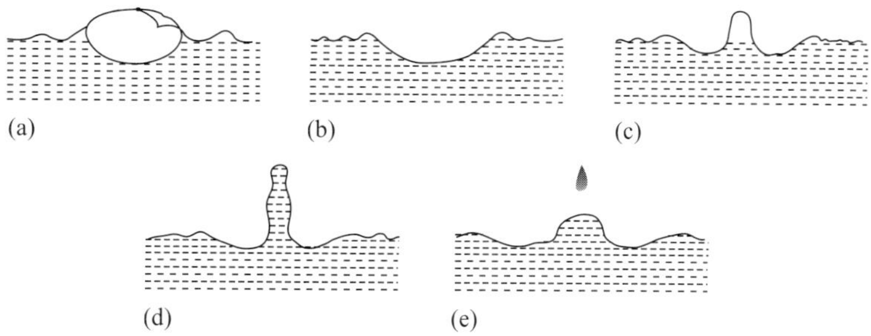

FIGURE 11.6 Schematic diagram of bubble bursting at the interface (from Newitt *et al.*, 1954).

and to specify gas phase velocity so as to ensure the desired net gas flow. However, it must be remembered that gas enters the solution domain in the form of bubbles, which rise with a velocity different than the superficial gas velocity. It is therefore advantageous to set the gas velocity at the sparger inlet equal to the estimated bubble rise velocity. The volume fraction at the inlet can then be specified in a way that ensures the desired net gas flow. Thus, if the sparger is assumed to distribute gas uniformly, the boundary conditions can be written as:

$$V_G = V_{b\infty} \qquad \alpha_G = \frac{\langle U_G \rangle}{V_G} \tag{11.21}$$

where $\langle U_G \rangle$ is superficial gas velocity over the sparged area. For special sparger configurations such as ring spargers, a similar approach can be used by considering appropriate sparger area in the computational grid. When sparger type and resistance is not adequate to ensure uniform distribution, it will be necessary to include a sparger model in the overall flow model in order to account for non-uniform gas sparging at the sparger. Ranade (1993b) developed a simple model to simulate non-uniform gas sparging. In this model, the gas velocity through any location in the sparged area is assumed to be a function of pressure drop across the sparger at that location. The plenum pressure (pressure below the sparger) can be assumed to be uniform. The pressure above the sparger, p_0, is the sum of the overhead pressure, p_{top}, and hydrostatic head above the sparger. Thus, the pressure balance across the sparger can be written:

$$p_S - p_0 = k_L V_G + k_T V_G^2 \quad \because \quad p_0 = p_{top} + \int_0^H (\rho_L \alpha_L + \rho_G \alpha_G) g \, dz \tag{11.22}$$

where k_L and k_T are characteristic laminar and turbulent resistance coefficients of the sparger, and p_S is the pressure below the sparger (plenum pressure).

For column walls, which are impermeable to fluids, standard wall boundary conditions may be specified. Whether the full column should be considered in the solution domain or symmetry or other boundary conditions may be invoked to reduce the extent of the solution domain, essentially depends on the objective and the proposed mathematical model. If the interest is in estimating long-time-averaged flow characteristics (as done by Ranade, 1997), invoking symmetry is often useful and can facilitate rapid results. However, when the interest is in capturing inherently unsteady flow characteristics, which are not symmetrical, it is essential to consider the whole column as the solution domain (as done by Ranade and Tayalia, 2001). Overall flow can be modeled using an axis-symmetric assumption, if and only if, the governing equations are derived in such a way as to represent the influence of local dynamic flow structures on time-averaged flow via additional terms. Ranade (1997) developed such a model based on two empirical coefficients to simulate long-term-averaged flow patterns. The two parameters were estimated from a data set of Yao *et al.* (1991). The same values of these parameters were used for subsequent simulations. Results show good agreement between predicted results and long-time-averaged experimental results of Hillmer *et al.* (1994), Grienberger and Hofmann (1992), Menzel *et al.* (1990) and Hills (1974). However, when the objective is to simulate inherently unsteady flow, which is asymmetric, it will be necessary to avoid imposing symmetry boundary condition. For a two-dimensional column, therefore, it will be necessary to consider the whole domain. For three-dimensional cylindrical columns, either a body-fitted grid should be used, which will avoid specification of boundary condition at the axis, or conventional axis boundary conditions should be modified to allow flow through the axis (the value of any variable at the axis location is set to average of all the computational cells surrounding it).

Boundary conditions for the top horizontal surface of the bubble column requires special attention. Following the experimental practice of keeping the height of the gas–liquid dispersion smaller than actual column height, the top surface of the column can be modeled as an outlet for gas and liquid phase. It is expected that the solution of the model equations will determine the height of the gas–liquid dispersion and only gas will exit from the inlet. In other words, it is expected that the model will predict a gas volume fraction of unity above the gas–liquid interface. Such an approach, however, has to ensure that the governing equations are capable of handling change in the prevailing continuous phase (liquid below the gas–liquid dispersion height and gas above it). This is seldom done and despite this, solution of the conventional two-fluid model using the top surface as an outlet is attempted. As expected, such an attempt always leads to non-physical velocity values at the region of the gas–liquid interface and encounters severe convergence difficulties. In many cases with high superficial gas velocity, the liquid mass of the column is lifted out of the column. In order to enhance convergence behavior, Padial *et al.* (2000) used a smoothly varying continuous phase density across the gas–liquid interface:

$$\rho_C = \frac{1}{2}\left\{\rho_L + \rho_G - (\rho_L - \rho_G)\tanh\left[\frac{2\left(\alpha_G - \frac{1}{2}\right)}{\alpha_G(1-\alpha_G)}\right]\right\} \tag{11.23}$$

Such an empirically adjusted smooth profile of continuous phase density helps to maintain a fairly stable interface. Some fraction of the liquid, however, may still escape the column during initial phases of solution development.

In most reactor engineering applications, it may not be necessary to include the gas–liquid interface in the solution domain. In an alternative approach, the solution domain is restricted to the height of gas–liquid dispersion. Of course, an exact value of dispersion height is not known *a priori*. However, in most cases, overall gas volume fractions and therefore, height of the gas–liquid dispersion can be estimated. Even if there is 40% error in the prediction of overall gas volume fraction, it will result in only 10% error in the estimation of height of gas–liquid dispersion, if the volume fraction is about 25%. Except for very shallow bubble columns, fluid dynamics is not sensitive to the 10% error in the height of gas–liquid dispersion. Thus, it is always possible to estimate a reasonable solution domain height to model gas–liquid flows in bubble columns. The top surface of the solution domain may then be assumed to coincide with the free surface of dispersion. This free surface may or may not be assumed to be flat. The normal liquid phase velocity, the tangential shear stress and the normal fluxes k, ε and ϕ are set to zero at the free surface. The gas bubbles are free to escape from the top surface. If source code is accessible, one can modify the code to implement these boundary conditions. In most commercial CFD codes, user-defined routines with options such as 'patch boundary conditions' may be used to implement this boundary condition. When direct implementation is not possible, Ranade (1998, 2000) proposed two approximate alternatives.

In the first alternative, if the terminal rise velocity of gas bubbles is known (or can be estimated with confidence), the top surface of the dispersion may be defined as an 'inlet'. Normal liquid velocity may be set to zero while normal gas velocity may be set to terminal rise velocity. The implicit assumption here is that gas bubbles escape the dispersion with terminal rise velocity. It should be noted that even after defining the top surface as an inlet, gas volume fraction at the top surface is a free variable. There is no implicit forcing of gas volume fraction distribution. Alternatively, the top surface of the dispersion can be modeled as a no shear wall. This will automatically set normal liquid velocity to zero. It will also set normal gas velocity to zero. In order to represent escaping gas bubbles, an appropriate sink may be defined for all the computational cells attached to the top surface (Figure 11.7):

$$S_G = -A_B \alpha_{GB} W_{GB} \rho_G \qquad (11.24)$$

where A_B is the area of the bottom surface of the computational cell attached to the top surface, W_{GB} and α_{GB} are the normal velocity of gas bubbles and gas volume fraction of the computational cells lying below the computational cell attached to the top surface. Such formulations of top surface avoid handling sharp gradients of gas volume fractions at the gas–liquid interface and are much more stable numerically.

To illustrate application of the Eulerian–Eulerian approach, some results of two-dimensional bubble columns are discussed here. Three-dimensional bubble columns and other reactor engineering applications are discussed in Section 11.3.

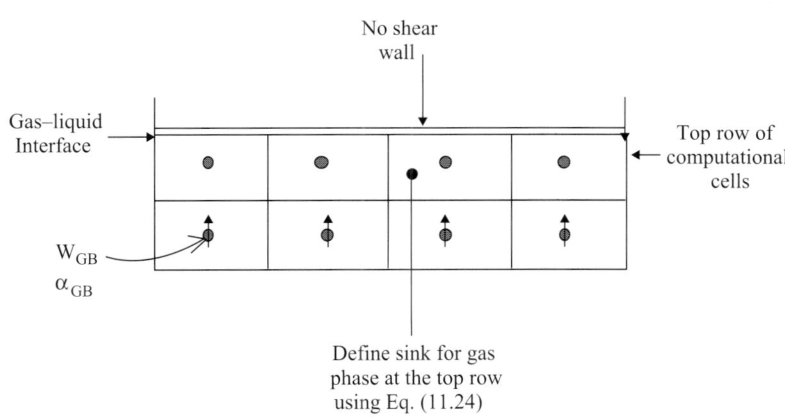

FIGURE 11.7 Top boundary condition for bubble column reactor.

Brief review of recent simulations of bubble columns

Rigorous experimental data is available for apparently two-dimensional bubble columns (Becker *et al.*, 1994, 1999). It is, therefore, useful to simulate the fluid dynamics of such a column to validate the underlying mathematical model. Pfleger *et al.* (1999) recently reported comparison of their simulated results with experimental data (Fig. 11.3). Sokolichin and Eigenberger (1999) also reported good agreement between predicted results and experimental data. To illustrate such simulations, we reproduce some of the results obtained by Ranade (2000). He simulated gas–liquid flow in a two-dimensional bubble column (0.2 m width, 0.45 m dispersion height and 0.04 m depth) having the same geometrical column configuration as used in the experiments by Becker *et al.* (1999). A solution domain and computational grid ($51 \times 90 \times 11$ computational cells for width $\times$ height $\times$ depth) is shown in Fig. 11.8. A two-fluid model was used to simulate gas–liquid flow in such a column. A standard k–ε model was used to simulate turbulence. A QUICK discretization scheme was used with a SUPERBEE limiter functions (see Chapter 6 for more details on discretization schemes). Modeled interphase coupling terms comprised drag force and virtual mass terms. For estimation of drag coefficient, a correlation of Schiller and Naumann (1935) was used. Governing equations were solved in a transient manner with a time step of 0.008 s. For each time step, 100 internal iterations were carried

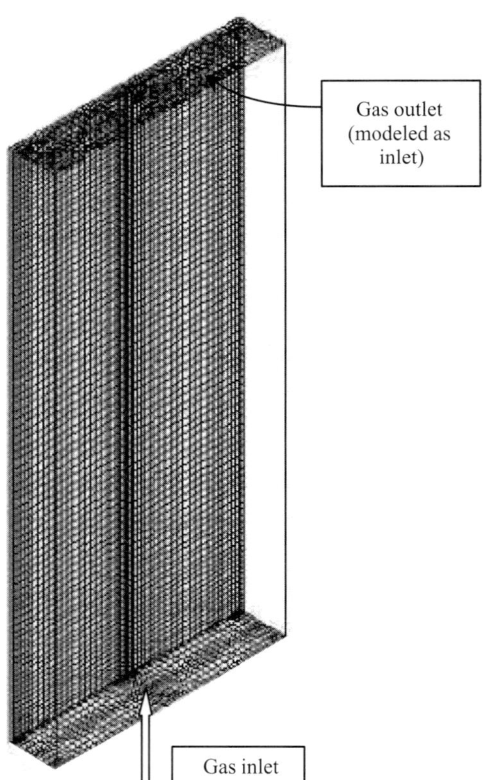

FIGURE 11.8 Solution domain and grid.

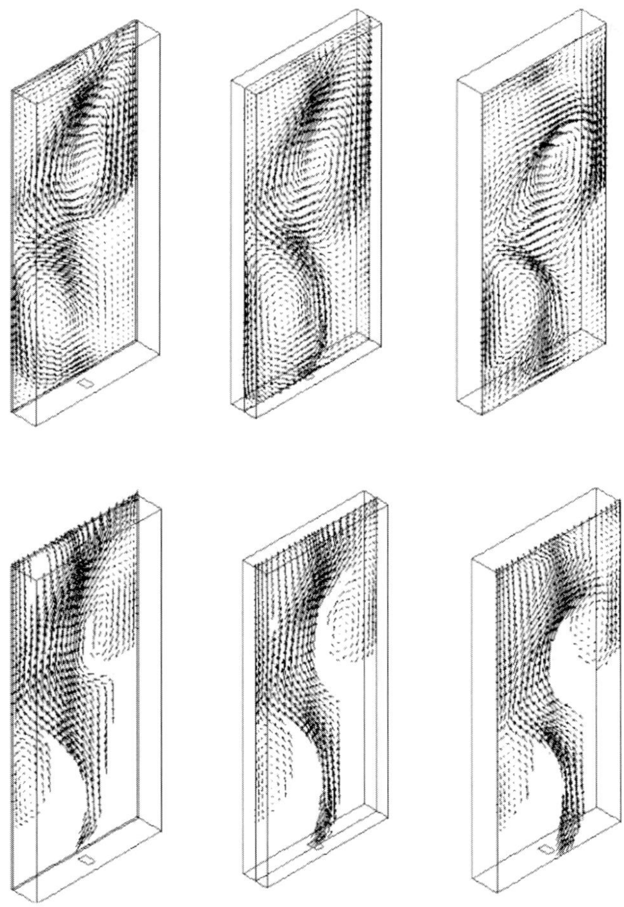

FIGURE 11.9 Predicted flow field, Top: liquid phase; Bottom: gas phase (from Ranade, 2000).

out. This number of internal iterations was sufficient to ensure an adequate degree of convergence of all the equations. Further refinement of time step did not affect the simulation results significantly.

Simulation results clearly showed the inherently unsteady flow characteristics of gas–liquid flows. The predicted instantaneous flow field is shown in Figs 11.9 and 11.10 at three different planes. It can be seen that gas bubbles rise in the column in a meandering way. Experiments by Becker *et al.* (1999) indicate that the bubble swarm moves laterally with a period of about 16 s. Eulerian–Eulerian simulations carried out by Ranade (2000) also show a meandering effect. The time history of the simulated velocity field at four locations within the column clearly shows the oscillatory nature of the flow (Fig. 11.11). It can be seen that simulation results somewhat underpredict the period of oscillations ($\sim$12 s). However, overall characteristics are in good agreement with experimental observations. Recent simulations by Pfleger *et al.* (1999) also show some underprediction of the period of oscillation. Despite this, time-averaged predictions agree quite well with experimental data. The predicted results shown in Figs 11.9 and 11.10 indicate the three-dimensional nature of the flow even in

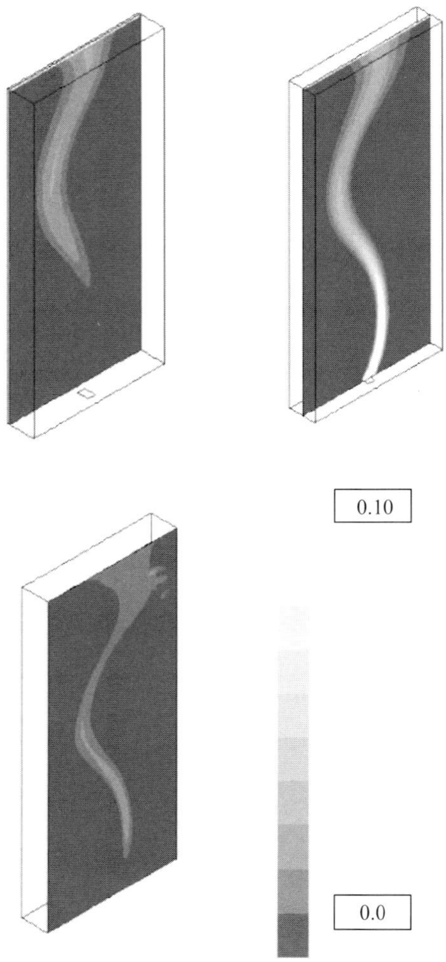

FIGURE 11.10 Predicted gas volume fraction distribution (from Ranade, 2000).

an apparent two-dimensional bubble column. If such three-dimensional effects are not considered, the meandering motion of the bubble swarm is not captured with adequate accuracy because of the overprediction of turbulent kinetic energy. Volume integration of the predicted turbulent energy dissipation rate indicates that about 30% of the input energy ($g\langle V_G \rangle$) is dissipated in the form of turbulent energy. The remainder of the energy must be dissipating at the gas–liquid interface. Predicted overall gas volume fraction is 0.63%. If we assume that average slip velocity is about 0.23 ms^{-1}, the amount of energy dissipated at the gas–liquid interface may be estimated as the product of the gravitational constant, gas volume fraction and slip velocity. This is about 68% of the total input energy. This value agrees quite well with the predicted overall turbulent energy dissipation (assuming that the laminar dissipation is negligible compared to turbulent dissipation). The simulated results can be examined in a variety of ways to understand the dynamic characteristics of gas–liquid flows in bubble columns. For example, three-dimensional iso-surface plots

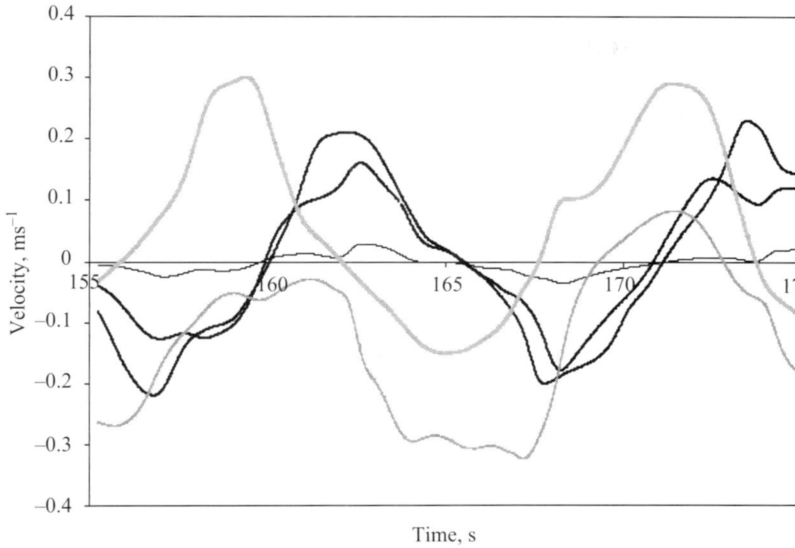

FIGURE 11.11 Transient velocity traces at different locations in rectangular 2D column (from Ranade, 2000).

may give more information about the prevalent flow structures. The iso-surface of gas volume fraction may also clearly show the meandering motion of the bubble swarm (not shown here). In order to identify streamwise vortices, it is useful to examine values of normalized helicity (which is a scalar quantity representing the cosine of the angle between the velocity and vorticity vectors). Near the vortex cores, the magnitude of normalized helicity will be near unity with its sign depending on the orientation of the velocity vector to the vorticity vector. A typical helicity iso-surface plot is shown in Fig. 11.12 and shows several regions high magnitude normalized helicity indicating the presence of vortex cores. Thus, Eulerian–Eulerian simulations are able to capture the inherently unsteady flow characteristics of gas–liquid flows in bubble columns.

For bubble columns with relatively low gas volume fractions, bubble size distribution is fairly narrow. As gas velocity and therefore, gas volume fraction increases, a heterogeneous or churn-turbulent regime sets in with much wider bubble size distribution than the homogeneous regime. With such a wide bubble size distribution, it is important to develop appropriate averaging methods and corresponding closure models. Use of governing equations, derived based on the assumption of a single bubble size, generally lead to significant overprediction of gas volume fraction, though comparison of liquid phase mean velocity is not bad (see Kumar *et al.*, 1994, for example). Recently, Krishna *et al.* (2000a) proposed use of a three-phase model to simulate the churn-turbulent regime of bubble columns. Basic concepts are shown schematically in Fig. 11.13. Based on experimental observations, the gas phase is divided into two separate phases, one with small bubbles of diameter of the order of a few millimeters, and the other with large spherical cap bubbles with diameter of a few centimeters. Large bubbles were introduced only in the central core, in their simulations. Drag coefficient values were calculated based on empirical correlations of observed bubble

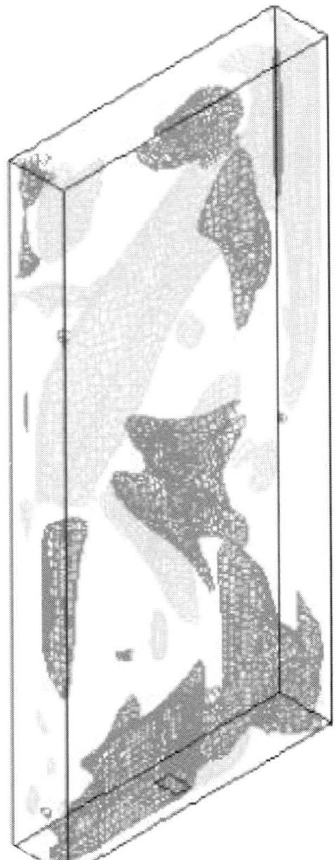

FIGURE 11.12 Iso-surface of normalized helicity. Normalized helicity = 0.5 (dark surface) and −0.5 (light surface) (from Ranade, 2000).

slip velocities. Krishna *et al.* (2000a) had introduced four adjustable parameters to tune the drag coefficient and diameter of the large bubbles. With these parameters, they were successful in simulating liquid velocity profiles and gas volume fractions as observed by Hills (1974). Treatment of the outlet boundary conditions was not discussed in their paper. Comparison of their simulated results and experimental data is shown in Fig. 11.14. The comparison looks quite adequate for most engineering applications. It must, however, be noted that these results may not be grid independent and the values of adjustable parameters may depend on grid size.

Instead of arbitrarily considering two bubble classes, it may be useful to incorporate a coalescence break-up model based on the population balance framework in the CFD model (see for example, Carrica *et al.*, 1999). Such a model will simulate the evolution of bubble size distribution within the column and will be a logical extension of previously discussed models to simulate flow in bubble columns with wide bubble size distribution. Incorporation of coalescence break-up models, however, increases computational requirements by an order of magnitude. For example, a two-fluid model with a single bubble size generally requires solution of ten equations (six momentum, pressure, dispersed phase continuity and two turbulence characteristics). A ten-bubble class model requires solution of 46 (33 momentum, pressure,

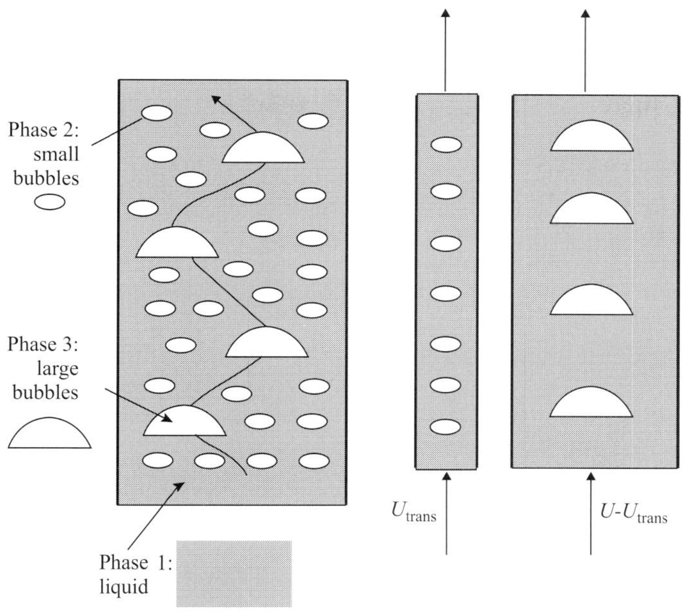

FIGURE 11.13 Three phase simulation of bubble columns (from Krishna *et al.*, 2000a).

10 continuity and two turbulence characteristics) equations. In such a model, each bubble class is considered as a separate phase and momentum and continuity equations are solved for each bubble class. If the bubble size distribution is relatively narrow and can be represented by a single velocity field, it is possible to reduce the computational requirements by solving the momentum equations for only one bubble class and assigning the same velocity field to all bubble classes (Lo, 2000). Separate continuity equations comprising terms pertaining to coalescence and break-up need to be solved for each bubble class. For such a case with the ten-bubble class model, the number of governing equations reduces from 46 to 19. This approach will be quite useful to simulate gas–liquid interfacial area and mass transfer with moderate increase in computational demands. Recently, Buwa and Ranade (2000) employed this approach to simulate evolution of bubble size distribution in a two-dimensional bubble column. Their model is briefly discussed in Appendix 11.1.

Bubble column reactors are also widely used as slurry reactors. The simplest way to simulate the fluid dynamics of slurry bubble column reactors is to treat the solid and liquid phases as a single slurry phase with effective slurry properties. This approach was used by Torvik and Svendsen (1990) and may give reasonable predictions for low solid volume fractions. The variation of solid volume fraction within the column is ignored in such an approach. For denser slurry applications, however, solid volume fraction may vary significantly within the column and solid and liquid phases need to be considered separately. The overall fluid dynamics can then be simulated using a three-fluid model (gas, liquid and solid). It is necessary to formulate appropriate inter-phase exchange terms for these three phases. When the solid volume fraction in slurry bubble column reactors increases even further and is more than 10%, it is necessary to use granular flow models to simulate flow of solid particles. Details of granular flow models are discussed in the next chapter when describing the modeling of fluidized

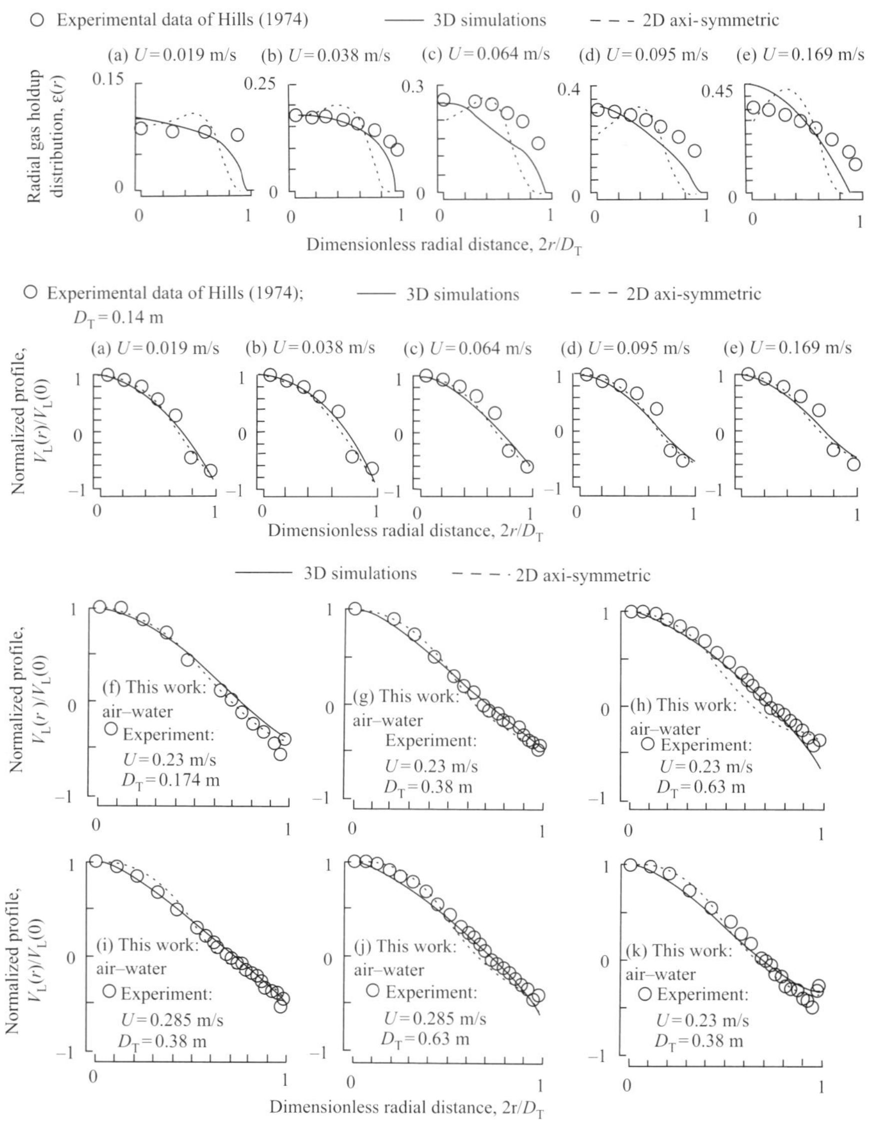

FIGURE 11.14 Comparison of predictions using three-phase model and experimental data (from Krishna *et al.*, 2000a).

bed reactors. Wu and Gidaspow (2000) used such a granular flow model to simulate the fluid dynamics of a methanol synthesis reactor. Their results show encouraging agreement with the pilot plant data. Further experimental and computational research on fluid dynamics of dense slurry bubble column reactors is essential to make further progress in predictions of such slurry reactors. Recent experimental techniques such as computer tomography (CT) and computer aided radioactive particle tracking (CARPT), which can 'look' into opaque, dense slurry bubble columns, may provide the necessary experimental data to guide further development.

In general, it may be concluded that it is possible to develop appropriate Eulerian–Eulerian models to simulate complex gas–liquid (solid) flows, with some support from the experimental data. Some of the possible applications of such models are discussed in the next section. Before discussing these applications, recent simulations carried out with Eulerian–Lagrangian and volume of fluid (VOF) approaches are briefly reviewed here.

11.2.2. Eulerian–Lagrangian and VOF Approach

Basic governing equations to apply Eulerian–Lagrangian and VOF approaches to simulate dispersed gas–liquid flows are discussed in Chapter 4. As mentioned therein, the major advantage of the Eulerian–Lagrangian approach is its greater flexibility with respect to incorporation of microscopic, particle-level phenomena. Bubble–bubble interaction and coalescence or break-up can be included in the model. The precise state of individual bubbles can be monitored, which has significant advantage in simulating gas–liquid reactors. However, this flexibility and knowledge of the precise state of individual bubbles comes with associated increase in computational costs. Simulation of large industrial bubble column reactors containing millions of gas bubbles often becomes computationally intractable. However, despite this limitation, Eulerian–Lagrangian simulations can provide very useful insight and can be used to validate the averaging procedure employed in developing Eulerian–Eulerian models.

In order to reduce the computational requirements, Lapin and Lubbert (1994) considered bubble clusters instead of individual bubbles while employing a Eulerian–Lagrangian approach to simulate bubble columns. However, they externally imposed bubble slip velocity rather than calculating it by solving momentum equations. Delnoij (1999) carried out more rigorous Eulerian–Lagrangian simulations of flow in bubble columns. Apart from solving momentum equations for individual bubbles, Delnoij also considered bubble–bubble collisions and their effect on bubble trajectories. Samples of their results are shown in Fig. 11.15. Delnoij (1999) did not consider coalescence and break-up. Ranade and Utikar (1999) used bubble tracking in a Lagrangian framework along with the coalescence models. They have, however, simplified the governing equations using the approximation of potential flow around bubbles. Despite such a simplistic approximation, their model could capture the key features of the dynamics of gas–liquid flows reasonably well. It is necessary to develop a comprehensive computational model based on a Eulerian–Lagrangian framework (with coalescence and break-up models) to simulate dispersed gas-liquid flows in bubble columns. Detailed comparisons of simulated results from Eulerian–Lagrangian approach and Eulerian–Eulerian approach will be very useful to validate averaging procedures employed to derive Eulerian–Eulerian models. Such detailed comparisons and analysis will lead to better formulations of Eulerian–Eulerian models, which may then be reliably used for reactor engineering applications.

It must be noted here that even for Eulerian–Lagrangian simulations, although there is no complexity of averaging over trajectories, the accuracy of simulations of individual bubble trajectories depends on lumped interphase interaction parameters such as drag force, virtual mass force and lift force coefficients. All of these interphase interaction parameters will be functions of bubble size and shape, presence of other bubbles or walls, surrounding pressure field and so on. Unfortunately, adequate information is not available on these aspects. To enhance our understanding of basic

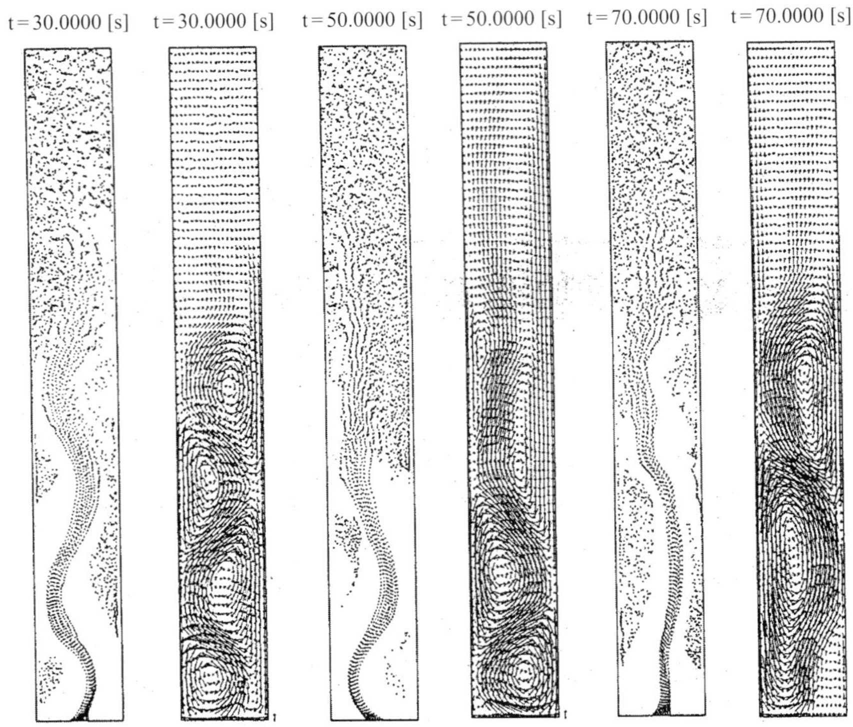

FIGURE 11.15 Results of simulations of Delnoij *et al.* (1997). Column width = 0.175 m; Column height = 1.3475 m; superficial gas velocity = 0.035 m/s^{-1}; uniform bubbles of diameter 0.002 m.

issues in bubble–bubble interaction and to obtain the required information for model development, it may be necessary to develop and to use volume of fluid (VOF) or interface tracking based simulations. As discussed in Chapter 4, the volume of fluid approach allows resolution of the small-scale flow field around individual bubbles (including possible deformation of bubbles). Such capability will provide valuable information about bubble–bubble interactions. Lin *et al.* (1996) applied VOF to simulate the motion of gas bubbles in two-dimensional columns. More recently, Li *et al.* (2000) and Krishna *et al.* (2000b) also carried out VOF simulations of the rise of single bubbles under different operating conditions. A sample of results from Li *et al.* (2000) is shown in Fig. 11.16. The agreement between simulated rise velocity and experimental data is quite encouraging. Krishna and van Baten (1999) also tried to simulate interaction between multiple bubbles while they are rising through the two-dimensional columns. However, agreement between predicted and experimentally observed rise velocity is not as good as observed in the case of single bubbles. It may be necessary to carry out detailed three-dimensional VOF simulations to get accurate predictions of bubble–bubble interactions. No such attempt has been published so far. Although the computational requirements of such an exercise will be huge, such VOF simulations will be very useful to develop appropriate sub-models for Eulerian–Eulerian and Eulerian–Lagrangian approaches.

A brief review of recent modeling attempts indicates several limitations of the current state of the art. However, with an appropriate dose of engineering judgment

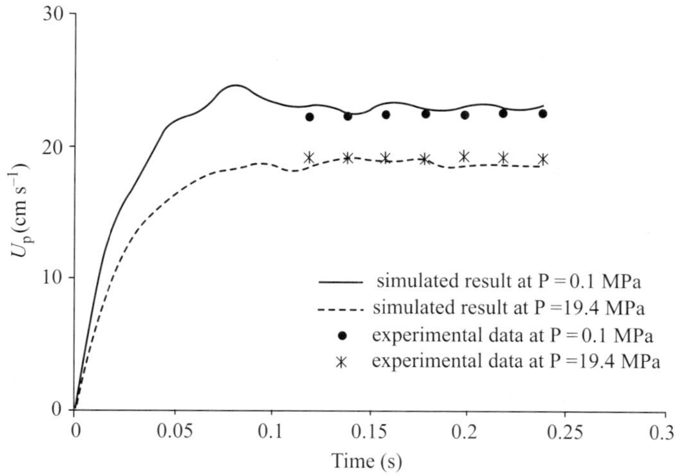

FIGURE 11.16 Comparison of simulated and experimental rise velocities at different pressures (from Li *et al.*, 2000).

and the necessary experimental back-up, it is possible to derive meaningful engineering results using these CFD models of bubble column reactors, which otherwise may not be possible. Some of the possible applications are illustrated in the following section.

11.3. APPLICATION TO REACTOR ENGINEERING

An overall procedure for reactor engineering is discussed in Chapter 1. Additional comments on the engineering of bubble column reactors are made in Section 11.1. Some of these are repeated here to emphasize their importance. As for any other reactor, conventional reaction engineering models are first used to evaluate the influence of various fluid dynamic characteristics (mixing, volume fraction, interfacial area, heat transfer coefficient and so on) on overall performance of a reactor. These studies lead to the formulation of specific duties for the reactor, which may be related to specific demands of the underlying fluid dynamics. After finalizing these demands on reactor fluid dynamics, the reactor engineer has to evolve a suitable hardware configuration to fulfill these demands. CFD-based models can make significant contributions at this stage.

After completing reaction-engineering work, it is first necessary to evolve a reactor configuration before one can start evaluating whether such hardware can perform the expected duties. In the case of bubble columns, evolving reactor hardware involves at least the following (also see Fig. 11.2):

- Bubble column configuration/dimensions: simple versus loop configuration, diameter, height to diameter ratio, internals (draft tube, radial baffles, cooling/heating coils, packings), feed inlet/outlet nozzles (for gas as well as liquid phase components), gas-liquid separator, foam breakers/entrainment reducers, necessary process monitoring sensors and so on. Each of these will further involve selection from various alternatives. Even for the very simple

bubble column reactor with no internals, it is necessary to select a suitable sparger in addition to the basic sizing.
- Design of sparger: type, sparger resistance, sparger holes, gas velocity and bubble size generated at sparger, operability of the sparger at varying gas loads, design of plenum chamber (if necessary) and so on.

More often than not, the reactor engineer evolves more than one configuration to meet the expected duties. It is necessary to examine these alternatives and to select a few short-listed configurations for further studies. Normally, this short-listing procedure involves various heuristic arguments based on prior experience and available information. CFD models can be used to quickly evaluate the various configurations to assist this short-listing procedure. To estimate commonly required reactor duties like liquid phase mixing and heat transfer coefficient, it may be sufficient to predict time-averaged liquid velocity profiles and corresponding time-averaged gas volume fraction profiles. For such cases, it may be adequate to use two-dimensional models. One example of such a model developed by Ranade (1997) was discussed in an earlier section. The work of Krishna *et al.* (2000a) also confirms that two-dimensional models may give adequately accurate estimations of overall gas volume fraction and liquid circulation velocities. Such two-dimensional models may also be used to qualitatively evaluate the influence of different reactor internals, such as draft tubes and radial baffles, on liquid phase mixing in the reactor. Ranade (1993b) demonstrated such an application to evaluate the influence of radial baffles on mixing in bubble column reactors.

The two-dimensional models are, however, unable to capture details of flow structures. If it is essential to capture such flow structures in the simulated results, it is necessary to use three-dimensional models. For example, to evaluate different spargers, it will be necessary to examine the role of unsteady structures on mixing. Ranade and Tayalia (2001) evaluated liquid phase mixing caused by single and double ring spargers using a computational model. They considered an axis-symmetric, two-dimensional domain as well as the full 3D domain (which does not require imposition of symmetry at the column axis). Though estimated volume-averaged quantities such as gas volume fraction, liquid velocity are within 10% for the 2D and 3D models, the details of flow structures are quite different. Typical results obtained for a double-ring sparger are shown in Fig. 11.17. Comparison of the predicted flow field for single and double ring spargers using a 3D model are shown in Fig. 11.18. The complete 3D computational model was able to differentiate between single and double ring spargers and can, therefore, be used to evaluate different spargers. Recently Padial *et al.* (2000) used a three-dimensional model to evaluate the influence of size and location of draft tube on the fluid dynamics of bubble column reactors. Such models can then be extended to simulate the influence of draft tube on mixing in bubble column reactors.

Once a small number of reactor configurations have been short-listed based on the CFD models discussed above, more rigorous simulations and rigorous experimental verification (and calibration, if necessary) of the computational models can be undertaken. The behavior of gas–liquid dispersions is known to be very sensitive to impurities and therefore it is essential to undertake a systematic experimental program at this stage. Scale-down methodologies should be used to arrive at a suitable experimental program. These small-scale experiments are invariably carried out in

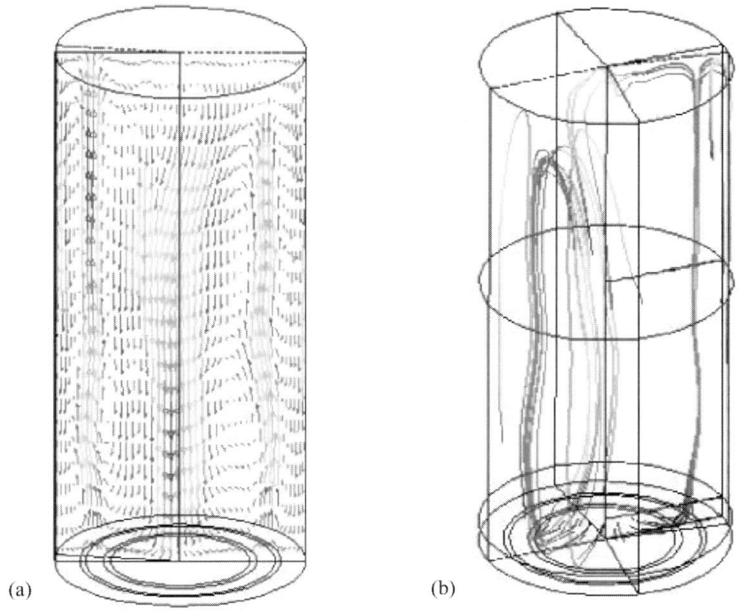

FIGURE 11.17 Typical results obtained for double ring sparger (From Ranade and Tayalia, 2001). (a) Vector plot, (b) particle streak lines.

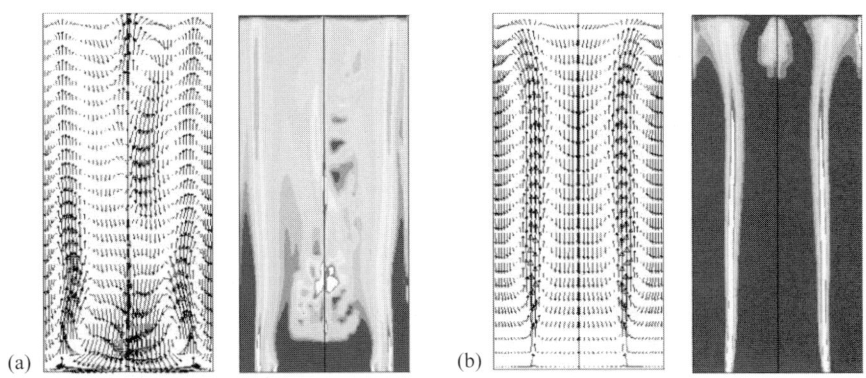

FIGURE 11.18 Comparison of predicted flow field for double (a) and single (b) ring spargers (from Ranade and Tayalia, 2001).

simple geometries and different conditions than actual operating conditions. Available information on the influence of pressure and temperature should be used to select appropriate model fluids for these experiments. Detailed CFD models should then be developed to simulate the fluid dynamics of a small-scale experimental set-up under representative conditions. The computational model is then enhanced further until it leads to adequately accurate simulations of the observed fluid dynamics. The validated CFD model can then be used to extrapolate the experimental data and to simulate fluid dynamics under actual operating conditions. An example of the application of such a methodology to a loop reactor is discussed in Chapter 9. Here we briefly discuss two recent examples from the published literature.

The first is concerned with optimization of an industrial ozonation reactor (Cockx *et al.*, 1999). Ozonation reactors are used to remove microorganisms or micropollutants from drinking water. The efficiency of these reactors depends on liquid phase mixing (since disinfection kinetics is approximately first order) and gas–liquid mass transfer. Cockx *et al.* (1999) developed a computational model using a Eulerian–Eulerian framework. The model was evaluated first by comparing predicted results with a pilot-scale airlift reactor. Different sub-models, such as drag coefficient, effective bubble diameter and so on, were calibrated to obtain adequate agreement between predicted and experimental results. The computational model was then used to simulate the fluid dynamics and performance of an industrial-scale (350 m^3) ozonation reactor. Although local measurements of flow variables were not available for the industrial-scale reactor, some local measurements of ozone concentrations and residence time distribution data were available. These data were used to validate predictions of the computational model. These comparisons are shown in Fig. 11.19. It can be seen that agreement is adequate for most reactor engineering applications. The validated CFD model was then used to optimize a larger ozonation reactor by suitably modifying internals. The model was used to evaluate alternative reactor configurations and to evolve a final configuration. Initial and modified configurations of

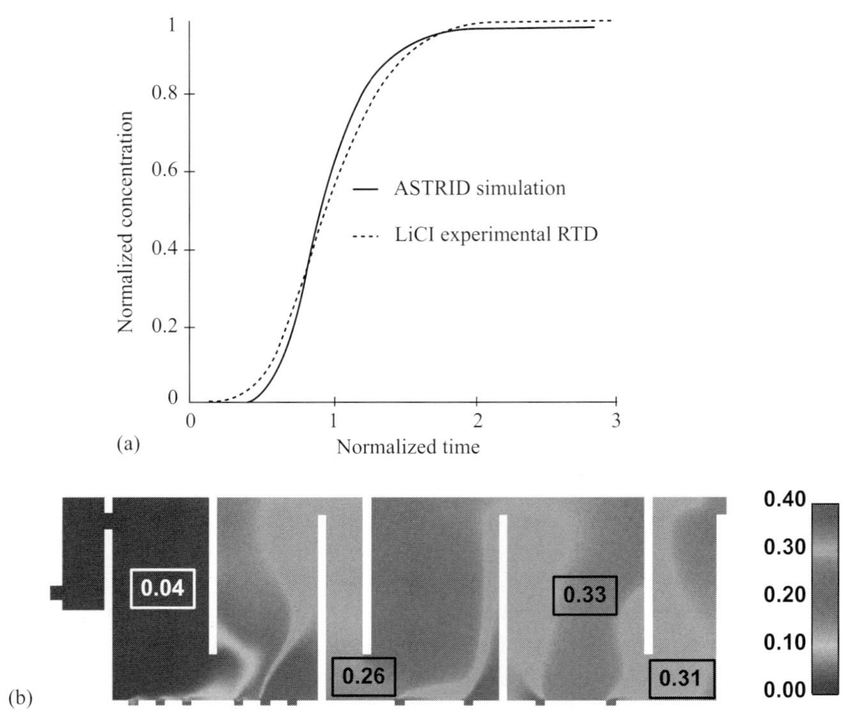

FIGURE 11.19 Validation of computational model (from Cockx *et al.*, 1999). (a) Predicted and measured cumulated tracer plots. (b) Predicted and measured concentration of dissolved ozone (numbers in squares indicate experimental data).

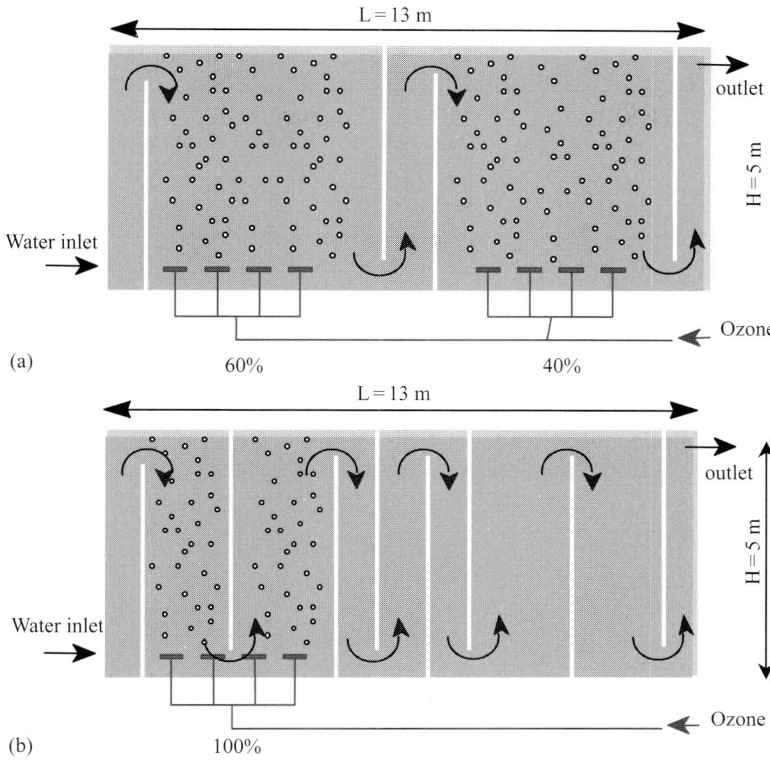

FIGURE 11.20 Initial (a) and modified (b) configurations of industrial ozonation reactor (from Cockx *et al.*, 1999).

ozonation reactor are shown in Fig. 11.20. The proposed modifications led to better hydraulics and a significant increase in ozone transfer efficiency.

The second application deals with simulation of methanol synthesis in gas–liquid slurry bubble column reactors, discussed by Wu and Gidaspow (2000). Most slurry bubble columns are designed using one-dimensional models with empirical correlations of gas volume fractions and other necessary fluid dynamic characteristics. Most of these one-dimensional models assume uniform solid (catalyst) volume fraction over the reactor. Wu and Gidaspow (2000) developed a detailed hydrodynamic model by considering a two-dimensional solution domain. The hydrodynamic model was coupled with the reaction model to simulate overall performance of the methanol synthesis reactor. The comparison of their predicted results and experimental data is shown in Table 11.2. The agreement between predicted results of such a detailed two-dimensional model with experimental data was much better than that observed with predictions of a one-dimensional model. Apart from predicting the realistic values of conversion, the detailed hydrodynamic model provides valuable information on flow structures and their sensitivity with respect to design and operating parameters. Such information is essential for guiding further developments in syn-gas to liquid fuels technology.

As discussed earlier, coalescence break-up models incorporated in detailed CFD models will allow accurate simulation of interfacial area and corresponding mass and

TABLE 11.2 Methanol Synthesis Reactor: Comparison of simulations and experimental data (from Wu and Gidaspow, 2000)

	CO Conversion, %	Gas hold-up, %	Slurry height, in	Total catalyst, kg	Methanol, gmol $h^{-1}kg^{-1}$
Simulation	14.24	26.9	215	740	16.93
RUN E-8.1	13.50	29.5	200	567	20.50

heat transfer. It may, however, be necessary to calibrate the parameters of coalescence and break-up models with the help of experimental data before the combined models can be used to estimate mass transfer performance. Even in the absence of adequate experimental data for calibration purposes, detailed CFD models can be used to qualitatively evaluate different configurations and can identify the most promising sparger and internal designs. The design of feed pipe and product outlets can be evaluated as well, as illustrated by the ozonation reactor case discussed here. Computational flow models and CFD tools play a crucial role in linking actual reactor hardware to reactor performance. These models allow extrapolation of cold flow results to actual operating conditions (high temperature and pressure) and provide detailed information and insight into the reactor flow field. In general, the reactor engineer has to ensure that the computational model contains adequate basic physics, that the numerical implementation is well within the set tolerances, and that simulations capture all the relevant flow features. Judicious use of such computational flow models, (1) to help understand basic phenomena and (2) to simulate complex industrial reactors (using a hierarchy of modeling layers), will lead to better engineering of bubble column reactors.

11.4. SUMMARY

Application of a Eulerian–Eulerian approach to modeling flow in bubble column reactors is discussed in detail. Some recent applications of this and Eulerian–Lagrangian and VOF approaches were reviewed to identify areas which need further research. Despite their limitations, CFD models are capable of predicting the detailed flow field within bubble columns. By devising effective methods to graphically display numerical solutions, many aspects of the flow structure can be carefully studied. Moreover, CFD models may be used to study various aspects of flow fields that are not easily amenable to experimental measurements. Some recent examples of using CFD models to simulate industrial bubble column reactors were discussed. Judicious use of computational models will be useful to qualitatively grade different configurations and may greatly assist the engineering decision-making process. Recent progress in the development of coalescence break-up models may enhance the ability of computational models to make quantitative predictions of mass transfer in bubble column reactors.

REFERENCES

Ahmadi, G. (1987), On the mechanics of incompressible multiphase suspensions, *Adv. Water Res.*, **10**, 32–43.

Auton, T.R. (1983), The dynamics of bubbles, drops and particles in motion in liquids. PhD thesis, University of Cambridge, UK.

Basset, A.B. (1888), "A Treatise on Hydrodynamics", Deighton-Bell, Cambridge.

Becker, S., Sokolichin, A. and Eigenberger, G. (1994), Gas-liquid flow in bubble columns and loop reactors: Part II: Comparison of detailed experiments and flow simulations, *Chem. Eng. Sci.*, **49**, 5747–5762.

Becker, S., De Bie, H. and Sweeney, J. (1999), Dynamic flow behavior in bubble columns, *Chem. Eng. Sci.*, **54**, 4929–4935.

Besnard, D.C. and Harlow, F.H. (1988), Turbulence in multiphase flow, *Int. J. Multiphase Flow*, **14**, 679–699.

Buwa, V. V. and Ranade, V. V. (2000), Modeling of bubble coalescence and breakage processes in gas-liquid flows, NCL Internal report, August 2000.

Carrica, P.M., Drew, D., Bonetto, F. and Lahey, R.T., Jr. (1999), A polydisperse model for bubbly two-phase flow around a surface ship, *Int. J. Multiphase Flow*, **25**, 257–305.

Chen, R.C., Reese, J. and Fan, L.-S. (1994), Flow structure in a three-dimensional bubble column and three-phase fluidized bed, *AIChE J.*, **40**, 1093–1104.

Clark, N.N., Atkinson, C.M. and Flemmer, R.L.C. (1987), Turbulent circulation in bubble columns, *AIChE J.*, **33**, 515.

Clift, R., Grace, J.R. and Weber, M.E. (1978), "Bubbles, Drops and Particles", Academic Press, New York.

Cockx, A., Do-Quang, Z., Line, A. and Roustan, M. (1999), Use of computational fluid dynamics for simulating hydrodynamics and mass transfer in industrial ozonation owers, *Chem. Eng. Sci.*, **54**, 5085–5090.

Cook, T.L. and Harlow, F.H. (1986), Vortices in bubbly two-phase flows, *Int. J. Multiphase Flow*, **12**, 35–43.

Delnoij, E. (1999), Fluid dynamics of gas-liquid bubble columns: A theoretical and experimental study, Doctoral dissertation, Twente University, Enschede, The Netherlands.

Delnoij, E., Lammers, F.A., Kuipers, J.A.M. and van Swaaij, W.P.M. (1997), Dynamic simulation of dispersed gas–liquid two-phase flow using a discrete bubble model, *Chem. Eng. Sci.*, **52**, 1429.

Drew, D.A. (1983), Mathematical modeling of two-phase flow, *Ann. Rev. Fluid Mech.*, **15**, 261.

Drew, D.A., Cheng, L. and Lahey, R.T. Jr. (1979), The analysis of virtual mass effects in two-phase flow, *Int. J. Multiphase Flow*, **5**, 233.

Elghobashi, S.E. and Abou-Arab, T.W. (1983), A two-equation turbulence model for two-phase flows, *Phys. Fluids*, **26**, 931–938.

Grienberger, J. and Hofmann, H. (1992), Investigations and modeling of bubble columns, *Chem. Eng. Sci.*, **47**, 2215–2221.

Hesketh, R.P., Etchells, A.W. and Russell, T.W.F. (1991), Bubble breakage in pipeline flows, *Chem. Eng. Sci.*, **46**, 1–9.

Hillmer, G., Weismantel, L. and Hofmann, H. (1994), Investigations and modeling slurry bubble columns, *Chem. Eng. Sci.*, **49**, 837–843.

Hills, J.H. (1974), Radial non-uniformity of velocity and voidage in a bubble column, *Trans. IChemE*, **52**, 1–9.

Hunt, J.C.R., Auton, T.R., Sene, K., Thomas, N.H. and Kowe, R. (1987), *ICHMT Intn. Seminar on Transient Phenomena in Multiphase Flow*, Dubrovnik, Yugoslavia, May 24–30, 103–125.

Ishii, M. and Zuber, N. (1979), Drag coefficient and relative velocity in bubbly, droplet or particulate flows, *AIChE J.*, **25**, 843–855.

Jakobsen, H.A., Sannaes, B.H., Grevskott, S. and Svendsen, H.F. (1997), Modelling of vertical bubble-driven flows, *Ind. Eng. Chem. Res.*, **36**, 4052–4074.

Johansen, S.T. (1988), On the modeling of dispersed two phase flow, PhD thesis, University of Trondheim, Norway.

Joshi, J.B. and Sharma, M.M. (1979), A circulation cell model for bubble column, *Trans. I. Chem. Eng.*, **57**, 244–251.

Kataoko, I., Besnard, D.C. and Serizawa, A. (1992), Basic equation of turbulence and modeling of interfacial terms in gas–liquid two phase flows, *Chem. Eng. Commun.*, **118**, 221.

Kim, W.K. and Lee, K.L. (1987), Coalescence behavior of two bubbles in stagnant liquids, *J. Chem. Eng. Jpn.*, **20**, 449.

Kirkpatrick, R.D. and Lockett, M.J. (1974), The influence of approach velocity on bubble coalescence, *Chem. Eng. Sci.*, **29**, 2363.

Krishna, R., Ursenau, M.I., van Baten, J.M. and Ellenberger, J. (1999), Rise velocity of swarm of large gas bubbles in liquids, *Chem. Eng. Sci.*, **54**, 171–183.

Krishna, R. and van Baten, J.M. (1999), Simulating the motion of gas bubbles in liquids, *Nature*, **398**, 208.

Krishna, R., van Baten, J.M. and Ursenau, M.I. (2000a), Three-phase Eulerian simulations of bubble column reactors operating in the churn-turbulent regime: a scale-up strategy, *Chem. Eng. Sci.*, **55**, 3275–3286.

Krishna, R., van Baten, J.M. and Urseanu, M.I. and Ellenberger, J. (2000b), Rise velocity of single circular-cap single bubbles in two-dimensional beds of powders and liquids, *Chem. Eng. Proc.*, **39**, 433–440.

Kumar, S.B., Devanathan, N., Moslemian, D. and Dudukovik, M.P. (1994), Effect of scale on liquid circulation in bubble columns, *Chem. Eng. Sci.*, **49**, 5637–5652.

Lahey, R.T. (1987), *ICHMT Int. Seminar on Transient Phenomena in Multiphase Flow*, Dubrovnik, Yugoslavia, May 24–30, pp. 139–177.

Lahey, R.T. and Drew, D.A. (1989), The three-dimensional tune and volume averaged conservation equations for two-phase flows, *Adv. Nucl. Sci. Technol.*, **20**, 1–69.

Lapin, A. and Lubbert, A. (1994), Numerical simulation of the dynamics of two-phase gas-liquid flow in bubble columns, *Chem. Eng. Sci.*, **49**, 3661–3674.

Launder, B.E. and Spalding, D.B. (1972), "Mathematical Models of Turbulence", Academic Press, London.

Lee, S.-Y. and Tsui, Y.P. (1999), Succeed at gas/liquid contacting, *Chem. Eng. Prog.*, **54**, 23–49.

Lehr, F. and Mewes, D. (2001), A transport equation for the interfacial area density applied to bubble columns, *Chem. Eng. Sci.*, **56**, 1159–1166.

Li Yong, Zhang, J. and Fan, L.S. (2000), Discrete-phase simulations of single bubble rise behavior at elevated pressure in a bubble column, *Chem. Eng. Sci.*, **55**, 4597–4609.

Lin, T.J., Reese, J., Hong, T. and Fan, L.S. (1996), Quantitative analysis of and computation of two-dimensional bubble columns, *AIChE J.*, **42**, 301–318.

Lo, S. (2000), Modeling of bubble break-up and coalescence with the MUSIG model, Report No. AEAT-4355, CFX International, UK.

Luo, H. and Svendsen, H.F. (1996), Theoretical model for drop and bubble break-up in turbulent dispersions, *AIChE J.*, **42**, 1225–1233.

Lumley, J.L. (1975), *Lecture Series No. 76*, Von Karmann Institute, Belgium.

Maxey, M.R. and Riley, J.J. (1983), Equation of motion for a small rigid sphere in nonuniform flow, *Phys. Fluids*, **26**, 883.

Menzel, T., Weide, T., Staudacher, O., Wein, O. and Onken, U. (1990), Reynolds shear stress for modelling of bubble column reactors, *Ind. Eng. Chem. Res.*, **29**, 988–994.

Newitt, M.D., Dombrowski, N. and Knelman, F.H. (1954), Liquid entrainment: 1. mechanism of drop formation from gas or vapor bubbles, *Trans. Inst. Chem. Eng.*, **32**, 244.

Padial, N.T., VanderHeyden, W.B., Rauenzahn, R.M. and Yarbro, S.L. (2000), Three-dimensional simulation of a three-phase draft-tube bubble column, *Chem. Eng. Sci.*, **55**, 3261–3273.

Pfleger, D., Gomes, S., Gilbert, N. and Wagner, H.-G. (1999), Hydrodynamic simulations of laboratory scale bubble columns fundamental studies of the Eulerian–Eulerian modeling approach, *Chem. Eng. Sci.*, **54**, 5091–5099.

Prince, M.J. and Blanch, H.W. (1990), Bubble coalescence and break-up in air sparged bubble columns, *AIChE J.*, **36**, 1485–1499.

Ranade, V.V. (1992), Flow in bubble columns: some numerical experiments, *Chem. Eng. Sci.*, **47**, 1857–1869.

Ranade, V.V. (1993a), Turbulent flow and mixing in bubble columns, *Proc. European Symposium on Computer Aided Process Engineering – 3*, Eds Moser, F., Schnitzer and Bart, H. J., pp. 27–31.

Ranade, V.V. (1993b), Numerical simulation of turbulent flow in bubble column reactors, *AIChE Symposium Series no. 293*, **89**, 61–71.

Ranade, V.V. (1997), Modeling of turbulence flow in a bubble column reactor, *Chem. Eng. Res. Des.*, **75**, 14–23.

Ranade, V.V. (1998), Modeling of flow in bubble columns. NCL internal report.

Ranade, V.V. (2000), Modeling of gas–liquid flows in stirred and bubble column reactors, *CPCFD Meeting*, Cincinnati, May 2000.

Ranade, V.V. and Joshi, J.B. (1987), Transport phenomena in multiphase reactors, *Proceedings of International Symposium on Transport Phenomena in Multiphase Systems*, BHU Press, Varanasi, pp. 113–196.

Ranade, V.V. and Mashelkar, R.A. (1993), Turbulent mixing in dilute polymer solutions, *Chem. Eng. Sci.*, **47**, 1619–1628.

Ranade, V.V. and Tayaliya, Y. (2001), Modeling of fluid mechanics and mixing in shallow bubble column reactors: influence of sparger design, *Chem. Eng. Sci.*, **56**, 1667–1675.

Ranade, V.V. and Utikar, R.P. (1999), Dynamics of gas–liquid flows in bubble column reactors, *Chem. Eng. Sci.*, **54**, 5237–5244.

Rietema, K. and van den Akker, H.E.A. (1983), On the momentum equations in dispersed two phase systems, *Int. J. Multiphase Flow*, **9**, 21–36.

Salcudean, M., Lai, K.Y.M. and Guthrie, R.I.L. (1985), Multidimensional heat, mass and flow phenomena in gas–liquid stirred reactors, *Can. J. Chem. Eng.*, **63**, 51–61.

Sato, Y., Sadatomi, M. and Sekoguchi, K. (1981), Momentum and heat transfer in two-phase bubble flow I, *Int. J. Multiphase Flow*, **7**, 167.

Schiller, L. and Naumann, Z. (1935), *Z. Ver. Deutsch. Ing.*, **77**, 318.

Spalding, D.B. (1978), *Second International Conference on Physicochemical Hydrodynamics*, Washington, pp. 421–436.

Sokolichin, A. and Eigenberger, G. (1999), Applicability of standard k–ε turbulence model to the dynamic simulation of bubble columns, *Chem. Eng. Sci.*, **54**, 2273–2284.

Svendsen, H.F., Jakobsen, H.A. and Torvik, R. (1992), Local flow structures in internal loop and bubble column reactors, *Chem. Eng. Sci.*, **47**, 3297–3304.

Thomas, N.H., Auton, S.K. and Hunt, J.C.R. (1983), *Int. Conference on Physical Modeling of Multiphase Flows*, Coventry, UK, pp. 169–181.

Torvik, R. and Svendsen, H.F. (1990), Modelling of slurry reactors: a fundamental approach, *Chem. Eng. Sci.*, **45**, 2325–2333.

Tsuji, Y.-, Morikawa, Y. and Shiomi, H. (1984), LDV measurements of an air-solid flow in a vertical pipe, *J. Fluid Mech.*, **139**, 417–434.

Wu, Y. and Gidaspow, D. (2000), Hydrodynamic simulation of methanol synthesis in gas–liquid slurry bubble column reactors, *Chem. Eng. Sci.*, **55**, 573–587.

Yao, B.P., Zheng, C., Gasche, H.E. and Hofmann, H. (1991), Bubble behavior and flow structure of bubble columns, *Chem. Eng. Proc.*, **29**, 65–75.

APPENDIX 11.1: MULTIGROUP MODEL TO SIMULATE BUBBLE SIZE DISTRIBUTION

In a multigroup model, bubble population is divided into a number of groups and each group is treated as a separate phase. In many cases, it is adequate to associate a single velocity field calculated based on an effective bubble diameter instead of associating separate velocity fields to each bubble group. This approximation significantly reduces the burden on computational resources. In order to simulate bubble size distribution, it is, however, necessary to solve mass balance equations for each bubble group. The multigroup model developed by Buwa and Ranade (2000) is described here.

Their formulation is based on the concept that the entire bubble population can be described in terms of mass (or diameter) of the smallest bubble. It is assumed that the mass of any bubble in the considered population will be an integer multiple of the mass of the smallest bubble, $m_{\min}$. The simplest way to describe the bubble size distribution in such circumstances will be to define $(m_{\max}/m_{\min})$ number of bubble groups, where $m_{\max}$ is the mass of the largest bubble that can be envisaged in the considered bubble population. However, it can be seen that such a description will require an inordinately large number of bubble groups (1000 groups to describe a population with smallest bubble of 1 mm and largest bubble of 10 mm). Fortunately such a high resolution

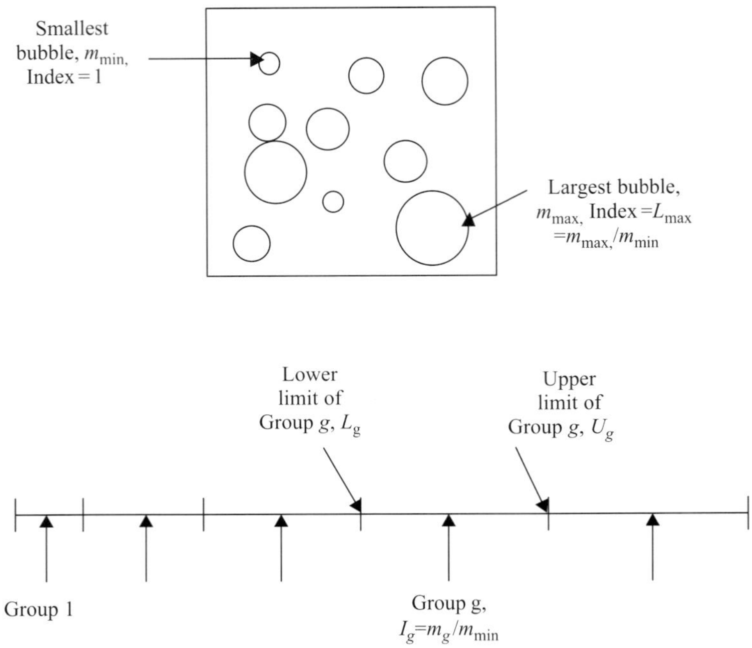

FIGURE 11A.1 Multigroup model to describe bubble population.
Notes: (1) Lower and upper limits are inclusive in a particular group and are integer (multiples of mass of minimum bubble). This means, $L_g = U_{g-1} + 1$. (2) Central index associated with the group, I_g is defined as algebraic mean of lower and upper limits.

of the bubble size distribution is seldom required. It is adequate to lump bubbles of different sizes into a single group and to describe the entire bubble population using 5 to 20 non-uniform sub-groups. The choice of boundaries between these sub-groups depends on bubble size distribution itself and may have to be finalized by examining the predictions (following a procedure similar to that for selection of grid distribution for flow simulations). The approach and notation used by Buwa and Ranade (2000) to describe classification of bubble population in terms of different groups is shown in Fig. 11A.1. The mass conservation equation for any individual bubble group, g, can then be written as:

$$\frac{\partial}{\partial t}(\rho_G \varepsilon_{Gg}) + \frac{\partial}{\partial x_j}(\rho_G \varepsilon_{Gg} U_{Ggj}) = m_g\{C_g^+ - C_g^- + B_g^+ - B_g^-\} \qquad (11A.1)$$

where C_g and B_g represent loss (superscript $-$) or gain (superscript $+$) in the number of bubbles of group 'g' due to coalescence and breakup respectively. Following the principles of population balance, the loss and gain terms can be expressed as

$$C_g^+ = \frac{1}{2}\sum_{k=1}^{g} K_{Ckl} P_{Ckl} n_k n_l X_{gkl} \quad \because \quad L_g \le I_k + I_l \le U_g, \;\; X_{gkl} = \frac{I_k + I_l}{I_g} \qquad (11A.2)$$

$$C_g^- = \sum_{k=1}^{NG} K_{Cgk} P_{Cgk} n_g n_k \quad \because \quad U_g < I_g + I_k \le U_{NG} \qquad (11A.3)$$

where n_g is bubble number density of group g, NG is total number of bubble groups, K_{Cgk} is rate of coalescence of bubbles of group g and k and P_{Cgk} is probability of coalescence of bubbles of group g and k. X_{gkl} accounts for the intergroup transfer due to coalescence.

$$B_g^+ = 2\sum_{k=g}^{NG} K_{\mathrm{B}k} n_k \phi_{gk} \quad \because \quad \phi_{gk} = \sum_{i=L_g}^{U_g} \frac{P_{\mathrm{B}ki}}{\sum_{j=1}^{I_k-1} P_{\mathrm{B}j,I_k-1-j}} \frac{im_{\min}}{m_g} \tag{11A.4}$$

$$B_g^- = K_{Bg} n_g \tag{11A.5}$$

where $K_{\mathrm{B}k}$ is the total breakage rate of bubbles of group 'k', $P_{\mathrm{B}ki}$ is the probability of formation of a bubble with mass '$im_{\min}$' from a bubble of group 'k'. The term $\sum_{j=1}^{I_k-1} P_{\mathrm{B}j,I_k-1-j}$ represents sum of probabilities of bubble of group 'k' breaking with breakage fraction varying from $m_{\min}/m_k$ to $(I_k-1)m_{\min}/m_k$. The term ϕ_{gk} signifies the number of group 'g' bubbles formed per number of group 'k' bubbles broken. Note that this formulation conserves mass but does not conserve bubble numbers. Suitable modifications may however be made to ensure conservation of bubble numbers and/or interfacial area while retaining the same overall structure.

Several authors have proposed different models to describe the bubble coalescence and breakage processes (Prince and Blanch, 1990; Hesketh *et al.*, 1991; Luo and Svendsen, 1996; Carrica *et al.*, 1999; Lehr and Mewes, 2001). Bubble coalescence and breakage may occur by different mechanisms. Local turbulence in the liquid phase, velocity gradients and shear flows are known to cause bubble coalescence. Similarly, collision of a bubble with energetic eddies in the liquid phase or other phenomena such as tip streaming are known to cause bubble breakage. In most gas–liquid reactors, turbulence-induced breakage and coalescence were found to be dominant in comparison with other mechanisms (Prince and Blanch, 1990). Buwa and Ranade (2000) compared magnitudes of different mechanisms and have recommended the turbulence induced collision model of Prince and Blanch (1990) to describe bubble coalescence, and the turbulent eddy interaction model of Luo and Svendsen (1996) to describe the bubble breakage process. These models were used to close the set of mass conservation equations of bubble groups described above:

$$K_{\mathrm{C}kl} = 0.35\pi(d_k + d_l)^{1/3}\varepsilon^{1/3}\left(d_k^{2/3} + d_l^{2/3}\right)^{1/2} \tag{11A.6}$$

$$P_{\mathrm{C}kl} = \exp\left\{\frac{-t_{kl}}{\tau_{kl}}\right\} \quad \because \quad t_{kl} = \left\{\frac{r_{kl}^3 \rho_l}{16\sigma}\right\}^{1/2} \ln\frac{h_o}{h_f},$$

$$\tau_{kl} = \left\{\frac{r_{kl}^{2/3}}{\varepsilon^{1/3}}\right\}, \quad r_{kl} = \frac{1}{4}\left(\frac{1}{d_k} + \frac{1}{d_l}\right)^{-1} \tag{11A.7}$$

$$K_{\mathrm{B}k} = 0.923(1-\alpha_{\mathrm{G}})\left(\varepsilon^{1/3} d_k^{-2/3}\right)\frac{1}{2}\left\{\int_{f_{\mathrm{BV,min}}}^{f_{\mathrm{BV,max}}}\int_{\xi_{\min}}^{1}(1+\xi)^2\xi^{-11/3}\exp\{-\chi_k\}\,d\xi\,df_{\mathrm{BV}}\right\} \tag{11A.8}$$

$$\chi_k = \left\{\frac{12\left[f_{\mathrm{BV}}^{2/3} - (1-f_{\mathrm{BV}})^{2/3} - 1\right]\sigma}{\beta\rho_c \varepsilon^{2/3} d_k^{5/3}\xi^{11/3}}\right\} \quad \because \quad f_{\mathrm{BV}} = \frac{im_{\min}}{m_k} \tag{11A.9}$$

$$P_{\mathrm{B}ki} = \int_{\xi_{\min}}^{1} \exp\{-\chi_k\}\,d\xi \tag{11A.10}$$

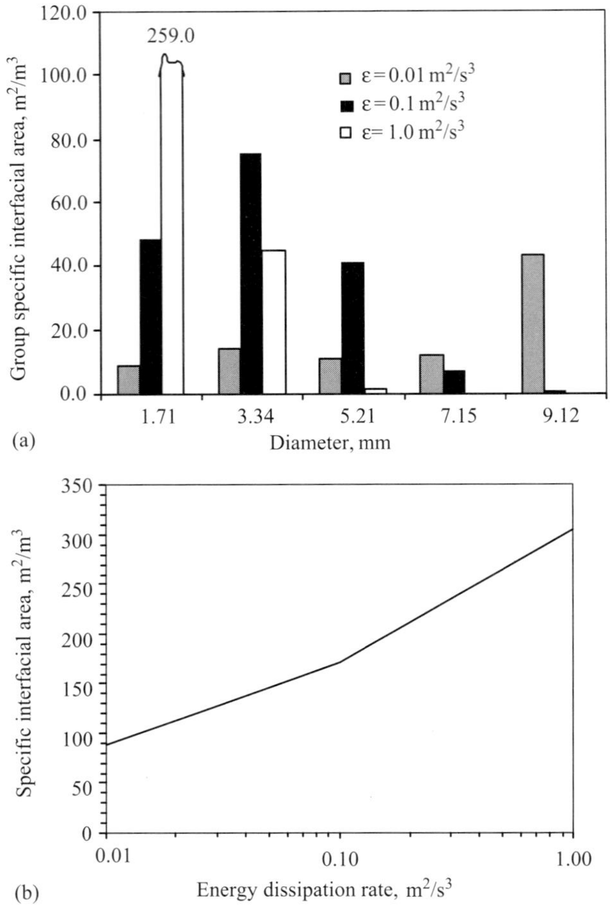

FIGURE 11A.2 Predicted equilibrium bubble size distribution at three values of turbulent energy dissipation rates. Effect of energy dissipation rate on (a) group mass fraction and (b) total surface area.

d_k and r_k denote the diameter and radius of bubbles of group k. f_{BV} is a breakage fraction and is defined in Eq. (11A.9), h_0 and h_f, used in Eq. (11A.7), denote initial and critical film (between two coalescing bubbles) thickness and are usually assumed to be 1×10^{-4} m (Kirkpatrick and Lockett, 1974) and 1×10^{-8} m (Kim and Lee, 1987). Typical equilibrium bubble size distributions predicted by this model at three different values of turbulent energy dissipation rates and corresponding total interfacial area are shown in Fig. 11A.2a and 11A.2b respectively. As expected, the model predicts the shift towards finer bubble sizes at higher values of turbulent energy dissipation rates. Ongoing and future experimental and modeling studies are expected to lead towards enhanced understanding and better predictive capabilities. For example, recently Lehr and Mewes (2001) have proposed a new model to describe bubble breakage process, which was found to improve the predictions of bubble size distribution. Such new models of coalescence and breakage can be incorporated in the overall framework discussed here.

12 FLUIDIZED BED REACTORS

Fluidized bed reactors offer the advantages of excellent solid mixing and heat transfer characteristics. These reactors find widespread applications in the chemical, petrochemical, metallurgical and energy industries. Some typical applications involving gas–solid fluidized bed reactors are listed in Table 12.1. Flow regimes prevailing in these fluidized bed reactors are also listed in this table. Despite the widespread use, the complex hydrodynamics of fluidized bed reactors is still not completely understood. Several different flow regimes may exist in the reactor as detailed in Table 12.1. Depending on these flow regimes and different configurations, several varieties of fluidized bed reactors are used in practice, as shown in Fig. 12.1. Application of computational flow modeling to the reactor engineering of these fluidized bed reactors is briefly discussed in this chapter.

Before we discuss reactor-engineering issues of fluidized bed reactors, we briefly describe flow regimes and their identification. A discussion on the basics of modeling multiphase flows and possible approaches was given in Chapter 4. With reference to that discussion, we include here a brief review of CFD modeling of fluidized bed reactors and guidelines for selection/development of appropriate flow models to simulate the most commonly encountered flow regimes in fluidized bed reactors. Despite the significant progress made in recent decades, several questions and issues concerning the rigorous modeling of gas–solid fluidized beds remain unanswered. The consequences and implications of not understanding some of these issues on reactor engineering applications are discussed. Despite these, ways of fruitfully using

TABLE 12.1 Some Industrial Applications of Fluidized Bed Reactors

Processes/applications	Operating regime
Fluidized bed catalytic cracking (FCC)	Riser reactor: fast-fluidized bed regime Regenerator: bubbling bed/turbulent fluidized bed regime
Maleic anhydride/phthalic anhydride	Turbulent fluidized bed regime
Acrylonitrile	Bubbling/turbulent bed regime
Ethylene dichloride	Bubbling/turbulent bed regime
Polymerization of olefins (polyethylene/polypropylene)	Bubbling/turbulent fluidized bed regime
Coal gasification	Turbulent fluidized bed regime
Fischer–Tropsch synthesis	Dense phase/fast-fluidized bed regime
Acrylonitrile/metacrylonitrile	Bubbling/turbulent bed regime
Calcination/roasting of ores	Bubbling/turbulent bed regime
Incineration of solid waste	Bubbling/turbulent bed regime

computational fluid dynamic models of gas–solid fluidized bed reactors are presented with the help of some examples.

12.1. ENGINEERING FLUIDIZED BED REACTORS

It must be noted that different flow regimes have quite different hydrodynamic characteristics and therefore, it is essential to identify the desired or prevailing flow regime in the fluidized bed reactor. An ideal situation is to have a comprehensive flow model which will *a priori* predict the prevailing flow regime. However, knowledge of the prevailing flow regime and development of a computational flow model specifically tailored to the prevailing regime leads to more reliable simulations. Such an approach is used to carry out most simulations of industrial fluidized bed reactors. Before we describe computational models for specific flow regimes, the characteristics of various flow regimes and their identification is discussed briefly below.

12.1.1. Gas–Solid Flows in Fluidized Bed Reactors

When gas is passed through a bed of solid particles, various types of flow regime, ranging from fixed bed to pneumatic conveying, are observed. The prevailing flow regime and quality of fluidization depend on several factors. Operating conditions, solids flow rate (flux), gas flow rate (flux) and system configuration affect the prevailing flow regime. In addition, the properties of solid particles (size distribution, shape, density, and restitution coefficient) significantly affect the quality of fluidization. Geldart (1973) suggested a simple, four-group classification of solids within which the range of bed behavior can be categorized based on particle density and particle size (Geldart's classification is shown in Fig. 12.2.):

- Group C: This class of solids includes very fine and cohesive powders, e.g. cement, flour, starch etc. With this class, normal fluidization is extremely difficult and channeling takes place when fluidized.

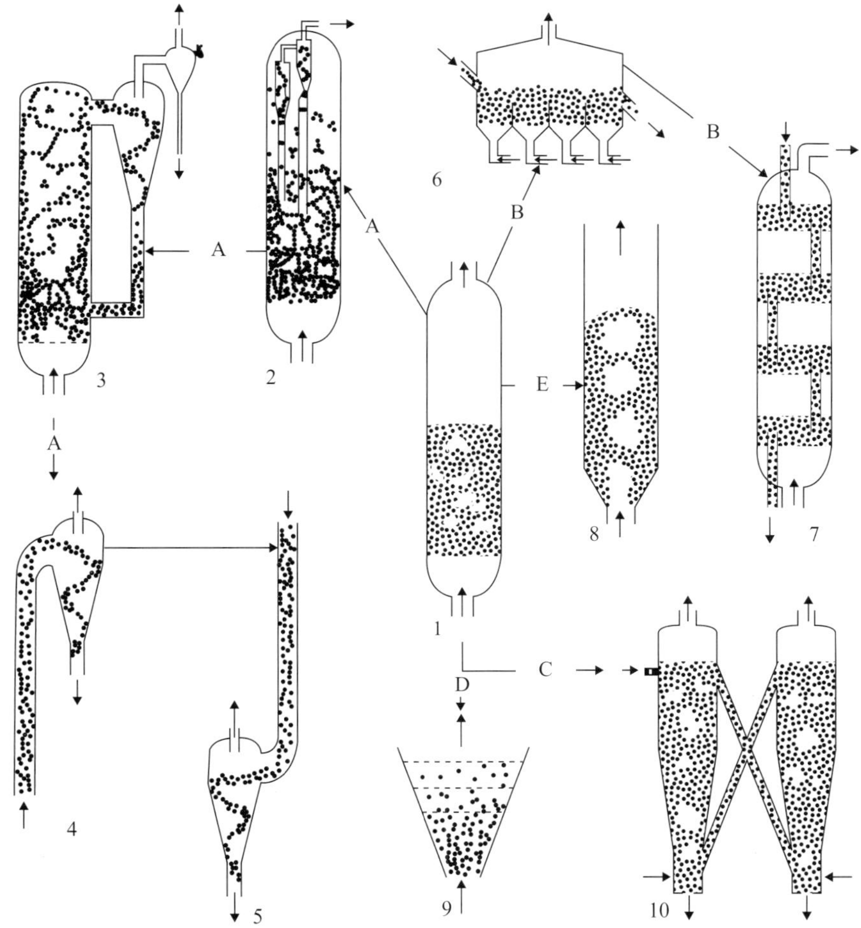

Reactor type

1: Bubbling fluidized bed reactor
2: Turbulent fluidized bed reactor
3: Circulating fluidized bed reactor
4: Riser reactor
5: Downer reactor
6: Cross-current fluidized bed reactor
7: Counter-current fluidized bed reactor
8: Spouted bed reactor
9: Floating fluidized bed reactor
10: Twin fluidized bed reactor

Key issues

A: Higher gas velocity
B: Counter-current contacting is beneficial
C: Incompatible differences in desired environment
D: Dusty environment
E: Large particles/low gas load

FIGURE 12.1 Types of fluidized bed reactors (from Kuipers *et al.*, 1998).

- Group A: Solid particles having a small mean particle size or low particle density ($<\sim 1500\,\mathrm{kg\,m^{-3}}$). Typical examples of this class are catalysts used for fluid catalytic cracking (FCC) processes. These solids fluidize easily, with smooth fluidization at low gas velocity and bubbling/turbulent fluidization at higher velocity.

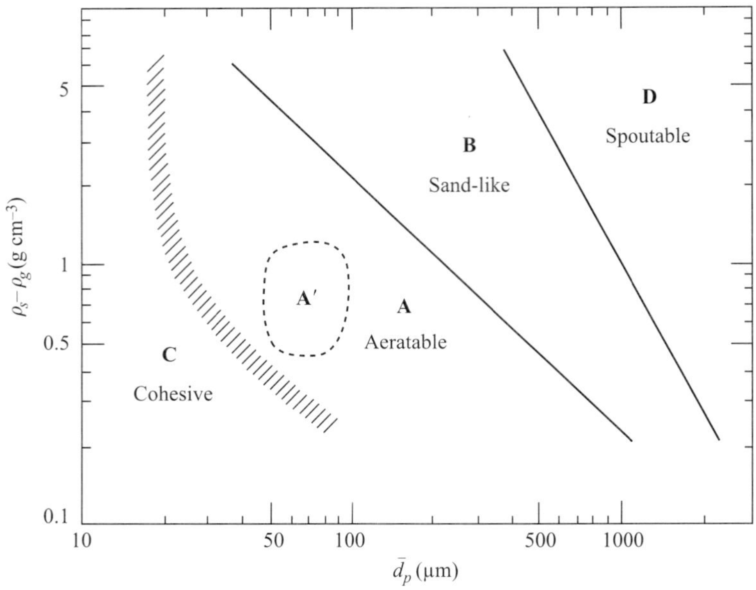

FIGURE 12.2 The Geldart classification of particles for air at ambient conditions. Region A′: Range of properties for well-behaved FCC catalyst (from Kunii and Levenspiel, 1991).

- Group B: Solids having particle size 40 μm $< d_p <$ 500 μm and density in the range $1400 < \rho_s < 4000\,\text{kg m}^{-3}$. These solids fluidize vigorously with formation of bubbles, which grow in size; e.g. sand particles.
- Group D: These solid particles are large and/or dense and are spoutable. Large exploding bubbles or severe channeling may occur in fluidization of group D solids.

Apart from density and particle size as used in Geldart's classification, several other solid properties, including angularity, surface roughness and composition may also significantly affect quality of fluidization (Grace, 1992 and references cited therein). However, Geldart's classification chart often provides a useful starting point to examine fluidization quality of a specific gas–solid system. Reactor configuration, gas superficial velocity and solids flux are other important parameters controlling the quality of fluidization. At low gas velocity, solids rest on the gas distributor and the regime is a fixed bed regime. Some commonly encountered gas–solid flow regimes are shown in Fig. 1.9. The relationship between these flow regimes, type of solid particles and gas velocity is shown schematically in Fig. 12.3. When superficial gas velocity increases, a point is reached beyond which the bed is fluidized. At this point all the particles are just suspended by upward flowing gas. The frictional force between particle and gas just counterbalances the weight of the particle. This gas velocity at which fluidization begins is known as minimum fluidization velocity (U_{mf}). The bed is considered to be just fluidized, and is referred to as a bed at minimum fluidization. If gas velocity increases beyond minimum fluidization velocity, homogeneous (or smooth) fluidization may exist for the case of fine solids up to a certain velocity limit. Beyond this limit (U_{mb}: minimum bubbling velocity), bubbling starts. For large solids, the bubbling regime starts immediately

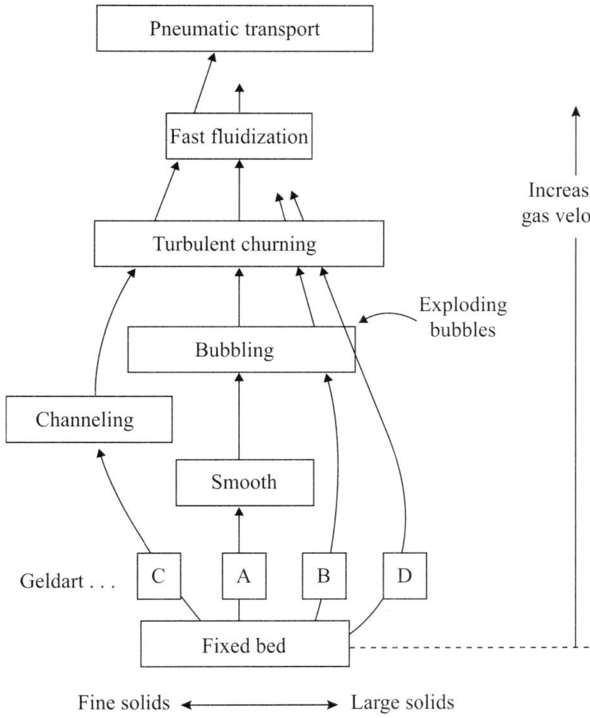

FIGURE 12.3 Progressive change in gas–solids contact (flow regimes) with change in gas velocity (from Kunii and Levenspiel, 1991).

if the gas velocity is higher than minimum fluidization velocity ($U_{mb} = U_{mf}$). With an increase in velocity beyond minimum bubbling velocity, large instabilities with bubbling and channeling of gas are observed. At high gas velocities, the movement of solids becomes more vigorous. Such a bed is called a bubbling bed or heterogeneous fluidized bed (Fig. 1.9). In this regime, gas bubbles generated at the distributor coalesce and grow as they rise through the bed. For deep beds of small diameter, these bubbles eventually become large enough to spread across the diameter of the vessel. This is called a slugging bed regime. In large diameter columns, if gas velocity increases still further, then instead of slugs, turbulent motion of solid clusters and voids of gas of various size and shape are observed. Entrainment of solids becomes appreciable. This regime is called a turbulent fluidized bed regime (Fig. 1.9, Fig. 12.3). With further increase in gas velocity, solids entrainment becomes very high so that gas–solid separators (cyclones) become necessary. This regime is called a fast fluidization regime. For a pneumatic transport regime, even higher gas velocity is needed, which transports all the solids out of the bed. As one can imagine, the characteristics of gas–solid flows of these different regimes are strikingly different. It is, therefore, necessary to determine the prevailing flow regime in order to select an appropriate mathematical model to represent it.

Several regime maps have been proposed in the literature. One widely used regime map developed by Grace (1986) is shown in Fig. 12.4. This map is developed

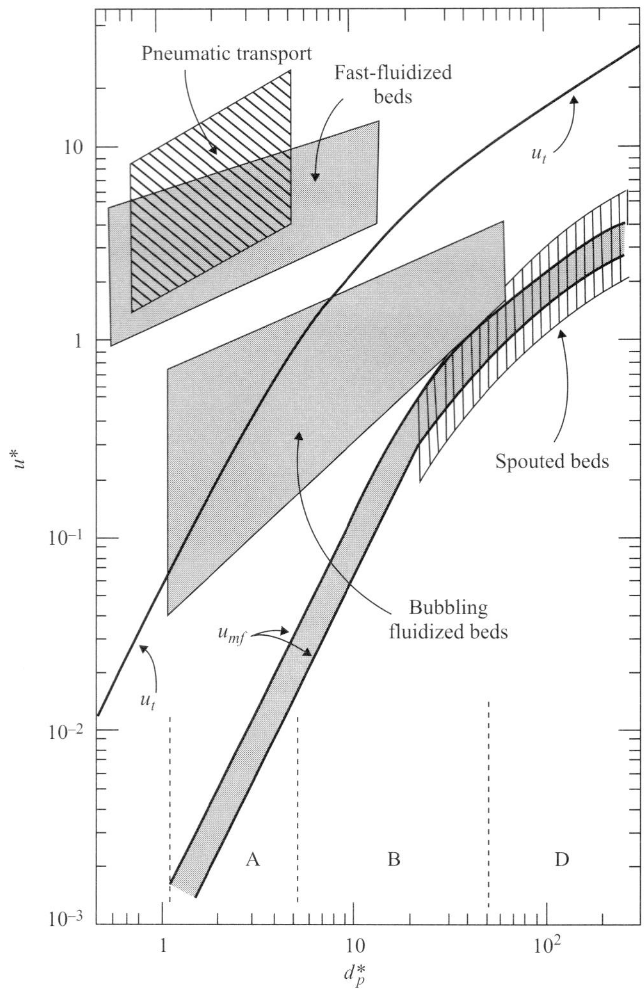

$$u^* = u\left[\frac{\rho_G^2}{\mu(\rho_S - \rho_G)g}\right]^{1/3} \qquad d_p^* = d_p\left[\frac{\rho_G(\rho_S - \rho_G)g}{\mu^2}\right]^{1/3}$$

FIGURE 12.4 General flow regime map for gas–solids flows (from Kunii and Levenspiel, 1991).

using two dimensionless numbers defined in Fig. 12.4. The main conclusions to be drawn from this regime map can be summarized as follows:

- For fine solids (class A and B), stable operation of a bubbling bed exists over a wide range of operating conditions. For larger particles (class D), the operating range is relatively narrow.
- For small particles, bubbling starts at a gas velocity much higher than minimum fluidization velocity (3–8 times U_{mf}) and continues way beyond the terminal velocity U_t. For large particles, bubbling occurs at a gas velocity close to U_{mf}.

- Fast fluidization is possible for small particles at very high gas velocity (around 1000 U_{mf}).

There are several empirical correlations to predict minimum fluidization velocity and minimum bubbling velocity, which can be used to examine whether bubbles will exist or not (see for example, correlations summarized by Kunii and Levenspiel, 1991). Generally, most of these correlations predict similar results for fine particles ($<100\ \mu m$). However, for large solid particles, there is a considerable scatter in the predictions of different published correlations. When there is a wide size distribution and non-spherical particles, it is often necessary to use experiments to make reliable estimates of minimum fluidization and minimum bubbling velocity. Bubbles in a bubbling bed can be quite irregular in shape and vary greatly in size. In beds of fine solid particles, bubbles grow quickly to a few centimeters in size and remain at that size as a result of equilibrium between coalescence and splitting. For larger particle beds, bubbles grow steadily in the bed and reach tens of centimeters in size. Several correlations have been proposed to estimate bubble sizes and bubble growth in fluidized beds (Mori and Wen, 1975; Darton *et al.*, 1977; Werther, 1978 and so on). Similarly several correlations have been proposed to estimate bubble rise velocity (Davidson and Harrison, 1963; Werther, 1983). Since the types of turbulent fluidized bed regime are not very well defined, the transition between bubbling bed and turbulent regime and that between turbulent and fast fluidization regime, are also not very clearly defined. A recent review by Bi *et al.* (2000) may be consulted to estimate these transition velocities. With this brief introduction to gas–solid flows in fluidized bed reactors, major reactor engineering issues, conventional design practices and the role of computational flow modeling to facilitate better reactor engineering are discussed below.

12.1.2. Reactor Engineering

For good reactor operation, it is desirable to realize effective gas and solid contact leading to maximum mass and energy exchange between gas and solid particles. The objective of a reactor engineer is to realize such an effective gas–solid contact without compromising other desirable characteristics such as residence time distribution (RTD), backmixing and so on. Prevailing flow regimes obviously play an important role in determining gas–solid contacting characteristics.

Bubbling fluid beds are generally used when excellent solids mixing and bed to wall heat transfer characteristics are desired. RTD and degree of backmixing is a strong function of such bubbling characteristics as mean bubble size, size distribution, bubble rise velocity, bubbling frequency and bubble shape. Knowledge of bubble size and rise velocity can then be used to estimate transport coefficient between bubble and dense phase and also to estimate solids circulation and mixing. Studies indicate that the fluidized bed reactor can be operated in different modes either to promote solid mixing or segregation. In bubbling fluidized beds, bubbling of gas causes gross circulation of solid particles. When a bed of wide particle size distribution and of widely varying density is fluidized, denser particles tend to settle at the bottom of the bed. This phenomenon is counter-balanced by circulation of solids. At very large gas velocity ($U_o \gg U_{mf}$, where U_o is superficial gas velocity) solids circulation dominates the process and at gas velocity close to U_{mf} solids segregation dominates the process. Mixing and segregation of solids in the bed is set up by the dynamic equilibrium between the two competing mechanisms.

From a reactor engineering point of view, macroscale circulation of solid particles enhances backmixing, which lowers the conversion and selectivity of the fluidized bed reactor. In bubbling fluidized beds, severe by-passing of reactant gas is possible through fast rising large gas bubbles. It is generally believed that gas by-passing can be avoided in high velocity fluidized beds (turbulent or fast-fluidization regimes). High velocity fluidized bed reactors are attractive for high-pressure applications, since the reactor diameter is reduced for the same gas throughput.

In riser reactors, which are operated in a fast-fluidized regime ($U_o > 20U_t$, where U_o is gas superficial velocity and U_t is terminal settling velocity of solid particles), solids backmixing and radial distribution of solids play a central role in determining overall performance. Fast-fluidized beds are characterized by downflow of solids in the near wall region and upflow of solids through the central core. Solid volume fractions exhibit distinct peaks near the walls. In order to make realistic simulations, it is essential to predict such wall peaking of solids volume fraction accurately. The possibility of formation of clusters and their influence on the efficiency of gas–solid contacting is also an important design issue. Clusters formation and their properties are not yet well understood and several conflicting reports about their significance have been published (see a review by Chen, 1995). Cluster formation may increase or decrease local transport coefficient and may alter the fluid dynamics of riser reactors. Compared to the large body of empirical information/correlations available for the case of bubbling beds, empirical information available for fast-fluidized bed reactors and turbulent fluidized bed reactors is much less and contains a significant amount of scatter (Zijerveld, 1998; Venderbosch, 1998; Bi *et al.*, 2000 for reviews of recent data).

Conventional design practices involve making use of such accumulated empirical information to develop reaction-engineering models (two- or three-phase models for bubbling beds and axial dispersion models for turbulent and fast fluidized beds). Such models are invariably based on very simplified fluid dynamics (Kunii and Levenspiel, 1991). These models are used to understand the sensitivity of reactor performance to operating and model parameters. In many cases, transition from bubbling to turbulent fluidization is not sharp and significant uncertainty exists about the location of the transition. Thompson *et al.* (1999) developed a generalized bubbling-turbulent (GBT) model based on a probabilistic approach to overcome such difficulties. Kunii and Levenspiel (2000) recently discussed a reaction-engineering model for circulating fluidized beds operated in a fast-fluidized regime. These models and sensitivity studies using these models, coupled with prior experience in designing fluidized bed reactors, are used to evolve an experimental program to collect the required information about hydrodynamics with adequate accuracy. Experimental data obtained at two or more scales is then used to develop an appropriate fluid dynamic basis for the specific gas–solid system under consideration. This information is used again with reactor performance models to evaluate designs of industrial fluidized bed reactors. Scale-up experiments need to be carried out to ensure that the hydrodynamics of large-scale industrial reactors (with different gas distributors and internals) is not very different from that of pilot-scale reactors showing satisfactory reactor performance. Obviously, such a procedure restricts options for reactor configurations and it also has a significant amount of uncertainty due to the empiricism employed.

Moreover, these conventional models are not useful to understand the influence of details of the hardware configuration on reactor performance. Detailed hydrodynamic models are necessary to resolve hardware-related issues. For example, distributor design of an industrial fluidized bed reactor involve several aspects including shape and location of distributor, number of holes, distribution of holes, orientation of holes and so on. Empirical information suggests that if pressure drop across the distributor is small (less than 20% of the pressure drop across the fluidized bed), gas mal-distribution and by-passing (due to formation of large bubbles at the distributor holes) may occur. This information is not adequate to optimize distributor design and to estimate its influence on gas and solid dynamics within the fluidized bed. Non-optimum distribution of holes may result in local settling of solids and may lead to erosion-related problems, as was mentioned for the OXY reactor case in Chapter 9. Similar comments are applicable to designing the feed nozzle system (diameter, shape, orientation, number of nozzles, location of nozzles and so on). Feed nozzle design affects local gas–(liquid–)solid contacting and therefore, overall performance. To design improved feed systems for riser or bubbling bed reactors, detailed knowledge of local fluid dynamics is necessary. Apart from the distributor and feed nozzle design, to resolve other reactor-engineering issues such as designing internals etc. it would be necessary to develop detailed fluid dynamic models. In analyzing important issues such as the formation of local hot spots, by-passing, solids entrainment in a free board and so on, CFD-based models can contribute uniquely. With such contributions, computational flow modeling may greatly accelerate the entire reactor development program with enhanced confidence levels and better performance. CFD models can significantly reduce the demands on pilot planting by providing efficient and effective interpolation and extrapolation tools. A typical reactor engineering program for fluidized bed reactors based on CFD models is shown in Fig. 12.5.

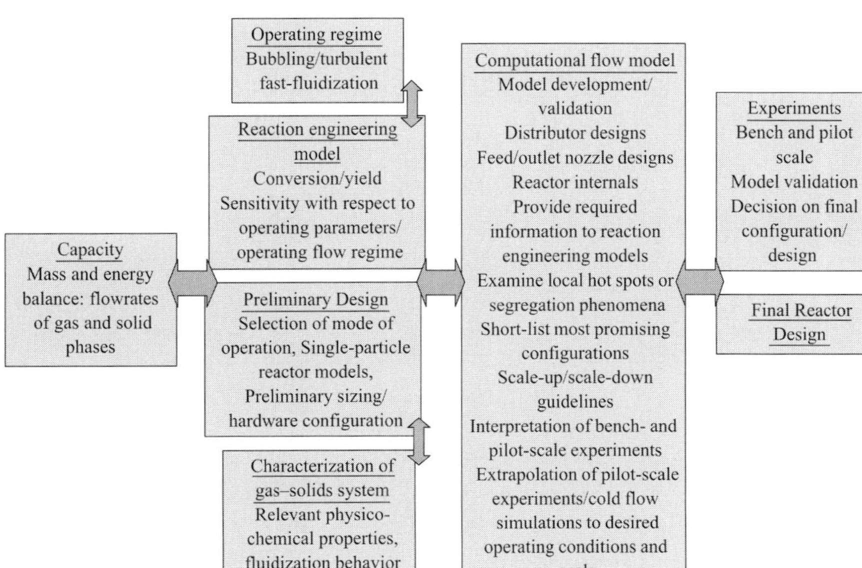

FIGURE 12.5 Reactor engineering of fluidized bed reactors.

It should, however, be noted that the physics of gas–solid contacting is extremely complex, and as yet, has defied rigorous representation in mathematical models. As shown in Fig. 12.5, some experimentation will be necessary. Keeping the specific objectives in mind, the reactor engineer has to judiciously formulate a model for the reactor. Key predictions of such a model need to be validated by comparison with experimental data before they can be used for reactor engineering applications (to evaluate different configurations, to short-list the most promising ones, to provide the relevant information of fluid dynamics to the reaction engineering models, to optimize distributor, feed system and reactor internals, to scale-up and to scale-down and so on). As mentioned in previous chapters, it is necessary to use different modeling approaches (hierarchy of models) to construct a useful picture of industrial fluidized bed reactors. A brief review of modeling strategies and some recent results are discussed in the following section. Some applications of CFD models to reactor engineering are then discussed.

12.2. CFD MODELING OF GAS–SOLID REACTORS

Basic approaches to modeling gas–solid flows, namely, Eulerian–Eulerian and Eulerian–Lagrangian, are discussed in Chapter 4. For gas–solid flow modeling, usually, Eulerian–Lagrangian models are called discrete particle models and Eulerian–Eulerian models are called granular flow models. Granular flow models (GFM) are continuum based and are more suitable for simulating large and complex industrial fluidized bed reactors containing billions of solid particles. These models, however, require information about solid phase rheology and particle–particle interaction laws. In principle, discrete particle models (DPM) can supply such information. DPMs in turn need closure laws to model fluid–particle interactions and particle–particle interaction parameters based on contact theory and material properties. The interrelationship between various models is schematically shown in Fig. 12.6. In principle, it is possible to work our way upwards from direct solution of Navier–Stokes

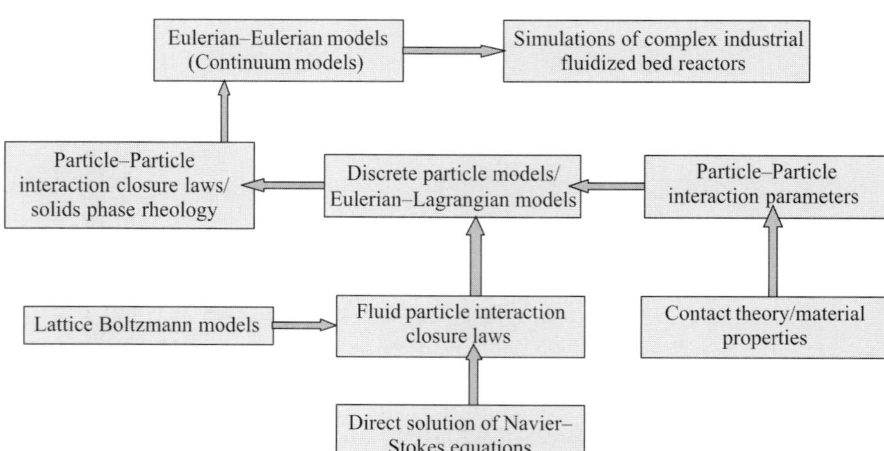

FIGURE 12.6 Hierarchy of models for the simulation of gas–solids fluidized bed reactors.

equations, lattice-Boltzmann models and contact theory to obtain all the necessary closure laws and other parameters required for granular flow models. However, with the present state of knowledge, complete *a priori* simulations are not possible. It is necessary to use these different models judiciously, combined with key experiments, to obtain the desired engineering information about gas–solid flows in industrial equipment. Direct solution of Navier–Stokes equations or lattice Boltzmann methods are too computation intensive to simulate even thousands of solid particles, rather than millions of particles. DPMs are usually used to gain an insight into various vexing issues such as bubble or cluster formations and their characteristics or segregation phenomena. A few hundred thousand particles can be considered in such DPMs. The understanding developed and simulation results are either directly or indirectly used to develop granular flow models. Applications of DPM and GFM to simulate gas–solid flows in riser and bubbling/turbulent bed reactors are discussed in the following sections.

12.2.1. Discrete Particle Models (DPM)

In discrete particle models, continuous phase (gas phase) is modeled using Eulerian framework. The trajectories of dispersed phase (solid phase) are then modeled in a Lagrangian framework. Acceleration of individual particles of dispersed phase is calculated from a force balance over that particle. Particle trajectories are then simulated using the flow field of gas phase. Basic governing equations are described in Chapter 4. Based on a large number of particle trajectories, desired characteristics of the gas–solid flow can be evaluated. The basic framework can be extended to include two-way coupling between gas and solid phases as well as four-way coupling to include particle–particle interactions. For most fluidized bed reactor applications, it is necessary to include the influence of particle collisions on the dynamics of gas–solid flows. To simulate particle–particle collisions, two approaches may be used: in the first approach, particle interaction times are assumed to be very small compared to the free flight times (hard-sphere approach) and in the second, interaction times are assumed to be large compared to the free flight times (soft-sphere approach). Hoomans (2000) applied a hard-sphere approach to model bubbling fluidized beds and riser flows; Kaneko (2000) applied a soft-sphere approach to simulate bubbling fluidized bed reactors. Some of these results illustrating the influence of key model parameters are discussed below.

Before implementing hard-sphere or soft-sphere models, several issues related to formulations of various terms need to be sorted out. For hard-sphere models, key parameters are coefficient of restitution, coefficient of tangential restitution and coefficient of friction. For soft-sphere models, key parameters are normal spring stiffness, tangential spring stiffness and damping coefficient (Hoomans, 2000). In principle, soft-sphere models reduce to hard-sphere models in the limit of very high spring stiffness. In practice, however, soft-sphere models cannot be applied for very high values of spring stiffness due to computational constraints. Higher values of spring stiffness require lower and lower values of time step and may inordinately increase demands on computational resources. For most simulations based on soft-sphere models, an arbitrary low value of spring stiffness is specified. Fortunately, the actual magnitude of the spring stiffness parameter does not significantly affect the simulated fluidization behavior and low value can be safely used for most simulations. Simulation results

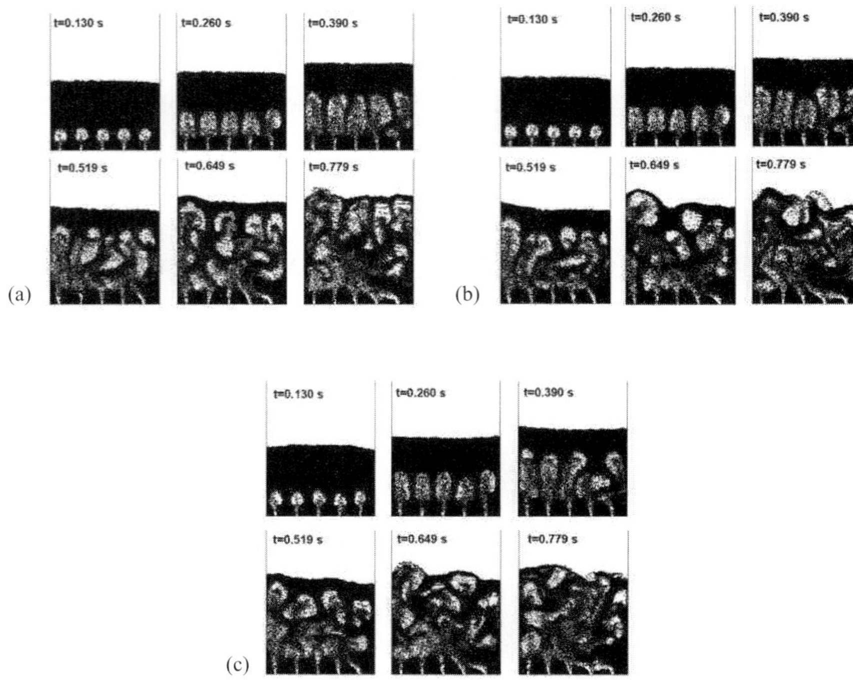

FIGURE 12.7 Simulated results for three values of spring stiffness ((a) 8 N m^{-1}; (b) 800 N m^{-1}; (c) 80 000 N m^{-1}). Soft sphere approach; number of particles = 14 000, $u = 3\,u_{mf}$ (from Kaneko, 2000).

(Kaneko, 2000) obtained for three values of spring stiffness constant (spread over four orders of magnitude) are shown in Fig. 12.7. It can be seen that if the objective is to understand the macroscopic behavior of the fluidized bed, low values of spring stiffness can be used for faster simulations. It must, however, be remembered that when such artificially low values of spring stiffness constant are used, the predicted values of contact time between solid particles are not realistic. When the objective is to understand local particle to particle heat or mass transfer, it is important to make accurate predictions of particle contact times. For such cases, it is necessary to use realistic values of spring stiffness constant at the expense of increased computational resources.

DPMs can also be used to understand the influence of particle properties on fluidization behavior. It has been demonstrated that ideal particles with restitution coefficient of unity and zero coefficient of friction, lead to entirely different fluidization behavior than that observed with non-ideal particles. Simulation results of gas–solid flow in a riser reactor reported by Hoomans (2000) for ideal and non-ideal particles are shown in Fig. 12.8. The well-known core-annulus flow structure can be observed only in the simulation with non-ideal particles. These comments are also applicable to simulations of bubbling beds. With ideal collision parameters, bubbling was not observed, contrary to the experimental evidence. Simulations with soft-sphere models with ideal particles also indicate that no bubbling is observed for fluidization of ideal particles (Hoomans, 2000). Apart from the particle characteristics, particle size distribution may also affect simulation results. For example, results of bubble formation simulations of Hoomans (2000) indicate that accounting

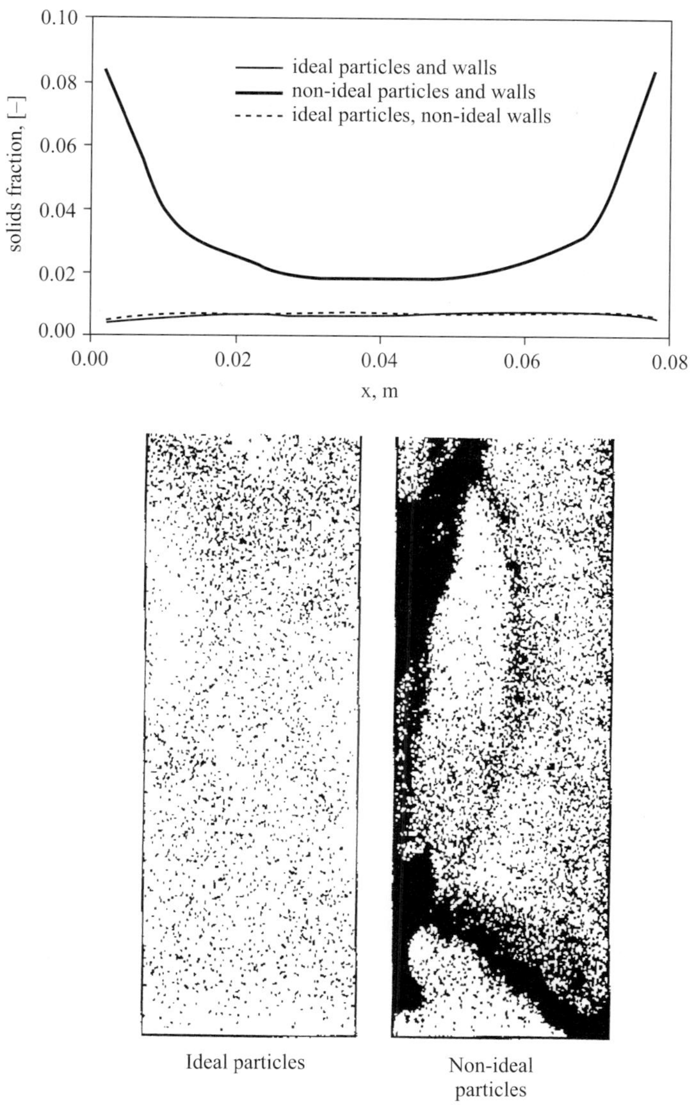

FIGURE 12.8 Simulated fluidization behavior for ideal and non-ideal particles in a Riser reactor (from Hoomans, 2000).

for non-uniform particle size leads to much better agreement with experimental data as shown in Fig. 12.9. During simulations with uniform particles, some small satellite bubbles appeared above and alongside the main bubble. Such satellite bubbles were not observed in the experiment nor in simulations with non-uniform particles.

When appropriate parameters are used, both, hard-sphere and soft-sphere models lead to similar predictions. Bubble formation results obtained from hard-sphere and soft-sphere models are shown in Fig. 12.10 (from Hoomans, 2000). The main bubble size and position in the bed observed in both simulations agree quite well with the experiment. The shape of the bubble observed in the experiment was more rounded than that observed in simulations. Thus, any of these, hard-sphere or soft-sphere

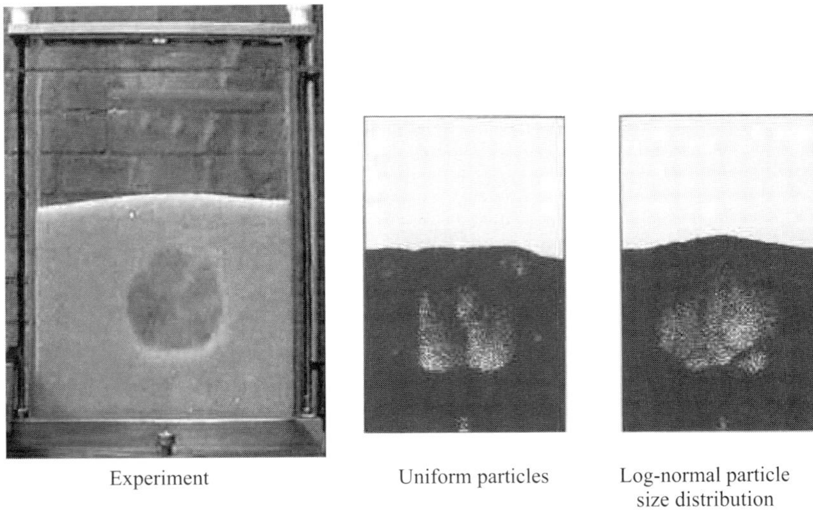

FIGURE 12.9 Comparison of simulation results with uniform and with log-normal particle size distribution and experimental observation (from Hoomans, 2000).

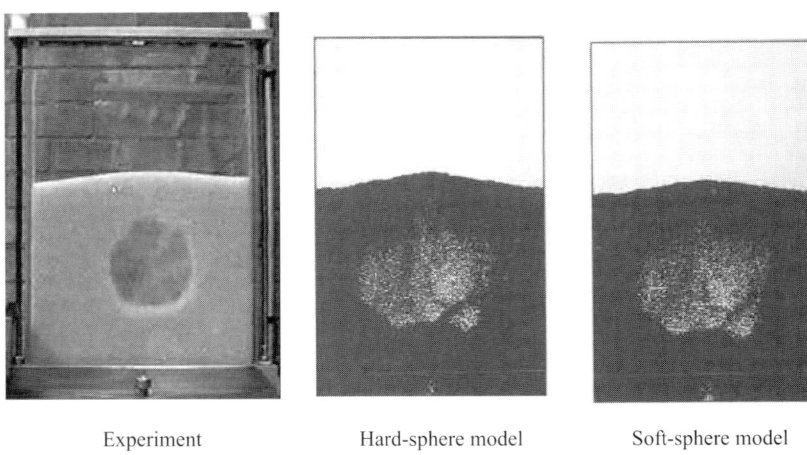

FIGURE 12.10 Comparison of simulation results for hard and soft sphere models with experimental results (from Hoomans, 2000).

models can be applied to gain insight into fluidization behavior. It should be noted that although predicted results of both approaches are almost the same, the computational efficiency of these two models might be different depending on the problem under consideration. Soft-sphere simulations progress at a constant speed (controlled by the time step, which in turn depends on the value of spring stiffness constant) whereas hard-sphere simulations are event driven and their speed depends strongly on system dynamics. More frequent collisions will slow down hard-sphere simulations (controlled by time interval between successive collisions).

DPMs may be used to understand the influence of particle characteristics on bubble formation, cluster formation and so on. These models may provide information regarding bubble size, cluster size, heat and mass transfer from such clusters to reaction engineering models. DPMs may also be used to extrapolate cold-flow data on bubble sizes/cluster sizes to high temperatures and high pressures. Interaction of gas distributor holes and gas–solid dynamics in the fluidized beds can also be examined with these models. Kaneko (2000) used DPMs to examine the behavior of fluidized polymerization reactors. These results are discussed in Section 12.3.

It must be noted here that most industrial fluidized bed reactors operate in a turbulent flow regime. Trajectory simulations of individual particles in a turbulent field may become quite complicated and time consuming. Details of models used to account for the influence of turbulence on particle trajectories are discussed in Chapter 4. These complications and constraints on available computational resources may restrict the number of particles considered in DPM simulations. Eulerian–Eulerian approaches based on the kinetic theory of granular flows may be more suitable to model such cases. Application of this approach to simulations of fluidized beds is discussed below.

12.2.2. Granular Flow Models (GFM)

Granular flow models are based on the interpenetrating continuum assumption. Both, gas and solid phases are modeled as a continuum. In this approach, individual particle trajectories are not simulated but an attempt is made to represent physics of those trajectories and particle–particle interactions using averaged form of governing equations. Because of use of such averaged equations, models based on this approach can be extended to simulate gas–solid flows comprising large number of solid particles. Basic equations of this approach are discussed in Chapter 4. Some recent work on development of CFD based models of fluidized bed reactors is briefly reviewed here. The discussion is divided into riser (fast fluidization regime) and dense bed (bubbling/turbulent bed regime) simulations.

Simulations of riser reactors

Riser reactors are used in a variety of applications, with fluid catalytic cracking (FCC) probably the most important one. Evolutionary design changes are constantly being introduced into all components of riser hardware to enhance the performance. Computational fluid dynamics has been used to understand the fluid dynamics of FCC systems and to evaluate alternative hardware configurations (Theologos *et al.*, 1997; Ranade, 1998). Several attempts have been made to model gas–solid flows in vertical pipes (Dasgupta *et al.*, 1998; Kuipers and van Swaaij, 1999 and references cited therein). Most of these attempts were based on the kinetic theory of granular flows (KTGF). Gao *et al.* (1999) simulated gas–solid flows in risers without using the kinetic theory of granular flows. Their results showed reasonably good agreement with two experimental data sets. However, in general, models based on KTGF require less ad hoc adjustments and have much wider applicability.

Sinclair and Jackson (1989) used the kinetic theory of granular flows to simulate gas–solid flows in risers. Their model was found to exhibit extreme sensitivity with respect to the value of restitution coefficient, e_s. Nieuwland *et al.* (1996) also observed such an extreme sensitivity. Bolio *et al.* (1995) reported that such extreme sensitivity could be overcome by including a gas phase turbulence model. Despite these studies, there are no systematic guidelines available to make appropriate selection of models and model parameters (such as laminar versus turbulent, values of restitution coefficients and specularity coefficient and interphase drag coefficients) to simulate gas–solid flow in industrial risers. It is observed from most of the available studies that the range of gas and solid fluxes investigated is not directly relevant to the operating range of industrial riser reactors. The influence of riser diameter, particle size and density, solids flux on various flow characteristics (pressure drop, solid volume fraction profiles and so on) has not been studied systematically. Here we report computational experiments discussed by Ranade (1999) to evolve possible guidelines for modeling gas–solid flows in riser reactors.

A two-fluid model with kinetic theory of granular flows was used to formulate the governing transport equations for gas–solid flows in riser. For details of the model equations, refer to the discussion in Chapter 4. Although in many industrial reactors, gas–solid flow in a riser may not be fully developed (except at the top region of the riser), it is always beneficial to start by developing relevant models to simulate fully developed gas–solid flow in a vertical riser. After adequate validation of such a base model, it can then be extended to simulate developing flow of gas and solid mixture. Ranade (1999) modeled fully developed flow by considering a very short riser with periodic (translationally) boundaries. With this approach, it is not necessary to model the large height of the riser reactor to ensure a fully developed state of flow. The computational grid used in his simulations is shown in Fig. 12.11. In order to resolve steeper gradients near the wall, a finer grid was used in the near wall region. The computational model was mapped on to a commercial CFD code, FLUENT version 4.5 (Fluent Inc., USA) with the help of user-defined subroutines.

For each simulation, superficial gas and solid velocities were specified as input parameters. Computations were started by setting the initial guess equal to these specified velocities. After each time step (of 0.001 s), all the variables except fluid pressure at the inlet, were set from the values calculated at the corresponding outlet computational cells. When setting the gas and solid axial velocity at the inlet, a correction was made to enforce the specified net gas and solid fluxes. At the riser wall, boundary conditions proposed by Sinclair and Jackson (1989) are recommended and were used for solids axial velocity and granular temperature. For the gas phase, the usual no slip boundary conditions (with wall functions) were used. To estimate the interphase drag force, a correlation proposed by Wen and Yu (1966) was used. For the gas–solid flows considered in this work, the contributions of lift and virtual mass forces were negligible. The kinetic theory of granular flows was used to calculate other relevant properties (such as solids viscosity and pressure). A standard k–ε model was used to simulate gas phase turbulence. In order to consider solid phase turbulence, the time-averaged granular temperature equation was solved. Additional terms including

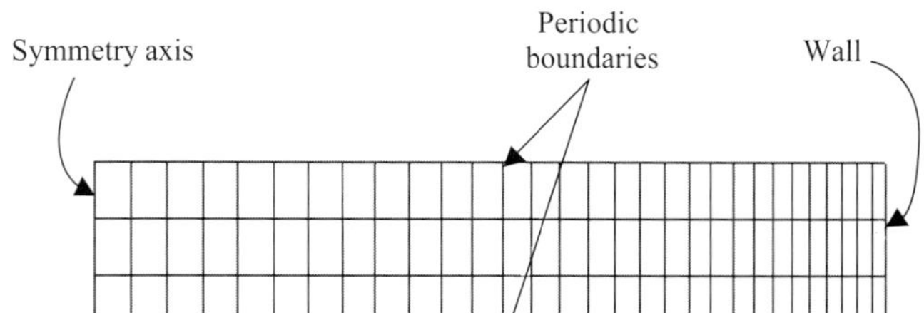

FIGURE 12.11 Computational grid for riser reactor (fully developed flow).

dissipation of solid phase turbulence, correlation between fluctuations of granular temperature and solids phase volume fraction were considered in the model. The basic governing equations are discussed in Chapter 4. Using these governing equations and the proposed boundary conditions, transient simulations were carried out until the fully developed steady state results were obtained.

Using a similar model, Bolio *et al.* (1995) reported good agreement between model predictions and the experimental data of Tsuji *et al.* (1984). Instead of repeating those simulations, we report here a comparison of simulated gas–solid flow with the experimental data of Yang (1991). The value of solid flux used in these experiments was also rather low (10 kg m^{-2} s^{-1}). The comparison is shown in Fig. 12.12. It can be seen that the centerline gas velocity predicted without considering the turbulence model, is significantly higher than that reported by Yang (1991). Predicted results after considering the turbulence model show much better agreement with experimental data (Fig. 12.12). The predicted radial profiles of solid hold-up are shown in Fig. 12.13. In order to verify that the predicted results are not unreasonably sensitive to the value of particle–particle restitution coefficient, gas–solid flow simulations were also carried out with a restitution coefficient of 0.95. Comparison of predicted radial profiles of gas and solid velocity for these two values of restitution coefficient indicate that predicted results are not unduly sensitive to the value of restitution coefficient.

It can be seen that lower values of particle–particle restitution coefficient predict higher values of centerline solids hold-up. Unfortunately, experimental data concerning solids hold-up was not available for the same operating conditions. The predicted profiles of granular temperature for the two values of restitution coefficient also show significant difference at the region near the symmetry axis. Despite these differences, it can be concluded that the model does not exhibit extreme sensitivity to the value of restitution coefficient. The influence of the value of the speculiarity parameter on

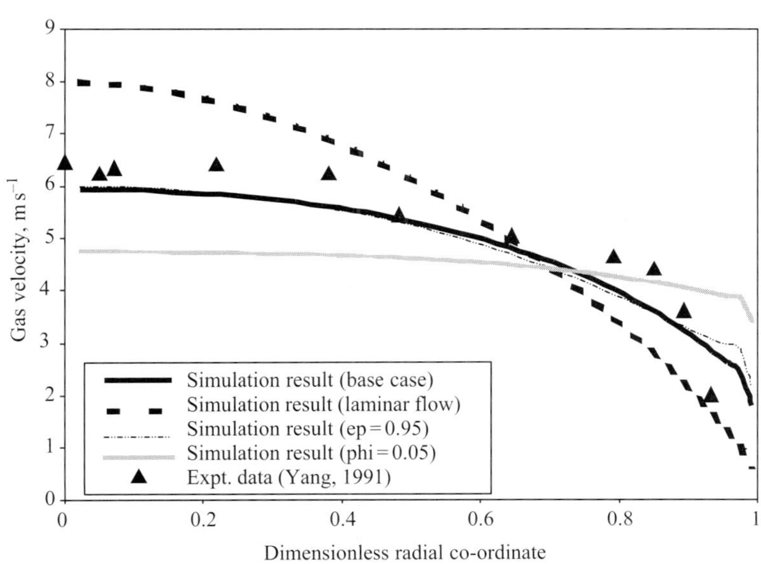

FIGURE 12.12 Comparison of simulation results with experimental data at low solids flux (d_p = 54 μm, ρ_s = 1545 kg m^{-3}, D = 0.14 m, U_g = 4.33 m s^{-1}, G_s = 10 kg m^2 s^{-1}) (from Ranade, 1999).

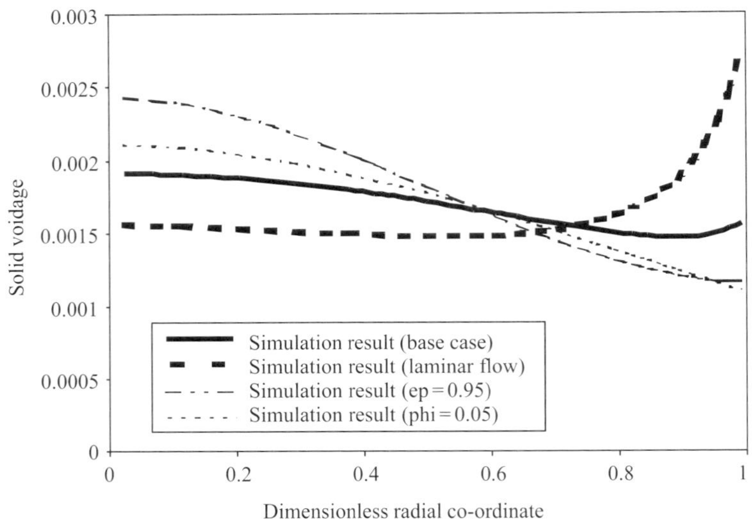

FIGURE 12.13 Sensitivity of simulation results to model parameters (d_p = 54 μm, ρ_s = 1545 kg m^{-3}, D = 0.14 m, U_g = 4.33 m s^{-1}, G_s = 10 kg m^{-2} s^{-1}) (from Ranade, 1999).

predicted results was also examined. Kuipers and coworkers (1991, 1998) used a value of speculiarity coefficient 0.5 while Bolio *et al.* (1995) used a very small value (0.002). The reduction in the value of speculiarity parameter causes flatter profiles of gas velocity (Fig. 12.12). An order of magnitude decrease in the value of speculiarity coefficient (0.05 from 0.5) increased the wall slip of solid particles from 0.9 to 3.2 m s^{-1}. It can be seen that the predicted results obtained with the value 0.5 showed much better agreement with experimental data (Fig. 12.12). In view of these results, for all subsequent simulations, particle–particle restitution coefficient, particle–wall restitution coefficient and speculiarity coefficients were set to 1.0, 0.9 and 0.5, respectively. With these parameter settings, the computational model was found to give satisfactory agreement with the experimental data of Yang (1991).

To simulate gas–solid flows in industrial FCC risers, it is necessary to simulate flows at high solids fluxes. At higher solids flux, radial segregation increases and a significant downflow of solids may occur in the near-wall region in the riser. Several authors have reported such downflow of solids near the wall (van Breugel *et al.*, 1969; Bader, 1988; Nieuwland *et al.*, 1996; Derouin *et al.*, 1997). We simulated the experimental conditions reported in these studies using the same computational model as was used to simulate the data of Yang (1991). Typical comparisons at higher solids fluxes are shown in Fig. 12.14. It can be seen that the agreement between predicted results and experimental data has significantly deteriorated and the model used in the present work failed to capture the significant downflow near the riser wall. It was interesting to note that the simulations showed the downflow at the wall if they were carried out without considering the gas phase turbulence model. Pita and Sundaresan (1991) showed reasonable agreement between predicted results and the experimental data of Bader *et al.* (1988) without including the turbulence model. Their

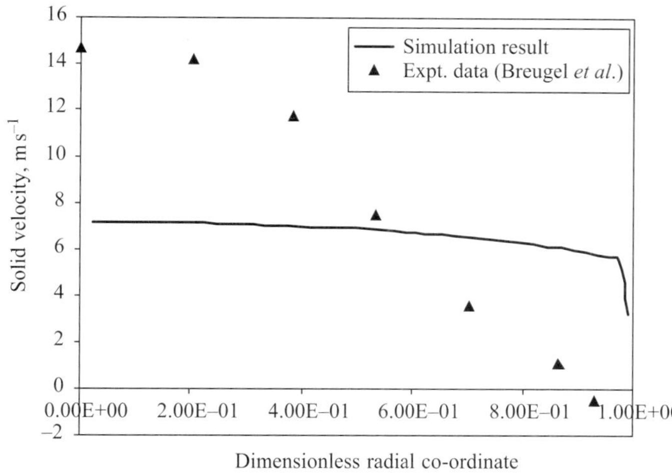

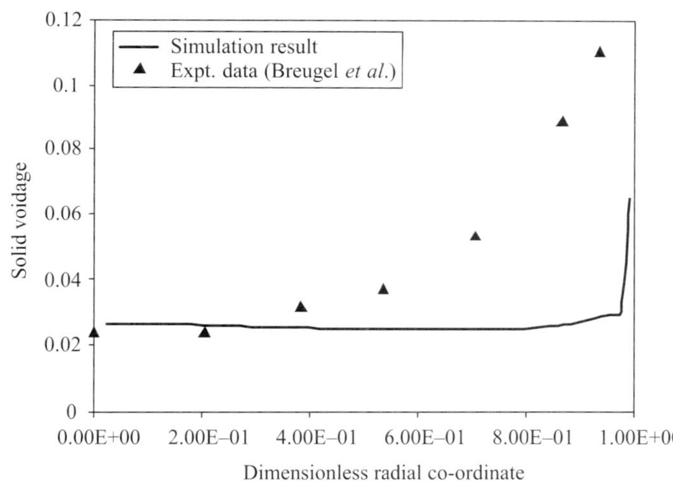

FIGURE 12.14 Comparison with experimental data from van Breugel *et al.*, 1969 ($d_p = 40\,\mu m$, $\rho_s = 2300\,kg\,m^{-3}$, $D = 0.30\,m$, $U_g = 6.30\,m\,s^{-1}$, $G_s = 390\,kg\,m^{-2}\,s^{-1}$). (From Ranade, 1999).

computational model, however, exhibits extreme sensitivity with respect to particle–particle restitution coefficient and therefore cannot be used to simulate practical riser flows.

Kuipers and van Swaaij (1999) also observed that it was not possible to simulate the downflow near the riser wall without modifying the underlying interphase momentum exchange model. The pronounced lateral segregation and solids downflow near the wall with velocities much higher than terminal-settling velocities may occur due to the formation of clusters. Typical size of these clusters and how these clusters affect the dynamics of gas–solid flows in vertical risers is not properly understood. Several ad hoc modifications based on fitting a limited set of experimental data have been attempted. Matsen (1982) proposed a correlation to estimate slip velocity of clusters as a function of single-particle terminal settling velocity and volume fraction of solids. The ratio of slip velocity to terminal settling velocity at 10% solids volume fraction is about 5. Kuipers and van Swaaij (1999) used a correlation proposed by Nieuwland *et al.* (1994) to correct the interphase drag coefficient to account for cluster formation in the riser flows. This correlation predicts the ratio of slip velocity to terminal settling velocity as about 30. Thus, these two correlations to account for the influence of clusters on the interphase drag force term differ significantly from each other. It appears that cluster formation, their size and slip velocity may be functions of more parameters than just the solids volume fraction and terminal settling velocity. In order to further understand various issues in the simulations of gas–solid flows in a riser, it will be instructive to examine the results of numerical experiments. Here we describe the results of some such numerical experiments to illustrate the influence of relevant variables such as riser diameter, particle diameter and solids flux on predicted results.

For these numerical experiments, a base case of gas–solid flow with the following parameters was considered: particle diameter 100 μm, particle density 2000 kg m^{-3}, gas density 5 kg m^{-3}, riser diameter 0.30 m, gas superficial velocity 10 m s^{-1} and solids flux of 400 kg m^{-2} s^{-1}. The model of Ranade (1999) was used along with the turbulence model to simulate the base case and various other cases with systematic variation of the main governing parameters of gas–solid flows in risers. The data used for these numerical experiments are listed in Table 12.2. Additional simulations were also carried out to examine the interaction between parameters by simultaneously varying more than one parameter. Unless otherwise mentioned, for all simulations, the particle–particle restitution coefficient was set to one, the particle–wall restitution coefficient was set to 0.9 and the speculiarity coefficient was set to 0.5. The influence of several parameters on the predicted values of solids velocity, slip velocity, solids volume fraction, solids granular temperature and gas phase turbulent kinetic energy was studied. Analysis of the results obtained by these numerical experiments will be useful to guide the development of a computational model to simulate industrial fluidized beds.

The influence of riser diameter on the predicted results is shown in Fig. 12.15. It can be seen that there are significant qualitative differences in the predicted radial

TABLE 12.2 Data Used for Numerical Experiments and Predicted Pressure Drop

No.	D, m	d_p, μm	ρ_s, kg m^{-3}	ρ_g, kg m^{-3}	U_g m s^{-1}	G_s, kg m^{-2} s^{-1}	$\Delta p/L$ Pa/m
1	0.30	100	2000	5	10.0	400	647.17
2	0.06	100	2000	5	10.0	400	1924.3
3	1.00	100	2000	5	10.0	400	488.35
4	0.30	200	2000	5	10.0	400	666.65
5	0.30	050	2000	5	10.0	400	617.35
6	0.30	100	2000	5	10.0	200	444.97
7	0.30	100	2000	5	10.0	100	375.74
8	0.30	100	2000	5	5.0	400	950.21
9	0.30	100	2000	5	5.0	200	528.21
10	0.30	100	1000	5	10.0	400	385.72
11	0.30	100	2000	1	10.0	400	546.67

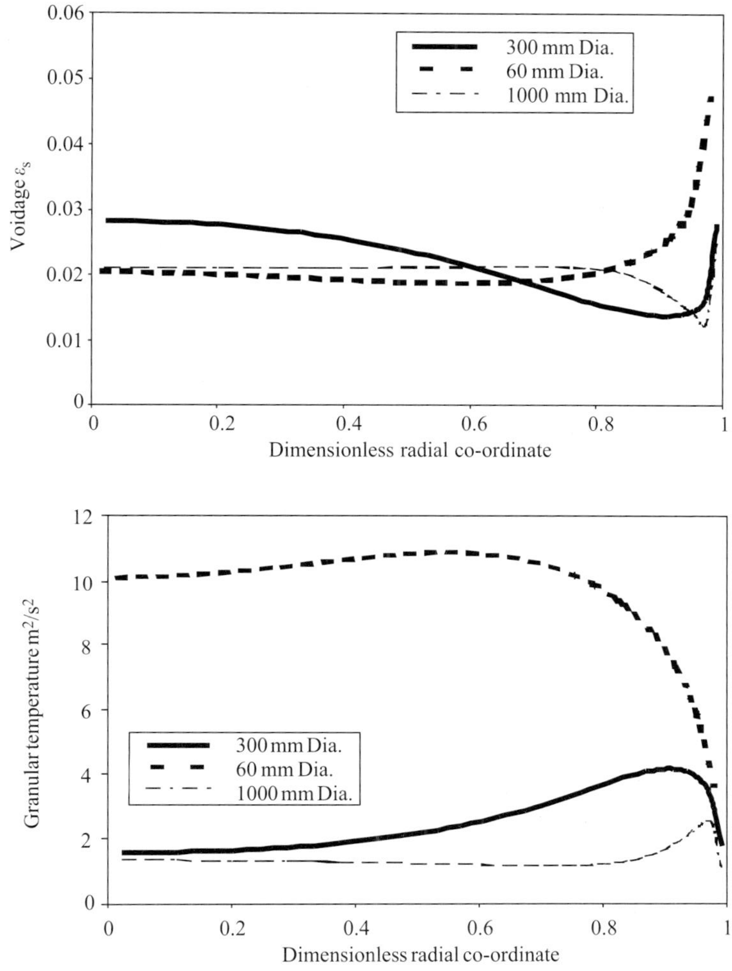

FIGURE 12.15 Influence of riser diameter (from Ranade, 1999).

profiles for the small diameter riser (0.06 m) and for larger diameter risers (0.3 and 1.0 m). For the small diameter riser, pronounced wall peaking was predicted even in the absence of cluster corrections. For the large diameter risers, the model predicts a qualitatively different profile with minima in solids hold-up near the wall. As the riser diameter increases, the location of the maximum in the predicted solids flux profile shifts towards the riser wall. In view of the significant influence of riser diameter on the characteristics of gas–solid flows in risers (especially on solids granular temperature), it is inappropriate to use empirical cluster corrections derived by fitting the experimental data obtained in a smaller diameter riser. The formation of clusters and the role of riser diameter in cluster formation need to be studied in detail to develop industrially useful models (Sunderesan, 2000). Simulations using DPMs may be useful in this regard.

Additional numerical experiments were carried out for three values of particle diameters and two values of solids density. These results are shown in Fig. 12.16a

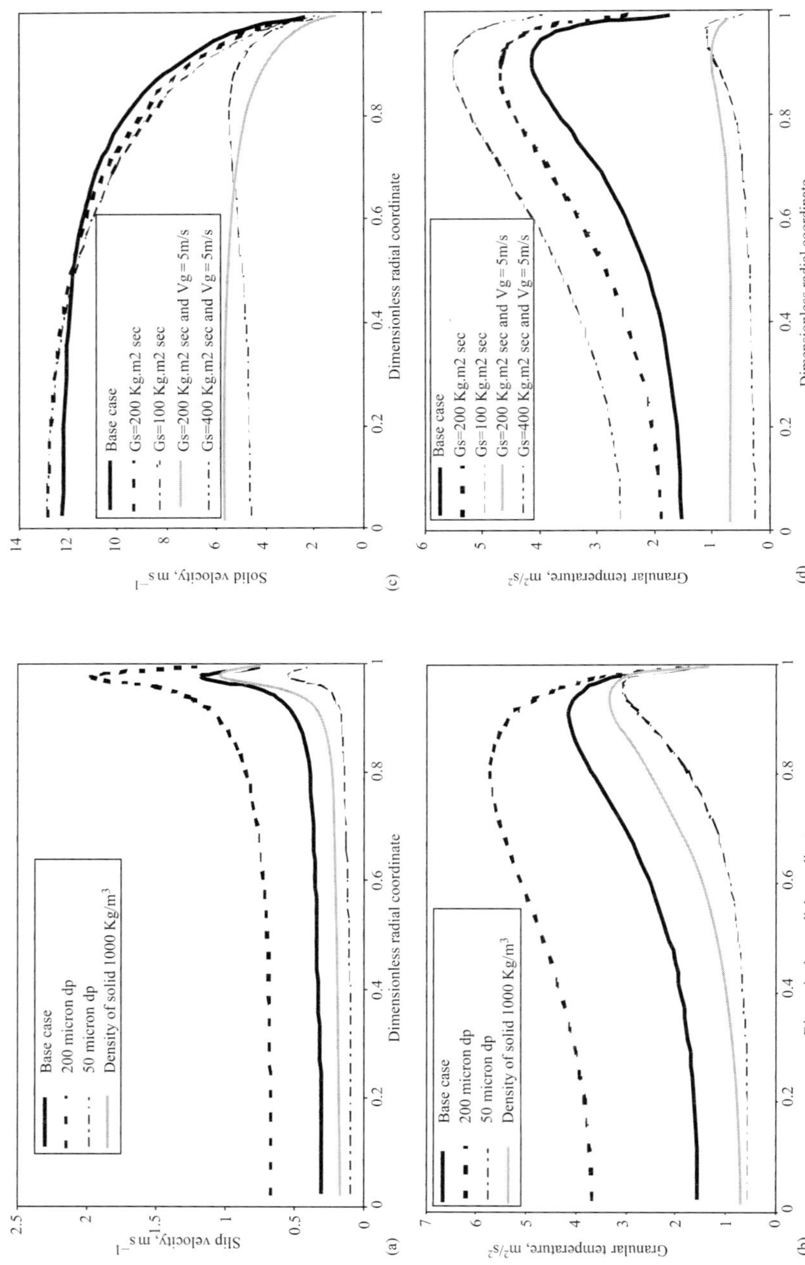

FIGURE 12.16 Influence of particle diameter, particle density, gas and solids flux (From Ranade, 1999).

and 12.16b. Smaller particle diameters lead to a flatter profile for solids velocity. As expected, the predicted slip velocity increases with particle diameter. All slip velocity profiles exhibit a sharp peak near the riser wall. The predicted solids hold-up profiles for all four cases are not significantly different. The predicted granular temperature increases with particle diameter and particle density, though the shape of the profile remains the same. Results of the numerical experiments to examine the influence of gas and solids flux are shown in Fig. 12.16c and 12.16d. It can be seen that for the same superficial gas velocity, the decrease in solids flux leads to higher granular temperature and higher slip velocities. For the same solids flux, a decrease in gas velocity significantly reduces the granular temperature. Predicted profiles of slip velocity exhibit a maximum in the near-wall region, the magnitude of which increases with increasing superficial gas velocity and decreasing solids flux. The computational model, however, failed to predict any significant downflow of solids even for the highest solids flux ($400\,\mathrm{kg\,m^{-2}\,s^{-1}}$) and lowest gas velocity ($5\,\mathrm{m\,s^{-1}}$) case. The role of gas phase and secondary solids phase turbulence on radial segregation of solids needs to be studied systematically to evaluate the currently used KTGF-based models. The predicted values of pressure drops (Table 12.2) show the expected trends. However, unless the downflow near the wall is captured, quantitative comparison with the experimental data will be difficult.

Pita and Sundaresan (1991) reported results of numerical experiments using their computational model (without including a turbulence model). They reported the existence of multiplicity for large diameter risers. In order to examine the possibility of multiple solutions, numerical experiments were initiated with several different initial guess fields. However, multiplicity was not detected in any of the cases discussed above. The computational model always converged to the same result from any initial guess field. The computational model used in the present work predicted monotonic decrease in pressure drop with increase in riser diameter for specific values of gas and solid fluxes. This trend is in line with the observations of Yerushalmi and Avidhan (1985). Pita and Sundaresan's model, however, predicted a reversal in the trend: it predicts an increase in pressure drop with increase in riser diameter, if it increases beyond a certain value (about 0.1 m). Such a reversal in trend may occur if the model predicts the downflow of solids near wall for the large diameter risers. The model used in the present work did not predict any downflow even for the 0.5 m riser. It is necessary to generate systematic data concerning radial segregation of solids and effective slip velocity of solids (clusters and particles) by conducting experiments at different riser diameters covering the range of particle diameters and gas and solid fluxes relevant to industrial riser flows. The data will also be useful to understand cluster formation and to quantify its influence on the dynamics of gas–solid flows. Understanding gained through interpretation of experimental data and the results of numerical experiments may be translated into appropriate sub-models to represent cluster formation and their effect on gas–solid dynamics. Such sub-models may be able to capture the downflow of solids near riser walls with adequate accuracy. Instead of empirically adjusting the values of restitution coefficient and speculiarity coefficient, independent measurements of these parameters should accompany the experimental data suggested above.

In light of these comments, some recent work (Kuipers *et al.*, 1998; Dasgupta *et al.*, 1998; Mathiesen *et al.*, 1999, 2000; Neri and Gidaspow, 2000) on the application of granular models to simulating gas–solid flows in riser reactors is briefly reviewed here. Mathiesen *et al.* (1999, 2000) developed a multifluid model to account for the particle size distribution. Each solid phase is characterized by a diameter, form factor, density and restitution coefficient. Their model was able to predict axial segregation by particle size quite well (Fig. 12.17a). The model was, however, not able to capture radial segregation by particle size adequately. This may be because the model ignored some of the external forces acting on solid particles. The predictions of solids volume fraction were also not very good (Fig. 12.17b). The model of Neri and Gidaspow (2000) could capture the oscillatory motion of dense clusters reasonably well. Predicted results show the well-known core-annulus flow regime in the time-averaged sense. The values of solid volume fraction near the wall, however, were underpredicted (Fig. 12.17c). Apart from the time-averaged results, the predicted dynamic characteristics were found to be in reasonable agreement with experimental data. Their results show that imposition of the symmetry boundary condition at the riser axis is not justified because of the strongly asymmetric instantaneous flows. Benyahia *et al.* (2000) also report simulations of oscillatory behavior and asymmetric flow in risers. The calculated solids volume fraction deviated from the experimental data at the wall region. These results indicate that state of the art CFD models are not yet able to capture the influence of clusters without empiricism. It is essential to establish a systematic database to develop useful empirical relationships for immediate use and to guide further development of computational models. Herbert *et al.* (1999) systematically stored data collected over the past several years at ETH in an Oracle relational database. Databases of this type will be valuable for further development and for fine tuning CFD-based models for reactor engineering applications. Some applications of such CFD models to reactor engineering are discussed in the next section.

Simulations of bubbling/turbulent bed reactors

Bubbling/turbulent fluidized bed reactors are characterized by excellent solids mixing and gas–solids contact. Most of these properties can be attributed to the presence of bubbles. An understanding of the formation and motion of gas bubbles and their influence on various transport rates is of crucial importance for reactor engineering of bubbling/turbulent bed reactors. In a bubbling bed, distinct gas voids or bubbles exist. In turbulent beds, voids and large clusters of solids particles are distributed all over the reactor. A Eulerian–Eulerian approach is particularly suitable to simulate industrial bubbling/turbulent bed reactors (which may contain billions of solid particles). Some of the key issues in developing computational models for such reactors are discussed below.

Bubbling/turbulent beds contain regions of steep voidage gradients, which are difficult to handle numerically. Most early work on the simulation of dense bubbling beds was restricted to simulation of a single or few bubbles in a two-dimensional fluidized bed for a short time (Kuipers *et al.*, 1991). Although this work is useful, for industrial applications it is more relevant to simulate vigorously bubbling fluidized beds and obtain predictions of bubble frequency, bubble volume fraction, bubble size and bubble rise velocities. When reviewing these attempts, Clift (1993) invoked the so-called 'Occam's razor' and recommended that such CFD models of dense bubbling beds may only be used as 'learning models', and conventional or discrete bubble Lagrangian models may be used for the design and scale-up of bubbling fluidized beds. His recommendation was mainly based on state of the art results in 1993. Since

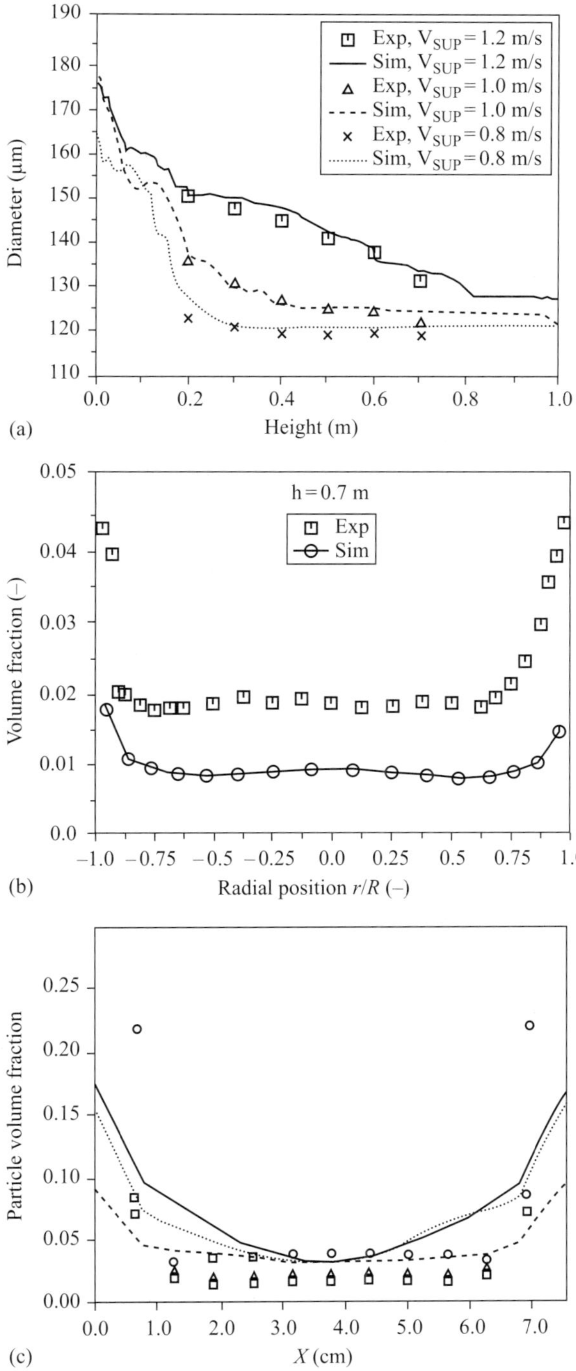

FIGURE 12.17 Some simulation results for gas–solids flows in a riser. (a) Axial particle diameter profiles for different superficial gas velocities (V_{SUP}) (from Mathiesen *et al.*, 2000). (b) Radial solid volume fraction profiles at 0.7 m from the bottom, $V_{SUP} = 1.0\,m\,s^{-1}$ (from Mathiesen *et al.*, 2000). (c) Radial solids volume fraction profiles at different heights: solid line and circles 1.86 m; short-dashed line and squares 4.18 m; long-dashed line and diamonds: 5.52 m (from Neri and Gidaspow, 2000).

then, significant progress has been made and it is now possible to simulate bubbling beds having a large number of bubbles. Ferschneider and Mege (1996) applied a two-fluid model to simulate bubbling fluidization of Geldart group A powders (particle diameter 100 μm) in a two-dimensional column. Comparison of their predicted results with experimental data is shown in Fig. 12.18. It can be seen that although predictions of bubble diameter and bubble rise velocity are reasonable, the model significantly overestimates bubble volume fraction. Such an overestimation may lead to carry-over of the entire dense bed as reported by Ranade (1998).

It should be noted that a two-fluid model along with the kinetic theory of granular flow contains several modeled terms (stress tensors, solid phase bulk and shear viscosity, radial distribution function and so on). Several different modeled versions of each of these have been used (Nieuwland *et al*., 1996). A general consensus on selection of an appropriate version has not yet emerged. Enwald *et al.* (1999) used two different stress tensor models to simulate bubbling beds, which led to quite similar results. Fortunately, the existence of bubbles is independent of which stress tensor model is used, since the mechanism of bubble formation originates from general two-fluid model formulation (Glasser *et al*., 1996). In addition to the selected model equations, numerical issues such as mesh refining and discretization schemes may also play a significant role. Syamlal (1998) reported significant influence of discretization scheme on simulated bubble shapes. His results are shown in Fig. 12.19. Studies by van Wachem *et al.* (1998, 1999) and Enwald *et al.* (1999) also indicate the strong influence of numerical parameters on simulated characteristics of bubbling fluidized beds. In both of these studies, bubbling beds of Geldart group B particles were simulated. van Wachem *et al.* (1998) report that a finer mesh is required to simulate bubbling at lower fluidization velocities. They had to use different mesh sizes for different velocities in order to get similar volume fractions inside bubbles at different fluidization conditions (0.007 m for two times minimum fluidization velocity and 0.01 m for four times minimum fluidization velocity). Their simulated results also indicate reasonably good predictions of bubble size and bubble rise velocity (Fig. 12.20). Enwald *et al.* (1999) report that as the operating pressure or the ratio of density of fluidizing medium to solid particles decreases, a finer mesh is required. A sample of simulated results reported by Enwald *et al.* (1999) is shown in Fig. 12.21. It can be seen that simulations with a granular flow model lead to very few bubbles near the distributor, unlike experimental observations. Simulations with constant particle viscosity models carried out with a fine mesh resulted in reasonable agreement with experimental data.

In light of these recent works and progress in the development of robust and efficient parallel solvers, it is now possible to use CFD models for the reactor engineering of bubbling/turbulent fluidized beds. The key issue in developing such models is that the reactor engineer should not focus on developing an all-encompassing model by including every conceivable term. Instead, the reactor engineer should make judicious use of accumulated knowledge about the considered fluidized bed reactor to construct a model which gives predictions consistent with the accumulated experience. For example, Ranade (1998) used an analogy between dense bubbling beds and bubble column reactors to simulate key issues regarding gas distributor and solids entry configuration in a FCC regenerator (as discussed in Chapter 9). Some of the recent applications of CFD models to reactor engineering of fluidized beds are discussed in the following section.

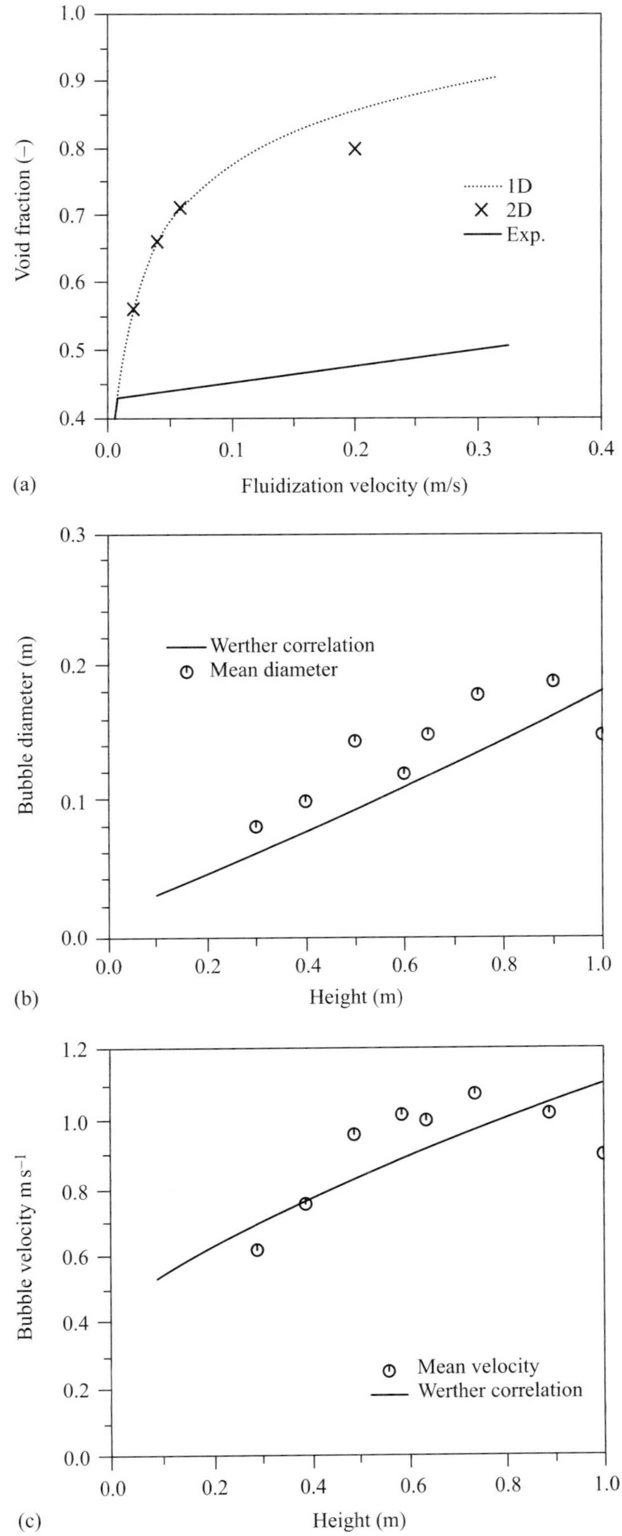

FIGURE 12.18 Comparison of simulated bubbling fluidization of Geldart group A particles with experimental data (from Ferschneider and Mege, 1996).

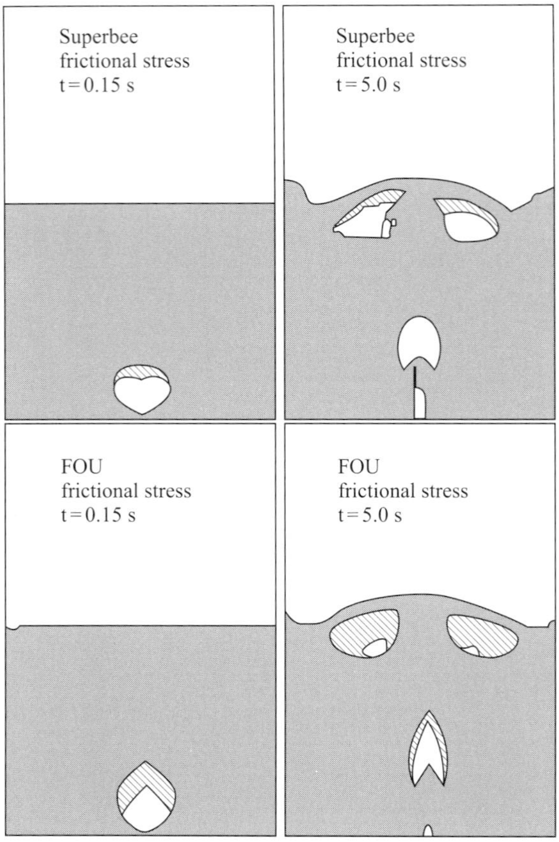

FIGURE 12.19 Influence of discretization schemes on bubble shape (from Syamlal, 1998). Contours of void fractions (white: more gas). Superbee: QUICK with superbee limiters FOU: First order upwind.

12.3. APPLICATIONS TO REACTOR ENGINEERING

General issues in reactor engineering are discussed in Chapter 1. Many of these issues are also discussed in Chapters 10 and 11 with reference to stirred tank and bubble column reactor. These discussions are also applicable to the engineering of fluidized bed reactors. As mentioned repeatedly in this book, it is first necessary to evolve a 'wish list' for the reactor to quantify demands on the reactor. Suitable reactor configurations and modes of operation can then be evolved. Krishna (1994) discussed a systematic approach for the selection of appropriate reactor and mode of operation. Available modeling tools can then be used to short-list the most promising configurations. Classical reaction engineering models give useful information about the overall behavior of the reactors. Usually two-phase or three-phase models are used to simulate bubbling fluidized bed reactors (Kunii and Levenspiel, 1991). These models are also extended to simulate turbulent beds. Grace *et al.* (1999) developed a generalized bubbling turbulent (GBT) bed model based on a probabilistic approach. Usually plug flow is assumed to simulate the behavior of riser reactors. An approach analogous to GBT can also be developed for the fast-fluidization regime in riser

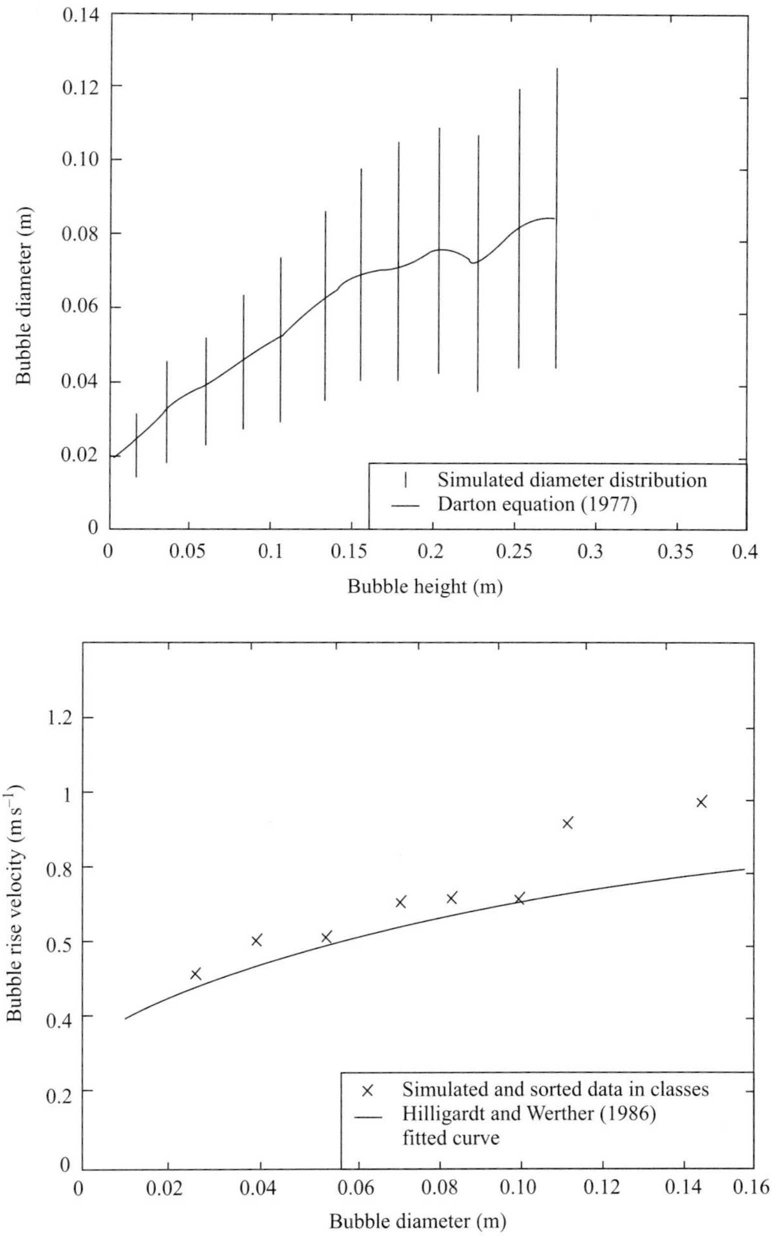

FIGURE 12.20 Simulations of bubbling fluidization of Geldart group B particles (from van Wachem *et al.*, 1998).

reactors. Through these developments in reactor modeling, it is becoming evident that unless the influence of the complex hydrodynamics of fluidized bed reactors is accounted for, it is not possible to develop a comprehensive model which can be used for reactor engineering purposes. CFD models can provide information about such complex hydrodynamics of fluidized bed reactors. It may not be efficient to

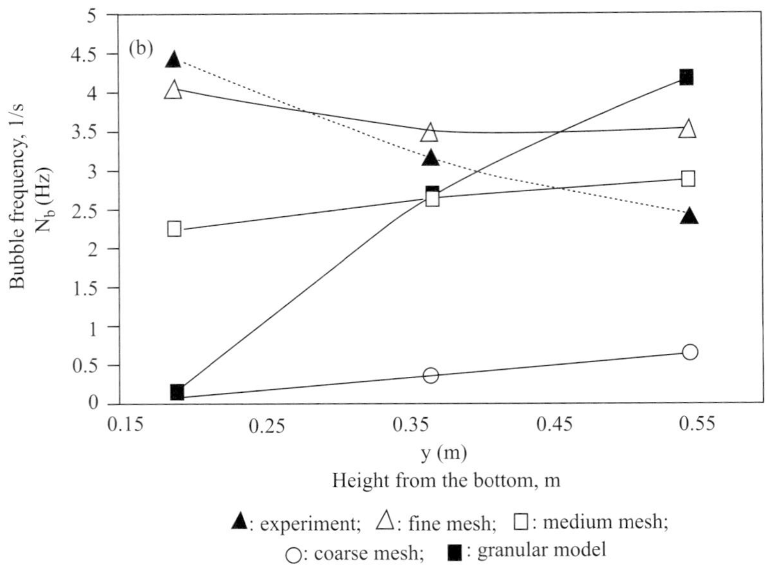

FIGURE 12.21 Comparison of simulated (constant viscosity or granular model) and experimentally observed bubble frequency (Pressure 0.8 Mpa, from Enwald *et al.*, 1999).

develop a comprehensive CFD model to simulate an entire reactor operation. Insight gained through application of CFD models may, however, lend significant help in engineering decision making. Two examples of the application of CFD-based models to enhance the performance of fluidized bed reactors are discussed in Chapter 9. Here we illustrate the potential by describing more applications from published literature.

Use of CFD models to understand mixing and mal-distribution issues in an oxy-chlorination reactor was discussed in Chapter 9. Samuelsberg (1994) used a two-fluid model with kinetic theory of granular flows to simulate a bubbling fluidized bed carrying out oxi-chlorination reactions. They simulated only a two-dimensional slice of the oxi-chlorination reactor. The internal heat transfer tubes were modeled as a porous block (volume blockage 0.75) assuming a constant bed-to-wall heat transfer coefficient. The simulated spatial distribution of ethylene di-chloride (EDC) is shown in Fig. 12.22. The highly dynamic behavior of bubbling beds is clearly evident from this figure. It can also be seen that the most significant EDC formation takes place in the bottom part of the reactor. Though this model employs a strongly simplified representation of a full-scale oxy-chlorination reactor and internal heat exchanger, it provides much more detailed information than conventional design and development models. The possibility of hot spot formation and interaction of gas mal-distribution on reactor performance can be understood using such a computational model. A discrete particle model was used by Kaneko *et al.* (1999) to understand similar issues in a bubbling polymerization reactor. This model was used to understand differences between porous and perforated plate gas distributors in terms of reactor performance and hot-spot formation. A sample of their results is shown in Fig. 12.23. It can be seen that simulations indicate the possibility of formation of a dead zone for the perforated distributor. The temperature of gas in such a dead zone may increase significantly during the course of the reaction.

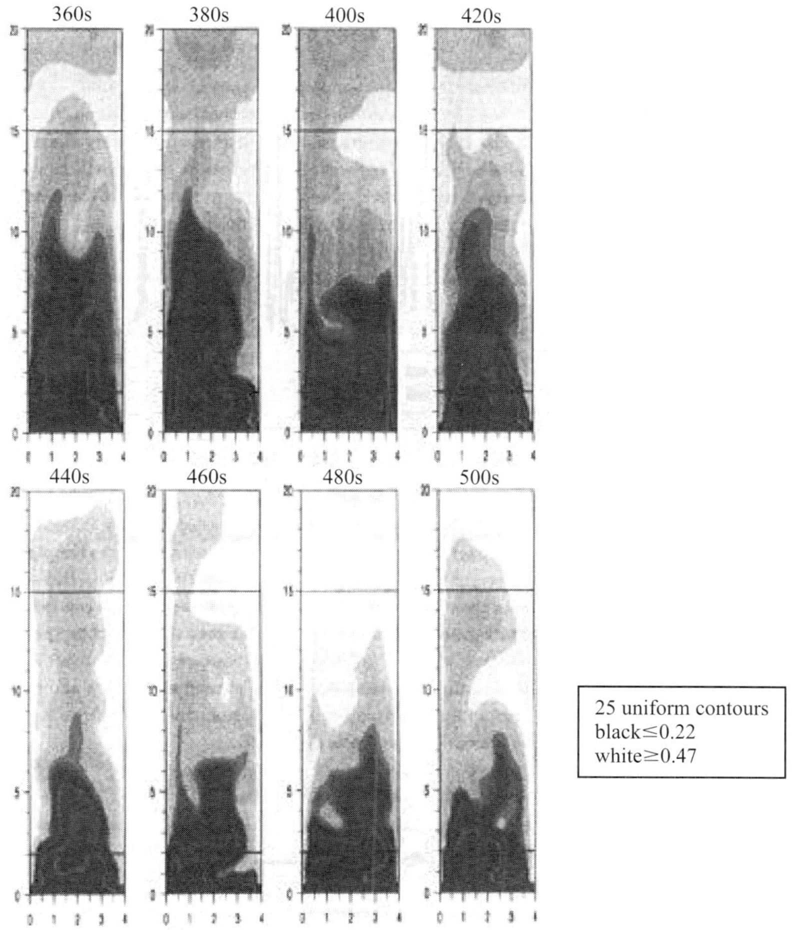

FIGURE 12.22 Simulated spatial distribution of ethylene di-chloride (from Samuelsberg, 1994).

CFD-based models have also been used to simulate the performance of riser reactors (Theologos and Markatos, 1993; Theologos *et al.*, 1997; Gao *et al.*, 1999). Gao *et al.* (1999) developed a three-dimensional two-phase turbulent flow model to simulate a FCC riser reactor. A thirteen-lump kinetic model was used to simulate cracking reactions taking place in the FCC riser. The computational flow model was first verified by comparing predicted results with the published experimental data of Bader *et al.* (1988) and Yang (1991). A sample of their results is shown in Fig. 12.24. It can be seen that their computational model was able to capture key flow characteristics of gas and solid phase quite adequately. This is crucial for extending the use of computational flow models for reactor engineering. Gao *et al.* (1999) then used this computational model to simulate the industrial riser reactor. In such a reactor, feed is usually introduced at the bottom of the riser via multiple nozzles. Conventional one-dimensional riser models cannot account for radial variation of catalyst and feed concentrations. The CFD-based three-dimensional model of Gao *et al.* (1999) could capture such radial as well as axial variations. Local fluid dynamics near feed nozzles

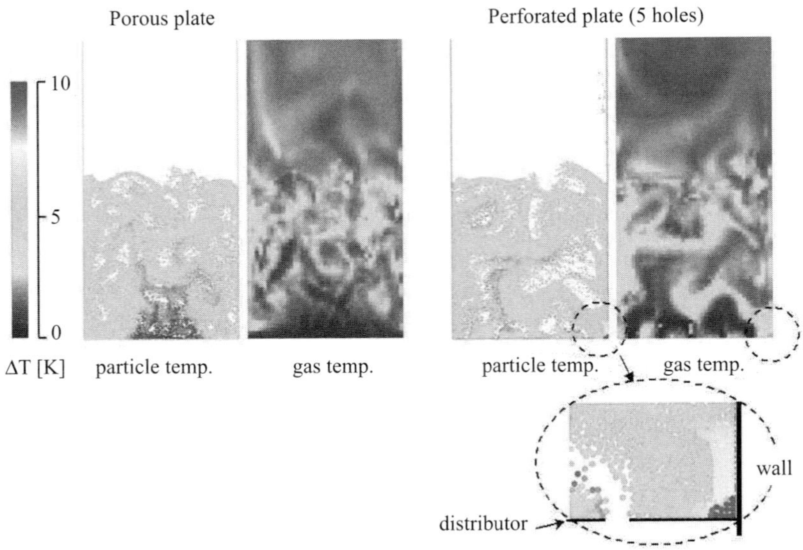

FIGURE 12.23 Influence of gas distributor on particle and gas temperatures (simulations of ethylene polymerization, 14000 particles, $u = 3u_{mf}$, $t = 6.25$, from Kaneko *et al.*, 1999).

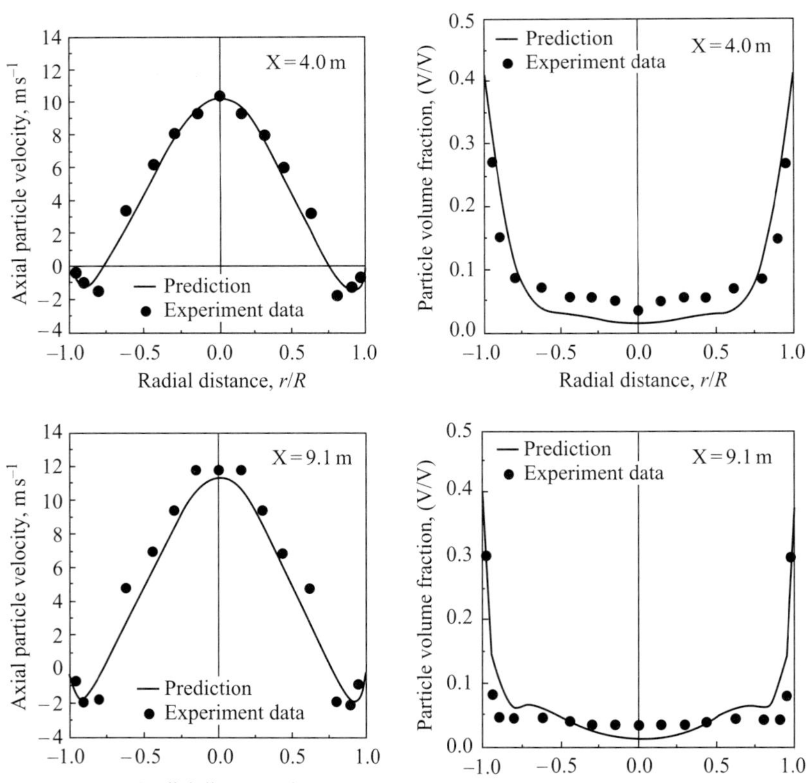

FIGURE 12.24 Comparison of simulation results with the experimental data of Bader *et al.*, 1988 (from Gao *et al.*, 1999).

is strongly affected by high velocity jets, leading to lower gasoline yields. Their computational model could correctly capture the performance of two commercial riser reactors. As observed in many commercial risers, the yield of gasoline attains a maximum at a certain height within the riser and then declines due to overcracking. Several operational modifications are proposed to avoid such overcracking. Gao *et al.* (1999) demonstrated application of their computational model to evaluate a reaction-terminating technique to eliminate overcracking. In this technique, water is injected into a riser reactor at a suitable height. The injected water reduces the temperature and thus, reduces overcracking. Various alternatives were evaluated by Gao *et al.* (1999) and the performance of their simulation is shown in Fig. 12.25. It can be seen that the detailed computational flow model coupled with an appropriate reaction model was able to identify the most promising operational strategy to enhance gasoline yield. Theologos *et al.* (1999) also included feed atomization effects in their CFD model of a FCC riser reactor. This model was able to simulate feed vaporization and the influence of feed droplet sizes on the vaporization zone. They, however, used a rather simplified kinetic scheme (3-lump model) to represent cracking reactions.

Even if the detailed chemistry is not incorporated in the flow model, computational flow models can be used to resolve such hardware related-issues as configuration of feed nozzles, reactor internals, erosion due to solids particles and so on. Gustavsson and Almstedt (2000) applied a two-fluid model to understand the erosion of heat exchanger tubes immersed in bubbling fluidized beds. The simulation results provide detailed information about how bubble passage, wake impact and wake passage affect local fluid dynamics around cooling tubes and thereby affect erosion. Predicted results qualitatively agree with the experimental evidence. Such CFD-based models allow extrapolation of bench- and pilot-scale data to larger scales and cold flow simulation data to actual operating conditions (high temperatures, high pressures). In general, the computational flow models can be used (1) to understand the basic phenomena and (2) to simulate the influence of complex reactor hardware (feed nozzles, distributor, internals and so on) on the performance of industrial reactors. Invariably, it will be

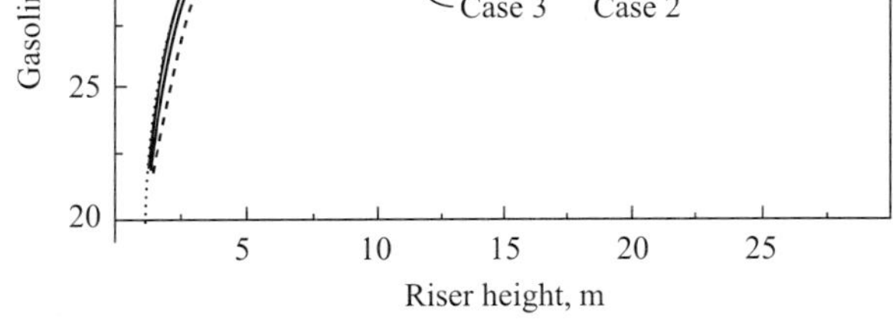

FIGURE 12.25 Evaluation of operating strategy to enhance gasoline yield (from Gao *et al.*, 1999). Unit II: Standard operation of riser reactor: Cases 1–3 represent water injected at a riser height of 11.4 m. Case 1: $T_{regen} = 602.3°C$, catalyst flux $= 9.93\ kg\ s^{-1}$. Case 2: Increased (3.5%) temperature of regenerated catalyst. Case 3: Increased (20%) catalyst flux.

necessary to use a hierarchy of modeling tools as discussed in Chapter 9 to achieve the reactor engineering objectives. A reactor engineer has to ensure that the computational model contains adequate basic physics, that the numerical implementation is well within set tolerances, and that simulations capture all the relevant flow features. Judicious use of such computational flow models will greatly reduce the burden on experimental studies and will lead to better-engineered configurations of fluidized bed reactors.

12.4. SUMMARY

Regimes of gas–solid flows in fluidized bed reactors have been discussed briefly. Two types of computational flow models, (1) discrete particle models and (2) granular flow models, are then discussed. Application of these models to fast-fluidized bed reactors (riser reactors) and bubbling/turbulent bed reactors has been discussed in detail. Recent computational work in this area has been reviewed. The importance of numerical issues such as grid refinement and discretization schemes have been highlighted with the help of examples. Some applications of computational flow models for reactor engineering of fluidized bed reactors were then discussed. Judicious use of computational models, coupled with other reaction engineering tools, will be useful to qualitatively grade different configurations and can greatly assist engineering decision-making processes. These models can substantially reduce the burden on experimental studies by providing efficient interpolation and extrapolation tools. Further work on parallelizing multifluid CFD codes will be necessary to carry out next generation, three-dimensional simulations of industrial fluidized bed reactors.

REFERENCES

Bader, R., Findlay, J. and Knowlton, T.M. (1988), Gas–solid flow patterns in a 30.5 cm diameter circulating fluidized bed, "Circulating Fluidized Bed Technology", Vol. II, P. Basu and J.F. Large, eds, Pergamon Press, New York.

Benyahia, S., Arastoopour, H., Knowlton, T.M. and Massah, H. (2000), Simulation of particles and gas flow behavior in the riser section of a circulating fluidized bed using the kinetic theory approach for the particulate phase, *Powder Technol.*, **112**, 24–33.

Bi, H.T., Ellis, N., Abba, I.A. and Grace, J.R. (2000), A state of the art review of gas–solid turbulent fluidization, *Chem. Eng. Sci.*, **55**, 4789–4825.

Bolio, E.J., Yasuna, J.A. and Sinclair, J.L. (1995), Dilute turbulent gas–solid flows in risers with particle–particle interactions, *AIChE J.*, **41**, 1375.

Chen, J.C. (1995), Clusters, *AIChE Symposium Series*, No. 313, **92**, 1–5.

Clift, R. (1993), An Occamist review of fluidized bed modeling, *AIChE Symposium Series*, No. 296, **89**, 1–17.

Darton, R.C., Lanauze, R.D., Davidson, J.F. and Harrison, D. (1977), Bubble growth due to coalescence in fluidized beds, *Trans. Inst. Chem. Eng.*, **55**, 274–280.

Dasgupta, S., Jackson, R. and Sundaresan, S. (1998), Gas particle flow in vertical pipes with high mass loading of particles, *Powder Technol.*, **96**, 6–23.

Davidson, J.F. and Harrison, D. (1963), "Fluidized Particles", Cambridge University Press.

Derouin, C., Nevicato, D., Forissier, M., Wild, G. and Bernard, J.R. (1997), Hydrodynamics of riser units and their impact on FCC operation, *I & EC Res.*, **36**, 4504.

Enwald, H., Peirano, E., Almstedt, A.E., and Leckner, B. (1999), Simulation of the fluid dynamics of a bubbling fluidized bed. Experimental validation of the two-fluid model and evaluation of a parallel multiblock solver, *Chem. Eng. Sci.*, **54**, 311–328.

Ferschneider, G. and Mege, P. (1996), Eulerian simulation of dense phase fluidized beds, *Revue de L'institut Francais du Petrole*, **51**(2), 301–307.

Gao, J., Xu, C., Lin, S., Yang, G. and Guo, Y. (1999), Advanced model for turbulent gas–solid flow and reaction in FCC riser reactors, *AIChE J.*, **45**, 1095–1113.

Geldart, D. (1973), Types of gas fluidization, *Powder Technol.*, **7**, 285–292.

Glasser, B.J., Kevrekidis, I.G. and Sundaresan, S. (1996), One- and two-dimensional traveling wave solutions in gas-fluidized beds, *J. Fluid Mech.*, **306**, 183–221.

Grace, J.R. (1986), Contacting modes and behavior classification of gas–solid and other two-phase suspensions, *Can. J. Chem. Eng.*, **64**, 353–363.

Grace, J.R. (1992), Characterization and interpretation of fluidization phenomena, *AIChE Symposium Series*, no. 289, **88**, 1–16.

Grace, J.R., Abba, I.A., Hsiaotao, Bi and Thompson, M.L. (1999), Fluidized bed catalytic reactor modeling across the flow regimes, *Can. J. Chem. Eng.*, **77**, 305–311.

Gustavsson, M. and Almstedt, A.E. (2000), Two-fluid modeling of cooling-tube erosion in a fluidized bed, *Chem. Eng. Sci.*, **55**, 867–879.

Herbert, P., Reh, L. and Nicolai, R. (1999), The ETH experimental database and results from the past eight years, *AIChE Symposium Series*, No. 321, **95**, 61–65.

Hilligardt, K. and Werther, J. (1986), Local bubble gas hold-up and expansion of gas/solid fluidized beds, *German Chem. Eng.*, **9**, 215.

Hoomans, B.P.B. (2000), Granular dynamics of gas–solid two-phase flows, PhD thesis, University of Twente, Enschede, The Netherlands.

Kaneko, Y., Shiojima, T. and Horio, M. (1999), DEM simulation of fluidized beds for the gas-phase olefin polymerization, *Chem. Eng. Sci.*, **54**, 5809–5821.

Kaneko, Y. (2000), Particle behavior and reaction in gas phase olefin polymerization reactors, PhD thesis, Tokyo University of Agriculture & Technology, Japan.

Krishna, R. (1994), A systems approach to multiphase reactor selection, *Adv. Chem. Eng.*, **19**, 201–250.

Kuipers, J.A.M., Prins, W. and van Swaaij, W.P.M. (1991), Theoretical and experimental bubble formation at a single orifice in a two-dimensional gas-fluidized bed, *Chem. Eng. Sci.*, **46**, 2881–2894.

Kuipers, J.A.M., Hoomans, B.P.B. and van Swaaij, W.P.M. (1998), Hydrodynamic models of gas fluidized beds and their role for design and operation of fluidized bed chemical reactors, in "Fluidization IX", Eds Fan, L.-S. and Knowlton, T.M., p. 15.

Kuipers, J.A.M. and van Swaaij, W.P.M. (1999), Simulation of three-dimensional riser flow using the KTGF, preprint.

Kunii, D. and Levenspiel, O. (1991), "Fluidization Engineering", Butterworth-Heinemann, Oxford.

Kunii, D. and Levenspiel, O. (2000), The K-L reactor model for circulating fluidized beds, *Chem. Eng. Sci.*, **55**, 4563–4570.

Mathiesen, V., Solberg, T. and Hjertager, B.H. (2000), An experimental and computational study of multiphase flow behavior in a circulating fluidized bed, *Int. J. Multiphase Flow*, **26**, 387–419.

Mathiesen, V., Solberg, T., Arastoopour, H. and Hjertager, B.H. (1999), Experimental and computational study of multiphase gas/particle flow in a CFB riser, *AIChE J.*, **45**, 2503–2518.

Matsen, J.M. (1982), Mechanisms of choking and entrainment, *Powder Technol.*, **31**, 21–33.

Mori, S. and Wen, C.Y. (1975), Estimation of bubble diameter in gaseous fluidized beds, *AIChE J.*, **21**, 109–117.

Neri, A. and Gidaspow, D. (2000), Riser hydrodynamics: simulation using kinetic theory, *AIChE J.*, **46**, 52–67.

Nieuwland, J.J., Huizenga, P., Kuipers, J.A.M. and van Swaaij, W.P.M. (1994), Hydrodynamic modeling of circulating fluidized beds, *Chem. Eng. Sci.*, **49**, 5803.

Nieuwland, J.J., Sint Annaland van, M., Kuipers, J.A.M. and van Swaaij, W.P.M. (1996), Hydrodynamic modeling of gas-particle flows in riser reactors, *AIChE J.*, **42**, 1569–1582.

Pita, J.A. and Sundaresan, S. (1991), Gas–solid flow in vertical tubes, *AIChE J.*, **37**, 1009–1018.

Ranade, V.V. (1998), Modeling of a FCC Regenerator, presented at *Third International Conference on Multiphase Flows*, Lyon, June.

Ranade, V.V. (1999), Modelling of gas–solid flows in FCC riser reactor: fully developed flow, *2nd International Conference on CFD*, Melbourne.

Samuelsberg, A. (1994), Modeling and simulation of fluidized bed reactors, PhD thesis, Telemark Institute of Technology, Norway.

Sinclair, J.L. and Jackson, R. (1989), Gas–particle flow in a vertical pipe with particle–particle interactions, *AIChE J.*, **35**, 1473–1486.

Sunderesan, S. (2000), Modeling the hydrodynamics of multiphase flow reactors: current status and challenges, *AIChE J.*, **46**(6), 1102–1105.

Syamlal, M. (1998), Higher order discretization methods for the numerical simulation of fluidized beds, *AIChE Symposium Series*, No. 318, **94**, 53–57.

Theologos, K.N. and Markatos, N.C. (1993), Advanced modeling of fluid catalytic cracking riser-type reactors, *AIChE J.*, **39**(6), 1007.

Theologos, K.N., Nikou, I.D., Lygeros, A.I. and Markatos, N.C. (1997), Simulation and design of fluid catalytic cracking riser-type reactors, *AIChE J.*, **43**, 486.

Theologos, K.N., Lygeros, A.I. and Markatos, N.C. (1999), Feedstock atomization effects on FCC riser reactors selectivity, *Chem. Eng. Sci.*, **54**, 5617–5625.

Thompson, M.L., Bi, H.T. and Grace, J.R. (1999), A generalized bubbling/turbulent fluidized bed reactor model, *Chem. Eng. Sci.*, **54**, 5175–5185.

Tsuji, Y., Morikawa, Y. and Shiomi, H. (1984), LDV measurements of an air–solid flow in a vertical pipe, *J. Fluid Mech.*, **139**, 417–434.

van Breugel, J.W., Stein, J.J.M. and Buurman, C. (1969), Vertical gas solid flow, Internal report Shell Laboratory, Amsterdam.

van Wachem, B.G.M., Schouten, J.C., Krishna, R. and van den Bleek, C.M. (1998), Eulerian simulations of bubbling behavior in gas–solid fluidized beds, *Comput. Chem. Eng.*, **22**, s299–s306.

van Wachem, B.G.M., Schouten, J.C., Krishna, R. and van den Bleek, C.M. (1999), Validation of the Eulerian simulated dynamic behavior of gas–solid fluidized beds, *Chem. Eng. Sci.*, **54**, 2141–2149.

Venderbosch, R.H. (1998), The role of clusters in gas-solid reactors, PhD thesis, University of Twente, The Netherlands.

Wen, C.Y. and Yu, Y.H. (1966), Mechanics of fluidization, *CEP Symposium Series*, **62**, 100–111.

Werther, J. (1978), Effect of gas distributor on the hydrodynamics of gas fluidized beds, *Ger. Chem. Eng.*, **1**, 166.

Werther, J. (1983), in "Fluidization IV", Eds Kunii, D. and Toei, R., Engineering Foundation, New York, p. 93.

Yang, Y.L. (1991), Experimental and theoretical studies on hydrodynamics in cocurrent upflow and downflow circulating fluidized beds, PhD diss., Tsinhua University, Beijing, China.

Yerushalmi, J. and Avidhan, A.A. (1985), in "Fluidization", Eds Davidson, J.F., Clift, R. and Harrison, D., Academic Press.

Zijerveld, R.C. (1998), Chaotic hydrodynamics of large and small circulating fluidized beds, PhD thesis, Delft University of Technology, The Netherlands.

13 FIXED BED AND OTHER TYPES OF REACTORS

Three major generic types of reactor, stirred, bubble column and fluidized bed reactors have been discussed in the previous three chapters. In this chapter, we briefly cover the other major generic reactor type, the fixed bed reactor. Apart from these four major reactor types, several special types of reactors are also used in practice. Newer reactor types are being invented to optimally carry out new processes (catalytic converters, chemical vapor deposition reactors, microreactors, membrane reactors and so on). It is not possible to cover all these types in detail in a single book. A brief review of some recent applications of CFD models to other types of reactor is included in this chapter. The review is not an exhaustive one but rather, is indicative of possible applications of computational flow modeling to different types of reactor. The general methodology of applying computational flow models to reactor engineering applications as discussed in this and preceding chapters may be extended to any other reactor type.

13.1. FIXED BED REACTORS

In a fixed bed reactor, gas phase reactions are generally carried out using a stationary bed of solid catalyst. In a typical reactor, suitable screens support the bed of catalyst particles, through which the gas phase flows. Gaseous reactants adsorb on the catalyst surface, reactions occur on this surface and reaction products desorb back to the gas phase. Two major types of fixed bed reactor are the conventional axial flow fixed bed reactor and the radial flow fixed bed reactor. These types are shown

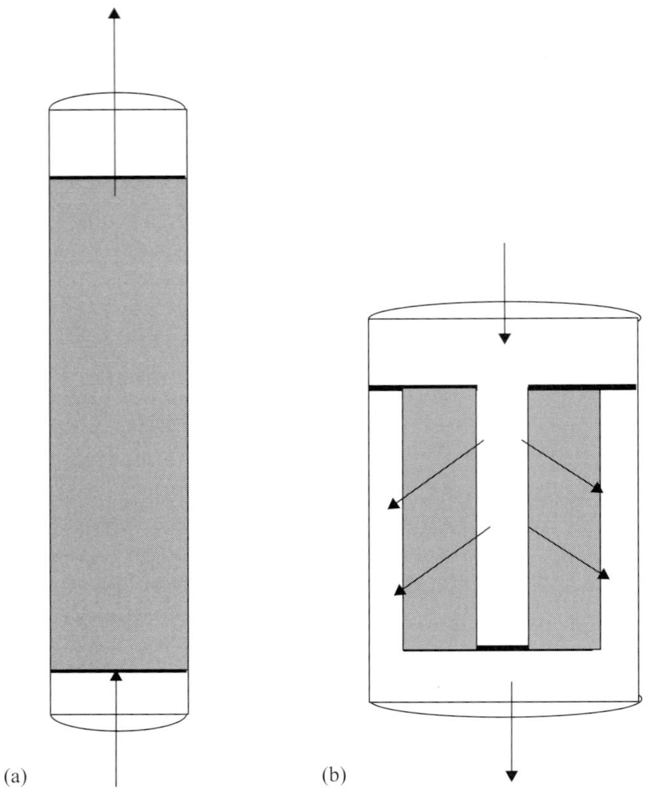

FIGURE 13.1 Types of fixed bed reactors. (a) Axial flow fixed bed reactor: Up or down flow, single or multi-stage, with or without inter-stage cooling, single or multi-tubular. (b) Radial flow fixed bed reactor: Radially inward or outward flow, straight or reverse flow (direction of inlet and outlet is same or opposite to each other).

schematically in Fig. 13.1. These reactors can be operated in various different modes as shown in this figure. The choice of reactor type depends on several issues including intrinsic reaction rate, heat of reaction, influence of external transport resistance on selectivity, molar change during the reaction, and so on. Several commercially important processes such as steam reforming (of methane or naptha), water gas shift reaction, methanol from synthesis gas, oxidation of sulfur dioxide, isomerization of xylenes, ammonia synthesis, alkylation of benzene, hydro de-waxing, reduction of nitrobenzene to aniline, manufacture of tetra-hydrofuran and butanediol from maleic anhydride, butadiene from ethanol, and so on, are carried out in fixed bed reactors.

Reaction engineering models for fixed bed reactors are well developed (Levenspiel, 1972). Generally, fixed bed reactors are modeled as plug flow or axial dispersed plug flow type models. All issues such as by-passing or channeling of gas while flowing through the catalyst bed is usually treated using a lumped parameter approach. Computational fluid dynamic models can make substantial contributions to enhancing our understanding of such complex flow behavior within the catalyst bed. If intrinsic reaction rates are fast, interphase heat and mass transfer characteristics become important design parameters. Accurate prediction of such interphase transport coefficients will require information about local fluid dynamics around catalyst pellets. It is very difficult to obtain such information under operating conditions. Computational flow models can be used to predict local fluid dynamics, from which the desired interphase transport coefficient values can be accurately estimated. These models can also be used to evaluate the influence of internals (bed supports, heat exchanger coils, gas distributors etc.) on flow distribution within the bed. Thus, computational fluid dynamics based models can make substantial contributions to linking actual hardware configuration with reactor performance. To illustrate possible applications of CFD models to fixed bed reactors, here we discuss an example of capacity enhancement of a radial fixed bed reactor (Ranade, 1997). Some recent publications on CFD models for fixed bed reactors are briefly reviewed to point out recent trends and the scope for using CFD models.

13.1.1. Radial Flow Fixed Bed Reactors

Radial flow fixed bed reactors were developed to handle large gas flow rates with minimum pressure drop and are most suitable for processes in which fluids need to be contacted with solid particles at high space velocity (Chang and Calo, 1981). Radial flow fixed bed reactors are used for a variety of processes including catalytic synthesis of ammonia, xylene isomerization and desulphurization.

The fluid dynamics of radial flow reactors (RFR) is very complex and involves severe changes in flow directions. In RFRs, feed enters parallel to the reactor axis either through the center pipe or the annulus and then flows radially through an annular catalyst basket (Fig. 13.1). It has been shown by Chang and Calo (1981) that perfect radial flow always results in the highest conversion. Axial flow through the bed, if present, decreases the conversion efficiency because it mixes fluids of different ages within the bed (similar to backmixing). Flow mal-distribution is, therefore, one of the most important variables controlling the performance of radial flow fixed bed reactors. Obviously, the capacity enhancement exercise for RFR must focus on elimination or minimization of flow mal-distribution. The flow modeling tools and methodology discussed earlier can lead to useful insights and can be used to evaluate various design solutions to minimize flow mal-distribution as discussed below. The discussion is organized in four sub-sections covering the major steps in the application of computational flow modeling to reactor engineering (problem definition, development of a suitable flow model, mapping the model onto a solver and application for process optimization).

Problem definition

The typical radial flow fixed bed reactor configuration shown in Fig. 13.1b is considered here. The reactor configuration is axis symmetric. Details of reactor construction are shown in Fig. 13.2 (only half of the reactor is shown since it is symmetric). The annular catalyst bed is supported by permeable cylindrical screens (inner and outer) and impermeable top and bottom cover plates. The top cover plate also comprises of a shroud as shown in Fig. 13.2. Such a shroud is generally provided to compensate for possible shrinkage in catalyst bed height with time. Reactants are fed to the reactor from the top end. The flow changes direction after hitting the cover plate. The feed enters the catalyst bed from the annular space between the catalyst bed and the reactor shell. The product stream exits through the outlet located at the bottom of the central pipe.

Because of the shroud in the cover plate, the active catalyst bed is limited to the annular zone A shown in Fig. 13.2. The extent of flow mal-distribution within the

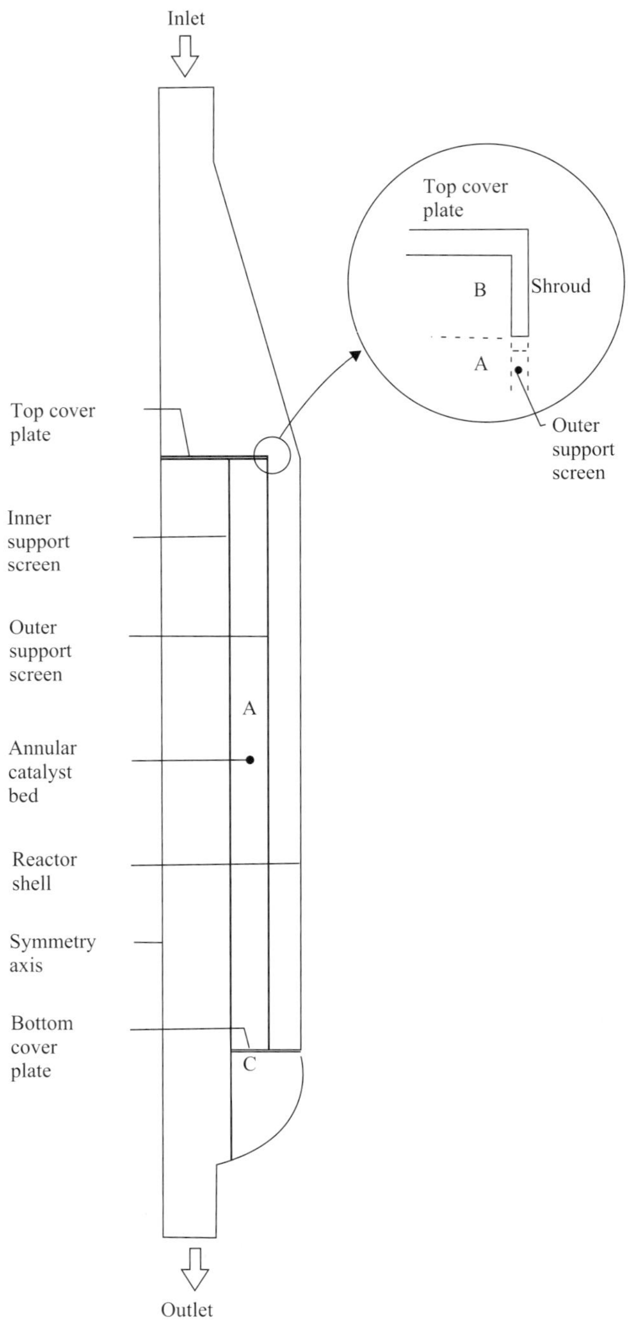

FIGURE 13.2 Details of considered radial flow fixed bed reactor (from Ranade, 1997).

active catalyst bed is essentially governed by the throughput, configuration details causing severe changes in the flow direction and the resistance offered by the support screens and the catalyst bed. It may be possible to control the resistance of the catalyst bed to some extent, by appropriately selecting the pellet size. However, the design of support screens and the overall configuration are the most important parameters governing fluid dynamics and, thereby, performance of the RFR under consideration. Designs of radial fixed bed reactors generally rely on conventional reaction engineering models (Chang and Calo, 1981). However, to realize the best possible operation and to enhance the performance of these reactors, a detailed knowledge of fluid dynamics and the extent of mal-distribution, is essential. Here we illustrate possible applications of CFD models to capacity enhancement of a typical radial flow fixed bed reactor.

For a radial flow fixed bed reactor, capacity enhancement will involve the following two aspects:

- assessment of fluid dynamics of the existing RFR configuration and identification of the scope for eliminating any flow mal-distribution;
- exploration of the possibility of loading more catalyst by increasing the volume of active catalyst bed. This may be achieved by eliminating the shroud and filling the catalyst up to the top cover plate (zone B in Fig. 13.2) and also by filling the catalyst up to the bottom of the reactor (zone C in Fig. 13.2).

It is, however, necessary to ensure that elimination of the shroud does not lead to flow mal-distribution by proper redesign of the screens. The support screens for the catalyst added in zone C also need to be properly designed to ensure uniform flow through the catalyst bed. It is, therefore, essential to develop a detailed flow model to evaluate these possibilities.

Development of a flow model

In order to understand the possible mal-distribution, it is essential to make an accurate prediction of flow in the upper region of the reactor, where severe changes in flow directions occur. Typical values of throughput for the RFR under consideration indicate that the flow is turbulent (for the specific case modeled here, feed velocity at the inlet was $40\,\mathrm{m\,s^{-1}}$). The selection of an appropriate turbulence model is, therefore, crucial. Anticipating recirculating flow in the upper region of the reactor with spatial variation of velocity and length scales of turbulence, it will be necessary to use at least a two-equation turbulence model. The standard k–ε model of turbulence, which has been tested and found to be useful for a variety of applications, may be used in absence of more specific information.

The next and most important step is to characterize the resistance offered by the porous catalyst bed and support screens. Several correlations relating the pressure drop through porous beds and velocity and bed characteristics are available (Carman, 1937; Ergun, 1952; Mehta and Hawley, 1969). The Ergun equation is one that is widely used to represent the resistance of a catalyst bed, and has the form:

$$\frac{\Delta P}{L} = \frac{150\mu}{D_\mathrm{p}^2\phi_\mathrm{p}^2}\frac{(1-\varphi)^2}{\varphi^3}V + \frac{1.75\rho}{D_\mathrm{p}\phi_\mathrm{p}}\frac{(1-\varphi)}{\varphi^3}V^2 \tag{13.1}$$

where $(\Delta P/L)$ is the pressure drop per unit length, μ is viscosity, D_p is the equivalent pellet diameter, ϕ_p is sphericity, φ is porosity and V is superficial velocity. The knowledge of pellet size, shape and voidage of the bed are thus sufficient to characterize the resistance of the catalyst bed. Equation 13.1 may be written in a compact form containing two parameters namely, permeability, β, and inertial resistance coefficient, C:

$$\frac{\Delta P}{L} = \frac{\mu}{\beta} V + C\left(\frac{1}{2}\rho V^2\right) \tag{13.2}$$

For the particular case investigated here, the values of permeability, β and inertial resistance coefficient, C were found to be $10^{-8}\,\text{m}^2$ and $10^4\,\text{m}^{-1}$, respectively. The resistance of the screens can be represented in terms of the contraction and expansion losses. The velocity heads lost during flow through screens can also be expressed in a form similar to that described in Eq. (13.2) by setting β to a very high value (10^{10}) with an appropriate value of C. The additional resistance offered by the fixed bed is usually included as additional body force terms in the governing equations. Compressibility of the gaseous feed may be ignored if the overall pressure drop is not large relative to the operating pressure of the reactor (as was the case in this particular example). The physical properties of the feed were therefore assumed to be constant (viscosity as 10^{-5} Pa.s and density $1\,\text{kg}\,\text{m}^{-3}$). In this exercise, since the objective was to evaluate possible flow mal-distribution, the development of additional specific sub-models for reactions or heat transfer, was not needed.

Mapping of flow model onto CFD solver

The geometry of the radial flow reactor was modeled and an appropriate grid generated using the 'preBFC' tool (Fluent Inc., USA). Since the reactor configuration is axis symmetric, axis symmetric two-dimensional geometry was considered. The porous media models discussed above were mapped onto a commercial CFD code, FLUENT (Fluent Inc., USA). Preliminary numerical experiments indicated that if the number of grids in the radial direction is more than 40 and in the axial direction is more than 100, the predicted results of pressure drop and flow mal-distribution become insensitive to the actual number of grids. The solution domain and grid used for all subsequent computations (50 grids in the radial direction and 116 grids in the axial direction) is shown in Fig. 13.3.

The standard k–ε model was used to simulate the turbulence. In view of the expected pore size distribution of the bed, turbulence generation in the porous catalyst bed was suppressed. Appropriate physical properties were specified in the CFD solver. Standard boundary conditions were used at all the impermeable walls and reactor outlet. The inlet boundary condition was specified using the known throughput of the RFR. It is necessary to specify the turbulence characteristics of the incoming stream at the inlet. These were specified using information about the turbulence in pipe flows. The model equations with the set boundary conditions were solved using the well-known SIMPLE algorithm (Patankar, 1980). To solve flow through porous media, it is always useful to specify a reasonably good initial guess for the pressure drop across the catalyst bed to facilitate speedy convergence. The use of zero as an initial guess for pressure necessitates the use of very low under-relaxation parameters. A few numerical experiments were carried out to select the appropriate solution

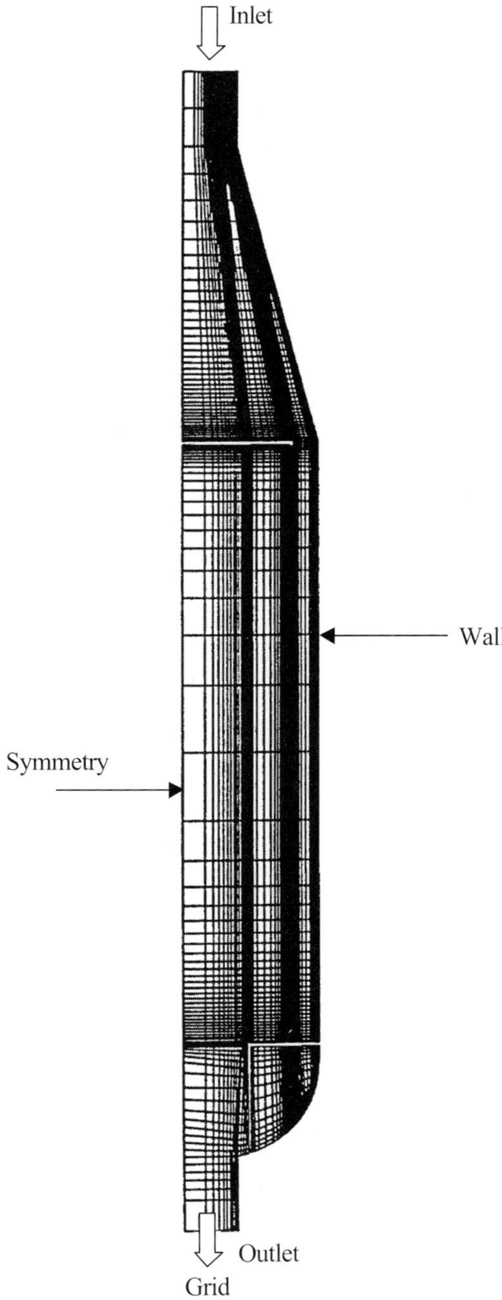

FIGURE 13.3 Solution domain and computational grid for radial flow fixed bed reactor (from Ranade, 1997).

parameters. Detailed optimization of the solution parameters (e.g. under-relaxation parameters and number of internal iterations) is difficult and often computationally expensive and is, therefore, not recommended unless several similar simulations need to be carried out.

Application for design and process optimization

Detailed experimental data for the velocity and pressure profiles in the industrial RFR under consideration was, unfortunately, not available for validation of the computational flow model. The available data of overall pressure drop across the bed could, however, be used to validate the flow model, to some extent. The predicted overall pressure drop across the bed (10 kPa) showed good agreement with the available data. In the absence of more data, this agreement was assumed to be adequate and the computational model was used to determine possible mal-distributions and to evaluate different options for capacity enhancement of the RFR under consideration.

The flow model generates detailed predictions of the flow field within the reactor. This allows rigorous scrutiny of the prevailing flow structures. For the case under consideration, details of flow at locations involving severe changes in the flow direction and the extent of mal-distribution within the active catalyst bed are of interest. In the first phase of analysis, the influence of screen resistance on the overall flow patterns and the mal-distribution was studied. The predicted profiles of inward radial velocity at the inner screen across the catalyst bed are shown in Fig. 13.4 for different screen resistance values (sign of radial velocity is negative since the fluid is flowing radially inward). It can be seen that higher screen resistance leads to more uniform flow, which agrees with intuitive expectations. The existing screens (with resistance coefficients C_2, of $2 \times 10^5\ m^{-1}$) seem to be satisfactory since the extent of non-uniformity is less than 10%. Contours of the stream function and a close-up of the flow field near the shroud and top cover plate are shown in Figs 13.5a and 13.6a, respectively. It can be seen that there is significant recirculation at the top end of the catalyst bed. The downward velocity field in the annular region between catalyst bed and reactor shell also exhibits some non-uniformity.

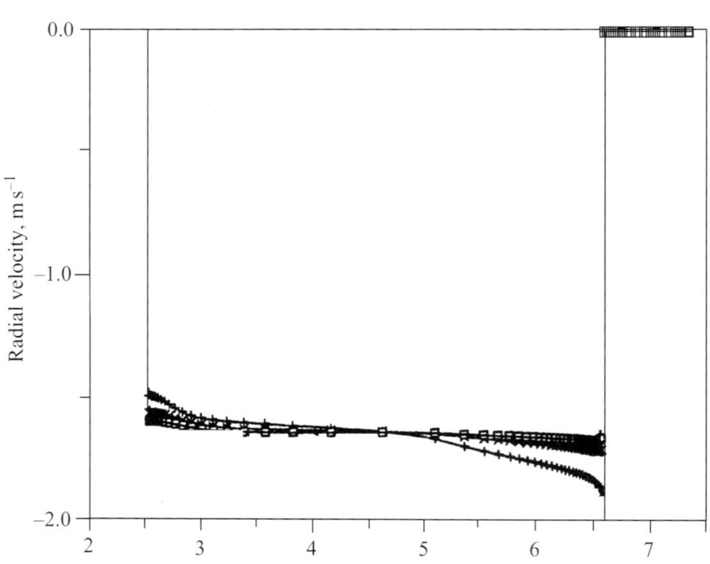

FIGURE 13.4 Predicted profiles of radial velocity at different values of screen resistance (from Ranade, 1997). RFR configuration: catalyst in zone A, top cover plate with shroud. Screen resistance coefficient, C/m for + = 0.0, × = 1.E5, □ = 2.E5.

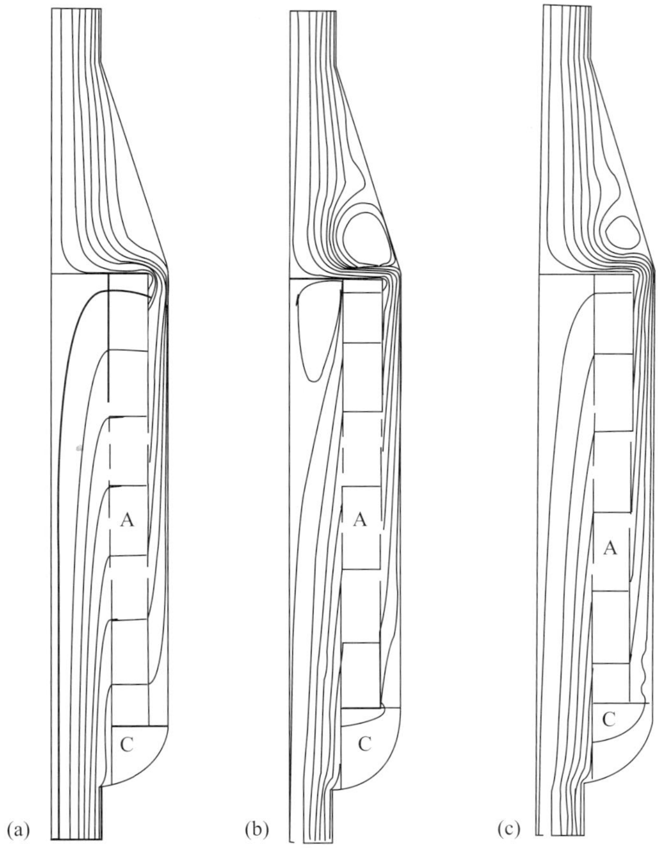

FIGURE 13.5 Predicted contours of stream function. (a) Catalyst in zone A, top cover plate with shroud ($C = 2 \times 10^5\,m^{-1}$). (b) Catalyst in zone A, B and C, top cover plate without shroud ($C = 2 \times 10^5\,m^{-1}$ for all the screens). (c) Catalyst in zone A, B and C, top cover plate without shroud ($C = 2 \times 10^5\,m^{-1}$ for inner screens of A and B and outer screen of A; $C = 1 \times 10^6\,m^{-1}$ for outer screen of B; $C = 5 \times 10^4\,m^{-1}$ for inner screen of zone C).

The flow from the catalyst bed into the central pipe is more or less uniform (Fig. 13.4) and indicates that there is not much scope to modify existing screen designs to enhance the capacity of the considered radial flow fixed bed reactor. One must, therefore, explore the second option of removing the shroud and increasing the active catalyst loading by adding catalyst in zones B and C (shown in Fig. 13.2). Fluid dynamics of the proposed RFR with active catalyst filled in zones B and C along with zone A was then simulated. As a first option, support screens for zones B and C were specified similar to the existing support screens for zone A. Contours of the predicted stream function and details of flow near the top cover plate, for this case, are shown in Figs 13.5b and 13.6b, respectively. It can be seen that removal of the shroud leads to increased circulation in the upper region of the RFR. The predicted profile of the radial velocity at the inner edge of the catalyst bed is shown in Fig. 13.7 (the corresponding profile of the base case is also shown in this figure as a reference). It can be seen that removal of the shroud, and filling with catalyst in zones B and C lead to significant non-uniformity of the flow through the catalyst bed.

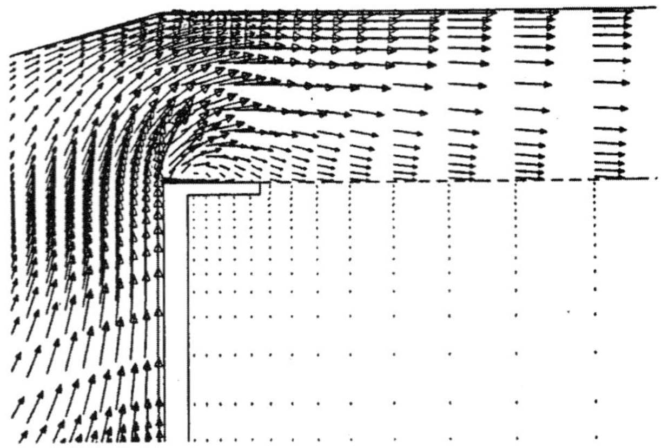

(a)

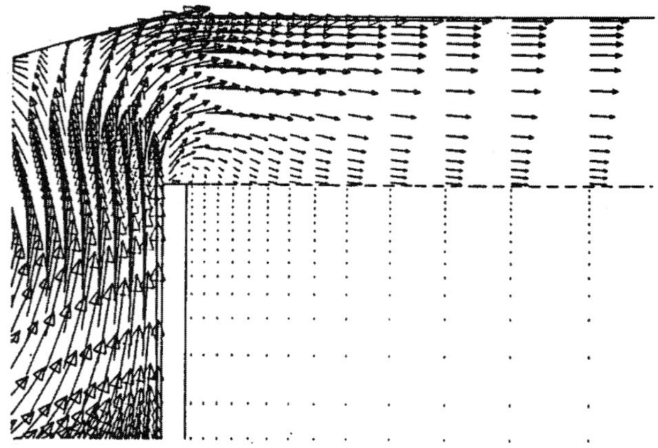

(b)

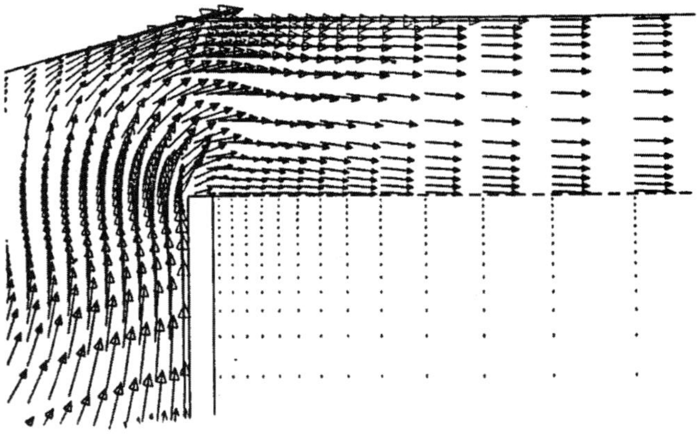

(c)

FIGURE 13.6 Predicted flow field near top cover plate (see Fig. 13.5 for details of configurations (a), (b) and (c)).

The high resistance offered by the support screens of zone C leads to very low flow through zone C and a re-circulating zone in the annular space between the catalyst bed and the reactor shell. The non-uniform flow through the catalyst bed also leads to significant re-circulation in the central pipe. Thus, mere removal of the shroud and

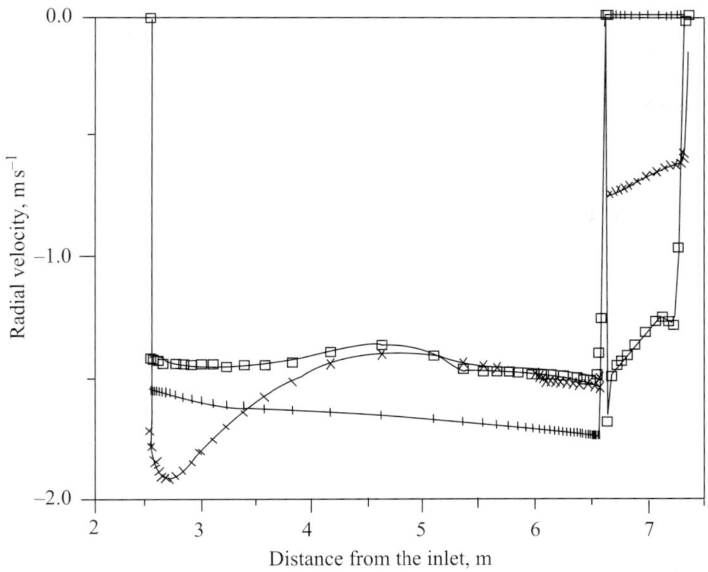

FIGURE 13.7 Predicted profiles of radial velocity at inner cylindrical screen of reactor (from Ranade, 1997). RFR configuration (as denoted in Fig. 13.5) for + − (a), × − (b), □ − (c).

filling with catalyst in zone B and C may not lead to capacity enhancements due to the associated problems of mal-distribution.

The analysis of simulated results, however, may suggest ways to redesign the support screens to improve the flow uniformity. In view of the role of the shroud in the fluid dynamics of RFR, a support screen with significantly higher resistance than the existing support screens may be installed in place of the shroud. To examine this, the resistance of the outer support screen for zone B was set to five times that for zone A. To facilitate more flow through zone C, the resistance of support screens for this zone needs to be reduced. Cover plate (screen) for zone C was, therefore, removed and the resistance of the inner support screen for the zone C was reduced to $5 \times 10^4\ m^{-1}$. Contours of the predicted streamlines and a close-up of the vector plot near the top cover plate are shown in Figs 13.5c and 13.6c, respectively. The corresponding profile of radial velocity at the inner edge of the catalyst bed is shown in Fig. 13.7. It can be seen that recirculation in the annular space between the catalyst bed and reactor shell has been eliminated by these changes. The size of the recirculating zone in the central pipe has also been considerably reduced. The flow non-uniformity caused by the removal of the shroud is more or less eliminated in this case. The flow through the zone C also has been considerably increased and is now of the same order as flow through zones A and B. Thus, the computational flow model provides quantitative guidelines to enhance the uniformity of the flow (in other words, enhancing the throughput or capacity) of the RFR under consideration.

13.1.2. Brief Review of Modeling of Fixed Bed Reactors

The methodology illustrated by the above example is fairly general and can be applied to any type of fixed bed reactor. For example, Ranade (1994) used a CFD model to optimize the design of a deflector plate in an axial fixed bed reactor. Foumeny and Benyahia (1993) also discuss the application of CFD models to optimizing internals for axial flow fixed bed reactors. It should be noted that the key issue in modeling fixed bed reactors is correct representation of the fixed bed (of solid particles). In most cases, such a fixed bed of solid particles can be modeled as an isotropic or anisotropic porous media. Additional resistance offered by such porous media can then be modeled by introducing an additional momentum sink in the momentum transport equations, as done for the case of RFR. Accuracy of such representation obviously depends on the accuracy of parameters used to represent porous media, namely, permeability, β and inertial coefficient, C. The best option to specify adequately accurate values of these parameters is, of course, experimental data.

However, it is not always possible to carry out experiments to determine values of these parameters, especially under the desired operating conditions of these fixed bed reactors (high pressure, high temperatures). In such cases, it is possible to develop rigorous computational models to characterize resistance of the fixed bed of solid particles. In these CFD models, an array of solid particles is considered. The geometry of these particles is modeled rigorously with an appropriate computational grid to cover the entire void between the solid particles. Rigorous momentum equations can then be solved to understand and to simulate details of fluid dynamics around each solid particle in the array. Such detailed simulations can be very educative about the small-scale phenomena occurring around particles in the bed and can also lead to realistic values of lumped parameters such as β and C under operating conditions. These detailed models can also be used to estimate external heat and mass transfer coefficients for the fixed bed flows. Logtenberg and Dixon (1998) and Logtenberg *et al.* (1999) developed detailed flow models by considering an array of solid particles. It is possible to solve mass, momentum and energy transport equations by considering intra-particle pores, if the pores are reasonably large. Some particles are specifically designed to generate macropores in addition to micropores, especially for bio-chemical applications involving large molecules. Knowledge of the intraparticle flow field is an important step in deriving predictive models of convective transport in these types of particles. Pfeiffer *et al.* (1996) simulated intraparticle flow in such macroporous (or gigaporous) particles. In some specialized applications, different types of fixed bed are used. For example, typical catalytic converters used by the automobile industry to reduce harmful emissions employ uniform, honeycomb like structures coated with active catalyst. It is better to use rigorous flow models of these intricate structures rather than representing them as extremely anisotropic porous media. Such detailed computational flow models are useful for understanding basic phenomena and may provide essential information to overall reactor engineering models. Such rigorous flow models may, however, become computationally intractable to use for large scale-industrial reactors. It is, therefore, necessary to develop a hierarchy of CFD models to collect the required information for design and optimization of large-scale industrial reactors.

So far, single-phase gaseous flow through fixed beds of solid particles has been discussed. When liquid flows through a fixed bed, it flows in the form of a film over solid surfaces. The flow, therefore, is entirely different than flow of gas through a fixed bed. In many cases, both, gas and liquid phases may flow through fixed beds. Modeling of these reactors involving flow of liquid over solid surfaces with a gas–liquid interface on the other side of the liquid film is discussed in the following section.

13.2. TRICKLE BED REACTORS/PACKED COLUMN REACTORS

A variety of packed columns are used either as trickle bed reactors (co-current downward flow of gas and liquid over catalyst pellets) or as column reactors (absorber/scrubbers or catalytic distillation towers, where gas and liquid phases flow counter-currently over a matrix of packings). Most conventional reaction engineering models assume drastically simplified flow patterns and are formulated as one-dimensional models. Recent experimental studies have shown the rich structure of multiphase flows through such equipment, which needs to be understood to develop reliable reactor engineering models. General volume-averaged conservation equations for multiphase flows are discussed in Chapter 4. These equations can also be applied to simulating gas–liquid flows through packed beds. It is, however, necessary to include appropriate closure models and models to account for bed heterogeneity in the overall computational model. Some recent approaches are briefly reviewed here.

Yin *et al.* (2000) developed a computational model to simulate flow and mass transfer in randomly packed distillation columns. It is necessary to develop appropriate models for interphase drag and dispersion coefficients. The general approach is to represent the overall pressure drop for gas–liquid flows in a packed column in two parts, namely wet and dry:

$$\frac{\Delta p}{\Delta z} = \left(\frac{\Delta p}{\Delta z}\right)_{\text{dry}} + \left(\frac{\Delta p}{\Delta z}\right)_{\text{wet}} \qquad (13.3)$$

The dry pressure drop can be accounted for by volume-averaged governing equations using the representation shown in Eq. (13.2). Generally for packed bed operations, only the second term on the right-hand side of this equation (corresponding to turbulent contributions) is adequate to represent dry pressure drop. The parameter C_2 appearing in this equation may be obtained by using available pressure drop correlations (Robins, 1991). Similar to gaseous flow through a fixed bed, the additional resistance offered by the bed is usually represented as an additional sink in the momentum equations (body force term). The presence of liquid phase in the packed bed reduces space for the gas phase and leads to higher pressure drop. Drag force exerted on the gas–liquid interface also contributes to the additional pressure drop. These two contributions (wet pressure drop) are usually modeled as interphase drag force. Available correlations of wet pressure drop (Robins, 1991) may be used to obtain expressions for a suitable interphase momentum exchange coefficient (refer Eq. (4.27)).

$$K_{\text{GL}} = \frac{(\Delta p/\Delta z)_{\text{wet}}}{|U_{\text{G}} - U_{\text{L}}|} \qquad (13.4)$$

In addition to these pressure drop models, models to represent spreading of liquid in packed beds because of spatial variation in flow resistance are needed. In a randomly packed bed, the void fraction is not uniform. This implies that some flow channels formed within a packed bed offer less resistance to flow than other channels of equal cross-sectional area. Liquid will tend to move toward channels of lower resistance, leading to higher liquid hold-up in such channels. Thus, even if the initial liquid distribution is uniform, inherent random spatial variation of the bed leads to non-uniform liquid flow. Yin *et al.* (2000) assumed that the dispersion coefficient for liquid phase volume fraction is linearly proportional to the adverse gradient of the axial flow resistance (the higher the resistance, the lesser the tendency for liquid flow):

$$\Gamma = -K_c \nabla R_z \tag{13.5}$$

where K_c is a proportionality constant and can be determined by fitting experimental data. R_z is axial flow resistance and can be estimated by considering the inertial term of the Ergun equation. The dispersion coefficient can thus be written:

$$\Gamma = 1.75\, K_c \frac{\rho U^2}{D_p \varphi^2} \nabla \varphi - 3.5\, K_c \frac{(1-\varphi)\rho U}{D_p \varphi} \nabla U \tag{13.6}$$

The first term on the right side of this equation represents the effect of bed structure (spatial variation of bed void fraction, φ) on liquid spreading, and the second term implies that even for homogeneous packed beds, the liquid spreading will occur if the initial distribution of liquid is non-uniform. The turbulent dispersion coefficient is modeled conventionally using the turbulent viscosity and turbulent Prandtl number. Yin *et al.* (2000) used the value of turbulent Prandtl number as 0.01, which is much lower than the generally used value (nearly 1). In order to close the model equations, it is necessary to provide information about spatial variation of voidage in packed beds. Yin *et al.* (2000) carried out measurements of voidage distribution and used an empirical correlation based on their own measurements. With such a model, Yin *et al.* (2000) were able to simulate pressure drop and height equivalent to a theoretical plate for a column packed with Pall rings. Their simulation results were able to capture the influence of size of packings and gas flow rate on pressure drop adequately (Fig. 13.8). The CFD model was also able to adequately simulate HETP (height equivalent to a theoretical plate) values of Pall rings. These results are shown in Fig. 13.9. It can be seen that the improvement of separation efficiency with increase in pressure (lower HETP) was correctly captured by the CFD simulations. Thus, the computational models can be used to understand the influence of packings size, operating pressure and other design and operating issues on performance.

It must be noted that the porosity and its distribution in a packed bed are the key parameters in determining the flow distribution within the bed. In recent years, numerous attempts have been carried out to provide quantitative information about porosity distribution (Mueller, 1991; Borkink *et al.*, 1992; Bey and Eigenberger, 1997). Mean porosity and its distribution are determined largely by particle size, shape, surface properties and method of packing. Generally, cross-sectional averaged porosity along the height of the bed is distributed randomly. The longitudinally averaged radial porosity profile exhibits a maximum near the wall. Recently, Jiang *et al.* (2000a, 2000b) considered such random distributions of porosity within the bed and developed a method to generate random distribution of bed porosity while satisfying the constraints on mean porosity and longitudinal averaged radial porosity profiles. A sample of random porosity distribution generated by their method is shown in Fig. 13.10. Such randomly distributed bed porosity may give more realistic results than assuming mean porosity all over the bed. It must be noted that the porosity distribution observed in a packed bed will be obviously dependent on scale of observation. It has been experimentally shown that at a scale of a cluster of particles, porosity has a Gaussian distribution (Jiang *et al.*, 2000a) while at a much smaller scale, porosity has a bi-modal distribution (Jiang *et al.*, 2001). This relationship between porosity

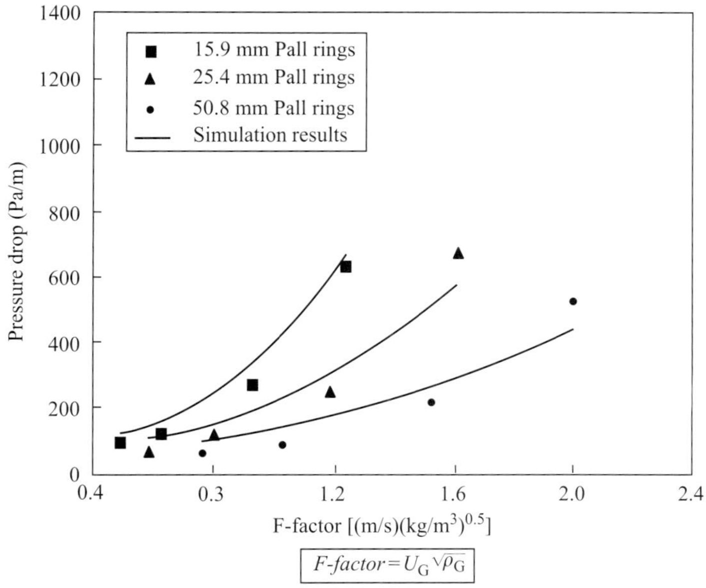

FIGURE 13.8 Comparison of predicted and experimental pressure drop for three Pall rings (from Yin *et al.*, 2000).

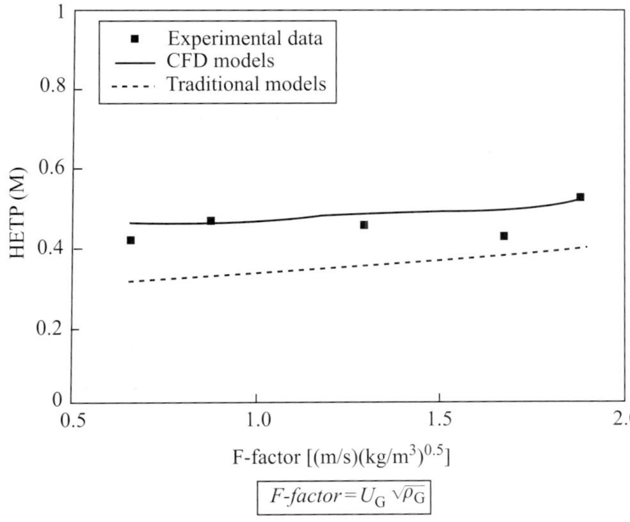

FIGURE 13.9 Comparison of predicted and experimental HETP values for 25.4 mm Pall rings (from Yin *et al.*, 2000).

distribution and size of bed section should be kept in mind when generating randomly distributed porosity within the bed.

Closure models, similar to those used by Yin *et al.* (2000), can also be used to simulate flows in trickle bed reactors. It must, however, be noted that in a packed column used for separations, packing element size is around 25 mm, while in trickle bed reactors, the particle sizes are typically in the range 0.5 to 6 mm. For large

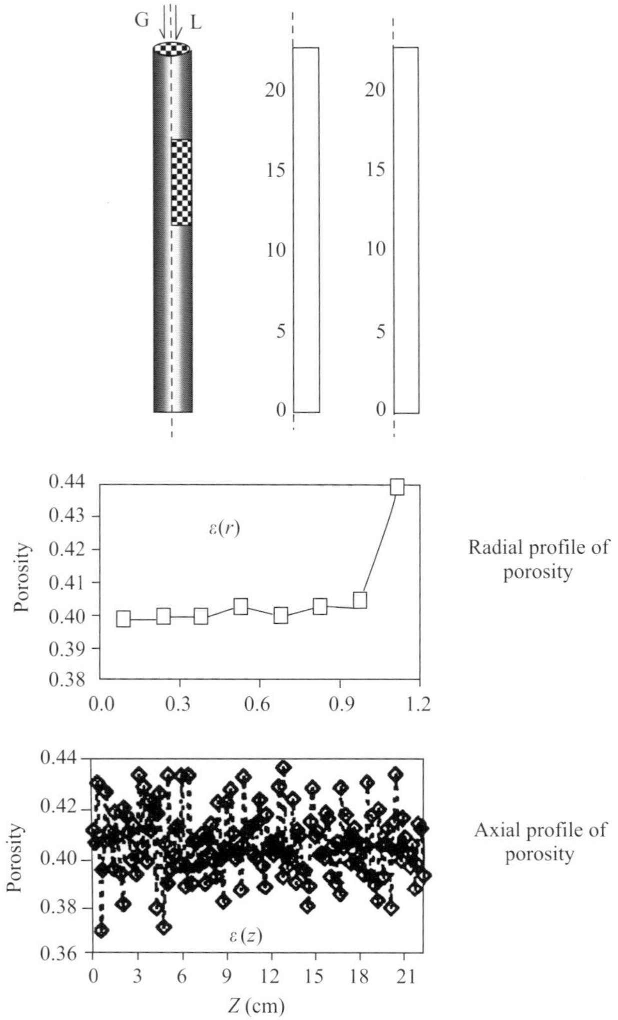

FIGURE 13.10 Computer generated 2D axis-symmetric solids volume fraction distribution (from Jiang *et al.*, 2000a).

particles, the gravity and inertial forces are important and the liquid distribution is not very sensitive to the wettability of the packing surface. Closure models used by Yin *et al.* (2000) to account for the gravity and inertial forces are discussed above. Jiang *et al.* (2000a, 2000b) also used the Ergun equation to account for these forces. In addition, it is necessary to account for interfacial tension and packing wettability in the physical sub-models to simulate gas–liquid flow through a bed of smaller particles. Based on the experimental data on liquid hold-up distribution with and without particle pre-wetting and an empirical relationship between particle wetting factor and velocity and pressure gradient (of Al-Dahhan and Dudukovik, 1995), Jiang *et al.* (2000a, 2000b) introduced an additional term representing capillary effect in their two-fluid model. When particles are completely wetted, these additional terms reduce to zero. These additional models are not yet sufficiently validated. It is, however, expected that further research along these lines will allow one to capture the influence of particle wetting on flow distribution within the packed beds.

Apart from these attempts to simulate macroscale flow distribution within the trickle bed, some attempts at understanding microscale flow phenomena using computational flow models have also been carried out. Higler *et al.* (1999) simulated counter-current flow of gas and liquid through a structured packed bed reactor. They simulated flow of liquid through a sandwich structure. One cross-over of tubes of triangular section was considered in their simulations. The results were useful to understand residence time distribution and the influence of cross-over on this distribution. Simulations of microscale flow phenomena may lead to better understanding of flow regimes of trickle bed reactors (co-current operations) or absorption columns. Casey *et al.* (1998) reported some of the early results of simulations of film flow over inclined surfaces with a gas flow in the opposite direction. They were able to capture the onset of wavy flow. Much more work is needed in these directions to enhance our understanding of flooding and regime transitions in gas–liquid flows in packed columns. Some of the applications of computational flow modeling to other chemical reactors are briefly reviewed in the following section.

13.3. OTHER REACTORS

One textbook reactor which also has several industrial applications, is a tubular reactor. For example, polymerization of ethylene is carried out in a tubular reactor. Although, a lot of information is available on global fluid dynamics of tubular reactors, when reactions and fluid dynamics are intimately connected via mixing, it is necessary to develop a comprehensive computational flow model including chemical reactions. Recently Kolhapure and Fox (1999) used such a computational flow model (based on a multi-environment reactive mixing model) to understand the effect of micromixing on LDPE (low density polyethylene) polymerization in a plant-scale tubular reactor. The relevant model equations and necessary numerical methods are already discussed in earlier chapters. The study by Kolhapure and Fox (1999) shows that imperfect mixing of species reduces monomer conversion, increases the polydispersity index and may cause local hot spots (with possible degradation and adverse product quality). Apart from giving important physical insights, such a computational flow model can also be used to carry out 'virtual experiments' to evaluate various design alternatives to minimize imperfect mixing in industrial LDPE reactors.

Another major application of computational flow modeling is for engineering chemical vapor deposition (CVD) reactors. Various types of CVD reactor are used in the microelectronics industry (Kleijn, 1991). In CVD reactors, fluid dynamics, transport processes and chemical reactions are again strongly interrelated and computational fluid dynamics based models can make substantial contributions to the design of industrial-scale CVD reactors. Recently, Komiyama *et al.* (1999) reported the application of computational flow models to simulate a tubular CVD reactor. The model was used to simulate growth rates and composition on a 5-inch wafer placed in a vertical, axis-symmetric, cold wall reactor. No fitting parameter was used for these simulations. Their predicted results are shown in Fig. 13.11a and 13.11b. It can be seen that CFD captured the growth rate and composition quite adequately. The simulation results indicate that decreasing mass transfer resistance near the wall led

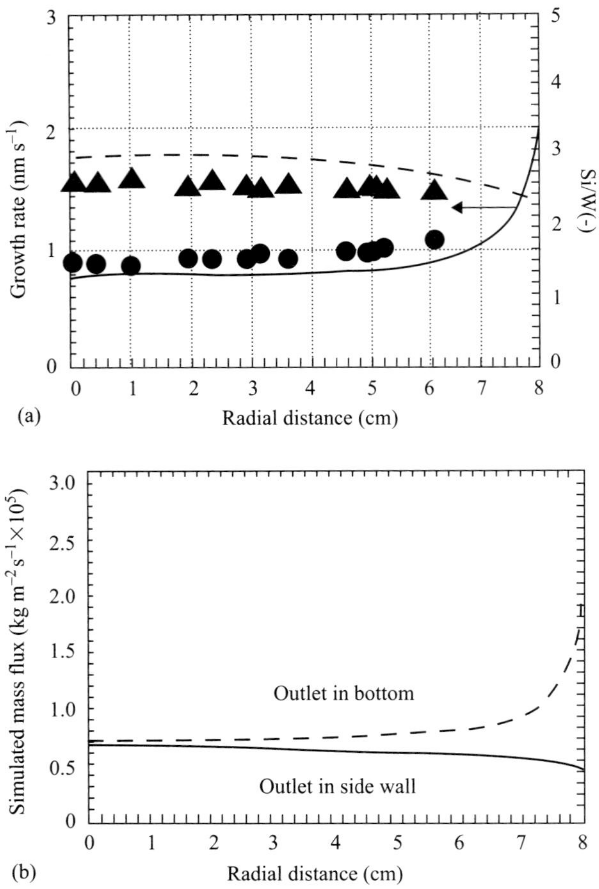

FIGURE 13.11 Application of computational flow model to simulate single-wafer CVD reactor (from Komiyama *et al.*, 1999). (a) Standard geometry, (b) evaluation of outlet configurations.

to higher growth rate near the wall region. The computational model was further used to evolve a suitable reactor configuration to reduce the non-uniformity in growth rate. These 'virtual' experiments on computer indicated that changing the position of the reactor outlet from bottom to sidewall leads to less non-uniformities in the growth rate (Fig. 13.11b). Thus, these comprehensive computational flow models can be used to accelerate the development of better CVD reactors with minimum prototyping.

Tubular reactors are also used to carry out some multiphase reactions. Warnecke *et al.* (1999) reported use of a computational flow model to simulate an industrial tubular reactor carrying out a gas–liquid reaction (propylene oxide manufacturing process). In this process, liquid is a dispersed phase and gas is a continuous phase. The two-fluid model discussed earlier may be used to carry out simulations of gas–liquid flow through a tubular reactor. Warnecke *et al.* (1999) applied such a model to evaluate the influence of bends etc. on flow distribution and reactor performance. The model may be used to evolve better reactor configurations. In many tubular reactors, static mixers are employed to enhance mixing and other transport processes. Computational flow models can also make significant contributions to understanding the role of static mixers and for their optimization. Visser *et al.* (1999) reported CFD simulations of flow and heat transfer in the Sulzer SMX static mixers. Such models can be used to evaluate newer options to efficiently carry out industrial mixing.

Catalytic converters used in the automobile industry are also a special class of tubular reactors. Many of these converters use monolith geometry in which unconverted hydrocarbons from exhaust gases are oxidized. Heat and mass transfer effects (including conjugate heat transfer and radiation) and flow mal-distribution are the crucial design issues. Detailed computational flow models can be used to understand these critical design issues and their influence on performance of the converter. Taylor (1999) developed a comprehensive CFD model to simulate heat and mass transfer in a monolithic catalytic converter. The models can be used to evaluate configurations leading to better heat transfer characteristics and therefore better converter durability at high temperatures. When catalyst does not deactivate rapidly, monolithic reactors may offer an attractive alternative to mechanically agitated slurry reactors, especially for fine chemicals (Cybulski *et al.*, 1999). CFD-based models can make substantial contributions to enhancing selectivity and optimization of monolithic reactors.

Apart from the conventional reactor types discussed so far, there are several special reactor types such as membrane reactors, jet loop reactors, microchannel reactors, furnaces and so on. It is virtually impossible to discuss or to describe these reactor types here. The basic principles discussed in this and previous chapters, however, allow the reactor engineer to identify and to address key design issues with the help of computational flow modeling. There is a growing trend to develop multifunctional reactors and compact reactors (see for example recent articles on process intensification by Green *et al.*, 1999 and Stankiwicz and Moulijn, 2000). For such cases, computational flow modeling will play an even more important role and will be used extensively for reactor engineering. The general approach of developing a hierarchy of modeling tools will allow reactor engineers to extend the range of computational models and to realize faster reactor development. In this book, we have discussed several examples of applying such a methodology for better reactor engineering based on tractable CFD models.

Computational flow models can also prove to be very useful for simulating a variety of reactor accessories, which may also significantly influence overall reactor performance. Reactor accessories may include distributors, instrumentation probes, safety mechanisms (vents), spargers, filters, cyclones and so on. There are several instances where minor problems such as clogging of the filter installed near the outlet nozzle, degradation (and subsequent contamination) at the relatively stagnant region near the instrument probes and so on, have caused unsatisfactory reactor performance. Computational flow models provide invaluable help to identify these problems, to identify the desired flow field and to evaluate various ways to realize the desired flow field in practice. Applications of CFD models to simulate various reactor accessories are increasing exponentially. This literature is not reviewed here explicitly, the general approach discussed in this book, however, might be used to carry out such simulations to enhance overall reactor performance.

13.4. SUMMARY

Application of a Eulerian–Eulerian approach to modeling flow in fixed bed as well as trickle bed reactors is discussed. A methodology of applying computational flow modeling to enhance the performance of a radial flow fixed bed reactor is discussed with the help of an example. Realistic representation of the characteristics of the fixed bed (porosity distribution, degree of anisotropy and so on) is crucial for carrying out simulations for engineering use. Most of the current work relies on empirical information and pressure drop data to calibrate computational flow models of fixed and trickle bed reactors. Such calibrated computational flow models will be useful to understand issues related to mal-distribution, channeling, formation of hot spots etc. in these reactors. Recent work on application of computational flow models for other miscellaneous reactors is briefly reviewed. Computational flow models are being increasingly used in designing newer and specialty reactors such as chemical vapor deposition reactors or catalytic converters. To realize process intensification and performance enhancement, accurate knowledge of the underlying flow field in chemical reactors is essential. The approach and computational models developed in this book will allow the reactor engineer to harness the power of computational flow modeling for better reactor engineering.

REFERENCES

Al-Dahhan, M.H. and Dudukovic, M.P. (1995), Catalyst wetting efficiency in trickle bed reactors at high pressures, *Chem. Eng. Sci.*, **50**, 2377–2389.

Bey, O. and Eigenberger, G. (1997), Fluid flow through catalyst filled tubes, *Chem. Eng. Sci.*, **52**, 1365–1376.

Borkink, J.G.H., van de Watering, C.G. and Westerterp, K.R. (1992), The statistical character of bed–scale effective heat transport coefficients for packed beds, *Trans. IChemE*, **70**(A), 610–619.

Carman, P.C. (1937), Fluid flow through granular beds, *Trans. Inst. Chem. Eng.*, **15**, 150–166.

Casey, M., Lang, E., Reiner, M., Schlegel, R. and Wehrli, M. (1998), Application of computational fluid dynamics for process engineering at Sulzer, *Speedup*, **12**, 43–51.

Chang, H.-C. and Calo, J.M. (1981), An analysis of radial flow packed bed reactors: how are they different?, in "Chemical Reactors", Ed. H.S. Foggler, ACS Symposium series 168, ACS, Washington DC.

Cybulski, A., Stankiewicz, A., Edvinsson Albers, R.K. and Moulijn, J.A. (1999), Monolithic reactors for fine chemicals industries: A comparative analysis of a monolithic reactor and a mechanically agitated slurry reactor, *Chem. Eng. Sci.*, **54**, 2351–2358.

Ergun, S. (1952), Flow through packed columns, *Chem. Eng. Prog.*, **48**(2), 89–94.

Foumeny, E.A. and Benyahia, F. (1993), Can CFD improve the handling of air, gas and gas–liquid mixtures?, *Chem. Eng. Prog.*, **21**, 91(1), 8–9.

Green, A., Johnson, B. and John, A. (1999), Process intensification magnifies profits, *Chem. Eng.*, **106**, December, 66–73.

Higler, A.P., Krishna, R., Ellenberger, J. and Taylor, R. (1999), Counter current operation of structured catalytically packed-bed reactor: liquid phase mixing and mass transfer, *Chem. Eng. Sci.*, **54**, 5145–5152.

Jiang, Y., Khadilkar, M.R., Al-Dahhan, M.H., Dudukovic, M.P. *et al.* (2000a), CFD modeling of multiphase flow distribution in catalytic packed-bed reactors: scale down issues, presented at *3rd International Symposium in Catalysis in Multiphase Reactors*, Naples (Italy) also published in Catalyst Today, **66**, 209–218 (2001).

Jiang, Y., Khadilkar, M.R., Al-Dahhan, M.H. and Dudukovic, M.P. (2000b), Statistical characterization of macroscale multiphase flow textures in trickle beds, presented at *16th International Symposium on Chemical Reaction Engineering*, Poland.

Jiang, Y., Khadilkar, M.R., Al-Dahhan, M.H. and Dudukovic, M.P. (2001), CFD modeling of multiphase flow in packed bed reactors: fluid flow, bed structure and modeling issues, *AIChE J.*, submitted for publication.

Kleijn, C. (1991), Transport phenomena in chemical vapor deposition reactors, PhD thesis, Delft University of Technology, The Netherlands.

Kolhapure and Fox, R. (1999), CFD analysis of micromixing effects on polymerization in tubular low-density polyethylene reactors, *Chem. Eng. Sci.*, **54**, 3233–3242.

Komiyama, H., Shimogaki, Y. and Egashira, Y. (1999), Chemical reaction engineering in the design of CVD reactors, *Chem. Eng. Sci.*, **54**, 1941–1958.

Levenspiel, O. (1972), "Chemical Reaction Engineering", 2nd edition, John Wiley & Sons, New York.

Logtenberg, S.A. and Dixon, A.G. (1998), Computational fluid dynamics studies of fixed bed heat transfer, *Chem. Eng. Processes*, **37**, 7–21.

Logtenberg, S.A., Nijemeisland, M. and Dixon, A.G. (1999), Computational fluid dynamics simulations of fluid flow and heat transfer at the wall-particle contact points in a fixed bed reactor, *Chem. Eng. Sci.*, **54**, 2433–2440.

Mehta, D. and Hawley, M.C. (1969), Wall effect in packed column, *Ind. Eng. Chem. Proc. Des. Dev.*, **8**, 280–282.

Mueller, G.E. (1991), Prediction of radial porosity distribution in randomly packed fixed beds of uniformly sized spheres in cylindrical containers, *Chem. Eng. Sci.*, **46**, 706.

Patankar, S.V. (1980), "Numerical Heat Transfer and Fluid Flow", Hemisphere, Washington DC.

Pfeiffer, J.F., Chen, J.C. and Hsu, J.T. (1996), Permeability of gigaporous particles, *AIChE J.*, **42**, 932–939.

Ranade, V.V. (1994), Modelling of flow mal-distribution in a fixed bed reactor using PHOENICS, *J. PHOENICS*, **7**(3), 59–72.

Ranade, V.V. (1997), Improve reactor via CFD, *Chem. Eng.*, **104**, May, 96–102.

Robins, L.A. (1991), Improve pressure-drop predictions with a new correlation, *Chem. Eng. Prog.*, **87**(5), May, 87–91.

Stankiwicz, A.I. and Moulijn, J.A. (2000), Process intensification: transforming chemical engineering, *Chem. Eng. Prog.*, **96**(11), January, 22–34.

Taylor, W. (1999), CFD prediction and experimental validation of high-temperature thermal behavior in catalytic converters, *SAE Special Publication*, **SP-1455**, 29–42.

Visser, J.E., Rozendal, P.F., Hoogstraten, H.W. and Beenackers, A.A.C.M. (1999), Three-dimensional numerical simulation of flow and heat transfer in the Sulzer SMX static mixer, *Chem. Eng. Sci.*, **54**, 2491–2500.

Warnecke, H.-J., Schafer, M., Pruss, J. and Weidenbach, M. (1999), A concept of simulate an industrial size tube reactor with fast complex kinetics and absorption of two gases on the basis of CFD modeling, *Chem. Eng. Sci.*, **54**, 2513–2521.

Yin, F.H., Sun, C.G., Afacan, A., Nandakumar, K. and Chuang, K.T. (2000), CFD modeling of mass transfer processes in randomly packed distillation columns, *Ind. Eng. Chem. Res.*, **39**, 1369–1380.

PART V
EPILOGUE

14 EPILOGUE

Almost all the processes relevant to the manufacturing industry (chemical, petrochemical, fertilizer, metallurgical, power, cement and so on) involve flow of fluids in some way or the other. Innovative and competitive edge in any manufacturing industry rests on how well these flow processes are designed and operated. In view of the central role of reactors in chemical process industries, there is tremendous potential for applying new flow modeling tools to chemical reactor engineering. Reactor engineering requires expertise from different fields ranging from chemistry and catalysis to fluid mixing and transport phenomena. Reactor engineering has to marry chemistry and catalysis with reactor hardware to evolve the best possible way to carry out the process under consideration. It is obvious that reactor engineers need to use several modeling tools to achieve their objectives. Computational flow modeling or CFD is being increasingly used for reactor engineering practice and research. In recent symposiums on reactor engineering (ISCRE and GLS conferences), more than 50% of the papers mentioned CFD. I hope that this book conveys the potential of computational flow modeling for reactor engineering applications and facilitates realization of this potential.

I have made an attempt to provide sufficient information to understand and to define the specific role of computational flow modeling in reactor engineering applications. Discussions on the main features of reactor engineering, computational flow modeling and their interrelationship will help to select appropriate models, and to apply these computational models to link reactor hardware to reactor performance. Mathematical modeling of flow processes (including turbulent flows, multiphase flows and reactive flows) and corresponding numerical methods to solve these model equations are discussed. Implementation of these mathematical models and corresponding numerical methods on computer, and key issues for evaluating available computational tools are also discussed. The overall methodology of achieving the objectives of reactor engineering via computational flow modeling is discussed with the help of practical examples. Aspects of the application of computational flow modeling to four major reactor types: stirred tank reactor, bubble column reactor, fluidized bed reactor and fixed (or trickle) bed reactor, and some other types of reactor are discussed. The selection of examples used in this book may appear somewhat biased since many of these are drawn from our own research and consulting experience. An attempt is, however, made to evolve general guidelines, which may be useful for solving practical reactor engineering problems.

At this juncture, it would be useful to re-examine the lessons learnt from our experience of the application of computational flow modeling to reactor engineering. From our experience, it is extremely important to correctly:

- identify and pose the problem;
- analyze key issues relevant to achieving the defined objectives; and
- select an appropriate modeling approach/tools which are consistent with the set objectives.

For any engineering discipline, the so-called Occam's razor always provides guidelines for selecting appropriate methods/tools. Occam's razor can be stated as, 'it is futile to do with more, what can be done with less'. There are many instances where simple, conventional models may provide elegant and adequate solutions. Even if complete solutions are not possible with simple, conventional models, conventional analysis and modeling is essential to understand the problem correctly and for appropriate formulation of the flow-modeling problem. If the time and space scale analysis indicates that a complete mixing assumption is more or less valid for the stirred reactor under consideration, it may not be necessary to use a computational flow model to simulate conversion obtainable in such a reactor. Conventional flow modeling and accumulated empirical knowledge about the equipment under consideration must be used to get whatever useful information that can be obtained, before undertaking rigorous CFD modeling.

It is, however, important to emphasize here the maxim that says 'one should always try to make things as simple as possible (following the Occam's razor) but not simpler'. It may be necessary to match the complexity of the problem with complexity of the analyzing tool. One may try to find simple solutions to complex problems, which may not be right all the time! Distinguishing the 'simple' (keeping the essential aspects intact and ignoring non-essential aspects) and 'simpler' (ignoring some of the crucial issues along with the non-essential issues; akin to throwing the baby away with the bath water) formulations is a very important step towards finding useful solutions to practical problems. One should have the expertise and skill to select an appropriate level of complexity of the analyzing tools to suit the set objectives. This is one of the most important prerequisites for successful execution of reactor-engineering projects. In many reactor-engineering applications, detailed fluid dynamic models may become necessary and may substantially contribute towards performance enhancement. Thus, playing with problem definition (evaluating symptoms/set objectives, identifying and separating essential and non-essential issues, reframing problem objectives in the light of such analysis) and selecting an appropriate modeling approach, is one of the most important tasks of a reactor engineer. More often than not computational flow modeling projects are likely to overrun the budget (of time and other resources) due to inadequate attention being paid to this initial step of the overall project. Inadequate attention to this step may even lead to failure in achieving the set objectives. Some of the examples discussed in Chapters 9 to 13 are useful to understand the importance of selecting an appropriate modeling approach using different sets of models.

Another important lesson is that it is beneficial and more efficient to develop mathematical and computational models in several stages, rather than directly working with and developing a one-stage comprehensive model. For example, even if the objective is to simulate non-isothermal reactive flows, it is always useful to undertake a stage-wise development and validation of computational models. Such stages could be: (1) simulate laminar flow; (2) examine these results and select an appropriate turbulence model; carry out simulation of turbulent flow; (3) evaluate isothermal turbulent simulations, verify existence of key flow features (go back to step 2 if results are not satisfactory), try to validate quantitatively wherever possible; (4) include non-isothermal effects (without reactions); (5) include reactive mixing models in the non-isothermal turbulent models; and (6) validate and apply. Development efforts and simulated results from each stage enhance understanding of the flow phenomena. For each stage of model development, quantitative evaluation of limiting solutions (may be with drastic simplifications) is often useful to enhance confidence in the developed computational model. The simulated results also provide information about the relative importance of different processes, which helps to make a judicious choice between 'simple' and 'simpler' representations. Such a multistage development process also greatly reduces numerical problems, as the results from each stage serve as a convenient starting point for the next stage.

Apart from appropriate model formulation, it is also essential to understand the influence of numerical issues (grid spacing, time step, degree of convergence and so on) on simulation results before one can use the results obtained from a computational flow model for engineering applications. One must resist the temptation to use physically realistic simulated results without quantitatively assessing grid dependence. This is true even when the objective is just to understand key flow features qualitatively. It is possible, in some cases, that a different grid spacing may show different key flow features. Sometimes it is observed that computational results obtained with a specific grid show good agreement with the available data. This acceptable agreement often encourages immediate application of the computational model to the problem under consideration. It must be remembered that no matter how good the agreement one finds between available data and results simulated on a specific grid, if the solution is not grid independent, the agreement is probably an artefact of the specific grid size. It is, therefore, necessary to make an attempt to obtain grid independent results before they are used for reactor engineering applications.

In many situations, however, it may not be possible to obtain grid independent solutions for flow in complex industrial equipment (due to the constraints on available time and computational resources). In such cases, the reactor engineer may still use these simulations for practical applications, provided some of the following precautionary steps are carried out:

- quantitative evaluation of special cases/limiting solutions;
- qualitative verification of key flow features;

- assessing dependence on grid spacing by extrapolating key results to zero grid spacing (results may not be grid independent even for the finest grid used in these simulations).

Another related issue is about finding some flow features in the simulation results, which are not really expected from the underlying mathematical model. For example, the Eulerian–Eulerian simulations of a bubble column containing finite vapor space above the liquid pool often show a gas–liquid interface when contours of gas volume fraction are plotted. Usually, in such simulations, the two-fluid model and the interphase drag coefficients suitable for regions in which gas is dispersed in a liquid are used. These models are not suitable to simulate the region in which the gas phase is continuous. Because of this and since by its very nature, Eulerian–Eulerian simulations are not suitable to simulate a gas–liquid interface, results near the interface are highly inaccurate. It is necessary to consider these aspects before one proceeds to use the simulated information about the pseudo-gas–liquid interface for engineering decision making. It is very important to understand the capabilities and limitations of the underlying mathematical model. Considerations of limiting solutions are often useful for this purpose. The necessity of verification and validation of computational flow models is repeatedly emphasized throughout this book. In many industrial applications, data required for adequate validation is not available and a reactor engineer has to rely only on 'indirect validation' of some gross quantities. Reactor engineers must, therefore, develop their skills in assessing the quality of simulations in the absence of direct validation. Such skills may be acquired by studying known case studies and through hands-on experience of applying computational flow modeling to reactor engineering. If some of these issues are properly taken care of, computational flow modeling (CFM) may be used to provide invaluable information for reactor engineering applications. CFM may be the only way to realize the 'wish list' of a reactor engineer in practice. CFM may also be used to study aspects of flow which are not amenable to experiments (due to high temperature/pressure or corrosive conditions). Detailed flow modeling of industrial processes offers new possibilities for performance enhancement and innovation in the design of industrial reactors. Because of these unique capabilities of computational flow modeling, CFM will have tremendous impact on current as well as future reactor engineering practices.

With the emergence of cheap, high speed computing platforms and the availability of commercial CFD codes and support, flow modeling needs to be harnessed to devise the best possible reactor hardware. Some comments on future trends and needs may be appropriate at this juncture. Each advance in the CFD community's capability to perform a particular class of computations, has led to a corresponding increase in the engineer's expectations. These expectations can be translated to define research and developmental requirements. These requirements may be classified into two categories: computational and physical. The most important areas of computational character, in which further work is needed, are:

- cheaper ways of conducting fine-grid computations;
- minimizing numerical diffusion without jeopardizing robustness;
- preserving the order and flexibility in CFD codes as the complexity of their physical content increases.

Further research on problems of physical character, needs to focus primarily on the development of better turbulence models, better multiphase flow models and better reactive flow models. Recent advances in applying renormalization group (RNG) theory to formulate turbulence models appear to be promising. However, much work is needed to understand the intricacies of turbulent, multiphase flows. Recent advances in direct numerical simulations and database of DNS results may provide useful guidelines for further development of physical models. Detailed and comprehensive experimental programs are needed to verify the applicability of the existing and new models. Quality experimental data collected through such programs and close communication between experimentalists and those developing numerical models and methods are essential to advance the applicability of multiphase CFD in practice. Experience of applying computational flow modeling to any practical reactor engineering problem may suggest several areas in which further studies are needed for development of better physical models. In view of the wide range of reactor engineering applications, it is practically impossible to make a comprehensive list of all such suggestions. Ranade (1995) listed some areas which need further research for better simulations of dispersed gas–liquid flows (in stirred and bubble column reactors). His list of important issues on which further work is needed may be generalized for any dispersed multiphase flow:

- interphase momentum exchange terms/influence of dispersed phase volume fraction;
- motion of dispersed phase particles near the wall, wall boundary conditions;
- role of particle wakes on dispersion/inter-phase momentum exchange;
- turbulent transport of dispersed phase particles/dependence on particle size;
- turbulence modification by dispersed phase particles;
- particle–particle interactions (collisions, coalescence/agglomeration, breakup);
- interphase heat and mass transfer/phase change models.

The list is merely suggestive. Complexity of reactive flows may greatly expand the list of issues on which further research is required. Another area which deserves mention here is modeling of inherently unsteady flows. Most flows in engineering equipment are unsteady (gas–liquid flow in a bubble column reactor, gas–solid flow in a riser reactor and so on). However, for most engineering purposes, all the details of these unsteady flows are not required to be known. Further work is necessary to evolve adequate representation of such flows within the CFD framework without resorting to full, unsteady simulations. This development is especially necessary to simulate inherently unsteady flows in large industrial reactors where full, unsteady simulations may require unaffordable resources (and therefore, may not be cost effective). Different reactor types and different classes of multiphase flows will have different research requirements based on current and future applications under consideration.

Apart from such research requirements to enhance the capabilities of CFD tools, more and more studies on the application of available tools to simulate engineering equipment are necessary. Accepting the limitations of knowledge of underlying physics and invoking model calibration whenever necessary, is mandatory to expand the application horizons of computational flow modeling. Such experience will provide invaluable information and may guide future developments. Besides this, such applications will significantly enhance the current reactor engineering practice.

Chemical and process engineers today routinely use process simulation tools to design and to optimize overall plant operations. Computational flow modeling tools are also expected to be used as widely as process simulators in the near future. Currently efforts are under way to integrate CFD and process simulation tools (for example, CFX and Hyprotech or FLUENT and Aspen). Several attempts are also being made to couple CFD tools with reactor simulation tools (with automated information flow between CFD and other simulation tools). Advances in software technology and enhanced computing resources allow efficient coupling of CFD codes with physical and chemical property databases (or predictive tools) on one hand and process or reactor simulation tools on the other hand. Such seamlessly integrated tools will allow evaluation of changes in the reactor hardware on overall process performance in the near future. Such capabilities will significantly influence the reactor-engineering practice of tomorrow.

Adequate attention to the key issues mentioned in this book and creative use of computational flow modeling will make significant contributions to enhancing chemical reactor engineering. The field of computational flow modeling for reactor engineering is evolving and being continuously updated. New advances may be assimilated using the framework discussed in this book. I hope that this book will stimulate applications of computational flow modeling to chemical reactor engineering.

NOTATION

A	Van Driest's constant
A_B	Area of bottom surface of the computational cell attached to top surface
A_{bc}	Projection of area of the interface between computational cell and impeller blade on a plane normal to the tangential velocity
a	Discretization coefficients
a_{pq}	Interfacial area per unit volume
B	Empirical constant in Eq. (3.26)
b	Discretization coefficients corresponding to outflow contributions
B_w	Blade width
C	Inertial resistance factors characterizing the porous media
C_1, C_2, C_μ	Parameters of k–ε model
C_D	Drag coefficient
C	Concentration
C_L	Empirical lift coefficient
C_p	Heat capacity
C_{VM}	Virtual mass coefficient
d	Diameter
D	Molecular diffusion coefficient or diameter or impeller diameter
D	Also used as diffusive contributions in discretized equations (Chapter 6)
D_{kT}	Thermal mass diffusion coefficient for species 'k'
E	Empirical constant in wall function, also used as a reciprocal of a characteristic micro-mixing time scale
$E(k)dk$	Turbulent kinetic energy contained in wave number range of k to $k+dk$
e	Restitution coefficient
f	Mixture fraction, Eq. (5.19)
f_B	Basset force coefficient
f_L	Transversal lift coefficient
f_n	Eulerian quantity at node 'n'
f_V	Virtual mass coefficient
F	External or inter-phase force or marker function
F	Also used as convective contributions in discretized equations (Chapter 6)
F_{ki}	Interface coupling terms except pressure
F_{SF}	Surface force
G	Generation of turbulent kinetic energy
G_{ke}	Extra generation of turbulence in phase 'k' due to presence of other phases
g	Acceleration due to gravity
g_{os}	Radial distribution function
h	Enthalpy
H	Hydrostatic head above the sparger
i_ξ	Unit vector in the ξ direction
j_k	Diffusive flux of species k
K	Inter-phase momentum exchange coefficient

k	Thermal conductivity of fluid or turbulent kinetic energy
k_a	Wave number of dissipative eddies
k_e	Wave number of energy containing eddies
k_0	Frequency factor
k_L, k_T	Resistance coefficients of the sparger (laminar and turbulent contributions)
l_T	Length scale of turbulence
L_B, L_P	Distance between centers of two moving spheres/bubbles
L_s	Segregation length scale
m	Mass fraction
N	Impeller rotational speed in revolutions per unit time
n	Moles or surface normal, Eq. (4.6) or unit normal vector or number of moles of oxidizer required to burn one mole of fuel
p	Pressure
p'	Pressure correction or fluctuating pressure
p_o	Total pressure at inlet boundary
p_s	Static pressure in solution domain
P	Pee function given by Eq. (3.39)
$P_{C,sn}$	Pressure due collision between solid phases 's' and 'n'
P_s	Solid phase pressure
q	Flux of enthalpy
Q_R	Circulatory flow in the reactor
Q_{pk}	Energy transfer between pth and kth phase
r	Radial co-ordinate
R	Reaction rate or radius
R'	Universal gas constant
Re_p	Reynolds number of particle
R_z	Axial flow resistance
S	Source or Surface of a computational cell
S_c	Mass source term
S_{cm}	Momentum source term
S_k	Source term of 'k'
S_M	Mass imbalance
S_{pk}	Rate of mass transfer from pth phase to kth phase
t	Time, time scale
T	Temperature
t_{DS}	Diffusion time scale
t_E	Characteristic time for engulfment step
u	Fluctuating velocity
u_T	Characteristic velocity
U	Velocity, radial velocity component
U_i	Local velocity in x_i direction
U_τ	Characteristic wall velocity, $\sqrt{\tau_w/\rho}$
V	Superficial velocity, tangential velocity component
V_b	Effective bubble velocity in a swarm
$V_{b\infty}$	Rise velocity of a single bubble
V_{cell}	Volume of computational cell
V_{ki}	Mean velocity of phase 'k' in direction 'i'

V_R	Volume of reactor
W_{BLD}	Tangential velocity of the blade
x, X	Mole fraction or co-ordinate direction
y	Distance from wall
y_P	Distance between wall and nearest node
z_{rk}	Molar stoichiometric coefficient of component '*r*' in reaction '*k*'

Greek notation

α	Volume fraction
α_P	Under-relaxation parameter
β	Permeability of porous media
δ_{ij}	Kronecker delta function
Δ	Characteristic filter scale
ΔE_n	Activation energy for reaction 'n'
p	Pressure drop
ε	Turbulent energy dissipation rate
ε_{rsl}	Levi-Cevita tensor
ϕ	General variable
ϕ_P	Sphericity
γ_{mj}	Rate of production of component '*m*' due to chemical reactions occurring in j^{th} environment
Γ	Effective diffusion coefficient
η_{pq}	Enhancement factor representing interaction of mass transfer and chemical reaction
φ	Porosity
κ	Coefficient of bulk viscosity or Van Karmann constant (Eq. (3.26)) or Local surface curvature, Eq. (4.8)
λ_k	Kolmogorov length scale where inertial sub-range ends
λ_s	Solid's bulk viscosity
λ_e	Linear interpolation factor
μ	Coefficient of viscosity
μ_{eff}	Effective viscosity
μ_s	Solids viscosity
ν	Kinematic viscosity of the fluid
ν_{eff}	Effective kinematic viscosity of the fluid
ω	Vorticity
π	Molecular flux of momentum, Eq. (2.5)
θ_s	Granular temperature
θ	Parameter controlling degree of implicitness or blade angle, Eq. (9.1)
ρ	Density of fluid
σ	Surface tension or turbulent Prandlt number
τ	Viscous stress tensor, residence time
τ_s	Solid stress tensor
τ_w	Wall shear stress
Ψ	Speculiarity coefficient
$\sum_k$	Sum over all *k*

Subscripts and superscripts

0	of isolated particle in an infinite fluid
b,B	of bubble
cell	of computational cell
C	of continuous phase
CD	Complete dispersion
D	drag, of dispersed phase
Dres	resultant drag
e	east face
ext	external
E	east node
f	of fuel
F	Flooding
g,G	gravity or of gas
i	direction i, or species i
k	of species k or phase k
kin	kinetic
km	of species k in mixture
k_n	of species k due to reaction n
l_s	of phases l and s
L	lift or of liquid
mb	minimum bubbling
mf	minimum fluidization
n	north face
ne	north-east
nw	north-west
N	north node
nb	neighboring nodes
o	of oxidant
p,P	of central node or particle or pellet or due to pressure gradient
ref	reference
R	of reactor, reference, recirculation
s	south face or of solid
sat	saturated
se	south-east
sw	south-west
S	south node
tip	impeller tip
top	over-head (pressure)
T	turbulent
VM	virtual mass
w	west face or of wall
W	west node
ϕ	of variable ϕ
θ	of granular temperature

Commonly used abbreviations

2D	Two-dimensional
3D	Three-dimensional
ASM	Algebraic stress models
CDS	Central differencing scheme
CFD	Computational fluid dynamics
CFM	Computational flow modeling
CRE	Chemical reactor engineering
CSF	Continuous surface force
CTO	Catalyst to oil ratio
CV	Control volume
DNS	Direct numerical simulations
DPM	Discrete particle models
DT	Disc turbine (Rushton turbine)
E	Engulfment model
EB	Eddy break-up model
EDD	Engulfment, deformation and diffusion model
EE	Eulerian–Eulerian
EL	Eulerian–Lagrangian
FCC	Fluid catalytic cracking
FD	Finite difference
FE	Finite element
FOU	First order upwind
FV	Finite volume
IEM	Interaction by exchange with the mean
IVP	Initial value problem
GFM	Granular flow models
KTGF	Kinetic theory of granular flows
LES	Large eddy simulations
LOR	Liquid phase oxidation reactor
MRF	Multiple reference frame
MSIP	Modified SIP
NVD	Normal variable diagram
ODE	Ordinary differential equations
PDE	Partial differential equations
PDF	Probability density function
PEA	Partial elimination algorithm
PISO	Pressure implicit with splitting of operator
PLIC	Piecewise linear interface calculation
PTD	Downflow pitched blade turbine
QUICK	Quadratic upstream interpolation for convective kinematics
RANS	Reynolds-averaged Navier–Stokes equations
RFR	Radial flow fixed bed reactor
RNG	Renormalization group
RSM	Reynolds stress models
RTD	Residence time distribution
SIMPLE	Semi-implicit method for pressure linked equations
SIMPLEC	SIMPLE consistent

SIMPLER	SIMPLE revised
SIP	Strongly implicit procedure
SLD	Sliding mesh approach
SLIC	Simple line interface calculation
SNP	Snapshot approach
SOR	Successive over-relaxation
TDMA	Tri-diagonal matrix algorithm
UD	User defined
UDS	Upwind differencing scheme
VOF	Volume of fluid

AUTHOR INDEX

SUBJECT INDEX